P9-DTD-824

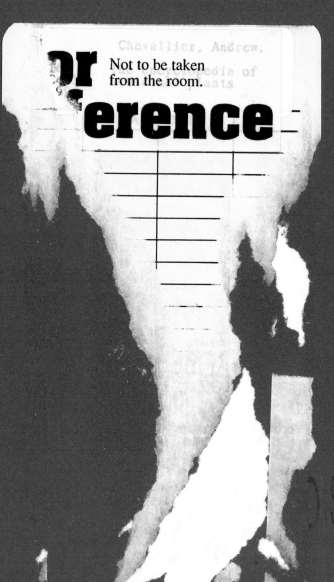

THE
ENCYCLOPEDIA
OF
MEDICINAL
PLANTS

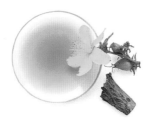

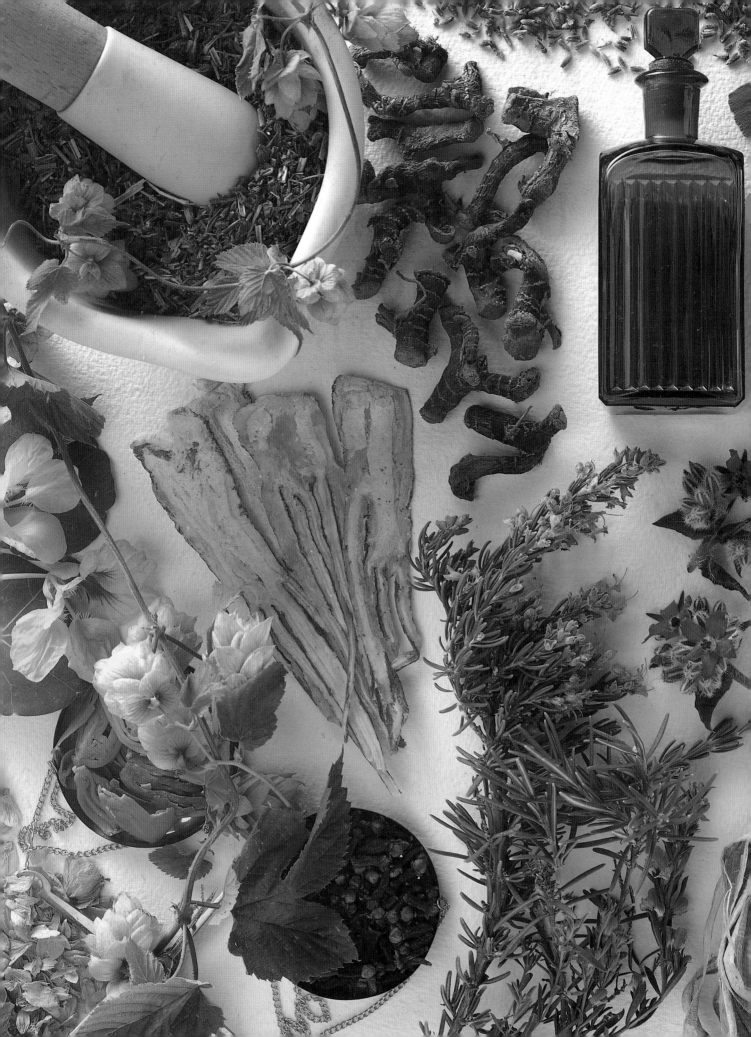

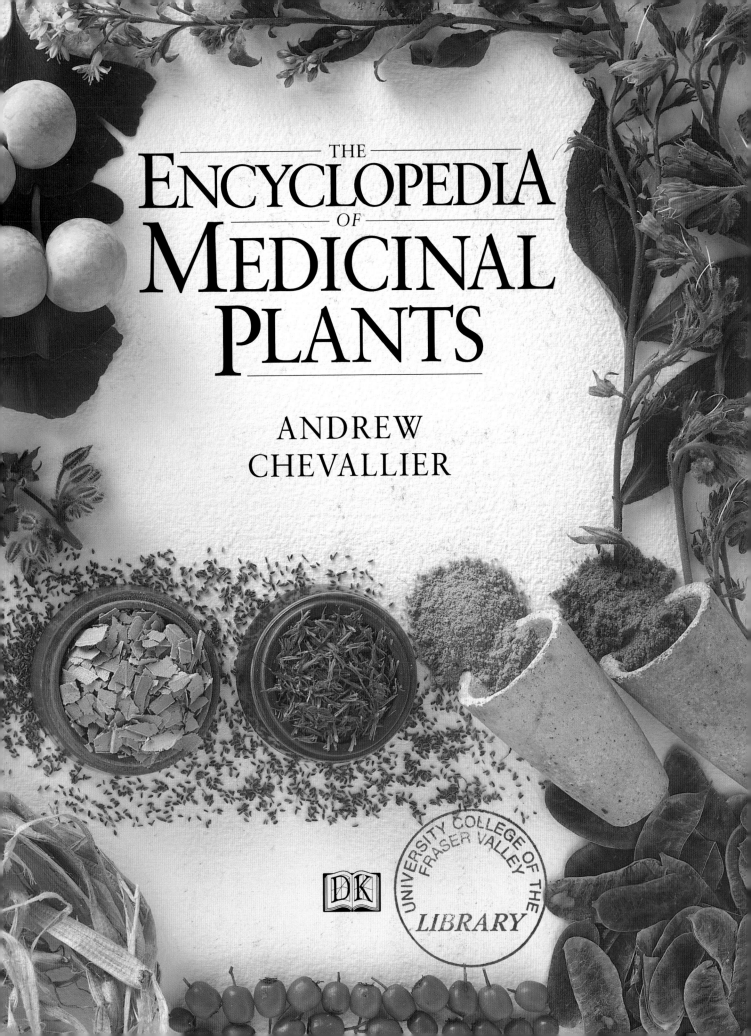

THE

ENCYCLOPEDIA
OF
MEDICINAL
PLANTS

ANDREW CHEVALLIER

A DK PUBLISHING BOOK

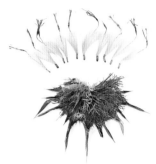

"First the word, then the plant, lastly the knife."
Aesculapius of Thassaly *c.* 1200 BC

Project Editor Penny Warren
Editors Valerie Horn, Christa Weil
Senior Editor Rosie Pearson
US Editor Mary Sutherland
Senior Art Editor Spencer Holbrook
Designers Robert Ford, Jeremy Butcher, Rachana Devidayal
Picture Researcher Jo Walton
Illustrator Gillie Newman
Main Photographers Andy Crawford, Steve Gorton
DTP Designer Karen Ruane
Managing Editor Susannah Marriott
Managing Art Editor Toni Kay
Production Antony Heller
US Consultant David Hoffmann

First American edition, 1996 2 4 6 8 1 0 9 7 5 3 1
Published in the United States by DK Publishing Inc.,
95 Madison Avenue, New York, New York 10016

Published in Great Britain by Dorling Kindersley Limited
Distributed by Houghton Mifflin Company, Boston

Library of Congress Cataloging-in-Publication Data
Chevallier, Andrew.
The Encyclopedia of Medicinal Plants / by Andrew Chevallier
p.   cm.
Includes bibliographical references and index
ISBN 0-7894-0672
1. Materia medica, Vegetable--Encyclopedias
2. Medicinal plants--Encyclopedias I. Title
RS164. C4437   1996   96-15192
615'.32'03--dc20   CIP

Reproduced in Italy by GRB Editrice, Verona
Printed and bound in Italy by New Interlitho, Milan

CONTENTS

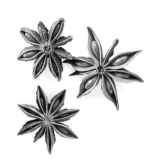

*A visual guide to 100 key herbs from around the world
with details of their habitat, constitutents, actions,
traditional and current uses, and information on
the latest research. Also included are key preparations
and practical self-help uses.*

*Over 450 other herbs from different herbal traditions
with descriptions of their therapeutic properties and
past and present uses.*

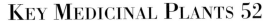

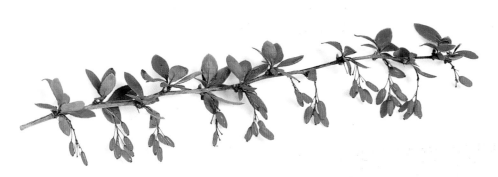

INTRODUCTION

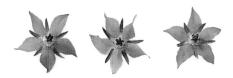

AFTER NEARLY TWO CENTURIES of inexorable decline in the use of herbal medicines, something quite unexpected has begun to happen. Herbs, which have always been the principal form of medicine in developing countries, are once again becoming popular throughout the developed world, as people strive to stay healthy in the face of chronic stress and pollution and to treat illness with medicines that work in concert with the body's own defenses. Statistics show that more and more people in Europe, North America, and Australasia are consulting trained herbal professionals and using the plant medicines that their grandparents or great-grandparents took. In Germany, for instance, the combined sales of herbal medicines, whether bought over the counter or prescribed, topped $3 billion in 1993. In the same year, from a much smaller base, sales of herbal medicines in the UK and Spain increased year on year by 10 and 35 percent, respectively. Growth figures elsewhere, in the US, for example, also show a similar rise.

PLANT MEDICINES

The variety and sheer number of plants with therapeutic properties are quite astonishing. It is estimated that around 70,000 plant species, from lichens to towering trees, have been used at one time or another for medicinal purposes. Today, Western herbal medicine still makes use of at least a thousand indigenous European plants, as well as many thousands of species native to the Americas, Africa, and Australasia. In Ayurveda – traditional Indian medicine – about 2,000 plant species are considered to have medicinal value, while the Chinese *Pharmacopoeia* lists over 5,700 traditional medicines, most of which are of plant origin.

About 500 herbs are still employed within conventional medicine, although whole plants are rarely used. In general, the herbs provide the starting material for the isolation or synthesis of conventional drugs. Digoxin, for example, which is used for heart failure, was isolated from common foxglove (*Digitalis purpurea*, p. 199), and the contraceptive pill was synthesized from constituents found in wild yam (*Dioscorea villosa*, p. 89).

ECOLOGICAL FACTORS

The increased use of medicinal herbs has a number of important implications. In the era of "set-aside" land, growing herbs as an organic crop offers new opportunities for farmers who find that their usual crops are no longer economical to grow.

The rise in popularity of herbal medicines, however, also directly threatens the survival of some wild species. Demand for American ginseng (*Panax quinquefolium*, p. 241) has become so great that it now brings around $733 a pound ($1,100 a kilo). It was a common plant in the woodlands of northern and eastern North America two centuries ago, but is now an endangered species and may become extinct in the wild. This example is by no means unique, and, sadly, many species are similarly threatened across the planet.

The extinction of plant species as a result of overintensive collecting is nothing new. The herb silphion, a member of the carrot family, was used extensively as a contraceptive by the women of ancient Rome. Silphion proved difficult to cultivate and was gathered from the wild in such large quantities that it became extinct during the 3rd century AD.

Today, if herbal medicine is to grow at its present rate, it is imperative that manufacturers, suppliers, practitioners, and the public use only produce that has been cultivated or wildcrafted in an ecologically sensitive manner.

About This Book

In the past, books on herbal medicine have tended to focus either on the traditional and folkloric use of plants *or* on their active constituents and pharmacology. *The Encyclopedia of Medicinal Plants*, which features more than 550 plants, aims to include both aspects. It discusses each plant's history, traditions, and folklore, and explains what is known from scientific research about the active constituents, key actions, and potential new uses.

It is easy when concentrating on the scientific aspect of herbal medicine to forget that much, in some cases *all*, that we currently know about a particular plant results from its traditional use. Moreover, even when a plant has been well researched, herbal medicines are so complex and variable that what is currently known is rarely definitive, but rather a sound pointer as to how it works. Sometimes the traditional use, in so far as it is based on the experience of practitioners, provides an insight into how best to use an herb that is missing from scientific knowledge alone. Herbal medicine is, after all, both a science *and* an art.

In choosing the plants profiled in the *Encyclopedia*, the aim has been to select herbs that are commonly used in different parts of the world and are considered to have particular health benefits. In addition, a small number are included because they are of significant historical interest. The index of key medicinal plants (pp. 54–153) contains many herbs that are readily available in health stores and pharmacies, for example, ginkgo (*Ginkgo biloba*, p. 98). It also includes herbs that are more commonly known as foods, such as lemon (*Citrus limon*, p. 81), but which, nonetheless, are valuable medicines. The index of other medicinal plants (pp. 156–281) contains some less commonly known but important medicinal herbs, such as tree of heaven (*Ailanthus altissima*, p. 161), a traditional Chinese remedy for many ailments, which is now being investigated for its potential in treating cancer.

A global overview of the history of herbal medicine puts the development of different herbal traditions from earliest origins to the present day into perspective. This is complemented with features on herbal medicine in Europe, India, China, Africa, Australia, and the Americas, providing a rounded picture of herbal medicine worldwide.

Herbal medicine is nothing if not practical in its approach, and the *Encyclopedia* has a detailed practical section with advice on preparing and using herbal medicines to treat a range of common health problems.

If more people come to appreciate the immense richness of the world of herbal medicine and are able to benefit from the curative properties of medicinal herbs, this book will have achieved its aim.

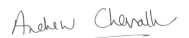

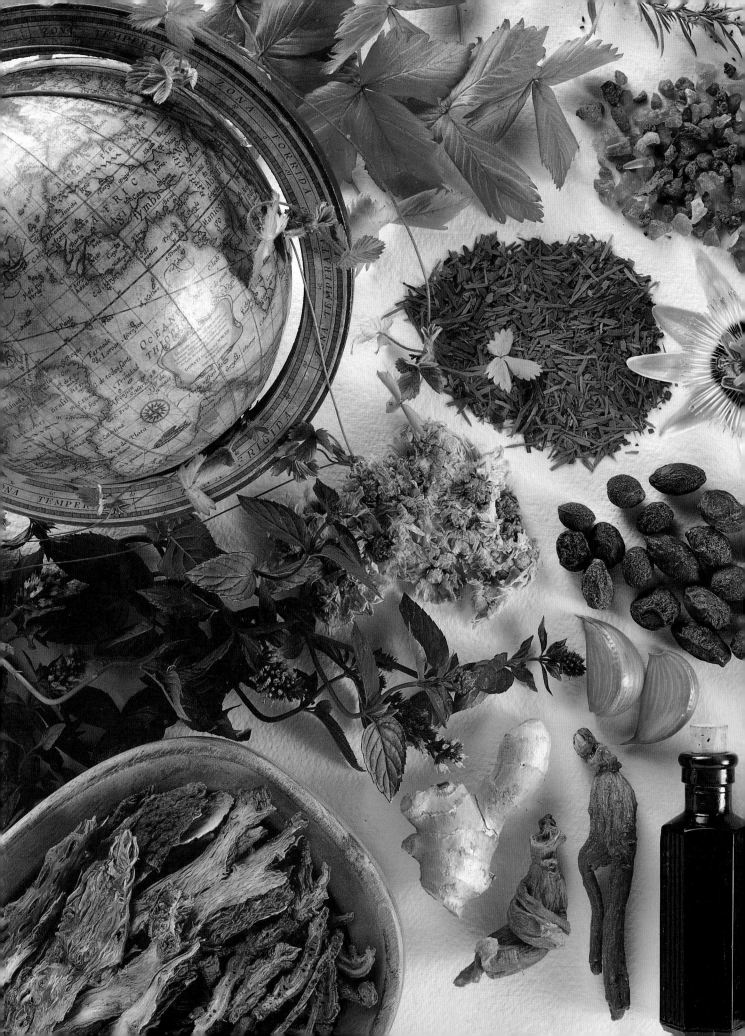

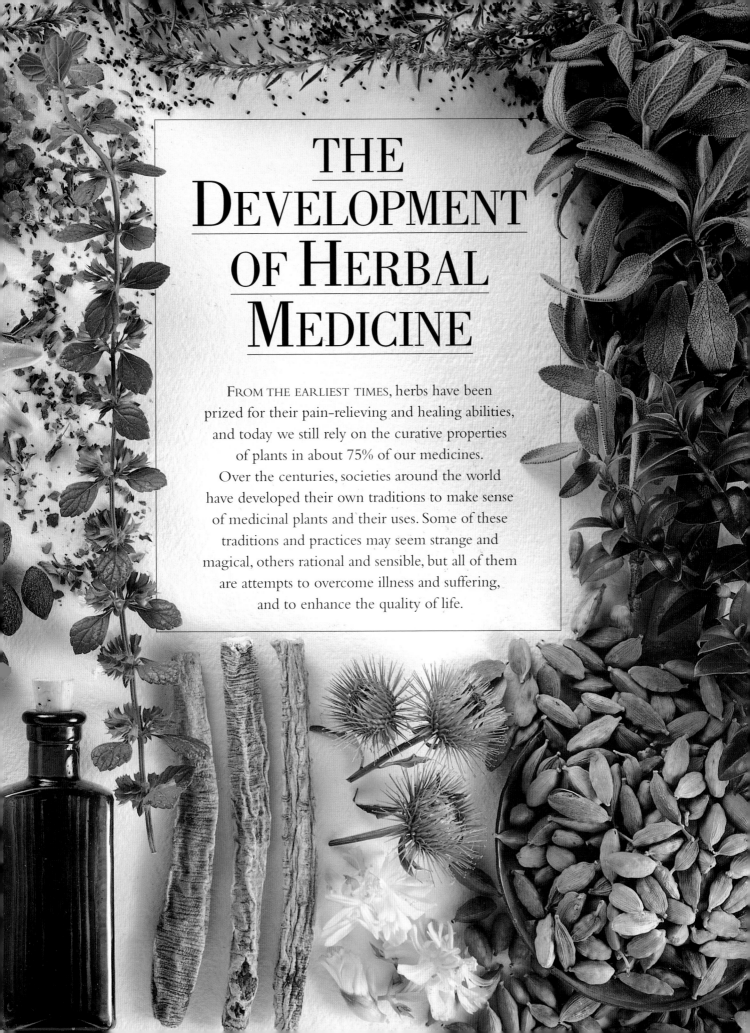

THE DEVELOPMENT OF HERBAL MEDICINE

FROM THE EARLIEST TIMES, herbs have been
prized for their pain-relieving and healing abilities,
and today we still rely on the curative properties
of plants in about 75% of our medicines.
Over the centuries, societies around the world
have developed their own traditions to make sense
of medicinal plants and their uses. Some of these
traditions and practices may seem strange and
magical, others rational and sensible, but all of them
are attempts to overcome illness and suffering,
and to enhance the quality of life.

HOW MEDICINAL PLANTS WORK

Many of the thousands of plant species growing throughout the world have medicinal uses, containing active constituents that have a direct action on the body. They are used both in herbal and conventional medicine and offer benefits that pharmaceutical drugs often lack, helping to combat illness and support the body's efforts to regain good health.

THERE IS NO DOUBT THAT in extreme situations the treatments devised by modern medicine can offer an unparalleled opportunity to relieve symptoms and save lives. A newspaper article in 1993 described the terrible conditions in a hospital in war-torn Sarajevo, the capital of Bosnia-Herzegovina. Deprived of conventional medical supplies and drugs, the doctors were forced to use a well-known European herb, valerian (*Valeriana officinalis*, p. 146), as a painkiller for the wounded and as an anesthetic. Valerian is an effective herbal medicine for anxiety and nervous tension, but it is woefully inadequate as an analgesic or anesthetic.

Orthodox pharmaceutical medicines sustain life and counter infections in situations where other types of treatment may have little to offer. Modern surgical techniques, such as keyhole surgery and plastic surgery, and the whole range of diagnostic and life-support machinery now available can all be used to improve the chances of recovery from serious illness or injury.

THE BENEFITS OF HERBAL MEDICINE

Yet despite the dramatic advances and advantages of conventional medicine, or biomedicine as it is also known, it is clear that herbal medicine has much to offer. We tend to forget that in all but the last fifty years or so, humans have relied almost entirely on plants to treat all manner of illnesses, from minor problems such as coughs and colds to life-threatening diseases such as tuberculosis and

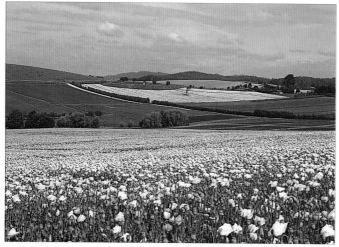

Opium poppy *fields in Tasmania. Opium, derived from the seed capsules of the opium poppy, yields the narcotic alkaloids morphine and codeine, powerful painkillers that are widely used in conventional medicine.*

malaria. Today, herbal remedies are coming back into prominence because the efficacy of conventional medicines such as antibiotics, which once had near-universal effectiveness against serious infections, is on the wane. Over the years, infectious organisms have developed resistance to synthesized drugs, and the herb *qing hao* (*Artemisia annua*, p. 64) and its active constituent artemisin, for example, are now being used to treat malaria in areas of the world where the protozoa causing the infection no longer respond to conventional treatment.

Herbal medicine often complements conventional treatments, providing safe, well-tolerated remedies for chronic illnesses. It is experiencing a dramatic renaissance in Western countries, partly because no effective conventional treatment as yet exists for many chronic illnesses, such as asthma, arthritis, and irritable bowel syndrome. In addition, concern over the side effects of biomedicine is encouraging people to look for more gentle forms of treatment. It is estimated that 10–20% of hospital patients in the West are there due to the side effects of conventional medical treatment.

USING HERBS WISELY

Most commonly used herbs are extremely safe to use. Some plants, however, can produce side effects, and, like all medicines, herbal remedies must be treated with respect. It is essential to take or use certain plants only under the guidance of a well-trained practitioner, to avoid adverse consequences. Ephedra (*Ephedra sinica*, p. 93), for example, can be extremely toxic at the wrong dosage, and comfrey (*Symphytum officinale*, p. 136), a very popular herb in the past, is thought to cause severe or even fatal liver damage in rare circumstances. When an herbal medicine is used correctly, however, the chances of developing a serious side effect are remote.

POTENT PLANT CHEMICALS

The ability of an herbal medicine to affect body systems depends on the chemical constituents that it contains. Scientists first started extracting and isolating chemicals from plants in the 18th century, and since that time, we have grown accustomed to looking at herbs and their effects in terms of the active constituents they contain. This *Encyclopedia* is no exception, providing details of all the main active constituents of the medicinal herbs featured and explaining their actions.

Research into isolated plant constituents is of great importance, for it has given rise to many of the world's most useful drugs. Tubocurarine, the most powerful muscle relaxant in existence, is derived from curare (*Chondrodendron tomentosum*, p. 187), and the strongest painkiller of all, morphine, comes from opium poppy (*Papaver somniferum*, p. 242). Many anesthetics are also derived from plants, for example, cocaine, which comes from coca plant (*Erythroxylum coca*, p. 204).

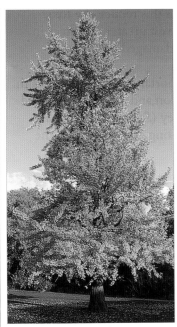

Ginkgo, one of the oldest known plant species, improves the circulation of blood to the head.

In the 1990s, biomedicine still relies on plants rather than the laboratory for at least 25% of its medicines, and many of these are among the most effective of all conventional drugs. It is hard to think of a world deprived of the antimalarial properties of quinine (derived from *Cinchona* spp., p. 79); or the heart remedy digoxin (from *Digitalis* spp., pp. 199–200); or the cough-relieving properties of ephedrine (from *Ephedra sinica*, p. 93), which is present in many prescription and over-the-counter cold remedies. These and many other conventional medicines are all derived from isolated plant constituents.

VALUE OF WHOLE PLANTS

Although it is important to understand the actions of individual active constituents, herbal medicine, unlike bio-medicine, is ultimately about the use and actions of whole plants – medicines that are literally god- or goddess-given – rather than developed in a laboratory. In the same way that taking a watch to bits and identifying its key parts will not show you how it works as a whole, dividing up a medicinal herb into its constituent parts cannot explain exactly how it works in its natural form. The whole herb is worth more than the sum of its parts, and scientific research is increasingly showing that the active constituents of many herbs, for example those in ginkgo (*Ginkgo biloba*, p. 98), interact in complex ways to produce the therapeutic effect of the remedy as a whole.

Plants contain hundreds, if not thousands, of different constituent chemicals that interact in complex ways. Frequently, we simply do not know in detail how a particular herb works – even though its medicinal benefit is well established. The pharmacological approach to understanding how whole herbs work is like working on a jigsaw where only some of the pieces have been provided. Furthermore, although it is very useful to know that a plant contains certain active constituents, such information can be misleading on its own. For example, tea (*Camellia sinensis*, p. 179) and coffee (*Coffea arabica*, p. 190) contain approximately the same levels of caffeine. Tea, however, contains a much greater quantity of tannins (which give tea its sour, astringent taste). These constituents reduce the amount of nutrients and drugs that are absorbed from the intestines into the blood-stream, and consequently less caffeine is absorbed. As a result, and true to most people's experience, tea is less stimulating than coffee.

This example reveals a couple of fundamental truths about herbal medicine. First, the experience of the herbal practitioner and of the patient often provide the most reliable guide to the medicinal effect of individual herbs. Second, the value of a medicinal herb cannot be reduced simply to a list of its active constituents.

PLANTS AS FOODS & MEDICINES

The human body is much better suited to treatment with herbal remedies than with isolated chemical medicines. We have evolved side-by-side with plants over tens of thousands of years, and our digestive system and physiology as a whole are geared to digesting and utilizing plant-based foods, which often have a medicinal value as well as providing sustenance.

The dividing line between "foods" and "medicines" may not always be clear. Are lemons, papayas, onions, and oats foods or medicines? The answer, very simply, is that they are both. Lemon (*Citrus limon*, p. 81) improves resistance to infection; papaya (*Carica papaya*, p. 181) is taken in some parts of the world to expel worms; onion (*Allium cepa*, p. 162) relieves bronchial infections; and oats (*Avena sativa*, p. 172) support convalescence. Indeed, herbal medicine comes into its own when the distinctions between foods and medicines are removed. *(continued)*

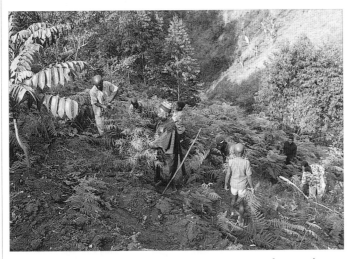

Cultivation of medicinal plants *in Cameroon. Scientific research indicates that whole plant preparations may often be gentler and more effective remedies than isolated plant chemicals.*

Although we might eat a bowl of porridge oblivious to the medicinal benefits, it will, nonetheless, increase stamina, help the nervous system to function correctly, provide a good supply of B vitamins, and maintain regular bowel function. A similar range of benefits is provided by many of the other gentler-acting herbs listed in the *Encyclopedia*.

HERBAL TREATMENTS

The strategies that herbal practitioners adopt to prevent illness or restore health in their patients are different in the many and varied herbal traditions across the planet, but the effects that herbal medicines have within the body to improve health do not vary. There are many thousands of medicinal plants in use throughout the world, with a tremendous range of actions and degrees of potency. Most have a specific action on particular body systems and are known to be suitable for treating certain types of ailments. *See* p. 13 for specific actions.

DIGESTION, RESPIRATION & CIRCULATION

Improving the quality of the diet is often an essential starting point in sustaining or regaining good health. The saying "You are what you eat" is by and large true, though herbalists prefer to qualify it, saying "You are what you *absorb* from what you eat." Herbal medicines not only provide nutrients but when needed they also strengthen and support the action of the digestive system, speeding up the rate of processing food and improving the absorption of nutrients.

The body requires another kind of "nutrient" to function – oxygen. The lungs and respiratory system can be helped with herbs that relax the bronchial muscles and stimulate respiration.

Once taken in by the body, nutrients and medicines are carried to the body's estimated three trillion cells. The circulatory system has a remarkable ability to adapt to an endlessly shifting pattern of demand. At rest, the flow of blood is mainly toward the center of the body; when active, the muscles in the limbs make huge demands. Herbal medicines work to encourage the circulation in particular ways. Some, for example, encourage blood to flow to the surface of the body; others stimulate the heart to pump more efficiently, and others relax the muscles of the arteries, lowering blood pressure.

CLEARING TOXICITY & SOOTHING SKIN

After the circulation has carried nutrients to the cells, waste matter must be removed. All too often in our polluted world, high levels of toxicity in the body are an underlying cause of ill health, and herbalists use a wide range of cleansing herbs that improve the body's ability to remove toxins. Perhaps the finest example of a detoxifying herb is burdock (*Arctium lappa*, p. 62), which is used extensively in both Western and Chinese

medicine. Once herbs such as this reduce the toxic "load," the body is able to invest greater resources in repairing and strengthening damaged tissue and weakened organs.

The skin also plays an important role in good health. Antiseptic plants fight infection, and vulnerary (wound-healing) herbs such as comfrey (*Symphytum officinale*, p. 136) encourage blood clotting and help speed the healing of wounds.

NERVOUS, ENDOCRINE & IMMUNE SYSTEMS

Good health depends on having a healthy balanced nervous system. In order to ensure long-term good health of the nervous system, it is important to adapt well to life's daily demands, to avoid excessive anxiety, worry, or depression, and to get sufficient rest and exercise.

The latest research suggests that the nervous system does not work in isolation. It is complemented by the endocrine system, which controls the release of a whole symphony of hormones, including the sex hormones, which control fertility and often affect vitality and mood. The nervous system is also intimately linked with the immune system, which controls the ability to resist infection and to recover from illness and injury.

This incredible complex of systems – part electrical, part chemical, part mechanical – must function harmoniously if good health is to be maintained. In health, the body has a seemingly infinite capacity, via its controlling systems, to adjust and change to external pressures. This ability to adapt to the external world while the body's internal workings remain constant is known as *homeostasis*. Many herbs work with the immune, nervous, and endocrine systems to help the body adapt more effectively to stresses and strains of all kinds – physical, mental, emotional, and even spiritual. They are effective because they work in tune with the body's processes.

Some herbs are *adaptogenic*, meaning that they have an ability to help people to adapt, either by supporting the nervous system and easing nervous and emotional tension, or by working directly with the body's own physiological processes to maintain health. The prime example of an adaptogenic herb is ginseng (*Panax ginseng*, p. 116), which is an effective remedy at times of great mental or physical stress, but in certain cases can also be taken when a relaxing effect is required, for example, to relieve headaches, or to ensure a good night's sleep.

COMPLEX NATURAL MEDICINES

As can be seen, an herb is not a "magic bullet" with a single action, but a complex natural medicine composed of many active constituents that work on different body systems. By combining scientific research into active constituents with clinical observation and traditional knowledge of the whole plant, we can develop a rounded picture of each herb's range of medicinal uses.

HERBS & BODY SYSTEMS

One of the most common ways of classifying medicinal plants is to identify their actions, for example, whether they are sedative, antiseptic or diuretic, and the degree to which they affect different body systems. Herbs often have a pronounced action on a particular body system, for example, a plant that is strongly antiseptic in the digestive tract may be less so in the respiratory tract. Examples of how herbs work on the body are given below.

SKIN

Antiseptics, e.g., tea tree (*Melaleuca alternifolia*, p. 110) disinfect the skin. *Emollients*, e.g., calendula (*Calendula officinalis*, p. 69) reduce itchiness, redness and soreness. *Astringents*, e.g., witch hazel (*Hamamelis virginiana*, p. 100) tighten the skin. *Depuratives*, e.g., burdock (*Arctium lappa*, p. 62) encourage removal of waste products. *Healing and vulnerary herbs*, e.g., self-heal (*Prunella vulgaris*, p. 122) and comfrey (*Symphytum officinale*, p. 136) aid the healing of cuts, wounds, and abrasions.

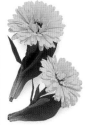

CALENDULA
(*Calendula officinalis*)

IMMUNE SYSTEM

Immune stimulants, e.g., echinacea (*Echinacea* spp. p. 90) and lapacho (*Tabebuia* spp., p. 137) encourage the immune system to ward off infection.

ECHINACEA
(*Echinacea* spp.)

RESPIRATORY SYSTEM

Antiseptics and antibiotics, e.g., garlic (*Allium sativum*, p. 56) help the lungs resist infection. *Expectorants*, e.g., elecampane (*Inula helenium*, p. 105) stimulate the coughing up of mucus. *Demulcents*, e.g., marsh mallow (*Althaea officinalis*, p. 163) soothe irritated membranes. *Spasmolytics*, e.g., visnaga (*Ammi visnaga*, p. 59) relax bronchial muscles.

GARLIC
(*Allium sativum*)

ENDOCRINE GLANDS

Adaptogens, e.g., ginseng (*Panax ginseng*, p. 116) help the body adjust to external pressures and stress. *Hormonally active herbs*, e.g., agnus castus (*Vitex agnus-castus*, p. 149) stimulate production of sex and other hormones. *Emmenagogues*, e.g., black cohosh (*Cimicifuga racemosa*, p. 78) encourage or regulate menstruation.

GINSENG
(*Panax ginseng*)

URINARY SYSTEM

Antiseptics, e.g., buchu (*Barosma betulina*, p. 67) disinfect the urinary tubules. *Astringents*, e.g., horsetail (*Equisetum arvense*, p. 202) tighten and protect the urinary tubules. *Diuretics*, e.g., cornsilk (*Zea mays*, p. 152) stimulate the flow of urine.

CORNSILK
(*Zea mays*)

MUSCULOSKELETAL SYSTEM

Analgesics, e.g., yellow jasmine (*Gelsemium sempervirens*, p. 214) relieve joint and nerve pain. *Anti-inflammatories*, e.g., white willow (*Salix alba*, p. 128) reduce swelling and pain in joints. *Antispasmodics*, e.g., cinchona (*Cinchona* spp., p. 79) relax tense and cramped muscles.

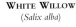

WHITE WILLOW
(*Salix alba*)

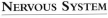

NERVOUS SYSTEM

Nervines, e.g., rosemary (*Rosmarinus officinalis*, p. 125) support and strengthen the nervous system. *Relaxants*, e.g., lemon balm (*Melissa officinalis*, p. 111) relax the nervous system. *Sedatives*, e.g., mistletoe (*Viscum album*, p. 281) reduce nervous activity. *Stimulants*, e.g., kola nut (*Cola acuminata*, p. 191) increase nervous activity. *Tonics*, e.g., oats (*Avena sativa*, p. 172) improve nerve function and tone, and help to restore the nervous system as a whole.

ROSEMARY
(*Rosmarinus officinalis*)

CIRCULATION & HEART

Cardiotonics, e.g., *dan shen* (*Salvia miltiorrhiza*, p. 129) vary in action. Some slow heart beat rate, while others increase it. Some improve the regularity and strength of the heart's contractions. *Circulatory stimulants*, e.g., cayenne (*Capsicum frutescens*, p. 70) improve the circulation of blood to the extremities. *Diaphoretics*, e.g., *ju hua* (*Chrysanthemum* x *morifolium*, p. 77) encourage blood flow to the surface of the body, promote sweating, and lower blood pressure. *Spasmolytics*, e.g., crampbark (*Viburnum opulus*, p. 148) relax the muscles, helping to lower blood pressure.

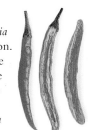

CAYENNE
(*Capsicum frutescens*)

DIGESTIVE ORGANS

Antiseptics, e.g., ginger (*Zingiber officinale*, p. 153) protect against infection. *Astringents*, e.g., bistort (*Polygonum bistorta*, p. 251) tighten up the inner lining of the intestines and create a protective coating over them. *Bitters*, e.g., wormwood (*Artemisia absinthum*, p. 63) stimulate secretion of digestive juices by the stomach and intestines. *Carminatives*, e.g., sweet flag (*Acorus calamus*, p. 55) relieve gas and cramps. *Cholagogues*, e.g., fringe tree (*Chionanthus virginicus*, p.186) improve the flow of bile into the intestines. *Choleretics*, e.g., artichoke (*Cynara scolymus*, p. 196) stimulate secretion of bile by the liver. *Demulcents*, e.g., psyllium (*Plantago* spp., p. 120) soothe the digestive system and protect against acidity and irritation. *Hepatics*, e.g., bupleurum (*Bupleurum chinense*, p. 68) prevent liver damage. *Laxatives*, e.g., senna (*Cassia senna*, p. 72) stimulate bowel movements. *Stomachics*, e.g., cardamom (*Eletteria cardamomum*, p. 91) protect and support the stomach.

SWEET FLAG
(*Acorus calamus*)

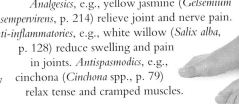

SENNA
(*Cassia senna*)

ACTIVE CONSTITUENTS

The medicinal effects of certain plants are well known. Senna, for example, has been taken as a laxative for thousands of years, and aloe vera was known to Cleopatra as a soothing skin remedy. It is only recently, however, that the active constituents responsible for the medicinal actions of plants have been isolated and observed. Knowing a little about the chemicals contained in plants helps you to understand how they work within the body.

MUCILAGE

Found in many plants, mucilage is made up of polysaccharides (large sugar molecules) that soak up water, producing a sticky jellylike mass. Mucilage lines the mucous membranes of the digestive tract, protecting against irritation, acidity and inflammation. This soothing and protective action appears to extend to other areas, including the mucous membranes of the throat, lungs, kidneys, and urinary tubules. Slippery elm (*Ulmus rubra*, p. 144) is a typical mucilaginous herb.

SLIPPERY ELM
(*Ulmus rubra*)

PHENOLS

This group of compounds includes salicylic acid – the natural forerunner of aspirin. Salicylic acid is found in many plants, for example wintergreen (*Gaultheria procumbens*, p. 213) and white willow (*Salix alba*, p. 128). Another phenol is thymol – a constituent of thyme (*Thymus vulgaris*, p. 142). Phenols are antiseptic and reduce inflammation when taken internally, yet they have an irritant effect when applied to the skin.

THYME
(*Thymus vulgaris*)

TANNINS

Tannins are produced to a greater or lesser degree by all plants. The harsh, astringent taste of tannin-laden bark and leaves makes them unpalatable to insects and grazing animals. Tannins contract the tissues of the body – hence their use to "tan" leather. They draw the tissues closer together and improve their resistance to infection. Oak bark (*Quercus robur*, p. 258) and black catechu (*Acacia catechu*, p. 157) are both high in tannins.

BLACK CATECHU
(*Acacia catechu*)

COUMARINS

Coumarins of different kinds are found in many plant species and have widely divergent actions. The coumarins in melilot (*Melilotus officinalis*, p. 232) thin the blood, bergapten, found in celery (*Apium graveolens*, p. 61), is used as a sunscreen, and khellin, found in visnaga (*Ammi visnaga*, p. 59), is a powerful smooth muscle relaxant.

CELERY
(*Apium graveolens*)

ANTHRAQUINONES

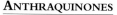

Anthraquinones are the main active constituents in herbs such as senna (*Cassia senna*, p. 72) and Chinese rhubarb (*Rheum palmatum*, p. 124), both of which are taken to relieve constipation. Anthraquinones have an irritant laxative effect on the large intestine, causing contractions of the intestinal walls and stimulating a bowel movement approximately 10 hours after being taken. They also make the stool more liquid, easing bowel movements.

CHINESE RHUBARB
(*Rheum palmatum*)

FLAVONOIDS

Found in many plants, flavonoids have a wide range of actions. They are anti-inflammatory and are especially useful in maintaining healthy circulation. Rutin, a flavonoid found in plants, including buckwheat (*Fagopyrum esculentum*, p. 208) and lemon (*Citrus limon*, p. 81), strengthens capillary walls.

LEMON
(*Citrus limon*)

ANTHOCYANINS

These pigments, which give flowers and fruits a blue, purple, or red hue, help to keep the blood vessels healthy. Blackberry (*Rubus fruticosus*, p. 261) and grapes (*Vitis vinifera*, p. 281) contain appreciable quantities of anthocyanins.

BLACKBERRY
(*Rubus fruticosus*)

GLUCOSILINATES

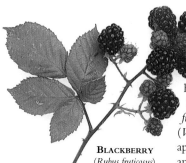

Found exclusively in species of the mustard family, glucosilinates have an irritant effect on the skin, causing inflammation and blistering. Applied as poultices to painful or aching joints, they increase blood flow to the affected area, helping to remove the build-up of waste products (a contributory factor in joint problems). Glucosilinates also help to reduce thyroid function. Both radish (*Raphanus sativus*, p. 258) and mustard (*Sinapis alba*) contain significant quantities of glucosilinates.

RADISH
(*Raphanus sativus*)

ACTIVE CONSTITUENTS

VOLATILE OILS

Volatile oils – which are extracted from plants to produce essential oils – are some of the most important plant constituents of all. Tea tree (*Melaleuca alternifolia*, p. 110), for example, is known to contain over 60 different volatile compounds within its volatile oil, many of them being strongly antiseptic. Some volatile oils contain sesquiterpenes, such as azulene, found in German chamomile (*Chamomilla recutita*, p. 76). These constituents have an anti-inflammatory effect.

GERMAN CHAMOMILE
(*Chamomilla recutita*)

SAPONINS

There are two types of saponins – triterpenoid and steroidal saponins. The latter get their name from their similarity to the human body's own naturally occurring steroid hormones. Many plants containing steroidal saponins have a marked hormonal activity, licorice (*Glycyrrhiza glabra*, p. 99) being one of the best known. Triterpenoid saponins, for example, those in cowslip root (*Primula veris*, p. 254), are often strong expectorants, and may also aid in the absorption of nutrients.

LICORICE
(*Glycyrrhiza glabra*)

CARDIAC GLYCOSIDES

Found in various medicinal plants, most famously in common foxglove (*Digitalis purpurea*, p. 199), yellow foxglove (*D. lutea*, p. 199), and wooly foxglove (*D. lanata*), cardiac glycosides such as digitoxin, digoxin, and gitoxin have a strong, direct action on the heart, helping to support its strength and rate of contraction when it is failing. Cardiac glycosides are also significantly diuretic. They help to transfer fluids from the tissues and circulatory system to the urinary tract, thereby lowering blood pressure.

COMMON FOXGLOVE
(*Digitalis purpurea*)

CYANOGENIC GLYCOSIDES

Though these glycosides are based on cyanide, a very potent poison, they have a helpful sedative and relaxant effect on the heart and muscles in small doses. Wild cherry bark (*Prunus serotina*, p. 255) and elder (*Sambucus nigra*, p. 131) both contain cyanogenic glycosides, which contribute to both plants' ability to suppress and soothe irritant dry coughs.

ELDERFLOWER
(*Sambucus nigra*)

VITAMINS

Some plants contain significant levels of vitamins. Watercress (*Nasturtium officinale*, p. 237), for example, contains an appreciable quantity of vitamin E, and the hips of dog rose (*Rosa canina*, p. 261) have particularly high levels of vitamin C. Most other medicinal plants contain at least some vitamins. While the content may be small it contributes to overall daily intake. For other plants that are rich in vitamins, *see* p. 297.

DOG ROSE
(*Rosa canina*)

BITTERS

Bitters are a varied group of constituents linked only by their pronounced bitter taste. The bitterness itself stimulates secretions by the salivary glands and digestive organs. Such secretions can dramatically improve the appetite and strengthen the overall function of the digestive system. With the improved digestion and absorption of nutrients that follow, the body is nourished and strengthened. Many herbs have bitter constituents, notably wormwood (*Artemisia absinthium*, p. 63) and chiretta (*Swertia chirata*, p. 135).

WORMWOOD
(*Artemisia absinthium*)

ALKALOIDS

A very mixed group, alkaloids mostly contain a nitrogen-bearing molecule (-NH₂) that makes them particularly pharmacologically active. Some are well-known drugs and have a recognized medical use. Vincristine, for example, derived from Madagascar periwinkle (*Vinca rosea*, p. 280), is used to treat some types of cancer. Other alkaloids, such as atropine, found in deadly nightshade (*Atropa belladonna*, p. 66), have a direct effect on the body, reducing spasms, relieving pain, and drying up bodily secretions.

DEADLY NIGHTSHADE
(*Atropa belladonna*)

MINERALS

Some herbs are particularly rich in minerals. Horsetail (*Equisetum arvense*, p. 202), for example, has high levels of silica. Dandelion (*Taraxacum officinale*, p. 140) has large quantities of potassium, and unlike other diuretics which flush this mineral out of the body, it helps to maintain high levels of potassium. These plants act as mineral supplements in their own right, while other herbs with a small concentration contribute to overall intake. For other plants with a high mineral content, *see* p. 297.

DANDELION
(*Taraxacum officinale*)

15

EARLY ORIGINS TO THE 19TH CENTURY

In an age of medical specialization in which an expert in neurology will know little about the latest developments in medicine for the ear, nose, and throat, it is difficult to imagine the practices of an earlier time, when healing was holistic in nature and heavily reliant on magic, mysticism, and age-old oral traditions.

FROM THE EARLIEST TIMES, medicinal plants have been crucial in sustaining the health and the well-being of mankind. Linseed (*Linum usitatissimum*, p. 226), for example, provided its harvesters with a nutritious cooking oil, fuel, a cosmetic balm for the skin, and fiber to make fabric. At the same time it was used to treat conditions such as bronchitis, congestion, boils, and a number of digestive problems. Given the life-enhancing benefits that this and so many other plants conferred, it is hardly surprising that most cultures believed them to have magical as well as medicinal abilities. It is reasonable to assume that for tens of thousands of years herbs were probably used as much for their ritual magical powers as

for their medicinal qualities. A 60,000-year-old burial site excavated in Iraq, for instance, was found to contain eight different medicinal plants, including ephedra (*Ephedra sinica*, p. 93). The inclusion of the plants in the tomb suggests they had supernatural significance as well as medicinal value.

In some cultures plants were considered to have souls. Even Aristotle, the 4th-century BC Greek philosopher, thought that plants had a "psyche," albeit of a lesser order than the human soul. In Hinduism, which dates back to at least 1500 BC, many plants are sacred to specific divinities. For example, the bael tree (*Aegle marmelos*, p. 159) is said to shelter Shiva, the god of health, beneath its branches.

In medieval Europe, the Doctrine of Signatures stated there was a connection between how a plant looked – God's "signature" – and how it might be used as a medicine. For example, the mottled leaves of lungwort (*Pulmonaria officinalis*, p. 256) were thought to resemble lung tissue, and the plant is still used to treat ailments of the respiratory tract.

Even in Western cultures, beliefs in plant spirits linger. Until this century, British farmworkers would not cut down elder trees (*Sambucus nigra*, p. 131) for fear of arousing the anger of the Elder Mother, the spirit who lived in and protected the tree.

In a similar vein, native peoples of the Andes in South America believe that the coca plant (*Erythroxylum coca*, p. 204) is protected by Mama Coca, a spirit who must be respected and placated if the leaves are to be harvested and used.

SHAMANISTIC MEDICINE

In many traditional societies today, the world is believed to be shaped by good and evil spirits. In these societies, illness is thought to stem from malignant forces or possession by evil spirits. If a member of the tribe falls ill, the shaman (the "medicine" man or woman) is expected to intercede with the spirit world to bring about a cure. Shamans often enter the spiritual realm with the aid of hallucinogenic plants or fungi, such as ayahuasca (*Banisteriopsis caapi*, p. 174), taken by Amazonian shamans, or fly agaric (*Amanita muscaria*), taken by traditional healers of the Siberian steppes. At the same time, the

Mistletoe, which the Druids called the "golden bough," had a central place in their shamanistic religious and healing ceremonies. The Druids had a well-developed knowledge of medicinal plants.

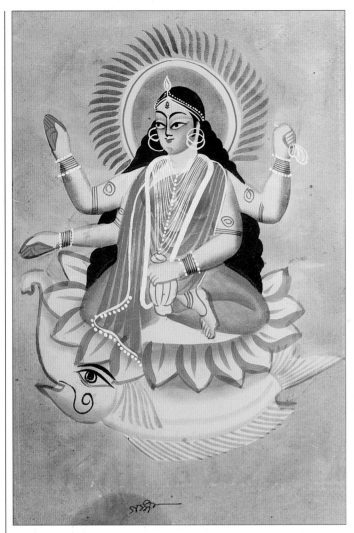

Shiva, the Hindu god who oversees health, is said to live under the bael tree, an important medicinal plant in India.

shaman provides medical treatment for the physical needs of the patient – putting salves and compresses on wounds, boiling up decoctions and barks for internal treatment, stimulating sweating for fevers, and so on. Such treatment is based on a wealth of acutely observed plant lore and knowledge, handed down in an oral tradition from generation to generation.

THE DEVELOPMENT OF MEDICINAL LORE

It is generally recognized that our ancestors had a wide range of medicinal plants at their disposal, and that they likewise possessed a profound understanding of plants' healing powers. In fact, up until the 20th century, every village and rural community had a wealth of herbal folklore. Tried and tested local plants were picked for a range of common health problems and taken as teas, applied as lotions, or even mixed with lard and rubbed in as an ointment.

But what were the origins of this herbal expertise? There are no definitive answers. Clearly, acute observation coupled with trial and error has played a predominant role. Human societies have had many thousands of years to observe the effects – both good and bad – of eating a particular root, leaf, or berry. Watching the behavior of animals after they have eaten or rubbed against certain plants has also added to medicinal lore. If one watches sheep or cattle, they almost unerringly steer a path past poisonous plants such as ragwort (*Senecio jacobaea*, p. 267) or oleander (*Nerium oleander*). Over and above such close observation, some people have speculated that human beings, like grazing animals, have an instinct that recognizes poisonous as opposed to medicinal plants.

ANCIENT CIVILIZATIONS

As civilizations grew from 3000 BC onward in Egypt, the Middle East, India, and China, so the use of herbs became more sophisticated, and the first written accounts of medicinal plants were made. The Egyptian Ebers papyrus of *c.* 1500 BC is the earliest surviving example. It lists dozens of medicinal plants, their uses, and related spells and incantations. The herbs include myrrh (*Commiphora molmol*, p. 84), castor oil (*Ricinus communis*, p. 260), and garlic (*Allium sativum*, p. 56).

In India, the *Vedas*, epic poems written in about 1500 BC, also contain rich material on the herbal lore of that time. The *Vedas* were followed in about 700 BC by the *Charaka Samhita,* written by the physician Charaka. This medical treatise includes details of around 350 herbal medicines. Among them are visnaga (*Ammi visnaga*, p. 59), an herb of Middle Eastern origin that has recently proven effective in the treatment of asthma, and gotu kola (*Centella asiatica*, p. 74), which has long been used to treat leprosy.

MEDICINE BREAKS FROM ITS MYSTICAL ORIGINS

By about 500 BC in developed cultures, medicine began to separate from the magical and spiritual world. Hippocrates (460– 377 BC), the Greek "father of medicine," considered illness to be a natural rather than a supernatural phenomenon, and he felt that medicine should be given without ritual ceremonies or magic.

In the earliest Chinese medical text, the *Yellow Emperor's Classic of Internal Medicine* written in the 1st century BC, the emphasis on rational medicine is equally clear: "In treating illness, it is necessary to examine the entire context, scrutinize the

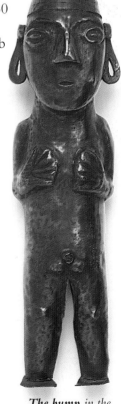

The bump in the right cheek of this figurine from Peru may represent coca, taken in that country to increase endurance.

symptoms, observe the emotions and attitudes. If one insists on the presence of ghosts and spirits one cannot speak of therapeutics."

FOUNDATION OF MAJOR HERBAL TRADITIONS 300 BC–AD 600

Trade between Europe, the Middle East, India, and Asia was already well established by the 2nd century BC, making trade routes available for many medicinal and culinary herbs. Cloves (*Eugenia caryophyllata*, p. 95), for example, native to the Philippines and the Molucca Islands near New Guinea, were imported into China in the 3rd century BC and first arrived in Egypt around AD 176. As the centuries passed, cloves' popularity grew. By the 8th century AD, their strong aromatic flavor and powerfully antiseptic and analgesic properties were familiar throughout most of Europe.

As trade and interest in herbal medicines and spices flourished, many writers attempted to catalog plants with a known medicinal action and record their properties systematically.

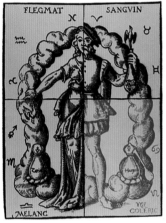

Galen's "Four Humors," *which he believed made up the human constitution.*

In China, the *Divine Husbandman's Classic (Shen'nong Bencaojing)*, written in the 1st century AD, has 364 entries, of which 252 are herbal medicines, including bupleurum (*Bupleurum chinense*, p. 68), coltsfoot (*Tussilago farfara*, p. 277), and *gan cao* (*Glycyrrhiza uralensis*, p. 215). This Daoist text laid the foundations for the continuous development and refinement of Chinese herbal medicine up to the present day.

In Europe, a 1st-century AD Greek physician named Dioscorides wrote the first European herbal, *De Materia Medica*. His intention was to produce an accurate and authoritative work on herbal medicines and in this he was dramatically successful. Among the many plants mentioned are juniper (*Juniperus communis*, p. 223), elm (*Ulmus carpinifolia*), peony (*Paeonia officinalis*, p. 241), and burdock (*Arctium lappa*, p. 62). The text, listing about 600 herbs in all, was to have an astonishing influence on Western medicine, being the principal reference used in Europe until the 17th century. It was translated into many languages as varied as Anglo-Saxon, Persian, and Hebrew. In AD 512, *De Materia Medica* became the first herbal to feature pictures of the plants discussed. Made for Juliana Arnicia, the daughter of the Roman emperor Flavius Avicius Olybrius, it contained nearly 400 full-page color illustrations.

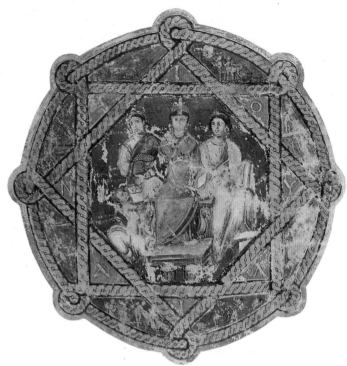

Frontispiece *decoration for the first illustrated herbal, Dioscorides' De Materia Medica, produced in Constantinople in AD 512.*

Galen (AD 131–200), physician to the Roman emperor Marcus Aurelius, had an equally profound influence on the development of herbal medicine. Galen drew inspiration from Hippocrates and based his theories on the "theory of the four humors" (*see* p. 30). His ideas shaped and, some would say, distorted medical practice there for the next 1,400 years.

In India and in China, elaborate medical systems somewhat resembling the theory of the four humors developed (*see* pp. 34–35 and pp. 38–39, respectively) that have endured to the present day.

Though European, Indian, and Chinese systems differ widely, they all consider that imbalance within the constituent elements of the body is the cause of illness, and that the aim of the healer is to restore balance, often with the aid of herbal remedies.

FOLK HEALING IN THE MIDDLE AGES

The theories of Galenic, Ayurvedic (Indian), and Chinese traditional medicine, however, would have meant practically nothing to most of the world's population. As is still the case today for some indigenous peoples who have little access to conventional medicines, in the past most villages and communities relied on the services of local "wise" men and women for medical treatment. These healers were almost certainly ignorant of the conventions of scholastic medicine, yet through apprenticeship and practice in treating illness, attending childbirth, and making use of locally growing herbs as a natural pharmacy, they developed a high level of practical medical knowledge.

We tend to underestimate the medical skills of apparently undeveloped communities – particularly during the so-called Dark Ages in medieval Europe – but it is evident that many people had a surprisingly sophisticated understanding of plant medicine. For example, recent excavations at an 11th-century monastic hospital in Scotland revealed that the monks were using exotic herbs such as opium poppy (*Papaver somniferum*, p. 242) and marijuana (*Cannabis sativa*, p. 180) as painkillers and anesthetics. Likewise, the herbalists in Myddfai, a village in South Wales, obviously knew of Hippocrates' writings in the 6th century AD and used a wide variety of medicinal plants. The texts that have been handed down from that herbal tradition are filled with an engaging blend of superstition and wisdom. Two prescriptions from a 13th-century manuscript illustrate the point. The first recipe could have been written by a modern, scientifically trained herbalist; the second, one must presume, is pure fancy as worms do not destroy teeth.

To Strengthen the Sight
Take Eyebright and Red Fennel, a handful of each, and half a handful of Rue, distil, and wash your eye daily therewith.

To Destroy a Worm in the Tooth
Take the root of a cat's ear, bruise, and apply to the patient's tooth for three nights, and it will kill the worm.

ISLAMIC & INDIAN MEDICINE AD 500–1500

Folk medicine was largely unaffected by sweeping forces of history, but Western scholastic medicine suffered greatly with the decline and fall of the Roman Empire.

It was thanks to the flowering of Arabic culture in AD 500–1300 that the gains of the classical Greek and Roman period were preserved and elaborated. The spread of Islamic culture along North Africa and into present-day Italy, Spain, and Portugal led to the establishment of renowned medical schools, notably at Cordoba in Spain. The Arabs proved to be expert pharmacists, blending and mixing herbs to improve their medicinal effect and their taste. Their contacts with both Indian and Chinese medicine meant that they had a remarkable range of medical and herbal knowledge to draw on and develop. Avicenna (980–1037), the author of *Canon of Medicine*, was the most famous physician of the day, but perhaps the most unusual herbal connection was made a century before his time by Ibn Cordoba, an intrepid Arab seafarer, who brought ginseng root (*Panax ginseng*, p. 116) with him from China to Europe. This valuable tonic herb was to be regularly imported into Europe from the 16th century onward.

Farther east, in India, the 7th century saw a golden age of medicine. Thousands of students studied Ayurveda in universities, especially at Nalanda. There, scholars recorded the medical achievements of the time, with advances such as the development of hospitals, maternity homes, and the planting of medicinal herb gardens.

CENTRAL & SOUTH AMERICAN CURES

On the other side of the world, the civilizations of Central and South America – Maya, Aztec, and Inca – all had herbal traditions with a profound understanding of local medicinal plants. One account tells how the Incas took local herbalists from what is now Bolivia back to their capital Cuzco in Peru because of the herbalists' great capabilities, which reputedly included growing penicillin on green banana skins.

At the same time there were cultures in which medicine and religion were still closely interwoven, possibly even more so than in Europe. In one gruesome example, Aztec sufferers of skin diseases sought to appease the god Xipe Totec by wearing the flayed skins of sacrificial victims. Fortunately, a supernatural appeal to the gods was not the sole means to relieve this and other afflictions. Many herbal remedies were available as alternative treatments, including sarsaparilla (*Smilax* spp., p. 268), a tonic and cleansing herb that was often used to treat psoriasis and similar conditions.

Galen and Hippocrates,
two of the preeminent
physicians of the classical era,
debate in this imaginary scene
depicted in a fresco.

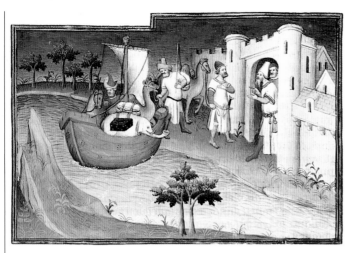

Marco Polo's voyage to China in the 14th century opened the door for a flourishing reciprocal trade in goods, including medicinal herbs, between East and West. Eventually, exotic herbs like ginger and cinnamon became staples in European medicine and cooking.

REBIRTH OF EUROPEAN SCHOLARSHIP AD 1000–1400

As European scholars slowly started to absorb the lessons of Arabic medical learning in the early Middle Ages, classical Greek, Roman, and Egyptian texts preserved in the libraries of Constantinople (later Istanbul) filtered back to Europe, and hospitals, medical schools, and universities were founded. Perhaps the most interesting among them was the medical school at Salerno on the west coast of Italy. It not only allowed students from all faiths – Christian, Moslem, and Jewish – to study medicine, but it also allowed women to train to become physicians. Trotula, a woman who wrote a book on obstetrics, practiced and taught there in about 1050. Herbs were, of course, central to the healing process. An adage from the Salerno school on sage (*Salvia officinalis*, p. 130) went as follows: *Salvia salvatrix, natura conciliatrix* (sage, the savior; nature, the conciliator).

By the 12th century, trade with Asia and Africa was expanding, and new herbs and spices were being regularly imported into Europe. Hildegard of Bingen (1098–1179), the famous German mystic and herbal authority, considered galangal (*Alpinia officinarum*, p. 58) – used in Asia as a warming and nourishing spice for the digestive system – to be the "spice of life," given by God to provide health and to protect against illness.

ASIAN UNIFICATION

Marco Polo's travels to China in the 14th century coincided with the unification of the whole of Asia from the Yellow Sea in China to the Black Sea in southeastern Europe by Genghis Khan and his grandson Kublai Khan, whose capital was in China, not far from Beijing. Neither the Chinese nor Ayurvedic medical traditions were directly threatened by this conquest. The Mongol rulers were strict in banning the use of certain toxic plants such as aconite (*Aconitum napellus*, p. 158), but their decree may have held an element of self-preservation, given aconite's alternative use as an arrow poison – one that could have been used against the ruling powers. Moreover, the Mongol unification may have helped to encourage greater communication between the two medical disciplines.

In other parts of Asia, such as Vietnam and Japan, Chinese culture and medicine exerted the primary influence. While *kampoh* – the traditional herbal medicine of Japan – is distinctive to that country, its roots stem from Chinese practices.

TRADE BETWEEN CONTINENTS 1400–1700

Trade routes had slowly expanded during the Middle Ages, bringing exotic new herbs in their wake. From the 15th century onward, an explosion in trade led to a cornucopia of new herbs becoming readily available in Europe. They included plants such as ginger (*Zingiber officinale*, p. 153), cardamom (*Eletteria cardamomum*, p. 91), nutmeg (*Myristica fragrans*, p. 113), turmeric (*Curcuma longa*, p. 88), cinnamon (*Cinnamomum verum*, p. 80), and senna (*Cassia senna*, p. 72).

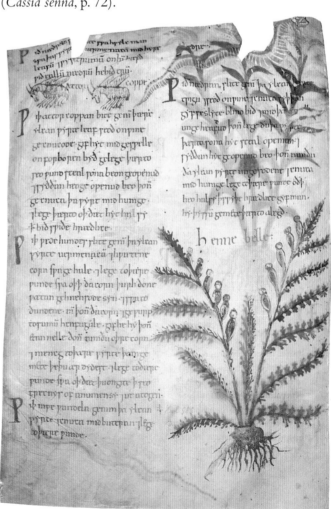

Manuscript page from an Anglo-Saxon herbal of about AD 1050, illustrating the aerial parts and root system of a medicinal plant.

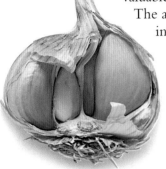

The trade in herbs was not entirely one way. The European herb sage, for example, was used in China, where it was considered to be a valuable *yin* tonic.

The arrival of Columbus's ships in the Caribbean in 1492 was followed by the rapid conquest and colonization of Central and South America by the Spanish and Portuguese. Along with their booty of plundered gold, the conquistadores returned to the Old World with previously unheard-of medicinal plants. Many

Garlic is native to Asia but was readily adopted for its medicinal and culinary qualities in the West.

of these herbs from the Americas had highly potent medicinal actions, and they soon became available in the apothecaries of the major European cities. Plants such as lignum vitae (*Guaiacum officinale*, p. 216) and cinchona (*Cinchona* spp., p. 79) with strong medicinal actions were used with greater and lesser degrees of success as treatments for fever, malaria, syphilis, smallpox, and other serious illnesses.

For most rural communities, however, the only foreign plants that were used medicinally were those that could also be grown locally as foods. Garlic offers one of the earliest and clearest examples. Originating in central Asia, over time it was cultivated farther and farther west and was grown in Egypt around 4500 BC. In Homer's 8th century BC epic poem *Ulysses*, the hero is saved from being changed into a pig, thanks to garlic! The herb was introduced into Britain after the Roman conquest in the 1st century AD, and by the time it reached the island its remarkable medicinal powers were well understood. In later centuries, potatoes (*Solanum tuberosum*, p. 269) and corn (*Zea mays*, p. 152), both native to South America, would become common foods. These plants have clear medicinal as well as nutritional benefits. Potato juice is a valuable remedy for the treatment of arthritis, while cornsilk makes an effective decoction for urinary problems such as cystitis.

HEALTH & HYGIENE 1400–1700

Between the 12th and 18th centuries, the influx of exotic medicinal plants added to an already large number of useful European herbs. Conceivably, an overall improvement of health in Europe might have resulted. After all, not only were new medicinal plants available but Europeans had the opportunity to observe the different medical practices of people in South America, China, Japan, and especially in India, where trade was well established.

But, in fact, the reverse was the case. People living in Europe during this period probably experienced some of the most unhealthy conditions the world has ever seen. In contrast, Native Americans before the arrival of Columbus lived longer, healthier lives than their counterparts in Europe. This fact is unsurprising given the cities of medieval Europe, with their open sewers, overcrowding, and ignorance of simple, basic hygiene.

Conditions such as these laid fertile ground for the spread of plague-infested rats from the ports of the Mediterranean throughout Western Europe. From the mid-14th century on, plague killed millions, in some cases close to 50 percent of the population. No medical treatment – herbal or mineral – was able to alter its fatal course. Epidemics continued to decimate the cities of Europe and Asia well into the 18th century. A recent outbreak in India in 1994 reawakened the terror inspired simply at the mention of the word "plague."

Syphilis was another disease spread by seafarers. It was reputedly brought back from the Caribbean to Naples by Columbus's crew in the 1490s, spreading quickly throughout Europe and to the rest of the world, reaching China in 1550.

European doctors had little success in combating diseases as devastating as plague. The medicine they practiced was based on the blind acceptance of Galen's humoral principles. Perhaps if, as in Chinese and Indian medicine, European medicine had continued to evolve, revising ancient medical texts and reinterpreting them in the light of new discoveries, it would have had greater success. As it was, European physicians were at least as likely to kill their patients with bloodletting and toxic minerals in misbegotten attempts to balance the humors as they were to cure. Indeed, the increasingly fashionable use of mineral cures, such as mercury, led to the growth of chemical formulations, culminating in scientific medicine's ultimate break away from herbal practices.

THE INFLUENCE OF PARACELSUS

One of the key European figures of the 16th century was Paracelsus (1493–1541), a larger-than-life character who rejected the tired repetition of Galen's theories in favor of detailed observation in medicine. "I have

17th-century doctor wearing a costume designed to protect against contamination by the plague.

not borrowed from Hippocrates, Galen or anyone else," he wrote, "having acquired my knowledge from the best teacher, that is, by experience and hard work." And again, "What a doctor needs is not eloquence or knowledge of language and of books, but profound knowledge of nature and her works." He also paid great attention to the exact dosage, saying that "it depends only on the dose whether a poison is a poison or not."

As a result, Paracelsus was an influential force in the future development of chemistry, conventional medicine, herbal medicine, and homeopathy. He is known as the "father of chemistry," but he also explored alchemy, which concerned itself with the transmutation of base materials to gold, and the search for immortal life. Paracelsus also revived interest in the Doctrine of

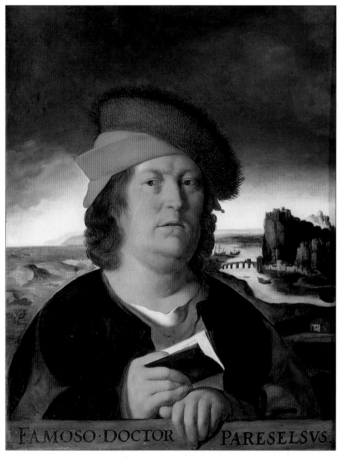

The iconoclastic Paracelsus, *an alchemist and chemist, was one of the greatest scientists of the 16th century, and advocated the use of minerals in healing but only in tightly controlled dosages.*

Signatures – the ancient theory that held that a plant's appearance indicated the ailments it would treat – and affirmed the value of locally grown medicinal herbs over expensive, imported specimens.

CULPEPER & PRINTED HERBALS

Paracelsus's advocacy of local herbs was later fiercely espoused by Nicholas Culpeper (1616–1654). The frontispiece to his *The English Physitian* has the memorable words: "Containing a Compleat Method of Physick,

whereby a Man may preserve his Body in Health, or Cure himself, being Sick, for three pence Charge, with such things only as grow in England, they being most fit for English Bodies."

Wounded during the English Civil War fighting for the Commonwealth, Culpeper championed the needs of the ordinary people who could afford neither the services of a doctor nor the expensive imported herbs and formulations that doctors generally prescribed. Drawing to some degree on Dioscorides, Arabian physicians, and Paracelsus, Culpeper developed a medical system that blended astrology and sound personal experience of the therapeutic uses of local plants. His herbal became an instant "bestseller" and appeared in many subsequent editions. The first herbal published in North America, in 1700, was an edition of his herbal.

While the popularity of *The English Physitian* was notable, other herbals also found a place in households. The development of the printing press in the 15th century brought herbal medicine into homes on a wide scale. Texts such as Dioscorides' *De Materia Medica* were printed for the first time, and throughout Europe herbals were published and ran through many editions.

DEADLY CURES 1700–1900

By the end of the 16th century, Paracelsus had become the figurehead of the new chemical medicine. However, where he had insisted upon caution in the use of metallic poisons – mercury, antimony, and arsenic – the new medical thinkers were not so inhibited. Larger and larger doses of the purgative known as calomel (mercurous chloride, Hg_2Cl_2) were given to those suffering from syphilis and many other diseases. The treatment was very often worse than the illness, with some patients dying and many more suffering from the long-term consequences of mercury poisoning.

Hippocrates' saying "Desperate cases need the most desperate remedies" was taken very literally, as is evident in the incredible excess of purging and bleeding that developed over the next three centuries in Europe and North America. These practices reached a peak in the "heroic" medicine of the early 19th century. Its leading proponent, Dr. Benjamin Rush (1745–1813), maintained that only bloodletting and calomel were required in medical practice. His position was obviously extreme, but it is clear that in this new climate, herbal medicines were becoming increasingly irrelevant.

THE NEW RATIONALISM

Along with the new emphasis on chemical cures, modern medicine came to look askance at the notion of the "vital force." Up until the end of the 16th century, nearly all medical traditions had been based on the concept of working with nature, with the body's healing capacities, which could be supported and strengthened

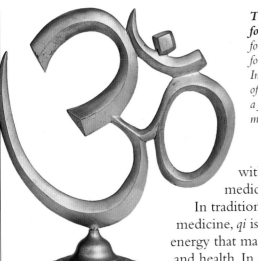

The symbol for "om" – life force – is used by followers of the Indian practice of Ayurveda as a focus for meditation.

with appropriate medicinal herbs.

In traditional Chinese medicine, *qi* is the primal energy that maintains life and health. In Ayurveda, it is *prana*, and in the Western tradition, Hippocrates writes about *"vis medicatrix naturae"* or the healing power of nature, while modern Western medical herbalists and homeopaths use the term "vital force."

The importance of the vital force was diminished in the West by the philosophy of René Descartes (1596–1650). This French mathematician divided the world into body and mind, nature and ideas. His philosophy ordained that the intangible vital force that maintains life and governs good health was the province of religion rather than of the newly self-aware "science" of medicine. To the new medical establishment, inching its way forward to scientifically sound medical practices, "supernatural" concepts, such as the vital force, were a reminder of the ignorance and superstition that were part and parcel of older healing practices.

Even before Descartes' theories, the rational approach to scientific and medical exploration was beginning to reap rewards. Slowly, medical understanding of bodily functions was gaining ground. William Harvey (1578–1657) made a detailed study of the heart and circulation, proving for the first time that, contrary to Galenic thought, the heart pumped blood around the body. Published in 1628, his study is a classic example of the revolution in medical science.

Since Harvey's time, science has had astounding success in revealing how the body works on a biochemical level and in distinguishing different disease processes. However, by comparison it has been altogether less successful in developing effective medical treatments for the relief and cure of diseases.

THE GAP IN THE SCIENTIFIC APPROACH

In hindsight, it seems as if the new science of medicine could only be born in separation from the traditional arts of healing, with which it had always been intertwined. As a result, even though traditional medicine has generally lacked scientific explanation, it has frequently been far ahead of medical science in the way it has been applied therapeutically. In *American Indian Medicine* (University of Oklahoma Press, 1970), Virgil Vogel provides a good example of "ignorant" folk medicine outstripping scientific understanding in therapeutic application:

"During the bitter cold winter of 1535–6, the three ships of Jacques Cartier were frozen fast in the fathom-deep ice of the St. Lawrence River near the site of Montreal. Isolated by four feet of snow, the company of 110 men subsisted on the fare stored in the holds of their ships. Soon scurvy was so rampant among them that by mid-March, 25 men had died and the others, 'only three or foure excepted,' were so ill that hope for their recovery was abandoned. As the crisis deepened Cartier had the good fortune to encounter once again the local Indian chief, Domagaia, who had cured himself of the same disease with 'the juice and sappe of a certain tree.' The Indian women gathered branches of the magical tree, 'boiling the bark and leaves for a decoction, and placing the dregs upon the legs.' All those so treated rapidly recovered their health, and the Frenchmen marvelled at the curative skill of the natives."

Naturally, the Native Americans had not heard of vitamin C deficiency, which causes scurvy, nor would they have been able to explain in rational terms why the treatment worked. Indeed, it was not until 1753 that James Lind (1716–1794), a British naval surgeon, inspired partly by Cartier's account, published *A Treatise of the Scurvy*, which showed conclusively that the disease could be prevented by eating fresh greens, vegetables, and fruit, and was caused by their lack in the diet. James Lind's work is a marvelous example of what can be achieved

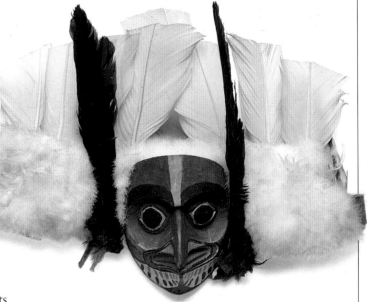

Mask of a northwestern Native American shaman.
The efficacy of techniques used by native healers often surpassed that of conventional medical practices of the time.

by combining a systematic and scientific approach with traditional herbal knowledge.

ISOLATING CHEMICALS

The discovery of the medicinal value of common foxglove (*Digitalis purpurea*, p. 199) is another case where traditional herbal knowledge led to a major advance in medicine. Dr. William Withering (1741–1799), a conventionally trained doctor with a long interest in medicinal plants, started to investigate foxglove after encountering a family recipe for curing dropsy (water retention). He found that in some regions of England, foxglove was traditionally used to treat this condition, which is often one of the indications of a failing heart. In 1785, he published *Account of the Foxglove*, documenting dozens of carefully recorded case histories, and showing how foxglove's powerful (and potentially dangerous) active constituents, now known as cardiac glycosides, made it a valuable plant medicine in the treatment of dropsy. Cardiac glycosides remain in common use to the present day. Yet despite this clearcut example of the possibilities inherent in a marriage of herbal medicine and scientific method, conventional medicine was to take another path in the 19th century.

LABORATORY VERSUS NATURE

From the early 19th century onward, the chemical laboratory began regularly to supplant Mother Nature as the source of medicines. In 1803, narcotic alkaloids were isolated from opium poppy (*Papaver somniferum*, p. 242). A year later, inulin was extracted from elecampane (*Inula helenium*, p. 105). In 1838, salicylic acid, a chemical forerunner of aspirin, was isolated from willow bark (*Salix alba*, p. 128), and was first synthesized in the laboratory in 1860. From this point on, herbal medicine and

In the 18th century, the physician William Withering documented foxglove's ability to restore a failing heart.

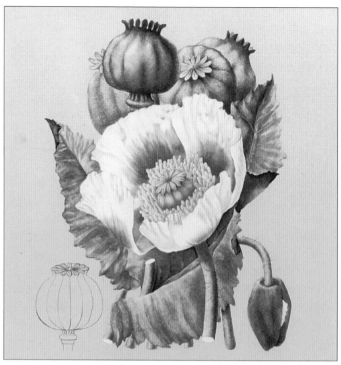

Opium poppy, *native to Asia, yields a resin that has long been smoked for its narcotic effect. The main active constituent, morphine, was first isolated in the laboratory in 1803.*

biomedicine were to take separate paths. Aspirin, an entirely new chemical formulation, was first developed in Germany in 1899. But this was still an early step. For the time being, the influence of the universities, medical schools, and laboratories of Europe would remain limited, and herbal medicine prevailed as the predominant form of treatment for most people around the world.

NEW FRONTIERS, NEW HERBAL MEDICINES

Wherever Europeans settled during the great migrations of the 18th and 19th centuries – North America, South America, southern Africa, or Australia – much of the European medicine familiar from home was either unavailable or prohibitively expensive. European settlers came to learn that native peoples were a wellspring of information about the medicinal virtues of indigenous plants. For example, settlers in southern Africa learned about the diuretic properties of buchu (*Barosma betulina*, p. 67) from native peoples, and Australian settlers came to understand the remarkable antiseptic properties of tea tree (*Melaleuca alternifolia*, p. 110) from observing the medicinal practices of the Aborigines. Mexican herbal medicine as it exists today is a blend of Aztec, Mayan, and Spanish herbs and practices.

In North America, native herbalists were particularly adept at healing external wounds and bites – being superior in many respects to their European counterparts in this area of medicine. This is not surprising, given the range of highly effective medicinal plants Native Americans had discovered – including well-known herbs such as echinacea (*Echinacea angustifolia*, p. 90), goldenseal (*Hydrastis canadensis*, p. 103), and lobelia (*Lobelia inflata*, p. 108).

European settlers learned much from observing native practices. Over the course of the 19th and early 20th centuries as pioneers moved west across the frontier territory, new plants were constantly being added to the official record of healing herbs. In addition to the three species mentioned above, about 170 native plants were listed in the *Pharmacopoeia of the United States*.

SAMUEL THOMSON & HIS FOLLOWERS

Lobelia was one of the key herbs, along with cayenne (*Capsicum frutescens*, p. 70), advocated by Samuel Thomson (1769–1843), an unorthodox herbal practitioner. He developed a drastically simple approach to medicine that was entirely at odds with the conventional practices of his time (*see* North America, p. 48). His approach was often extremely effective and was well suited to the needs of people living in frontier territory. His system of medicine, which was really the earliest form of naturopathy (a form of healing in which symptoms are treated with herbs, naturally grown food, sunlight, and fresh air) became extraordinarily popular, with millions of people across North America following his methods. Thomson's success waned as other more sophisticated herbal approaches were developed – those of the Eclectics and Physiomedicalists, for example – in the fertile medical world of 19th-century America, which also saw the birth of osteopathy (a system of healing based upon the manipulation of bones) and chiropractic (a similar system primarily involving manipulation of the spine).

WESTERN INFLUENCES ON ASIAN MEDICINE

Across the world in China, Thomson's practices might have been looked on with a measure of surprise, but they would have been familiar. In Chinese medicine, there has always been a debate as to what degree illness arises from cold, and to what degree it arises from heat. The *Shanghanlun (On Cold-Induced Maladies)*, written in the 2nd century AD and revised and reinterpreted in commentaries over the last 1,800 years,

Ginseng has been used as a tonic remedy in Chinese medicine for at least 5,000 years.

recommends the herb cinnamon (*Cinnamomum verum*, p. 80) as a principal remedy when the patient "shivers with fever, breathes heavily, and feels nauseous." In the 14th century, Wang Lu distinguished between cold-induced illness and febrile illness, and treated them in different ways; this distinction was elaborated in greater and greater detail by different Chinese herbalists right up to the 19th century.

During the early 19th century, the influence of Western biomedicine was beginning to affect traditional practices in both China and India. This was certainly beneficial in many respects. The judicious incorporation of scientific principles and methods into traditional herbal healing offered the possibility of greatly refining the effectiveness of traditional treatment.

However, in India under British rule, Western medicine eventually became the only alternative. Ayurveda was seen as inferior to biomedicine (*see* India, p. 37). Western practice was introduced not as a complement to traditional medicine but rather as a means to supplant it. According to one authority, "before 1835 Western physicians and their Indian counterparts exchanged knowledge; thereafter only Western medicine was recognised as legitimate and the Eastern systems were actively discouraged" (Robert Svoboda, *Ayurveda, Life, Health and Longevity*, 1992).

In China, the influx of Western ideas was less traumatic. Increasing numbers of Chinese medical students studied Western medicine, but this did not stop the continuing development of traditional herbal practice. By and large, each tradition was recognized as having both advantages and disadvantages.

HERBALISM OUTLAWED 1850–1900

In Europe, conventional medicine was seeking to establish a monopoly for its own type of practice. In 1858, the British Parliament was asked to impose legislation banning the practice of medicine by anyone who had not been trained in a conventional medical school. Fortunately, this proposal was rejected but in countries such as France, Spain, Italy, and the US, it became illegal to practice herbal medicine without an orthodox qualification. Herbalists were forced to risk fines or imprisonment simply for providing herbal medicine to patients who had sought their help.

In Britain, concerns such as these, combined with a desire to establish Western herbal medicine as an alternative to conventional practices, particularly in the industrial cities of the North of England, led to the formation in 1864 of the National Institute of Medical Herbalists, the first professional body of herbal practitioners in the world. Its history is an example of how tenacious herbal practitioners have had to be simply to retain their right to give safe, gentle, and effective herbal medicines to their patients.

20TH CENTURY & THE FUTURE

For most of us, medicine in the 20th century is exemplified by drugs, such as antibiotics, and highly technical methods of diagnosis and treatment. However, many might be surprised to discover that, for much of this century, herbal medicines have been the primary form of treatment, even in Western countries.

AS LATE AS THE 1930s, around 90 percent of medicines prescribed by doctors or sold over the counter were herbal in origin. It is only during the last 50 years that laboratory-produced medicines have become the norm. During World War I (1914–1918), for example, garlic (*Allium sativum*, p. 56) and sphagnum moss (*Sphagnum* spp.) were used by the ton in the battle trenches to treat and dress wounds and infections. Garlic is an excellent natural antibiotic and was the most effective antiseptic available at the time, and sphagnum moss, gathered from moorlands, makes a natural aseptic dressing.

SCIENCE & MEDICINE

The development of new medicines in the laboratory – either extracted from medicinal plants or synthesized – stretches back to the early 19th century, when chemists first isolated constituents such as morphine, from opium poppy (*Papaver somniferum*, p. 242), and cocaine, from coca (*Erythroxylum coca*, p. 204). From that time on, scientists made tremendous progress in understanding how isolated chemicals affect the body, as well as how the body works in both health and disease. From the 1860s onward, scientists – notably Louis Pasteur (1822–1895) – began to identify the micro-organisms that were ultimately responsible for causing infectious diseases, such as tuberculosis and malaria.

Louis Pasteur was a pioneer in the identification of bacteria.

Naturally enough, the first aim of those engaged in medical research was to seek out medicines that would act as "magic bullets," directly attacking the micro-organisms concerned and ridding the body of the threat. This eventually led to the discovery, or more accurately, the rediscovery of penicillin by a number of medical researchers, most notably Alexander Fleming (1881–1955) in 1929. However, while 20th-century scientists were the first to scientifically evaluate antibiotics as medicines, they were not the first to employ them for healing purposes. Antibiotic molds had been grown and used to combat infection in ancient Egypt, 14th-century Peru, and in recent European folk medicine.

In the decades following World War II (1939–1945), when antibiotics first came into use, it seemed as though a new era had dawned in which infection could be conquered, and life-threatening diseases such as syphilis, pneumonia, and tuberculosis would cease to be major causes of death in the developed world. Modern medicine also provided other highly effective drugs such as steroid anti-inflammatories, and it seemed only a question of time until cures for most illnesses were found.

ASCENDANCY OF BIOMEDICINE

As Americans and Europeans became accustomed to medication that led to an almost instant short-term improvement in symptoms (if not in underlying health), herbal medicines came to be seen by the public as outmoded and ineffective. Increasingly, the practice of herbal medicine was outlawed in North America and most of Europe, and the wealthy in developing countries abandoned herbal medicine in favor of the new treatments available.

This was in no small part due to the medical profession itself, which saw herbal medicine as a throwback to the superstitions of the past. From the late 19th century on, the aim of organizations such as the American Medical Association and the British Medical Association had been to monopolize conventional medical practice. Herbal medicine thus neared extinction in many countries, especially in the US and Britain. In Britain, for example, from 1941 until 1968 it was illegal to practice herbal medicine without medical qualifications.

THE TIDE TURNS

Although there were spectacular successes with modern chemical medicines, there were also horrific disasters, most notably the thalidomide tragedy in 1962 in Britain and Germany, when 3,000 deformed babies were born to mothers who had taken the drug as a sedative during pregnancy. This event

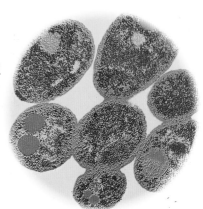

An electron micrograph of the parasite Plasmodium. *Transmitted to man by infected mosquitoes, it causes the disease malaria.*

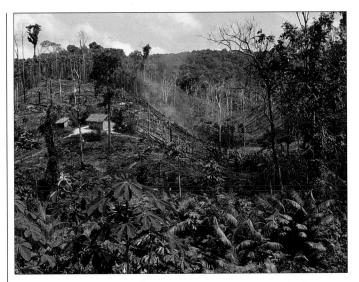

"Slash and burn" farming in the rainforest of Brazil results in the eradication of native medicinal plants. Efforts are now under way to provide local farmers with alternative means of profiting from the land.

marked a turning point in the public's opinion of chemical medicines. People began to realize that a serious cost could accompany the benefits of modern drug treatment. Together with the factors described below, this has brought about a sea change in public perceptions of the value of herbal medicine.

THE CHINESE EXAMPLE

Herbal medicine experienced a major gain in fortune in 1949 in China, when Mao Zedong and the Communist Red Army gained control of the country.

Traditional Western medicine was by then well established in China, but most of the population had little hope of access to modern hospitals, let alone to the new pharmaceutical drugs. Of necessity, traditional Chinese medicine – essentially herbal medicine and acupuncture – once more began to be used alongside Western medicine. The authorities aimed to provide the best of both worlds. Five teaching hospitals for traditional Chinese medicine (TCM) were established, where it was taught on a scientific basis, and great efforts were made to improve the quality of plant medicines.

Contrary to the trend in conventional Western medicine that makes the patient ever more dependent upon the doctor and high-tech machinery, TCM, like other forms of complementary medicine, stresses the patient's personal responsibility for his or her own cure, encouraging a holistic approach to treatment.

In the 1960s, China also established a system of "barefoot doctors." After a period of basic medical instruction that blended herbal medicine, acupuncture, and Western practices, these practitioners were sent out to provide health care to the millions of rural Chinese too remote from cities to benefit from the facilities available there. The barefoot doctors in the late 1960s became a model for the World Health Organization,

which created a strategy of including traditional herbal practitioners in planning for the health care needs of developing countries.

WESTERN MEDICINE & HERBAL PRACTICES

Further to the initiative by the World Health Organization, experience has shown that traditional (usually herbal) and Western medicine can indeed work well in tandem, although the relationship is often quite complex. J. M. Janzen's *The Quest for Therapy in Lower Zaïre* (University of California Press, 1978) describes one such interaction in Africa:

"The people of Zaïre recognize the advantages of Western medicine and seek its surgery, drugs, and hospital care, but contrary to what might have been expected, native doctors, prophets, and traditional consultations among kinsmen do not disappear with the adoption of Western medicine. Rather a [working relationship] has developed in which different forms of therapy play complementary rather than competitive roles in the thoughts and lives of the people."

The high cost of Western medical treatment is another factor that has encouraged people and governments to reexamine traditional healing. In China, Mexico, Cuba, Egypt, Ghana, India, and Mongolia, to give a few examples, herbal medicines are being cultivated in greater quantities and are being used to some degree by conventional as well as traditional practitioners.

Likewise, different types of treatment have evolved to meet the variety of needs within a population. India offers an extraordinary example of the kind of choices now available in types of medical care. Alongside conventional Western physicians, there are medically trained Ayurvedic practitioners, traditional Ayurvedic practitioners, healers and herbalists, and homeopaths.

CHANGING ATTITUDES

Perhaps the most important factor behind the growing interest in complementary medicine is the poor state of health in Western societies. Conventional medicine has by and large brought serious infectious diseases under control, although there are worrying signs that infectious organisms are becoming resistant to antibiotic treatment, largely as a result of their indiscriminate use. Chronic illness, however, seems to be on the increase. Probably around 50 percent of people in Western countries daily take one or more conventional medicines – for conditions as diverse as high blood pressure, asthma, arthritis, and depression. Many Western countries such as the US and France spend vast sums on health care, yet despite this massive investment much of the population remains demonstrably unhealthy. Even the significant increase in life expectancy in developed countries is starting to go into reverse, perhaps a result of environmental pollutants and toxic accumulation within the body.

Over the years, changes in public awareness have led to a renewed interest in herbal medicine. In fact, some herbal preparations are now so commonly used that they are accepted as a part of everyday life. One of many possible examples is evening primrose oil, which is used by hundreds of thousands of women in Britain to help relieve premenstrual tension. It is extracted from the seeds of *Oenothera biennis* (p. 239), a North American plant. Peppermint oil (*Mentha* x *piperita*, p. 112), prescribed for irritable bowel syndrome and other digestive problems, is another example, and senna (*Cassia senna*, p. 72), a simple, effective treatment for short-term constipation, is one of the most frequently used medicines throughout the world.

The growing awareness of how our lives as human beings are interwoven with the fate of our planet also reinforces the value of herbal medicines. As long as care is taken to prevent overharvesting, herbal medicine is ecologically in tune with the environment.

HERBALISM & HOLISM

The "germ theory of disease," which holds that illness springs from contact with an infectious organism, is still widely held in conventional medicine. Medical herbalists, however, believe that this is only part of the picture. While illnesses such as cholera and typhoid are highly infectious and are indeed likely to be caught by almost anyone, many infectious diseases are not transmitted automatically from one person to another. The question arises, therefore, what weakness within the patient has allowed the "seed" of infection to find fertile ground? Unlike much conventional medical practice, which focuses on eradicating the "bug" or abnormal condition, herbal medicine has a more balanced approach, seeking to treat the weakness that gave rise to ill health, and setting this in the context of the patient's life as a whole. Herbalists identify a variety of factors behind the onset of illness. While bodily signs and symptoms are the most important indicators (and sometimes the only significant ones), dietary, emotional, and even spiritual factors are also taken into account.

Our bodies contain over three trillion cells, which collectively must function in harmony if good health is to be maintained. Used wisely, herbs work in tune with our bodies, stimulating, supporting, or restraining different sets of cells in their allotted tasks within the body, and encouraging a return to normal balanced function. Remedies aim to strengthen the patient's own resistance, improve the vitality of weakened tissue, and encourage the body's innate ability to return to good health.

Of course, in severe acute illness, it may be too late to use an herbal approach to treatment. In these circumstances, strong-acting medicines such as heart drugs, antibiotics, painkillers, and even surgery can be lifesavers. However, a health-care system attuned to the needs of

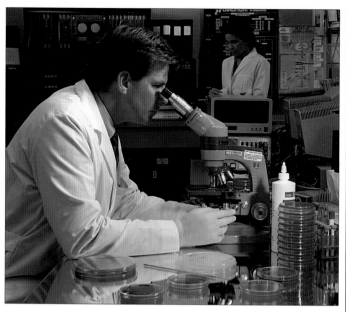

Thanks to increased research *into the composition and properties of plant medicines, herbalists are able to prescribe herbs, formulations, and dosages in a precise, effective manner.*

the patient might well provide herbal remedies as a first line of treatment, with conventional medicines held in reserve to be used only when necessary.

EVIDENCE IN SUPPORT OF HERBAL CURES

Many medical scientists have found it impossible to accept that natural medicines can be as good as or better than chemical cures in treating illness. Fortunately, as more and more research reveals just how effective herbal medicines can be, this attitude is beginning to change.

St. John's wort (*Hypericum perforatum*, p. 104) is a native European herb, valued for its healing properties. In his *Herball* (1597), John Gerard commended the oil as "a most pretious remedie for deep wounds and those that are thorow the body, for the deep sinuses that are prickt, or any wound made with a venomed weapon … *I know that in the world there is not a better* [italics added]." Four centuries later, in a contemporary trial, St. John's wort was shown to be powerfully antiviral, offering up hope that it may be valuable in the treatment of many conditions, including HIV and AIDS.

St. John's wort is also a time-honored remedy for mild depression and nervous exhaustion. A 1993 hospital-based research study in Austria showed that it is every bit as effective as conventional treatments, and unlike many of them has a very low incidence of side effects.

St. John's wort is an example of how modern research often confirms what has been known for centuries to herbal practitioners. Today's practitioners, however, have one important advantage – the method by which the plant works within the body is now better understood, so that it is possible to be precise about dosages, aware of side effects, and confident in what form the herb should be taken as a medicine.

In addition to St. John's wort, many other herbs are being investigated in the search for effective treatments for people suffering from HIV and AIDS. To give but two examples, the Australian Moreton Bay chestnut (*Castanospermum australe*), which was used as an Aboriginal arrow poison, and the Japanese white pine (*Pinus parviflora*) are currently under investigation. We can expect to see a dramatic increase in the number of herbs being investigated for medicinal use in the near future.

MEDICINAL HERBS & BIG BUSINESS

The major pharmaceutical companies have realized that rainforests, grasslands, thickets, and fields are sources of potentially invaluable medicines. As a result, they are investing large sums to try to find new plant chemicals that can be marketed as medicines. Glaxo, the largest pharmaceutical company in the world, trawls 13,000 plant chemicals a week searching for potentially useful constituents. It is in the process of automating its research in this area and will shortly have the capacity to investigate about two million plant chemicals a week.

If this is a taste of what is to come, we can expect remarkable discoveries from the world of plant medicine. There is, however, a key problem in the pharmaceutical industry's approach. It is geared to the development of isolated plant chemicals, which can then be synthesized and patented. With a patent, a company can make a profit, recouping the massive investment required to research and develop new medicines. Herbs, however, are whole, naturally occurring remedies. They cannot and should not be patented. Even if the major pharmaceutical companies were able to find an herb such as St. John's wort, which proved to be more effective and safer than conventional medicines, they would prefer to develop synthetic chemical drugs rather than plant medicines.

HERBAL SYNERGY

One word more than any other separates herbal from conventional medicine, and this word is synergy. When the whole plant is used rather than extracted constituents, the different parts interact, often, it is thought, producing a greater therapeutic effect than the equivalent dosage of isolated active constituents

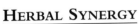

St. John's wort's traditional use as a remedy for nervous exhaustion and depression has been confirmed by clinical trials.

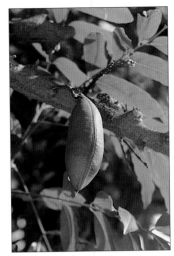

The Moreton Bay chestnut is being investigated as a treatment for AIDS.

generally preferred in conventional medicine.

Increasingly, research shows that herbs such as ephedra (*Ephedra sinica*, p. 93), hawthorn (*Crataegus oxyacantha*, p. 86), ginkgo (*Ginkgo biloba*, p. 98), and lily of the valley (*Convallaria majalis*, p. 192) have a greater-than-expected medicinal benefit, thanks to the natural *combination* of constituents within the whole plant. In some cases, the medicinal value of the herb may be due entirely to the combination of substances and cannot be reproduced by one or two "active" constituents alone.

THE FUTURE OF HERBAL MEDICINE

The main issue for the future of herbal medicine is whether medicinal plants, and the traditional knowledge that informs their use, will be valued for what they are – an immense resource of safe, economical, ecologically balanced medicines – or whether they will be yet another area of life to be exploited for short-term profit.

Another issue is convincing sceptics in the medical world that herbal medicine is not just a poor substitute for conventional medicine but a valuable form of treatment in its own right. In trials into the effect of certain Chinese herbs on patients with eczema at London's Royal Free Hospital in the early 1990s, conventional medical specialists were astonished when the addition of one extra herb to a Chinese formula containing 10 others resulted in a dramatic improvement in a previously unresponsive patient. This story offers evidence of the skill and art involved in herbal practice. In tailoring the remedy to suit the individual needs of the patient and in treating the underlying cause, significant improvements were made. This kind of approach is a far cry from the standard medical view of employing a single drug to treat a single disease.

In India and China, there have been university courses in herbal medicine for decades. In the Western world this process has been slower, although the first undergraduate course in herbal medicine in Western Europe started at Middlesex University in London in 1994. In its combination of traditional herbal knowledge and the medical sciences, it parallels large-scale developments in China, and points toward a future where patients might be able to choose between conventional and herbal approaches when considering what medical treatment will suit them best.

EUROPE

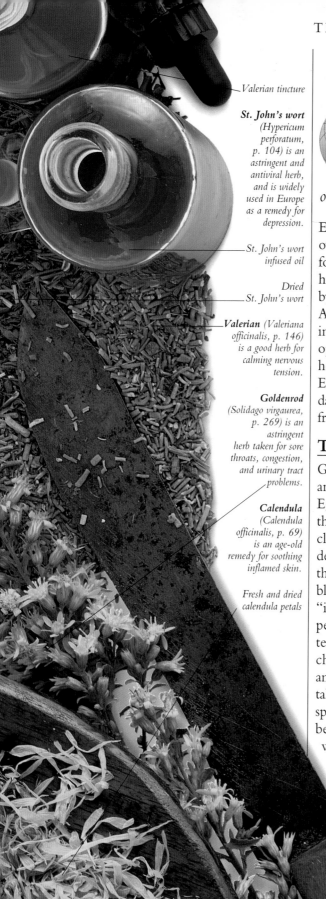

Despite regional variations, European herbal practices largely arose from the common root of the classical tradition. Today, herbalism is increasingly popular in Europe, and in some countries it is widely practiced by orthodox medical practitioners as well as by qualified herbalists.

EACH OF THE WORLD'S MAJOR herbal traditions has developed its own framework for making sense of illness. In Europe, the model for understanding and explaining illness was the "theory of the four humors," which persisted well into the 17th century. It was laid down by Galen (AD 131–201), physician to the Roman emperor Marcus Aurelius. Galen was born in Pergamum and part of his medical practice involved caring for the gladiators of the city, which gave him the opportunity to learn about anatomy and the remedies best suited to healing wounds. He wrote hundreds of books, and his influence on European conventional and herbal medicine has been immense. To this day, plant medicines are sometimes called Galenicals to distinguish them from synthesized drugs.

THE THEORY OF THE FOUR HUMORS

Galen developed his ideas from the texts of Hippocrates (460–*c.* 377 BC) and Aristotle (384–322 BC), who in turn had been influenced by Egyptian and Indian ideas. Hippocrates, expanding on the early belief that the world was made up of the elements fire, air, earth, and water, classified herbs as having hot, dry, cold, and moist properties. Aristotle developed and endorsed the theory of the four humors. According to the theory, four principal fluids – or humors – exist within the body: blood, choler (yellow bile), melancholy (black bile), and phlegm. The "ideal" person bore all four in equal proportion. However, in most people, one or more humors predominate, giving rise to particular temperaments or characters. For instance, excess choler produced a choleric-type person, who was likely to be short-tempered, sallow, ambitious, and vengeful. Galen also believed that *pneuma* (spirit) was taken in with each breath, and processed in the body to form the "vital spirit." Vitality and good health depended upon the proper balance between the four humors and the four elements and the correct mix with the inspired *pneuma*.

INFLUENCE OF CLASSICAL HERBALISTS

Two other classical writers strongly influenced the European herbal tradition. Dioscorides (AD 40–90), a Greek-born Roman army surgeon, wrote the classical world's most comprehensive book on herbal medicines, *De Materia Medica*, based on observations of nearly 600 plants. Pliny the Elder (AD 23–79) drew together writings from over 400 authors in his *Natural History*, recording, among other things, herbal lore of the time. Much traditional European knowledge of medicinal herbs comes from Dioscorides and Pliny. One of the most interesting herbs mentioned by both is

Valerian tincture

St. John's wort *(Hypericum perforatum, p. 104) is an astringent and antiviral herb, and is widely used in Europe as a remedy for depression.*

St. John's wort infused oil

Dried St. John's wort

Valerian *(Valeriana officinalis, p. 146) is a good herb for calming nervous tension.*

Goldenrod *(Solidago virgaurea, p. 269) is an astringent herb taken for sore throats, congestion, and urinary tract problems.*

Calendula *(Calendula officinalis, p. 69) is an age-old remedy for soothing inflamed skin.*

Fresh and dried calendula petals

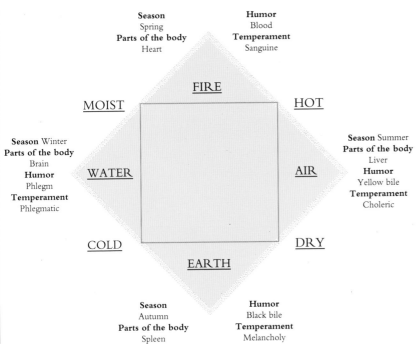

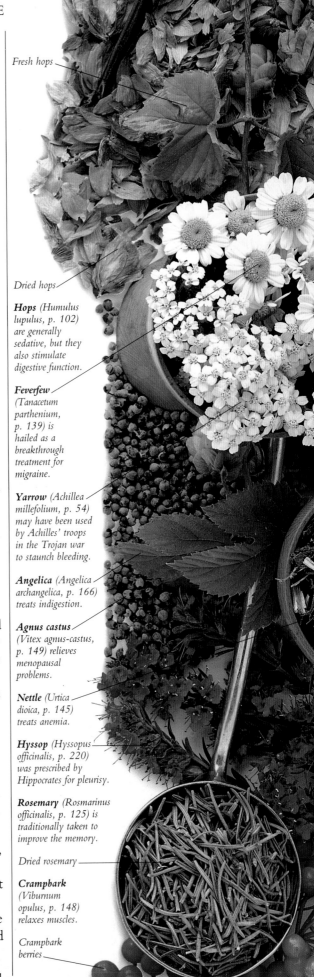

Fresh hops

Dried hops

Hops (*Humulus lupulus, p. 102*) *are generally sedative, but they also stimulate digestive function.*

Feverfew (*Tanacetum parthenium, p. 139*) *is hailed as a breakthrough treatment for migraine.*

Yarrow (*Achillea millefolium, p. 54*) *may have been used by Achilles' troops in the Trojan war to staunch bleeding.*

Angelica (*Angelica archangelica, p. 166*) *treats indigestion.*

Agnus castus (*Vitex agnus-castus, p. 149*) *relieves menopausal problems.*

Nettle (*Urtica dioica, p. 145*) *treats anemia.*

Hyssop (*Hyssopus officinalis, p. 220*) *was prescribed by Hippocrates for pleurisy.*

Rosemary (*Rosmarinus officinalis, p. 125*) *is traditionally taken to improve the memory.*

Dried rosemary

Crampbark (*Viburnum opulus, p. 148*) *relaxes muscles.*

Crampbark berries

The ancient theory of the four humors holds that four fluids within the body – black bile, phlegm, yellow bile, and blood – correspond to the four elements (earth, water, air, and fire), the four seasons, and other aspects of the natural world. Until the 17th century, physicians believed that an imbalance of the humoral system caused mental and physical illness.

mandrake (*Mandragora officinarum*, p. 230). With a forked root that resembles the human shape, mandrake was credited with great magical and healing powers. It was recommended by Dioscorides for many ailments including sleeplessness and inflammation of the eyes.

With the collapse of the Roman empire in the 4th century AD, the debate about how illness arose and how it should be treated shifted to the East. By the 9th century, Islamic physicians had translated much of Galen's work into Arabic, and his ideas affected the development of Arabic medicine into the Middle Ages, influencing Avicenna (980–1037). Later in the Middle Ages, Galen's writings were translated back into Latin from the Arabic and, for 400 years, his ideas held sway and were diligently applied in European medical practice. Even in the 16th and 17th centuries, students in university medical schools were given an academic training in the principles of the humoral system, as established by Galen. They learned how to diagnose an imbalance of the humors and the methods of restoring equilibrium, primarily bloodletting and purging (*see pp. 21–22*).

PRINTING & HERBAL MEDICINE

The invention of printing in the 15th century changed the face of herbal medicine in Europe. Before that time, European folk medicine had been handed down from generation to generation. Even though some early herbals were written in Anglo-Saxon, Icelandic, and Welsh, for example, for the most part the tradition was orally based.

During the following centuries, herbals were published throughout Europe in different languages, making standardized catalogs of herbs and their applications accessible to the general public, not just to those who understood Latin. As literacy rates rose, women in particular used the advice in the herbals to treat their families. *(continued)*

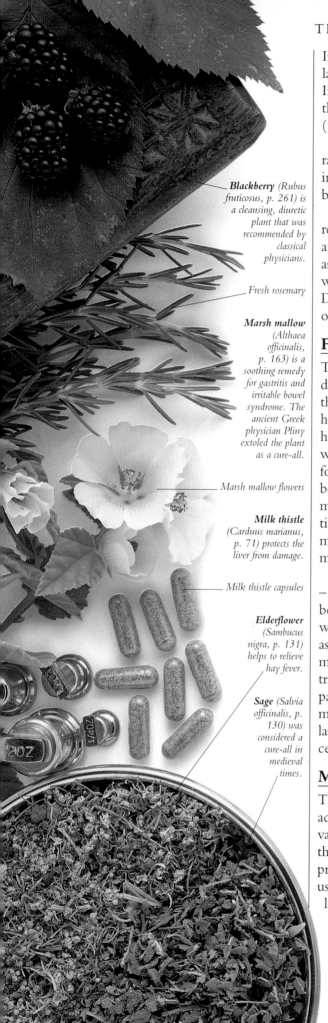

Blackberry (Rubus fruticosus, p. 261) is a cleansing, diuretic plant that was recommended by classical physicians.

Fresh rosemary

Marsh mallow (Althaea officinalis, p. 163) is a soothing remedy for gastritis and irritable bowel syndrome. The ancient Greek physician Pliny extoled the plant as a cure-all.

Marsh mallow flowers

Milk thistle (Carduus marianus, p. 71) protects the liver from damage.

Milk thistle capsules

Elderflower (Sambucus nigra, p. 131) helps to relieve hay fever.

Sage (Salvia officinalis, p. 130) was considered a cure-all in medieval times.

In some cases, the printed herbals were written by physicians, and largely reflected the writings of classical authors such as Dioscorides. In other instances they were based directly on first-hand experience – the English herbals of John Gerard (1597) and Nicholas Culpeper (1652) are good examples.

John Gerard's *The Herball* is clearly the work of a horticulturist, rather than an herbal practitioner, but is nonetheless a mine of information. The book includes many plants that had been recently brought back to Europe by explorers and traders.

Culpeper's *The English Physitian* has been used as a practical reference book ever since its publication. It is a rich blend of personal and practical experience, traditional European medicine, and astrological thought. Each herb is assigned a "temperature," a use within the humoral system, and a ruling planet and star sign. Like Dioscorides' *De Materia Medica* it has the merit of being based on close observation and extensive experience in the use of herbal medicines.

FOREIGN HERBS & SYNTHESIZED DRUGS

The growing use of foreign herbs in the 17th century prompted heated debate about the relative value of indigenous European herbs, but for the majority of the population this was irrelevant, since the imported herbs were well out of their price range. In the end, it created a rift in herbal medicine. Poor and rural peoples used locally available herbs, while the affluent city-dwellers and aristocrats purchased plants of foreign origin, prescribed by university-trained physicians. By the beginning of the 18th century, approximately 70 percent of plant medicines stocked by European apothecaries were imported. Over time, this city-based herbalism evolved into conventional scientific medicine, which in turn rejected its herbal roots and regarded plant medicines as inferior or spurious.

Once conventional medicine established its monopoly of practice – in most European countries by the end of the 19th century – it became (and in many cases remains) illegal to practice herbalism without medical certification. In Greece, traditional herbalists, known as *komboyannites*, were persecuted, and the word itself became an insult meaning "trickster" or "quack." In France and Italy, experienced traditional herbalists were imprisoned for providing treatment to their patients. The renaissance in herbal medicine that has occurred in the last 25 years offers hope that official censure will change.

MODERN PRACTITIONERS

The pattern of herbal medicine across Europe today is remarkably varied, but a common thread runs through the different traditions and practices. Most European herbalists use orthodox methods of diagnosis, looking for signs of infection and inflammation. However, most also try to establish a broad or holistic picture, placing the illness in the context of the patient's life as a

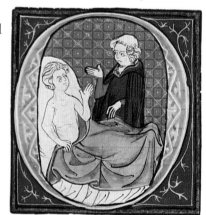

Healers in medieval Europe frequently sought to restore physical imbalance with bloodletting, purges, and preparations that caused vomiting.

whole. Herbalists then choose plant medicines and recommend suitable dietary and lifestyle changes that will allow the body's self-regenerating powers – the modern equivalent of the "vital spirit" – to establish good health once again. Recovery may take longer than it would if treated with conventional medicine, but relief is generally longer-lasting and free from side effects.

A patient with a stomach ulcer, for example, may be treated with herbs such as meadowsweet (*Filipendula ulmaria*, p. 96), German chamomile (*Chamomilla recutita*, p. 76), marsh mallow (*Althaea officinalis*, p. 163), and deadly nightshade (*Atropa belladonna*, p. 66) to soothe inflammation, astringe and protect the inner lining of the stomach, and reduce excess acid production. In addition, herbal practitioners also address poor dietary habits, stress, and poor posture – conditions that may undermine the body's ability to heal itself. Problems such as these are reversed with herbs to help relieve stress, and with advice on taking exercise, and following a diet rich in nonacidic vegetables and fruits.

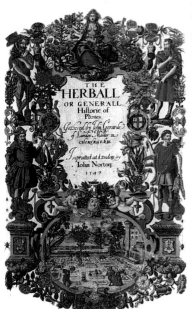

John Gerard's 1597 Herball *is one of the classic texts on healing plants.*

POPULAR HERBS

In European herbal medicine, native herbs are still highly popular. Alpine plants such as arnica (*Arnica montana*, p. 170) and pulsatilla (*Anemone pulsatilla*, p. 165) are much used in Swiss, German, Italian and French herbal medicine, while comfrey (*Symphytum officinale*, p. 136) is particularly well liked in Britain. There has also been a surge in demand for exotic herbs. The Chinese ginkgo tree (*Ginkgo biloba*, p. 98), which improves circulation of blood to the head and helps the memory, is now cultivated on large plantations in France. It was the bestselling medicine of all in Germany in 1992.

EUROPEAN TRADITIONS & THE FUTURE

Sales of over-the-counter herbal medicines in Europe are increasing at a dramatic rate. In the UK between 1990 and 1995, sales climbed by 25 percent. Herbal medicine or "phytotherapy" is so esteemed in Germany that conventionally trained doctors routinely prescribe herbs along with orthodox drugs. In contrast, herbalism in the UK is practiced by those who have trained in herbal rather than conventional medical schools, providing treatment that is complementary to conventional medicine. The picture is again different in Spain. Some doctors prescribe herbal medicine, but traditional herbalists, *curanderos*, still practice. They learn by apprenticeship, gathering herbs from the wild and preparing their own medicines.

How the European Union will manage to legislate the safe practice of each of these three types of herbalism remains to be seen, but each has a significant contribution to make in a future in which people are free to choose the treatment that accords with their ideas and wishes.

Dried feverfew

Hawthorn (*Crataegus oxyacantha*, p. 86) has a marked tonic effect on the heart.

Dried hawthorn flowers and berries

Cowslip (*Primula veris*, p. 254) is a sedative plant that helps calm what herbalist John Gerard called "the frensies."

Thyme (*Thymus vulgaris*, p. 142) is a good antiseptic and tonic herb. It is particularly effective as a treatment for chest infections.

Common foxglove (*Digitalis purpurea*, p. 199) is the source of digitalis, a widely used cardiac stimulant.

Heartsease (*Viola tricolor*, p. 280) gained its name from its former use in love potions. It is an effective expectorant, treating coughs and colds.

Lavender (*Lavandula officinalis*, p. 107) yields an essential oil that is a good first-aid remedy for insect bites and sunburn.

INDIA

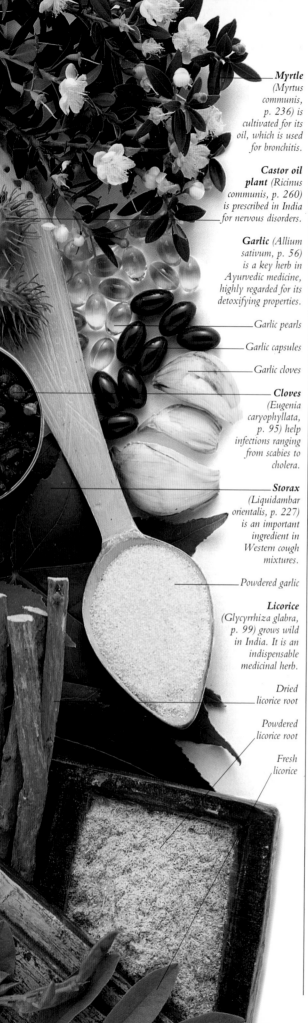

Myrtle (Myrtus communis, p. 236) is cultivated for its oil, which is used for bronchitis.

Castor oil plant (Ricinus communis, p. 260) is prescribed in India for nervous disorders.

Garlic (Allium sativum, p. 56) is a key herb in Ayurvedic medicine, highly regarded for its detoxifying properties.

Garlic pearls

Garlic capsules

Garlic cloves

Cloves (Eugenia caryophyllata, p. 95) help infections ranging from scabies to cholera.

Storax (Liquidambar orientalis, p. 227) is an important ingredient in Western cough mixtures.

Powdered garlic

Licorice (Glycyrrhiza glabra, p. 99) grows wild in India. It is an indispensable medicinal herb.

Dried licorice root

Powdered licorice root

Fresh licorice

In India and the surrounding regions, Ayurvedic medicine is the dominant herbal tradition. It is thought to be the oldest system of healing in the world, predating even Chinese medicine. Today it is actively promoted by the government as an alternative to conventional Western medicine.

THE NAME AYURVEDA DERIVES FROM two Indian words: *ayur*, meaning life, and *veda*, meaning knowledge or science. Ayurvedic medicine is more than a system of healing. It is a way of life encompassing science, religion, and philosophy that enhances well-being, increases longevity, and ultimately brings self-realization. It aims to bring about a union of physical, emotional, and spiritual health, known as *swasthya*. This state enables the individual to enter a harmonious relationship with cosmic consciousness.

EARLY ORIGINS

Ayurveda evolved over 5,000 years ago in the far reaches of the Himalayas from the deep wisdom of spiritually enlightened prophets, or *rishis*. Their wisdom was transmitted orally from teacher to disciple, and eventually set down in Sanskrit poetry known as the *Vedas*. These writings, dating to approximately 1500 BC, distilled the prevailing historical, religious, philosophical, and medical knowledge, and form the basis of Indian culture. The most important of these texts are the *Rig Veda* and the *Atharva Veda*.

In about 800 BC, the first Ayurvedic medical school was founded by Punarvasu Atreya. He and his pupils recorded medical knowledge in treatises that would in turn influence Charaka, a scholar who lived and taught around 700 BC. His writings, the *Charaka Samhita*, describe 1,500 plants, identifying 350 as valuable medicines. This major reference text is still consulted by Ayurvedic practitioners. The second major work was the *Susruta Samhita*, written a century later, which forms the basis of modern surgery and is still consulted today.

THE INFLUENCE OF AYURVEDA

Other systems of medicine such as the Chinese, Tibetan, and Islamic (Unani Tibb) traditions have their roots in Ayurveda. For example, the Buddha (born *c.* 550 BC) was a follower of Ayurveda, and the spread of Buddhism into Tibet during the following centuries was accompanied by increased practice of Ayurveda.

The ancient civilizations were linked to one another by trade routes, campaigns, and wars. Arab traders spread knowledge of Indian plants, and Ayurvedic medicine was studied by Arab physicians, who included Indian plants in their *materia medica*. This knowledge was passed on to the

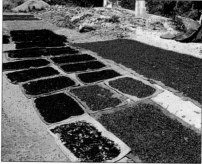

Cloves have been used medicinally for thousands of years in India. The flower buds are dried in the open air.

ancient Greeks and Romans, whose practices were eventually to form the basis of European medicine.

THE FIVE ELEMENTS

Ayurveda is a unique holistic system, based on the interaction of body, mind, and spirit. In Ayurveda, the origin of all aspects of existence is pure intellect or consciousness. Energy and matter are one. Energy is manifested in five elements – ether, air, fire, water, and earth – which together form the basis of all matter. In the body, ether is present in the cavities of the mouth, abdomen, digestive tract, thorax, and lungs. Air is manifested in the movements of the muscles, pulsations of the heart, expansion and contraction of the lungs, the workings of the digestive tract, and the nervous system. Fire is manifested in the digestive system, metabolism, body temperature, vision, and intelligence. Water is present in the digestive juices, salivary glands, mucous membranes, blood, and cytoplasm. Earth exists in the nails, skin, and hair, as well as in the elements that hold the body together: bones, cartilage, muscles, and tendons.

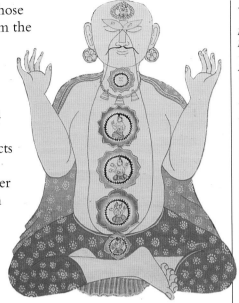

The chakras are represented in this figure. India's medical system, Ayurveda, identifies seven energy centers, chakras, sited along the spinal column from the head to the base of the spine. If they are blocked, illness results.

The five elements manifest in the functioning of the five senses, and they are closely related to our ability to perceive and interact with the environment in which we live. In Ayurveda, ether, air, fire, water, and earth correspond to hearing, touch, vision, taste, and smell, respectively.

THE DOSHAS & HEALTH

The five elements combine to form three basic forces, known as the *tridoshas*, which exist in everything in the universe and influence all mental and physical processes. From ether and air, the air principle *vata* is created; fire and water yield the fire principle *pitta*; earth and water produce the water principle *kapha*. The principles correspond closely to the three humors of Tibetan medicine and somewhat resemble Galen's theory of the four humors (see p. 31).

According to Ayurveda, we are all born with a particular balance of *doshas*. The proportions are largely determined by the balance of *doshas* in our parents at the time of our conception. Our body type, temperament, and susceptibility to illnesses are largely governed by the predominant *dosha*. In this way we inherit our basic constitution, called the *prakruti*, which remains unaltered throughout our lives.

The first requirement for health in Ayurveda is a proper balance of the *doshas*. If the balance is upset, illness, *ryadhi*, results. The disruption may be manifested in physical discomfort and pain, or in mental and emotional suffering, including jealousy, anger, fear, and sorrow. While our balance of *doshas* influences vulnerability to certain kinds of illness, the principles do not work in a vacuum. *(continued)*

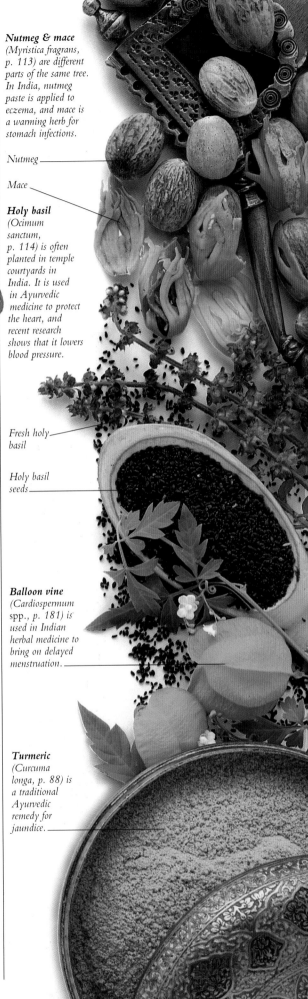

Nutmeg & mace (*Myristica fragrans*, p. 113) are different parts of the same tree. In India, nutmeg paste is applied to eczema, and mace is a warming herb for stomach infections.

Nutmeg

Mace

Holy basil (*Ocimum sanctum*, p. 114) is often planted in temple courtyards in India. It is used in Ayurvedic medicine to protect the heart, and recent research shows that it lowers blood pressure.

Fresh holy basil

Holy basil seeds

Balloon vine (*Cardiospermum* spp., p. 181) is used in Indian herbal medicine to bring on delayed menstruation.

Turmeric (*Curcuma longa*, p. 88) is a traditional Ayurvedic remedy for jaundice.

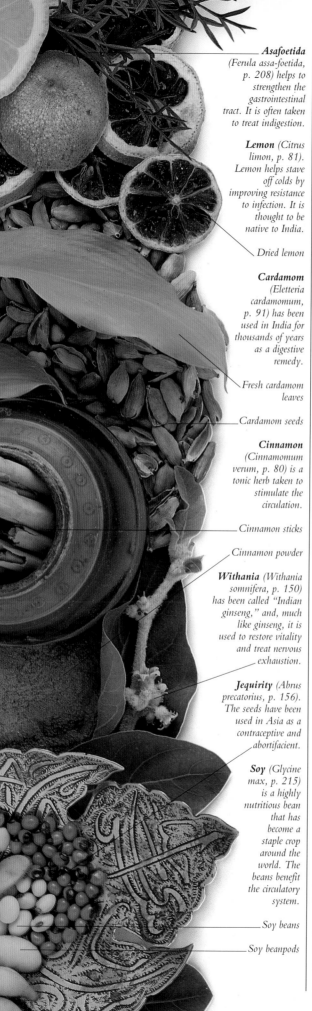

Asafoetida
*(Ferula assa-foetida,
p. 208) helps to
strengthen the
gastrointestinal
tract. It is often taken
to treat indigestion.*

Lemon *(Citrus
limon, p. 81).
Lemon helps stave
off colds by
improving resistance
to infection. It is
thought to be
native to India.*

Dried lemon

Cardamom
*(Eletteria
cardamomum,
p. 91) has been
used in India for
thousands of years
as a digestive
remedy.*

Fresh cardamom
leaves

Cardamom seeds

Cinnamon
*(Cinnamomum
verum, p. 80) is a
tonic herb taken to
stimulate the
circulation.*

Cinnamon sticks

Cinnamon powder

Withania *(Withania
somnifera, p. 150)
has been called "Indian
ginseng," and, much
like ginseng, it is
used to restore vitality
and treat nervous
exhaustion.*

Jequirity *(Abrus
precatorius, p. 156).
The seeds have been
used in Asia as a
contraceptive and
abortifacient.*

Soy *(Glycine
max, p. 215)
is a highly
nutritious bean
that has
become a
staple crop
around the
world. The
beans benefit
the circulatory
system.*

Soy beans

Soy beanpods

The effect our lifestyle has on our *prakruti – vakruti –* has a strong effect upon overall health, and it may easily disrupt *dosha* balance.

Illness may also result if the flow of energy, *prana*, around the body is interrupted. The flow is relayed via the seven *chakras* (psychic energy centers), situated at various points along the spinal column, from the crown of the head to the tailbone. If the energy flowing between these centers is blocked, the likelihood of ill health increases.

VISITING AN AYURVEDIC PRACTITIONER

An Ayurvedic practitioner first carefully assesses *prakruti* and *vakruti –* constitution and lifestyle. This involves taking a detailed case history and carefully examining the body, paying attention to the build, the lines in the face and hands, and skin and hair type – all of which point to more profound aspects of the patient's condition. However, the main foundations on which diagnosis rests are the appearance of the tongue and the pulse rate. In these respects, Ayurveda has much in common with Chinese and Tibetan medicine, in which these two indicators are also of the greatest importance. A very complex technique for taking the patient's pulse has been developed by Ayurvedic practitioners, requiring many years' experience.

When a *dosha* imbalance has been diagnosed, medical treatment and lifestyle advice are provided. The first step is eliminating toxins and the main cleansing and rejuvenation program, known as *panchakarma*, includes therapeutic vomiting, purging, enemas, nasal administration of medication, and purification of the blood.

ATTRIBUTES OF REMEDIES

Subsequent treatments fall into three main categories: medicines from natural sources, dietary regimens, and behavioral modifications. Medicines, foods, and lifestyle activities are all classified according to their effect on the three *doshas*. For instance, a health problem associated with an excess of *kapha*, the water principle, is characterized by congestion, excess weight, fluid retention, and lethargy. The practitioner might prescribe the consumption of warm, dry, light foods because the quality of *kapha* is cool and damp. Avoidance of cold damp foods (such as wheat, sugar, and milk products), which increase *kapha*, would also be advised. Herbal remedies would include warming spices such as ginger (*Zingiber officinale*, p. 153), cinnamon (*Cinnamomum verum*, p. 80), and cayenne (*Capsicum frutescens*, p. 70), as well as bitters such as turmeric (*Curcuma longa*, p. 88) and aloe vera (*Aloe vera*, p. 57).

The specific choice of herbal remedy depends on its "quality" or "energy," which Ayurveda determines according to twenty attributes (*vimshati guna*), such as hot, cold, wet, dry, heavy, or light. Ayurveda also classifies remedies according to six tastes – sweet, sour, salty, bitter, pungent, and astringent. Sweet, sour, and salty substances increase water (*kapha*) and decrease air (*vata*); bitter, pungent, and astringent remedies increase air and decrease water; and sour, salty, and pungent herbs increase fire (*pitta*).

PREPARATIONS & TREATMENTS

In addition to plant extracts, Ayurvedic medicines include honey and dairy produce, and sometimes minute doses of minerals such as salt are added. Remedies take the form of pills, powders, balms, and infusions, and most contain several different ingredients, all carefully balanced to

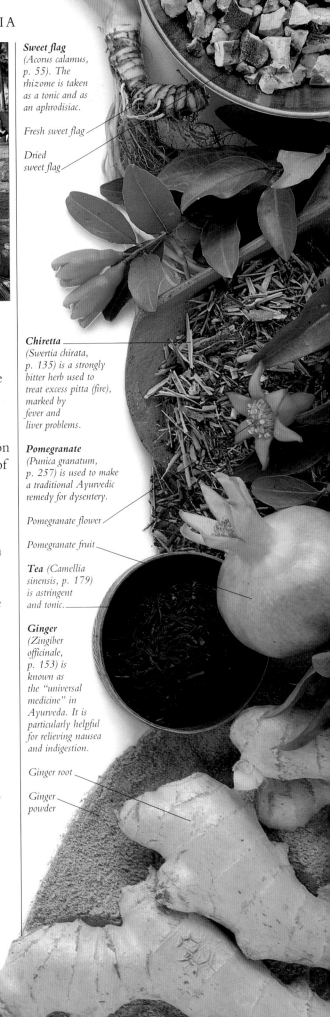

Sweet flag
(*Acorus calamus*,
p. 55). *The
rhizome is taken
as a tonic and as
an aphrodisiac.*

Fresh sweet flag

*Dried
sweet flag*

Chiretta
(*Swertia chirata*,
p. 135) is a strongly
bitter herb used to
treat excess pitta (fire),
marked by
fever and
liver problems.

Pomegranate
(*Punica granatum*,
p. 257) is used to make
a traditional Ayurvedic
remedy for dysentery.

Pomegranate flower

Pomegranate fruit

Tea (*Camellia
sinensis*, p. 179)
is astringent
and tonic.

Ginger
(*Zingiber
officinale*,
p. 153) is
known as
the "universal
medicine" in
Ayurveda. It is
particularly helpful
for relieving nausea
and indigestion.

Ginger root

*Ginger
powder*

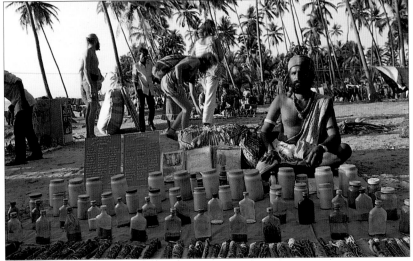

Ayurvedic market doctor. *Practitioners prescribe herbal remedies on the basis of their attributes — "warm" and "cool" are but two of them. The aim is to balance the patient's* doshas, *the principles that regulate sickness and health.*

individual needs. Treatment might include washes and enemas or the application of poultices as well as massage with warm herbal oil, burning incense, the use of precious stones and metals, and ritual purification for imbalanced mind and emotions. The chanting of mantras (incantations based on sacred texts), breathing, and meditation exercises may be advised, due to the power of sound and the effect of vibration and meditation on the body, mind, and spirit.

THE VALUE OF AYURVEDIC MEDICINE

The importance of Ayurveda is proved in part by its timelessness, since it has existed as an unbroken tradition for thousands of years, in spite of a number of obstacles. Following the rise of the Mogul empire in the 16th century, the dominance of Islamic medicine, Unani Tibb, led to the partial repression of Ayurveda in India. In the 19th century, the British dismissed it as nothing more than native superstition, and in 1833 they closed all Ayurvedic schools and banned the practice. Great centers of Indian learning thus fell apart, and Ayurvedic knowledge retreated into villages and temples. At the turn of the century, however, Ayurvedic medicine was reevaluated, and by the time India gained her independence in 1947 it had regained its reputation as a valid medical system. Today, Ayurveda flourishes side by side with Unani and Western medicine and is actively encouraged by the Indian government as an inexpensive alternative to Western drugs. In recent years, Ayurveda has attracted increasing attention from medical scientists in the West and in Japan, and the World Health Organization has resolved to promote its practice in developing countries.

Ayurveda's value lies in the fact that it is not a medical science that deals solely with treatment of disease. Instead, it offers practical guidelines for living, applicable to every facet of daily existence. It also seeks to reconcile health and lifestyle with the universal aspects of existence, and thus it enhances the well-being, longevity, and harmony of all those who practice it. For these reasons, Ayurveda is of lasting benefit to anyone seeking an alternative to traditional Western practices.

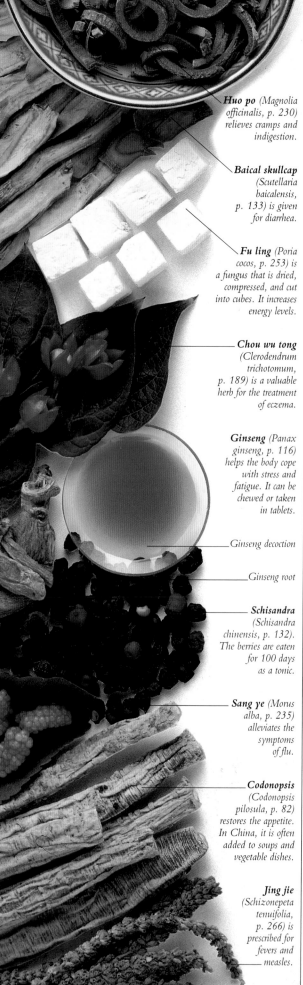

Huo po (Magnolia officinalis, p. 230) relieves cramps and indigestion.

Baical skullcap (Scutellaria baicalensis, p. 133) is given for diarrhea.

Fu ling (Poria cocos, p. 253) is a fungus that is dried, compressed, and cut into cubes. It increases energy levels.

Chou wu tong (Clerodendrum trichotomum, p. 189) is a valuable herb for the treatment of eczema.

Ginseng (Panax ginseng, p. 116) helps the body cope with stress and fatigue. It can be chewed or taken in tablets.

Ginseng decoction

Ginseng root

Schisandra (Schisandra chinensis, p. 132). The berries are eaten for 100 days as a tonic.

Sang ye (Morus alba, p. 235) alleviates the symptoms of flu.

Codonopsis (Codonopsis pilosula, p. 82) restores the appetite. In China, it is often added to soups and vegetable dishes.

Jing jie (Schizonepeta tenuifolia, p. 266) is prescribed for fevers and measles.

CHINA

China's ancient herbal tradition has survived intact into the 20th century, and in China it is accorded equal status with Western conventional medicine. Many Chinese universities now teach and research herbal medicine, a factor of crucial importance in the reemergence of herbalism worldwide.

TRADITIONAL CHINESE MEDICINE (TCM) and the herbal tradition that is part of it developed separately from Chinese folk medicine. It arose from ideas recorded between 200 BC and AD 100 in the *Yellow Emperor's Classic of Internal Medicine (Huang Di Nei Jing).* This text is based on detailed observations of nature and a deep understanding of the way that all life is subject to natural laws. It contains concepts that are fundamental to TCM, including *yin* and *yang*, the five elements (*wu xing*), and the theory of the effect of nature upon health.

In TCM, living in harmony with these principles is the key to good health and longevity. According to the *Yellow Emperor's Classic*, members of previous generations lived for a hundred years, and had constitutions so strong that illness was cured by incantations alone. Only later, as human vitality, or *qi*, declined and people became "overactive … going against the joy of life," did herbal medicine, acupuncture, and other branches of TCM become necessary.

KEY THEORIES

Unlike other herbal traditions that have a unified theory for making sense of illness and disease (for example, the European theory of the four humors), TCM has two different systems – the *yin* and *yang* theory and the five elements. They developed quite separately in China, and the five elements system was only accepted and fully incorporated into Chinese medicine during the Song dynasty (AD 960–1279).

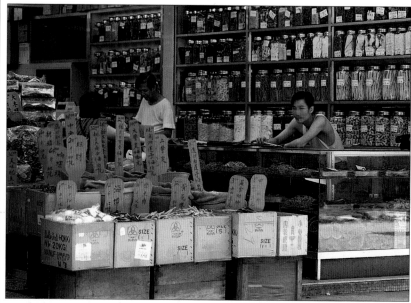

On the streets of Hong Kong herbal chemists are a familiar sight. Prescriptions are formulated during a consultation with an herbalist, and the patient then obtains the appropriate herbs.

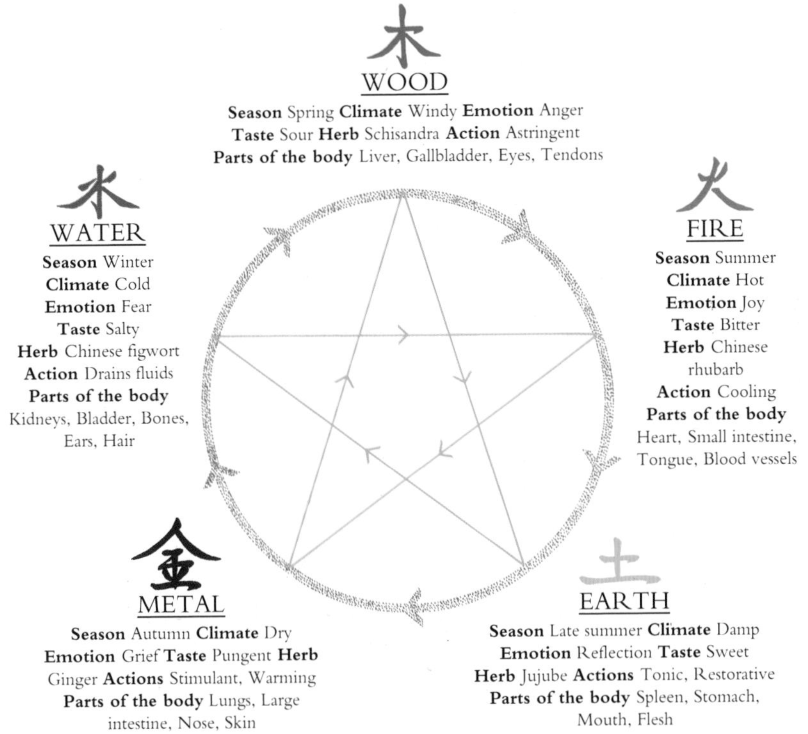

WOOD
Season Spring **Climate** Windy **Emotion** Anger
Taste Sour **Herb** Schisandra **Action** Astringent
Parts of the body Liver, Gallbladder, Eyes, Tendons

WATER
Season Winter
Climate Cold
Emotion Fear
Taste Salty
Herb Chinese figwort
Action Drains fluids
Parts of the body
Kidneys, Bladder, Bones,
Ears, Hair

FIRE
Season Summer
Climate Hot
Emotion Joy
Taste Bitter
Herb Chinese
rhubarb
Action Cooling
Parts of the body
Heart, Small intestine,
Tongue, Blood vessels

METAL
Season Autumn **Climate** Dry
Emotion Grief **Taste** Pungent **Herb**
Ginger **Actions** Stimulant, Warming
Parts of the body Lungs, Large
intestine, Nose, Skin

EARTH
Season Late summer **Climate** Damp
Emotion Reflection **Taste** Sweet
Herb Jujube **Actions** Tonic, Restorative
Parts of the body Spleen, Stomach,
Mouth, Flesh

The ancient five elements theory *is used by the Chinese when writing prescriptions. It associates herbs with the natural world, including elements, seasons, and parts of the body. In the circular movement, each element gives rise to the next (for example, winter gives rise to spring). The five-angled movement is a controlling one, in which each element restrains another.*

To this day, differences between these two theories are reflected in practitioners' approach to diagnosis and treatment.

In Chinese thought, everything in the universe is composed of *yin* and *yang* – words that were first used to denote the dark and light side of a valley. Everything has *yin* and *yang* aspects, or complementary opposites – such as day and night, up and down, wet and dry. Every *yin* or *yang* category can itself also be subdivided – so that while the front of the body is *yin* relative to the back, which is *yang*, the abdomen is *yin* relative to the chest, which is *yang*.

The five elements theory associates constituents of the natural world – wood, fire, earth, metal, and water – with other fundamentals such as seasons, emotions, and parts of the body. Each element gives rise to the next in a perpetual fashion (*see* diagram above). For this reason, the system might be more accurately described as the five phases, representing the process of continual movement in life. The five elements have a central role in Chinese herbal medicine, especially in the grouping of tastes of herbs and parts of the body.

DIAGNOSIS & TREATMENT

Instead of looking for causes of illness, Chinese practitioners seek patterns of disharmony, which are expressions of imbalance between *yin* and *yang*. Particular attention is given to reading the pulse and tongue, both of which are very important for an accurate diagnosis. Ill health results from a deficiency or excess of either *yin* or *yang*. A cold, for example, is not just the result of a virus (though this clearly is a cause), but a sign that the body is not adapting to exernal factors such as "wind-heat," "wind-cold," or "summer-heat." *(continued)*

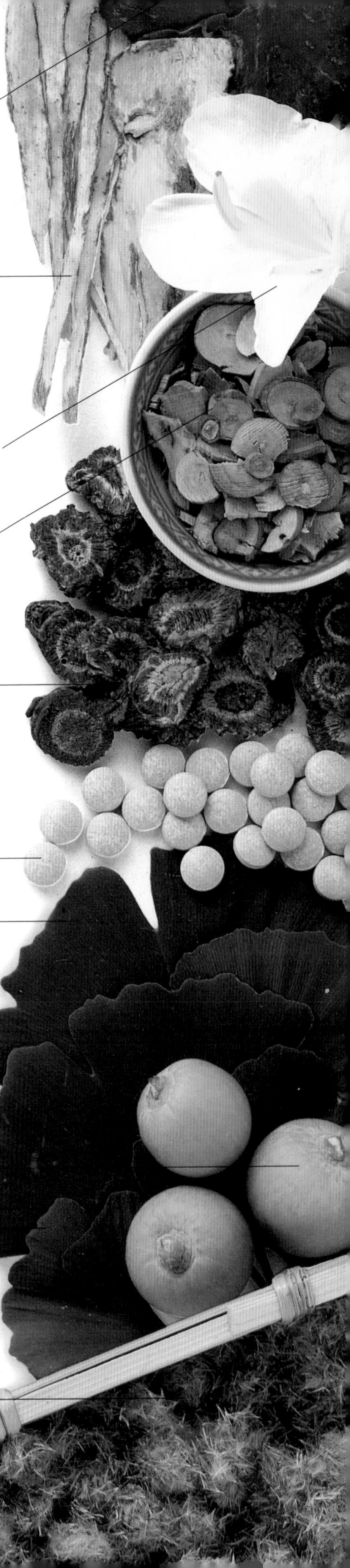

He shou wu
(Polygonum multiflorum, p. 121), the oldest Chinese tonic herb, is used to prevent aging.

Chinese angelica
(Angelica sinensis, p. 60) is taken by millions of Chinese women as a nourishing blood tonic.

Galangal *(Alpinia officinarum, p. 58) is a warming herb used for abdominal pain.*

Gui zhi
(Cinnamomum cassia, p. 80) is a warming herb that helps the circulation.

Qiang huo
(Notopterygium incisium, p. 238) is used in China for colds, especially those accompanied by aching muscles and joints.

Ginkgo tablets

Ginkgo
(Ginkgo biloba, p. 98) improves the memory and the circulation. Tablets, made from the leaves, are a bestselling herbal remedy in Europe.

Ginkgo seeds

Ginkgo leaves

Su xian hua
(Jasminum officinale, see J. grandiflorum, p. 222) is an aromatic herb used to treat depression.

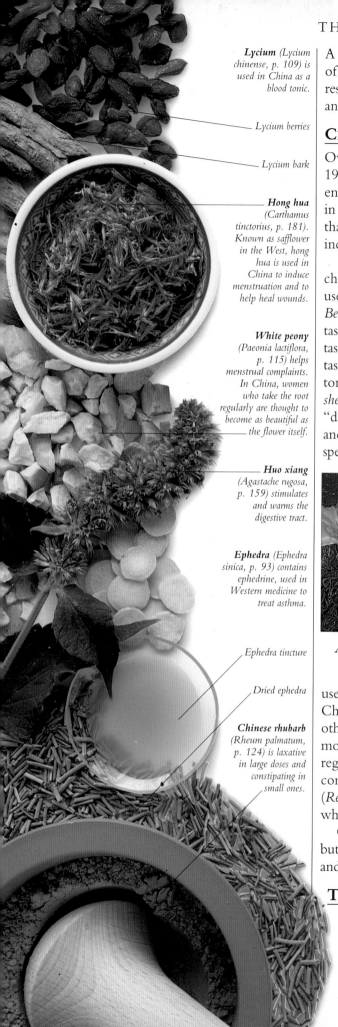

Lycium (*Lycium chinense*, p. 109) is used in China as a blood tonic.

— Lycium berries

— Lycium bark

Hong hua (*Carthamus tinctorius*, p. 181). Known as safflower in the West, hong hua is used in China to induce menstruation and to help heal wounds.

White peony (*Paeonia lactiflora*, p. 115) helps menstrual complaints. In China, women who take the root regularly are thought to become as beautiful as the flower itself.

Huo xiang (*Agastache rugosa*, p. 159) stimulates and warms the digestive tract.

Ephedra (*Ephedra sinica*, p. 93) contains ephedrine, used in Western medicine to treat asthma.

Ephedra tincture

Dried ephedra

Chinese rhubarb (*Rheum palmatum*, p. 124) is laxative in large doses and constipating in small ones.

A high temperature denotes too much *yang* and shivering is the result of an excess of *yin*. The art of the Chinese herbal practitioner is to restore harmony between *yin* and *yang* both within the patient's body and between the patient and the world at large.

CHINESE HERBS

Over the centuries, the number of medicinal herbs has grown and the 1977 *Encyclopedia of Traditional Chinese Medicinal Substances* has 5,757 entries, the majority of which are herbs. The Communist Revolution in 1949 helped swell the number of plants used in TCM, because herbs that had previously only been employed in folk medicine were incorporated into the tradition.

As the herbal tradition developed within TCM, the taste and other characteristics of herbs became closely linked with their therapeutic uses. *The Divine Husbandman's Classic of the Materia Medica* (*Shen'nong Bencaojing*, 1st century AD) lists 252 herbal medicines specifying their tastes and "temperatures," and today, Chinese herbalists still relate the taste and temperature of an herb directly to its therapeutic use. Sweet-tasting herbs such as ginseng (*Panax ginseng*, p. 116) are prescribed to tone, harmonize, and moisten, while bitter-tasting herbs such as *dan shen* (*Salvia miltiorrhiza*, p. 129) are employed to drain and dry excess "dampness." Hot-tasting herbs are used for treating "cold" conditions, and vice versa. Together, an herb's taste and temperature link it to specific types of illness. For example, Baical skullcap (*Scutellaria baicalensis*,

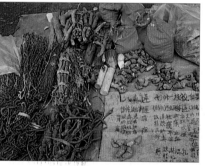

p. 133), which is bitter-tasting and "cold," is a drying, cooling herb for conditions such as fever and irritability, brought on by patterns of excess heat.

TAKING MEDICINES

The Chinese tradition relies heavily on formulas, which are set mixtures of herbs that have proven effectiveness as tonics or remedies for specific illnesses. Many are available over the counter and are

A vast array of herbal preparations is available to Chinese practitioners.

used by millions of people every day in China and around the world. Chinese herbalists often take a formula as a starting point and then add other herbs to the mixture. There are hundreds of formulas, one of the most famous being "Four Things Soup," a tonic given to women to regulate the menstrual cycle and tone the reproductive system. It consists of Chinese angelica (*Angelica sinensis*, p. 60), rehmannia (*Rehmannia glutinosa*, p. 123), *chuang xiong* (*Ligusticum chuangxiong*), and white peony (*Paeonia lactiflora*, p. 115).

Chinese herbal medicine uses tinctures or alcoholic extracts of herbs, but only infrequently. Generally, patients are given mixtures of roots and bark to take as decoctions two or three times a day.

THE CHINESE INFLUENCE IN JAPAN & KOREA

Japan and Korea have been strongly influenced by Chinese medical ideas and practices. *Kampoh*, traditional Japanese medicine, traces its origins back to the 5th century AD, when Buddhist monks from Korea introduced their healing arts, largely derived from Chinese medicine, into Japan. In the following century, the Empress Suiko (AD 592–628) sent envoys to China to study that country's culture and medicine. Direct Chinese influence on Japanese medicine, which was practiced for the most part by the monks, continued for 1,000 years. In the 16th century, Japan started to assert its cultural identity and *kampoh* developed its own characteristic traits, emphasizing the Japanese ideals of simplicity and naturalness. However, certain Chinese concepts, such as *yin* and *yang* and *ki* (*qi*), continued to have a central role.

In 1868, the Japanese embraced Western conventional medicine. Formal training in *kampoh*

*The **tai chi** symbol illustrates the harmony of* yin *and* yang. *In Chinese medicine, an imbalance of these principles in the body results in illness.*

officially ceased in 1885, but a few committed practitioners passed their knowledge on to younger generations, keeping the tradition alive. In the last 20 years the number of practitioners has greatly increased, and *kampoh* is currently taught at Toyama University in Honsu.

Korean herbal medicine is very similar to mainstream Chinese herbal medicine, and almost all the Chinese herbs are used in Korea. Ginseng (*Panax ginseng*, p. 116) has been cultivated in Korea for home use and export since 1300.

IMPORTANCE OF CHINESE HERBAL MEDICINE

Since 1949 when the Communists gained control, the herbal tradition has flourished in China (*see* p. 27) and today it is recognized as a valid medical system, available to the Chinese on an equal footing with conventional Western medicine. As is often the case elsewhere, herbs seem to be used mainly for chronic conditions, while Western medicine is more frequently employed for serious acute illness.

Chinese herbal medicine, however, is not just of significance in China and the surrounding regions. Many Chinese universities now teach and research herbal medicine, and this development (and the massive input of resources involved) has helped revitalize herbalism worldwide during the last 20–30 years.

Chinese herbal medicine is now practiced by trained practitioners in every continent and even has official government recognition in some countries. For example, in 1995 the French government signed an agreement with the Chinese to establish a hospital in Paris, offering acupuncture and traditional Chinese herbal medicine. In the same way that ephedra (*Ephedra sinica*, p. 93) was discovered to be such an excellent medicine for allergies and asthma, so increasing numbers of Chinese herbs will be found to have major health benefits, and there is little doubt that over the next few decades Chinese herbal medicine will continue to grow in popularity around the world.

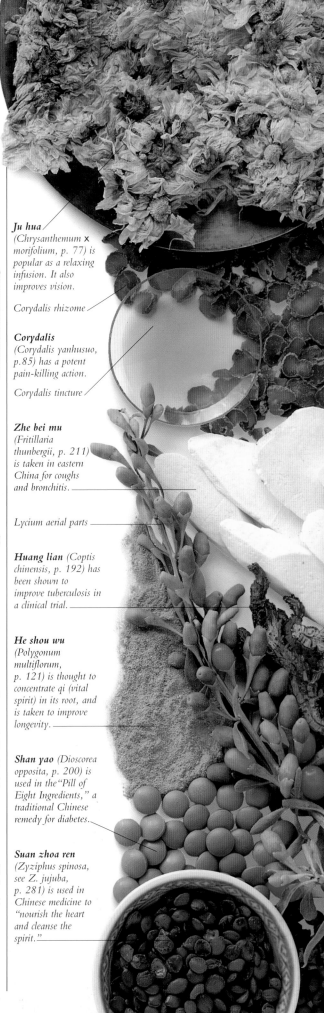

Ju hua (*Chrysanthemum* × *morifolium*, p. 77) is popular as a relaxing infusion. It also improves vision.

Corydalis rhizome

Corydalis (*Corydalis yanhusuo*, p.85) has a potent pain-killing action.

Corydalis tincture

Zhe bei mu (*Fritillaria thunbergii*, p. 211) is taken in eastern China for coughs and bronchitis.

Lycium aerial parts

Huang lian (*Coptis chinensis*, p. 192) has been shown to improve tuberculosis in a clinical trial.

He shou wu (*Polygonum multiflorum*, p. 121) is thought to concentrate qi (vital spirit) in its root, and is taken to improve longevity.

Shan yao (*Dioscorea opposita*, p. 200) is used in the "Pill of Eight Ingredients," a traditional Chinese remedy for diabetes.

Suan zhoa ren (*Zyziphus spinosa*, see Z. jujuba, p. 281) is used in Chinese medicine to "nourish the heart and cleanse the spirit."

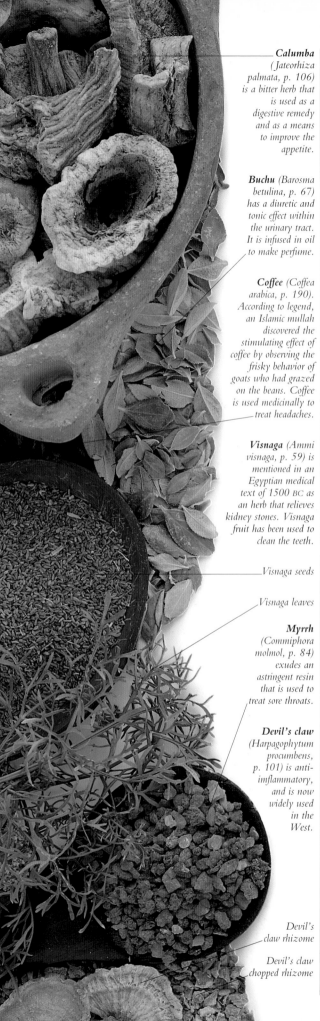

AFRICA

In Africa there is a greater variety of herbal traditions than in any other continent. During the colonial period, native herbal practices were largely suppressed, but today, in a marked turnaround, practitioners of conventional medicine often work closely with traditional healers.

THE THERAPEUTIC USE of medicinal plants in Africa dates back to the earliest times. Ancient Egyptian writings confirm that herbal medicines have been valued in North Africa for thousands of years. The Ebers papyrus (c. 1500 BC), one of the oldest surviving medical texts, includes over 870 prescriptions and formulas, 700 medicinal herbs – including gentian (*Gentiana lutea*, p. 97), aloe (*Aloe vera*, p. 57), and opium poppy (*Papaver somniferum*, p. 242) – and covers conditions ranging from chest complaints to crocodile bite. The medicinal arts put forward in this and other Egyptian texts formed the intellectual foundation of classical medical practice in Greece, Rome, and the Arabic world.

TRADE & THE ARABIAN INFLUENCE

Herbal medicines have been traded between the Middle East, India, and northeastern Africa for at least 3,000 years. Herbs widely used in the Middle East, such as myrrh (*Commiphora molmol*, p. 84), originally came from Somalia and the Horn of Africa. From the 5th century AD to the 13th century, Arab physicians were at the forefront of medical advancement and in the 8th century, the spread of Arabic culture across northern Africa had an influence on North African medicine that lasts to this day. In the mid-13th century, the botanist Ibn El Beitar published a *Materia Medica* that considerably increased the range of North African plant medicines in common use.

ANCIENT BELIEFS & INDIGENOUS HERBS

In the more remote areas of Africa, nomadic peoples, such as the Berber of Morocco and the Topnaar of Namibia, have herbal traditions that remain largely unaffected by changes in medicine in the world at large. For these peoples, healing is linked to a magical world in which spirits influence illness and death. In Berber culture, possession by a *djinn* (spirit) is a major cause of sickness, and herbs with "magical" properties are given to restore health. If the patient fails to recover, their condition is likely to be attributed to a curse or to the "evil eye."

The Topnaar formerly depended completely on their environment for medicines, using the few medicinal plants that grow in such harsh and arid conditions. Although they are now greatly influenced by the Western way of life and have lost much of their plant lore, they continue to employ many indigenous plants medicinally. The stem of the seaweed *Ecklonia maxima*, for example, is roasted, mixed with petroleum jelly, and rubbed into wounds and burns to speed healing, while *Hoodia currori*, a low-lying cactus, is stripped of its thorns and outer skin and eaten raw to treat coughs and colds.

Throughout Africa, thousands of different wild and locally grown medicinal plants are sold in the markets. Some are prescribed as medicines for home use. Others, such as kanna (*Membryanthemum*

Calumba (*Jateorhiza palmata*, p. 106) is a bitter herb that is used as a digestive remedy and as a means to improve the appetite.

Buchu (*Barosma betulina*, p. 67) has a diuretic and tonic effect within the urinary tract. It is infused in oil to make perfume.

Coffee (*Coffea arabica*, p. 190). According to legend, an Islamic mullah discovered the stimulating effect of coffee by observing the frisky behavior of goats who had grazed on the beans. Coffee is used medicinally to treat headaches.

Visnaga (*Ammi visnaga*, p. 59) is mentioned in an Egyptian medical text of 1500 BC as an herb that relieves kidney stones. Visnaga fruit has been used to clean the teeth.

Visnaga seeds

Visnaga leaves

Myrrh (*Commiphora molmol*, p. 84) exudes an astringent resin that is used to treat sore throats.

Devil's claw (*Harpagophytum procumbens*, p. 101) is anti-inflammatory, and is now widely used in the West.

Devil's claw rhizome

Devil's claw chopped rhizome

spp.) and iboga (*Tabernanthe iboga*), are chewed to combat fatigue and are taken as intoxicants in religious ceremonies. According to local accounts in the Congo and Gabon, iboga's stimulant effect was discovered when observers saw wild boars and gorillas dig up and eat the roots and subsequently become frenzied.

TRADITIONAL & CONVENTIONAL CARE

Conventional Western medicine is well established throughout Africa, but in rural areas, far from medical and hospital services, traditional medicine remains the only form of health care available. Even in urban areas conventional health care services can be limited and in this situation, traditional providers of care, such as spiritualists, herbalists, and midwives, are the main source of treatment available for the majority of the population. The World Health Organization aims to achieve a level of health care by the year 2000 that will permit all people to lead socially and economically productive lives. In an attempt to meet this, African countries have pioneered training traditional medical practitioners in simple medical techniques and basic hygiene procedures. In one center in Ghana, conventionally trained medical staff work hand-in-hand with traditional herbal practitioners, encouraging the safer use of herbal medicines and researching them in detail. This represents a remarkable change in attitude. In the 19th and much of the 20th centuries, colonial governments and Christian missionaries viewed traditional herbalists as witch-doctors practicing black magic and whose treatments and herbal remedies were best suppressed.

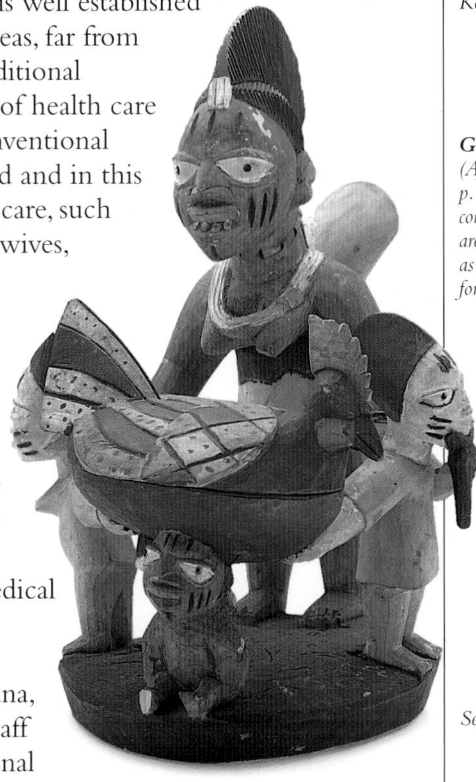

This Nigerian divination bowl was used by traditional healers in the diagnosis of illness via the interpretation of magical signs.

THE DISCOVERY OF NEW HERBAL CURES

Along with encouraging the safer use of herbal medicines, medical centers are researching their use in detail. The benefits of pygeum (*Pygeum africanum*, p. 257) have been conclusively established. This tree, which grows in Angola, Mozambique, Cameroon, and South Africa, was traditionally used in central and southern Africa to treat urinary problems. Today, it is regularly prescribed in conventional French and Italian medicine for prostate problems. Of the plants currently under investigation in Africa, two shrubs, *Bridelia ferruginea* (found in eastern and western grasslands) and *Indigofera arrecta* (found in tropical areas), show promise in the treatment of diabetes.

The reevaluation of traditional herbal medicine in Africa may result in the acceptance of additional plant-based medicines. Today, the opportunity exists to combine the best of traditional practice with conventional medical knowledge, for mutual gain.

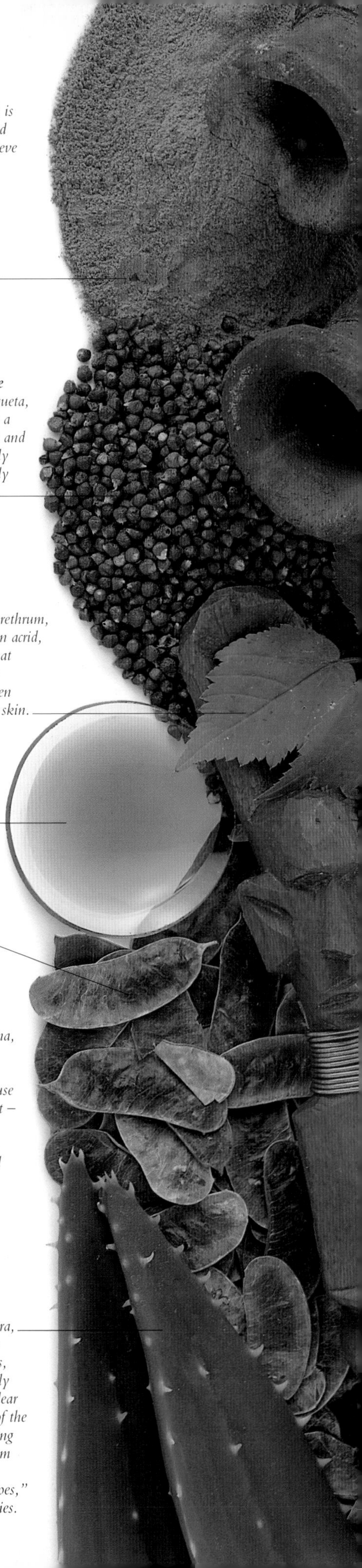

Kola nut (*Cola acuminata*, p. 191) is taken in western and central Africa to relieve headaches.

Kola nut powder

Grains of paradise (*Aframomum melegueta*, p. 159) are used as a condiment in Africa and are taken medicinally as a warming remedy for nausea.

Pellitory (*Anacyclus pyrethrum*, p. 164) has an acrid, irritant root that stimulates the circulation when applied to the skin.

Senna decoction

Senna pods

Senna (*Cassia senna*, p. 72) contains anthraquinones — constituents that cause the bowel to contract — hence the plant's laxative effect. The plant's first recorded medicinal use was in Arabia in the 9th century.

Aloe vera (*Aloe vera*, p. 57) contains two medicinal substances, each with a markedly different use. The clear gel from the center of the leaf speeds the healing of wounds. Juice from the base of the leaf, known as "bitter aloes," has laxative properties.

43

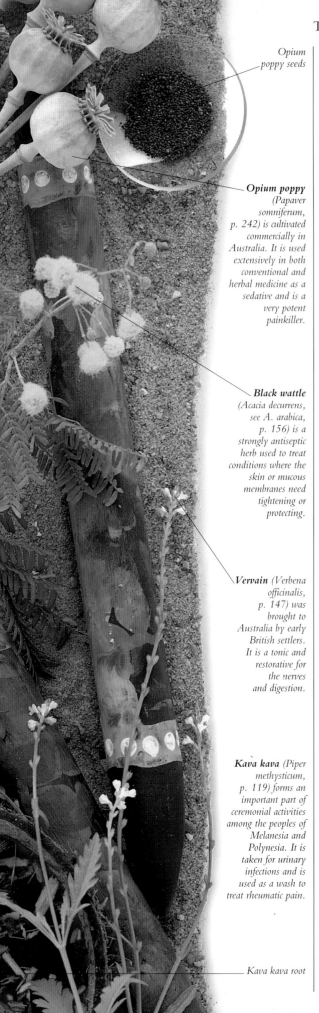

AUSTRALIA

Regrettably, much of the herbal knowledge of the Australian Aborigines was lost after the arrival of the Europeans. The predominant strains of Australian herbalism today derive from the West, China, and, increasingly, from other countries on the Pacific Rim.

THE CRADLE OF THE OLDEST continuous culture on earth, Australia is also the home of an ancient herbal tradition. The Aborigines, believed to have settled in Australia over 60,000 years ago, developed a sophisticated empirical understanding of indigenous plants, many of which, such as eucalyptus (*Eucalpytus globulus*, p. 94), are unique to Australia. While much of this knowledge has vanished with its keepers, there is currently a high level of interest in native herbal traditions.

ABORIGINAL HERBAL MEDICINE

The Aborigines probably had more robust health than the early European settlers who displaced them. They had very different ideas concerning health, disease, and illness, in which the influence of the spirit world played a major role. In common with other hunter-gatherer societies, the Aborigines devoted much time to ritual, reinforcing the sense of place and purpose in the lives of each individual. Healing plants and the laying on of hands were used in a complex weave of culture and medicine.

The influx of Europeans in the 18th century was disastrous for the Aborigines. They were exploited and driven off the land, and their population was decimated by killings and infectious Western diseases. Not only did the Europeans fail to discern any value in native customs but much of the orally based herbal tradition was lost through death of the elders and the dispersal of tribal groupings.

Nevertheless, a little is known of Aboriginal medicine. Aromatic herbs, such as eucalpytus, were often crushed and inhaled to treat many common illnesses, including respiratory diseases such as flu. Without metal technology, water could not be boiled, but decoctions were made by heating water with hot stones. The decoctions were drunk or applied externally. It is known that skin eruptions, such as boils and scabies, were common and that they were treated with acacia (*Acacia* spp.), while acute diarrhea was treated with eucalyptus or kino (*Pterocarpus marsupium*, p. 256). In Queensland, fever bark (*Alstonia* spp., p. 163), also called Australian quinine, was used to treat fevers.

INDIGENOUS & FOREIGN HERBS

Over the last 200 years, many native Australian plants have become popular around the world. Research into fever bark resulted in the discovery of the alkaloid reserpine, which markedly lowers blood pressure. The substance is now prescribed by herbalists and conventional practitioners alike. Eucalyptus and tea tree (*Melaleuca alternifolia*, p. 110) yield essential oils that are employed worldwide as antiseptics. Other native Australian plants are now used in Australian herbalism because of their medicinal use elsewhere, for example gotu kola (*Centella asiatica*, p. 74) and visnaga (*Ammi visnaga*, p. 59), which have a long

Opium poppy seeds

Opium poppy (*Papaver somniferum*, p. 242) is cultivated commercially in Australia. It is used extensively in both conventional and herbal medicine as a sedative and is a very potent painkiller.

Black wattle (*Acacia decurrens*, see A. arabica, p. 156) is a strongly antiseptic herb used to treat conditions where the skin or mucous membranes need tightening or protecting.

Vervain (*Verbena officinalis*, p. 147) was brought to Australia by early British settlers. It is a tonic and restorative for the nerves and digestion.

Kava kava (*Piper methysticum*, p. 119) forms an important part of ceremonial activities among the peoples of Melanesia and Polynesia. It is taken for urinary infections and is used as a wash to treat rheumatic pain.

Kava kava root

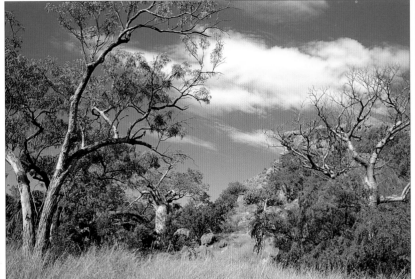

***Red river gum* (Eucalyptus camaldulensis)** *has aromatic, astringent leaves. When it is taken internally, generally to treat diarrhea, it turns the saliva red.*

history of medicinal use in India and the Middle East.

Early British settlers imported European medicinal plants, such as vervain (*Verbena officinalis*, p. 147), hawthorn (*Crataegus* spp., p. 86), mullein (*Verbascum thapsus*, p. 279), and dandelion (*Taraxacum officinale*, p. 140), which have now all become naturalized. Native American plants have also found their way to Australia, including prickly pear (*Opuntia ficus-indica*, p. 240) and Canadian fleabane (*Erigeron canadensis*, p. 203). Since Australian herbalists generally follow the Anglo-American herbal tradition, these plants are often employed in local practice.

CHINESE INFLUENCE

Traditional Chinese medicine has substantially influenced herbalism in Australia. Following the arrival of Chinese immigrants in the 19th century, the herbal formulas gained a reputation for effectiveness, and Chinese medicine maintained a small but loyal following in all the major cities. During the 1980s, a renaissance in all branches of herbal medicine began, and today Australia has three colleges of traditional Chinese medicine. Chinese herbs are also quite frequently used by Australian herbalists, and Chinese patent medicines are widely available in health food shops.

THE FUTURE

Australia is the center of growing interest in Indonesian, New Zealand, and Ayurvedic medicines. The potential of many native herbs is also being explored – the most notable example being the Moreton Bay chestnut tree (*Castonospermum australe*) – one of the many plant medicines with potential in treating AIDS (*see* p. 29).

Commercial cultivation of medicinal plants is expanding, with herbs such as tea tree and opium poppy (*Papaver somniferum*, p. 242) becoming major crops. In Tasmania, trials are under way to try to grow ginseng (*Panax ginseng*, p. 116) and goldenseal (*Hydrastis canadensis*, p. 103), two plants that are very difficult to cultivate.

With its ancient culture, ties to Western herbalism, and location on the Pacific Rim, Australia is host to many different herbal traditions. The next 20 years of Australian herbal medicine should be very exciting.

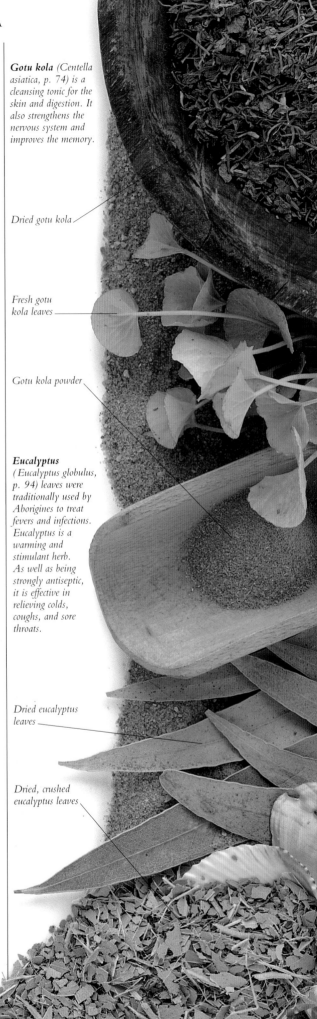

Gotu kola *(Centella asiatica, p. 74) is a cleansing tonic for the skin and digestion. It also strengthens the nervous system and improves the memory.*

Dried gotu kola

Fresh gotu kola leaves

Gotu kola powder

Eucalyptus *(Eucalyptus globulus, p. 94) leaves were traditionally used by Aborigines to treat fevers and infections. Eucalyptus is a warming and stimulant herb. As well as being strongly antiseptic, it is effective in relieving colds, coughs, and sore throats.*

Dried eucalyptus leaves

Dried, crushed eucalyptus leaves

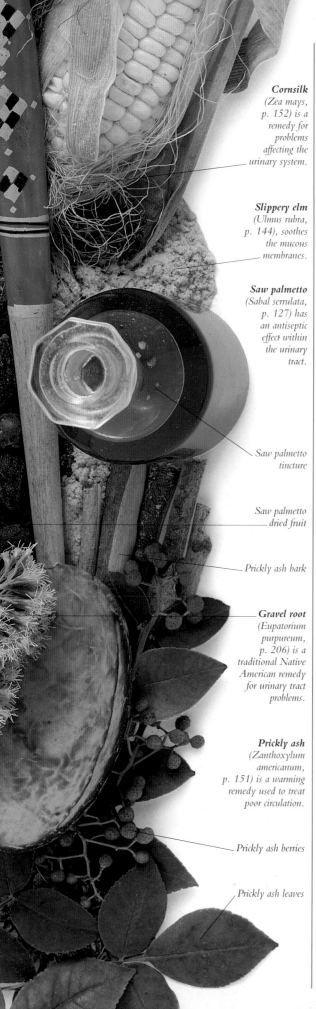

Cornsilk
(Zea mays,
p. 152) is a
remedy for
problems
affecting the
urinary system.

Slippery elm
(Ulmus rubra,
p. 144), soothes
the mucous
membranes.

Saw palmetto
(Sabal serrulata,
p. 127) has
an antiseptic
effect within
the urinary
tract.

Saw palmetto
tincture

Saw palmetto
dried fruit

Prickly ash bark

Gravel root
(Eupatorium
purpureum,
p. 206) is a
traditional Native
American remedy
for urinary tract
problems.

Prickly ash
(Zanthoxylum
americanum,
p. 151) is a
warming
remedy used to treat
poor circulation.

Prickly ash berries

Prickly ash leaves

NORTH AMERICA

Many ancient herbal traditions in North and Central America not only withstood the influx of European settlers but helped to reinvigorate Western herbalism. In parts of Central America herbal medicine is widely practiced, and in the US and Canada it is slowly regaining popularity.

STRETCHING FROM THE ARCTIC WILDS of Canada and Alaska to the tropical regions of Panama, North and Central America covers diverse geographical regions and harbors an immense variety of medicinal plants. Most of them are indigenous, but others – such as nutmeg, ginger, and tamarind – were introduced from the Old World from the 16th century onward. Likewise, native American medicinal plants – such as corn, cocoa, cayenne, and sunflower – were introduced to Europe, Asia, and Africa. This trade of species was an important part of the interplay between the Old and New World's herbal traditions.

HERBAL TRADITIONS IN CENTRAL AMERICA

Herbal medicine is commonly practiced in rural areas of Central America, especially in Guatemala and Mexico. In the Mexican tradition, loss of "balance" between hot and cold elements within the body is thought to be the underlying cause of illness, and the healer's art is to restore balance and vitality.

Mexican herbal medicine is not a static tradition but has evolved from a shifting blend of Aztec, Mayan, and Spanish influences. Long before Hernando Cortez and his conquistadors came ashore in 1519, the Mayan and Aztec cultures had a well-developed understanding of plant medicines. The *Badianus Manuscript*, the first American herbal (written by an Aztec, Martin de la Cruz, in 1552), lists the medicinal uses of 251 Mexican species. They include damiana (*Turnera diffusa*, p. 143), taken by the Maya as an aphrodisiac, and mesquite (*Prosopis juliflora*), used by the Aztecs as an eye lotion. Both species are still used medicinally, alongside European herbs such as pennyroyal (*Mentha pulegium*, p. 233) and thyme (*Thymus vulgaris*, p. 142). It is thought that approximately 65 percent of the plants used by traditional Mexican herbalists originated in Europe.

In other Central American countries efforts are being made to encourage people to use herbal medicine as the first line of treatment for illness. Projects in the Dominican Republic and Nicaragua, for example, are teaching women how to use local herbs within their communities, and in Cuba doctors increasingly prescribe medicinal herbs to make up for the scarcity of conventional medicines.

CARIBBEAN HERBAL MEDICINE

Throughout the Caribbean, domestic herbal medicine remains popular. Some of the widely used herbs include fever grass or lemon grass (*Cymbopogon citratus*, p. 196), which, as its name suggests, is used to treat fevers, and cerasee (*Momordica charantia*, p. 234), a creeping vine that is prized as a "cure-all" on many of the islands. Cerasee has been shown to have an ability to lower blood sugar levels and may help to slow down the onset of diabetes, a relatively common illness among Afro-

Caribbeans. The medical and religious customs on each Caribbean island vary; on many they reflect the African traditions of transported slaves, especially of the Yoruba people shipped from West Africa, who carried on the practices of their homelands. In some of these traditions, herbs are valued for their magical as well as for their medicinal properties. Tobacco (*Nicotiana tabacum*, p. 237), for example, is used for divination in many native cultures, including in Santeria and voodoo religious rituals, as are other herbs, including garlic (*Allium sativum*, p. 56) and cayenne (*Capsicum frutescens*, p. 70).

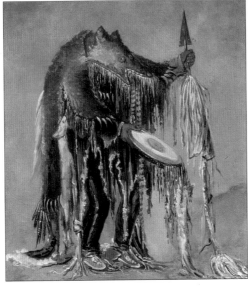

A Native American medicine man *performing a healing ritual intended to drive out evil spirits, as depicted by the 19th-century artist George Catlin.*

SHAMANISM

Moving north, Native American herbal medicine in what is now the United States and Canada was and is primarily shamanistic in nature, involving herbal lore, ritual, and magic. Shamanistic societies from Siberia to the Amazon believe that, in serious illness, the soul of the sick person has been taken over by malignant forces. The shaman's role is to heal both the physical *and* the spiritual dimension of the illness. The patient cannot be truly cured until his or her soul has been freed from the influence of evil spirits. Shamanistic ceremonies and rites to heal the sick person's spirit include dancing, chanting, drumming, playing games, and the stirring of ashes or sprinkling of water. By taking hallucinogens such as peyote (*Lophophora williamsii*, p. 228), the shaman is able to reach out to the spirit world and heal both the individual and the community as a whole.

POWER OF HERBS

In all Native American cultures from Canada to Chile, herbs are thought to have spiritual energy, and many of them are invested with great magical power. The Iroquois believe that cardinal lobelia (*Lobelia cardinalis*, see *L. inflata*, p. 108) and morning glory (*Ipomoea pandurata*) have the ability to heal or harm, and should be picked, stored, and used with great care. Morning glory is considered so powerful that even touching it could cause harm. The Iroquois use the plant as a remedy for coughs, tuberculosis, and other ailments, and also take it as a decoction with sunflower seeds (*Helianthus annuus*) as a sacrament in spring and autumn rituals.

Tobacco, now considered an addictive drug, was a sacred shamanistic herb for most Native American peoples. It was smoked in pipes and "thrown into fires as an offering, cast into the wind and water to abate storms, scattered about a fish weir to improve the catch and offered *(continued)*

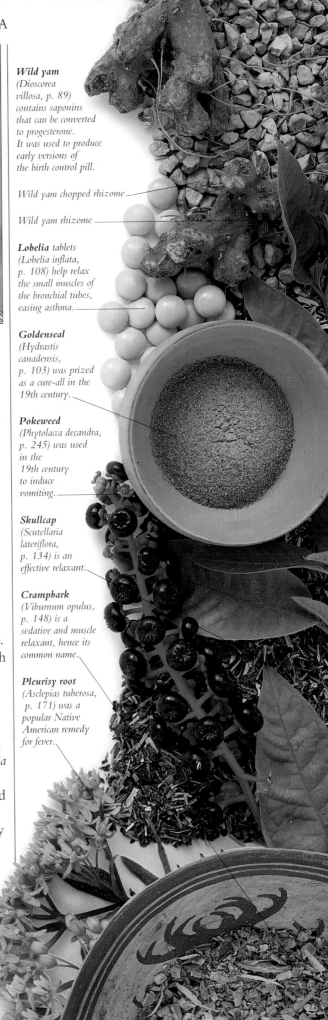

Wild yam *(Dioscorea villosa, p. 89) contains saponins that can be converted to progesterone. It was used to produce early versions of the birth control pill.*

Wild yam chopped rhizome

Wild yam rhizome

Lobelia *tablets (Lobelia inflata, p. 108) help relax the small muscles of the bronchial tubes, easing asthma.*

Goldenseal *(Hydrastis canadensis, p. 103) was prized as a cure-all in the 19th century.*

Pokeweed *(Phytolacca decandra, p. 245) was used in the 19th century to induce vomiting.*

Skullcap *(Scutellaria lateriflora, p. 134) is an effective relaxant.*

Crampbark *(Viburnum opulus, p. 148) is a sedative and muscle relaxant, hence its common name.*

Pleurisy root *(Asclepias tuberosa, p. 171) was a popular Native American remedy for fever.*

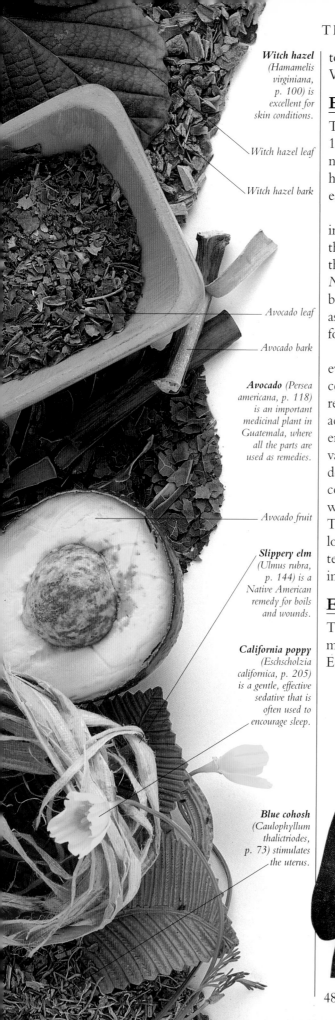

Witch hazel (Hamamelis virginiana, p. 100) is excellent for skin conditions.

Witch hazel leaf

Witch hazel bark

Avocado leaf

Avocado bark

Avocado (Persea americana, p. 118) is an important medicinal plant in Guatemala, where all the parts are used as remedies.

Avocado fruit

Slippery elm (Ulmus rubra, p. 144) is a Native American remedy for boils and wounds.

California poppy (Eschscholzia californica, p. 205) is a gentle, effective sedative that is often used to encourage sleep.

Blue cohosh (Caulophyllum thalictriodes, p. 73) stimulates the uterus.

to the air in thanksgiving for escape from danger," according to Virgil Vogel's *American Indian Medicine* (1970).

EUROPEAN SETTLERS

The first European settlers in North America, arriving in the early 17th century, tended to dismiss Native American medical practices as no more than primitive savagery. The settlers relied largely on imported herbal medicines, or on European plants hardy enough to grow in eastern North America.

As time went by, however, the settlers' increased contact with indigenous peoples in the frontier regions fostered a healthy respect for their healing skills. Sometimes settlers adopted not just the plants but the harvesting and therapeutic methods as well. Joseph Doddridge, in *Notes on the Settlement and Indian Wars* (1876), relates that butternut bark (*Juglans cinerea*, p. 222) was peeled downward if it was to be used as a purgative (acting "downward" by purging the bowels), and upward for use as an emetic (acting "upward" by provoking vomiting).

The types of healing regimens practiced by Native Americans eventually gained widespread popularity. Toward the end of the 18th century, Samuel Thomson (1769–1843) developed a simple therapeutic regimen based on Native American herbal practice. Thomson never acknowledged the debt, but it is clearly evident – from the use of emetics, purgatives, and stimulants, to the central role of sweating and vapor baths (based in part on Native American sweat lodges), to the deep knowledge of North American medicinal plants. Thomson considered that "all disease is caused by cold" and his system worked well for those with robust health struck down by infection or injury. The two main herbs in his system – cayenne, a stimulating herb, and lobelia, an emetic, relaxant, and stimulant – act to raise body temperature and dilate the blood vessels. Taking these plants helps to increase resistance to infection and speeds the healing of wounds.

ECLECTICISM & ITS INFLUENCE

The fertile marriage between Native American and Western herbal medicine led to more sophisticated herbal systems, such as Eclecticism, founded by Dr. Wooster Beech (1794–1868) in the 1830s. Beech studied both herbal and conventional medicine and tried to combine the new scientific knowledge of physiology and pathology with the best of the herbal tradition. Beech rejected Thomson's theories as being oversimplistic, and aimed to use the lowest dosages possible to achieve good results. His approach was so successful that at Eclecticism's height in 1909, more than 8,000 members were in practice, all with recognized medical qualifications. Another significant medical movement, inspired by Thomson's regimen and influenced by the Eclectics, was Physiomedicalism.

Samuel Thomson, who inspired the 19th-century Physiomedicalists, advocated Native American remedies.

48

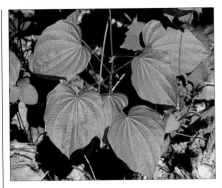

Wild yam *is found growing in Mexico. Its rhizome relaxes smooth muscle and it is used as an antispasmodic.*

Using many herbs, these practitioners sought to harmonize "the organic tissues with the vital force," with the aim of restoring equilibrium within the body. Believing the stomach was the source of disease, Physiomedicalists used herbs that induced vomiting, such as pokeweed (*Phytolacca decandra*, p. 245), to cleanse the organ. Other herbs, such as echinacea (*Echinacea* spp., p. 90), now recognized as an excellent immune-stimulant, and golden-seal (*Hydrastis canadensis*, p. 103), a tonic and anti-inflammatory, were then prescribed to aid recovery.

The second half of the 19th century was an extraordinary time for North American natural medicine. In addition to engendering osteopathy and chiropractic at the turn of the century, it also reinvigorated herbal medicine in Britain to such a degree that Physiomedicalism became an Anglo-American herbal tradition. To this day, British herbalists still use a far wider variety of North American medicinal herbs than do their European counterparts.

NORTH AMERICAN HERBALISM TODAY

In the US, herbal medicine went into steep decline after 1907 because of the government's decision to limit financial support for medical training to conventional medical schools. Since that time, herbal medicine in both the US and Canada has existed only on the fringes of conventional health care. In much of the US, it is illegal to practice herbal medicine without medical qualifications, but courses in herbalism are not offered at medical schools. Some Canadian colleges offer diplomas in herbalism.

Herbs are viewed primarily as a source of new phamacologically active chemicals rather than as medicines in their own right. The wild yam (*Dioscorea villosa*, p. 89) is a good example. The plant was used medicinally in Mexico from the time of the Aztecs as a treatment for rheumatic complaints and as an analgesic. In 1942, researchers discovered that it contains a steroid, diosgenin, that mimics the effect of progesterone – one of the female sex hormones – in the body. In the 1950s, the Mexican pharmaceutical company Syntex produced the first contraceptive pill from diosgenin, extracted from wild yam. Few people realize the role that plants have played in the development of modern pharmaceutical drugs, and fewer still question whether the body might be better served sometimes by the use of whole plants rather than with single chemicals.

With the passing of relatively liberal legislation in 1994, herbal remedies are more readily available in the US but they can only be sold as food supplements. This lags behind developments in the rest of the world, where herbs are recognized as medicines in their own right. Nevertheless, with the growing number of herbalists in North America, and with the opening of many schools of Western herbal medicine, herbalism is now stronger and more popular than ever could have been dreamed of 10 years ago.

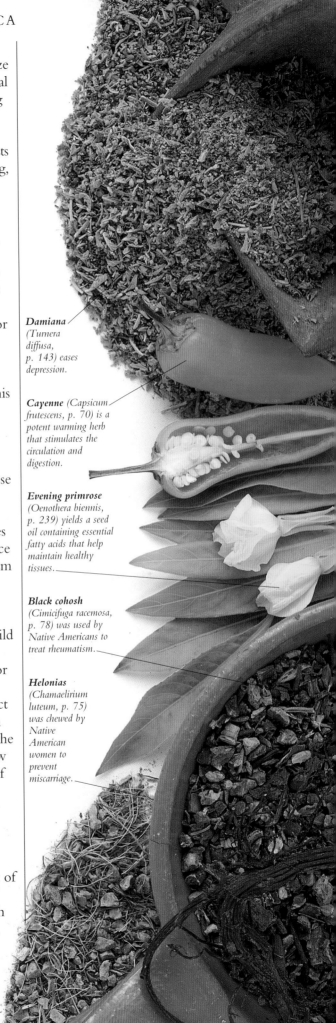

Damiana (*Turnera diffusa*, p. 143) eases depression.

Cayenne (*Capsicum frutescens*, p. 70) is a potent warming herb that stimulates the circulation and digestion.

Evening primrose (*Oenothera biennis*, p. 239) yields a seed oil containing essential fatty acids that help maintain healthy tissues.

Black cohosh (*Cimicifuga racemosa*, p. 78) was used by Native Americans to treat rheumatism.

Helonias (*Chamaelirium luteum*, p. 75) was chewed by Native American women to prevent miscarriage.

SOUTH AMERICA

Herbal medicine is a part of the struggle for survival for the indigenous peoples of South America, as they seek to protect their culture and natural habitats. As the great rainforests disappear we are losing thousands of plant species, some of which may have had great medicinal value.

HERBAL MEDICINE IN SOUTH AMERICA conjures up images of shamanistic rituals and a collection of thousands of as yet unclassified plants under the thick canopy of the rainforest. But these are only two facets of the continent's herbal tradition – those of the Amazon and Orinoco regions. Distinctly different plants and practices are found in other areas, for example, on the Bolivian Andes plateau, on the humid plains of Paraguay, and in cities such as Rio de Janeiro.

WEALTH OF NATIVE PLANTS

Ever since the Spanish conquest in the early 16th century, European writers have remarked on the huge variety of plant medicines used by native peoples. The most important of these was cinchona (*Cinchona* spp., p. 79), a traditional Andean fever remedy, which the Spaniards first discovered around 1630. Quinine, produced from this plant, became the most effective treatment for malaria for nearly 300 years and is still widely used as a tonic, bitter, and muscle relaxant. Other important plants originating in South America include the potato (*Solanum tuberosum*, p. 269), which was cultivated in more than 60 different varieties by the Inca. Its uses are wide-ranging, but it is particularly effective as a poultice for skin conditions. Ipecac (*Cephaelis ipecacuanha*, p. 184) – now commonly found in over-the-counter cough preparations – was taken by Brazilian native peoples to treat amebic dysentery. Maté (*Ilex paraguariensis*, p. 220), which grows in western regions of the continent, makes a stimulating beverage that is prepared and drunk like tea. Maté has become so popular it is now cultivated in Spain and Portugal as well as in South America.

Since the 1950s, specialist ethnobotanists have lived within native communities, particularly in the Amazon region, where most tribes have a highly developed herbal lore. Their work has resulted in a wealth of knowledge about Amazonian species. Pareira (*Chondrodendron tomentosum*, p. 187), a climbing vine of the rainforest, for example, yields the poison curare used in hunting, and is taken medicinally to treat water retention, bruising, and insanity. Sadly, however, the herbal medicine of many indigenous groups is now under threat as the rainforests disappear.

MIND-ALTERING REMEDIES

Notorious in the West as the source of cocaine, coca (*Erythroxylum coca*, p. 204) is an important medicine in South America for nausea and vomiting, toothache, and asthma. It is also completely interwoven into the culture of indigenous Amazonian and Andean peoples and serves as a precise

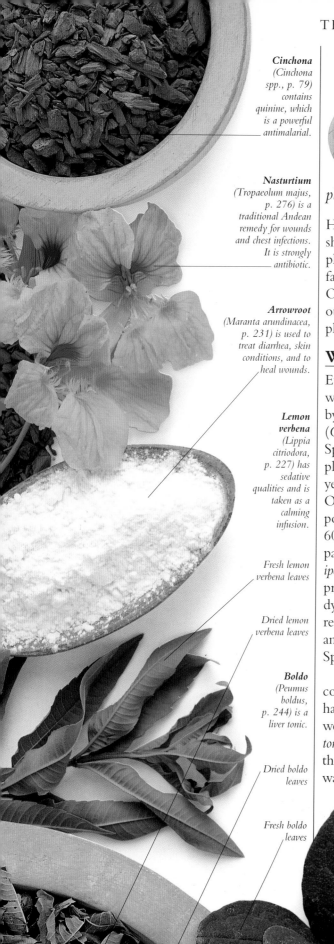

Cinchona *(Cinchona spp., p. 79) contains quinine, which is a powerful antimalarial.*

Nasturtium *(Tropaeolum majus, p. 276) is a traditional Andean remedy for wounds and chest infections. It is strongly antibiotic.*

Arrowroot *(Maranta arundinacea, p. 231) is used to treat diarrhea, skin conditions, and to heal wounds.*

Lemon verbena *(Lippia citriodora, p. 227) has sedative qualities and is taken as a calming infusion.*

Fresh lemon verbena leaves

Dried lemon verbena leaves

Boldo *(Peumus boldus, p. 244) is a liver tonic.*

Dried boldo leaves

Fresh boldo leaves

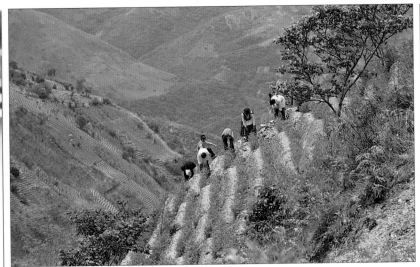

Coca harvest in Bolivia. *The leaves are picked when they begin to curl. They have been used as a stimulant for centuries by the indigenous peoples of the Andes.*

example of the unique relationship that traditional peoples have with the plant world. Many different myths confirm coca's sacred and ancient origins in South America, and great ritual and significance is attached to the leaves, which, when mixed with lime and chewed, reduce appetite and increase endurance.

Many hallucinogenic plants are used within South American shamanistic societies, notably ayahuasca (*Banisteriopsis caapi*, p. 174). This powerful "medicine" enables the shaman (priest) to communicate with the spirit world and cure the patient's ill health.

THE EUROPEAN INFLUENCE

In more westernized areas of South America, herbal medicine is often a blend of Spanish and local traditions (as is the case in Central America, *see* p. 46). Large herb markets exist in some cities, such as La Paz and Quito, which provide an astonishing variety of indigenous and European herbs. In Ecuadorian markets, for example, anise (*Pimpinella anisum*, p. 246), a digestive remedy for colic and cramping, which originally came from the Mediterranean, is sold alongside unusual native medicines such as arquitecta (*Culcitium reflexum*), a diuretic and detoxifying herb traditionally used in treatments for toxicity and infections, including syphilis.

RESEARCH & NEW HOPES

Research into native herbs has led to the use of certain plants in conventional medicine. Brazilian investigation into lapacho (*Tabebuia* spp., p. 138) indicates significant therapeutic potential for fungal infections, inflammation of the cervix, HIV, and cancer. While lapacho's effectiveness in treating cancer is controversial, it is currently prescribed both by local doctors and in hospitals.

Research into herbal medicine is expanding, with a hospital-based center in Santa Fe de Bogotá exploring the properties of indigenous medicinal herbs. Such studies are important for the world as a whole. The locally based researchers, unlike most multinational drug companies, are willing to develop medicines based on simple extracts, which may ultimately prove more effective than the isolated constituents often used in conventional drugs.

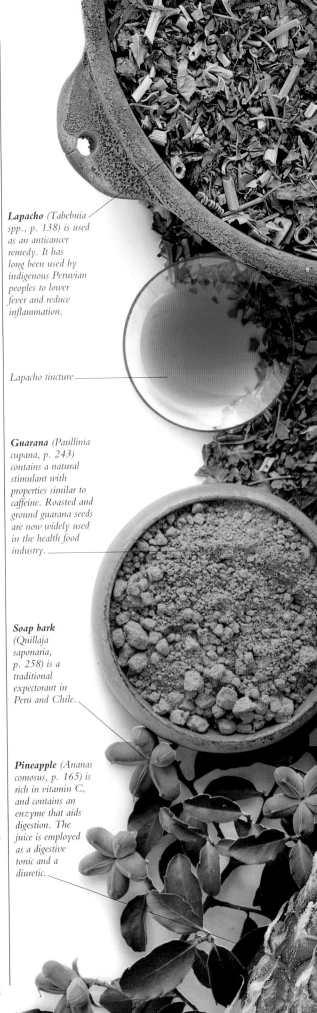

Lapacho (*Tabebuia* spp., p. 138) is used as an anticancer remedy. It has long been used by indigenous Peruvian peoples to lower fever and reduce inflammation.

Lapacho tincture

Guarana (*Paullinia cupana*, p. 243) contains a natural stimulant with properties similar to caffeine. Roasted and ground guarana seeds are now widely used in the health food industry.

Soap bark (*Quillaja saponaria*, p. 258) is a traditional expectorant in Peru and Chile.

Pineapple (*Ananas comosus*, p. 165) is rich in vitamin C, and contains an enzyme that aids digestion. The juice is employed as a digestive tonic and a diuretic.

51

KEY MEDICINAL PLANTS

OF THE ESTIMATED 500,000 plants on our planet, it is thought that around 10,000 are used regularly for medicinal purposes. The index of Key Medicinal Plants features 100 of the best-known medicinal plants in Latin name order. Many are commonly available and widely used in different herbal traditions around the world, for example German chamomile (*Chamomilla recutita*, p. 76) and ginger (*Zingiber officinale*, p. 153). Others such as the East African calumba (*Jateorhiza palmata*, p. 106) are key herbs within their native region. A significant proportion of these herbs have been well researched and most are excellent for home use.

ABOUT THE ENTRIES

PLANT NAMES
The Latin name given is the one by which the plant is most generally known in medical herbalism. If the plant has a Latin synonym this is provided. The first part of the Latin name designates the plant's genus (sub-family). The second part specifies the species name. In brackets after the Latin name(s) comes the plant's family name, the broader class to which the genus belongs. The plant's common name(s) are beneath the family name. If more than one common name is in popular use, they are listed in order of importance. Where appropriate, the origins of common names are given in brackets.

HABITAT & CULTIVATION
Gives information on where the plant is indigenous, its current distribution, how it is cultivated and harvested, and any preferred growing conditions.

RELATED SPECIES
Provides cross-references and information on related species that are used medicinally or are well known.

KEY CONSTITUENTS & KEY ACTIONS
Lists the key active constituents and the key medicinal actions of the plant on the body in order of importance. *Note* For more information on plant constituents and their actions, *see* pp. 10–15.

RESEARCH
Provides details of scientific research including results of any clinical trials. If appropriate, includes herbal practitioners' observations of the plant's known actions and potential new medicinal uses for the herb.

TRADITIONAL & CURRENT USES
Reveals how the plant was used medicinally in the past and how it is used today in different herbal traditions. Examines differences between traditional and current uses, and shows how scientific research is sometimes confirming the validity of the traditional use and sometimes uncovering completely new applications for the herb. *Note* See *Glossary* p. 321 for unfamiliar terms.

PARTS USED
Illustrates the parts of the plant used medicinally.

KEY PREPARATIONS & THEIR USES
Features key preparations with details of how they are taken or applied. Gives cautions about using the herb as a medicine and about the plant in general. States if the plant, its constituents, or its extracts are legally restricted. *Note* A self-help use is provided for many preparations. Before attempting any self-help use it is essential to read the cautions and the information on pp. 289 & 298–299.

SELF-HELP USES
Cross-refers to self-help treatments in *Remedies for Common Ailments*. *Note* Always read the cautions in *Key Preparations & Their Uses* and the information on pp. 289 & 298–299 before using any herb.

Achillea millefolium (Compositae)
YARROW, MILFOIL

YARROW
A creeping perennial, growing to 3 ft (1 m), with white flower heads and finely divided leaves.

YARROW IS A NATIVE EUROPEAN PLANT, with a long history as a wound healer. In classical times, it was known as *herba militaris* because it was used to staunch war wounds. It has long been taken as a strengthening bitter tonic, and all kinds of bitter drinks have been made from it. Yarrow helps recovery from colds and flu and is beneficial for hay fever. It is also helpful for menstrual problems and circulatory disorders.

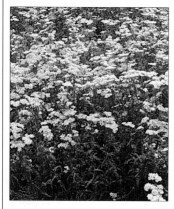

Yarrow was once known as "nosebleed," because its leaves were used to staunch blood.

HABITAT & CULTIVATION
Native to Europe and western Asia, yarrow can be found growing wild in temperate regions throughout the world, in meadows and along roadsides. The herb spreads via its roots, and the aerial parts are picked in summer when in flower.

KEY CONSTITUENTS
- Volatile oil with variable content (linalool, camphor, sabinene, chamazulene)
- Sesquiterpene lactones
- Flavonoids
- Alkaloids (achilleine)
- Polyacetylenes
- Triterpenes
- Salicylic acid
- Coumarins
- Tannins

KEY ACTIONS
- Antispasmodic
- Astringent
- Bitter tonic
- Increases sweating
- Lowers blood pressure
- Reduces fever

- Mild diuretic and urinary antiseptic
- Stops internal bleeding
- Promotes menstruation
- Anti-inflammatory

RESEARCH
Despite its many uses, yarrow has been poorly researched.

TRADITIONAL & CURRENT USES
- **Healing wounds** Achilles reputedly used yarrow to heal wounds, hence its botanical name. It has been used for this purpose for centuries, and in Scotland a traditional wound ointment was made from yarrow.
- **Therapeutic properties** Chamazulene, present in some volatile oils, is markedly anti-inflammatory and antiallergenic. Sesquiterpene lactones are bitter and tonic, and achilleine helps arrest internal and external bleeding. The flavonoids are probably responsible for yarrow's antispasmodic effect.
- **Gynecological herb** Yarrow helps regulate the menstrual cycle, reduces heavy bleeding, and eases menstrual pain.
- **Other uses** Combined with other herbs, yarrow helps colds and flu. Its bitter tonic properties make it useful for weak digestion and colic. It also helps hay fever, lowers high blood pressure, improves venous circulation, and tones varicose veins.

SELF-HELP USES
- **Cleansing wounds**, p. 304.
- **Colds & flu**, p. 311.
- **Digestive infections**, p. 305.
- **Fever**, p. 311.
- **Varicose veins**, p. 302.

✜ PARTS USED

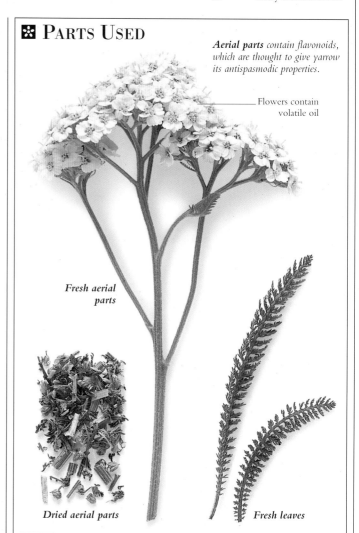

Aerial parts contain flavonoids, which are thought to give yarrow its antispasmodic properties.

Flowers contain volatile oil

Fresh aerial parts

Dried aerial parts

Fresh leaves

✍ KEY PREPARATIONS & THEIR USES

Cautions May cause allergic reaction in rare cases. Use the essential oil only under professional supervision. Do not take during pregnancy.

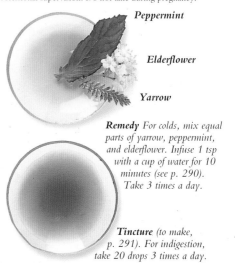

Peppermint

Elderflower

Yarrow

Remedy For colds, mix equal parts of yarrow, peppermint, and elderflower. Infuse 1 tsp with a cup of water for 10 minutes (see p. 290). Take 3 times a day.

Tincture *(to make, p. 291). For indigestion, take 20 drops 3 times a day.*

Essential oil extracted from the flowers is used by herbalists to treat congestion.

▱ POULTICE (to make, p. 294). Apply to scrapes, cuts, and bruises.

SWEET FLAG
An herbaceous, aquatic reedlike plant with tall, sword-shaped leaves. It grows to 3 ft (1 m).

Acorus calamus (Araceae)
SWEET FLAG, CALAMUS, BACC (HINDI)

SWEET FLAG HAS A LONGSTANDING reputation as a tonic and stimulant. An important herb in Ayurvedic medicine, it is also widely used in Europe and the US. The rhizome is a valuable remedy for the digestion, and is a tonic for the nervous system. It stimulates the appetite and soothes the digestion, relieving gas and calming indigestion and colic. Sweet flag has a strongly aromatic, bitter taste.

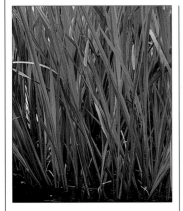

Sweet flag is an aquatic plant, similar in appearance to the iris. It has yellow flowers in summer.

HABITAT & CULTIVATION

Sweet flag, believed to originate from India, now grows in many parts of the world. It prefers wet soil and is found in ditches, beside lakes and rivers, and in marshy places. Propagation is carried out in autumn or early spring by dividing the clumps of rhizomes and replanting them in shallow water. The rhizomes are harvested as needed.

RELATED SPECIES

A. gramineus (*shi chang pu*) is a Chinese herb and a close relative that is used medicinally for much the same range of conditions as *A. calamus*.

KEY CONSTITUENTS

- Volatile oil – sesquiterpenes (*A. calamus* var. *americanus* only); asarone (except *A. calamus* var. *americanus*)
- Saponins
- Bitter principle (acorin)
- Mucilage

KEY ACTIONS

- Carminative
- Relieves muscle spasm
- Increases sweating
- Stimulant
- Tonic

RESEARCH

- **Asarone** Research attention has focused on the constituent asarone in the volatile oil, which has a carcinogenic action when isolated. Sweet flag grown in the US, known as *A. calamus* var. *americanus*, however, does not contain asarone, and only preparations made from this variety should be used.
- **Whole herb** In India, sweet flag powder has been taken for thousands of years with no reports of cancer arising from its use. This suggests that use of the whole herb may be safe, but more research is needed.

TRADITIONAL & CURRENT USES

- **Early uses** Sweet flag has been regarded as an aphrodisiac in India and Egypt for at least 2,500 years. In Europe, it was valued as a stimulant, bitter herb for the appetite (if not for the appetites), and as an aid to the digestion. In North America, the decoction was used for fevers, stomach cramps, and colic; the rhizome was chewed for toothache, and powdered rhizome was inhaled for congestion.
- **Ayurvedic medicine** Sweet flag is an important herb in Ayurvedic medicine, and is valued as a "rejuvenator" for the brain and nervous system, and as a remedy for digestive disorders.
- **Western herbalism** In Western herbal medicine the herb is chiefly employed for digestive problems such as gas, bloating, colic, and poor digestive function. Sweet flag, particularly *A. calamus* var. *americanus*, which is the most effective antispasmodic, relieves spasm of the intestines. It helps distended and uncomfortable stomachs, and headaches associated with weak digestion. Small amounts are thought to reduce stomach acidity, while larger doses increase deficient acid production – a good example of how different doses of the same herb can produce different results.

✤ PARTS USED

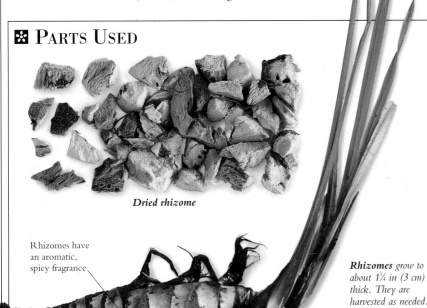

Dried rhizome

Rhizomes have an aromatic, spicy fragrance

Rhizomes grow to about 1¼ in (3 cm) thick. They are harvested as needed.

Fresh rhizome

KEY PREPARATIONS & THEIR USES

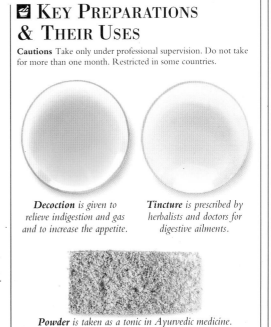

Cautions Take only under professional supervision. Do not take for more than one month. Restricted in some countries.

Decoction is given to relieve indigestion and gas and to increase the appetite.

Tincture is prescribed by herbalists and doctors for digestive ailments.

Powder is taken as a tonic in Ayurvedic medicine.

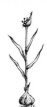

GARLIC
A bulbous perennial
growing to 1–3 ft
(30 cm–1 m) with
pale pink or green-
white flowers.

Allium sativum (Liliaceae)

GARLIC

KNOWN FOR ITS PUNGENT odor and taste, garlic is an ideal herbal medicine, being completely safe for home use and a powerful treatment for a host of health problems. It counters many infections, including those of the nose, throat, and chest. It also reduces cholesterol, helps circulatory disorders, such as high blood pressure, and lowers blood sugar levels, making it a useful dietary addition in late-onset diabetes.

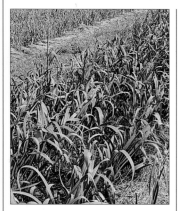

***Garlic** is widely cultivated commercially for use in cooking.*

HABITAT & CULTIVATION

Originally from central Asia, garlic is now grown worldwide. It is grown by dividing the bulb and is harvested late the following summer.

RELATED SPECIES

Onion and ramsons (*A. cepa* and *A. ursinum*, p. 162) are both important medicinal herbs.

KEY CONSTITUENTS

- Volatile oil (alliin, alliinase, allicin)
- Scordinins
- Selenium
- Vitamins A, B, C, and E

KEY ACTIONS

- Antibiotic
- Expectorant
- Increases sweating
- Lowers blood pressure
- Reduces blood clotting
- Antidiabetic
- Expels worms

RESEARCH

- **Antibiotic** Garlic has been researched in Germany, Japan, and the US from the 1980s onward, but authorities still disagree on how it achieves its remarkable antibiotic action. When the fresh clove is crushed, alliin is broken down by alliinase into allicin. Allicin and other constituents of the volatile oil are highly antiseptic and antibiotic, explaining why garlic is effective even in severe infections such as dysentery.
- **Blood pressure** Clinical trials in the 1980s have confirmed that garlic reduces blood lipid (fat) levels and lowers blood pressure.

TRADITIONAL & CURRENT USES

- **Traditional remedy** Garlic has always been esteemed for its healing powers and before the development of antibiotics it was a treatment for all manner of infections, from tuberculosis to typhoid. It was also used to dress wounds in the First World War.
- **Bronchial infections** Garlic is an excellent remedy for all types of chest infections. It is good for colds, flu, and ear infections, and it helps to reduce mucus.
- **Digestive tract** Digestive infections respond well to garlic. The herb can also rid the body of intestinal parasites.
- **Circulatory remedy** Garlic prevents circulatory problems and strokes by keeping the blood thin. It lowers cholesterol levels and blood pressure.
- **Other uses** Garlic is used for infections, and may be taken with conventional antibiotics to support their action and ward off side effects. Also, garlic reduces blood sugar levels and can help in late-onset diabetes.

✴ PARTS USED

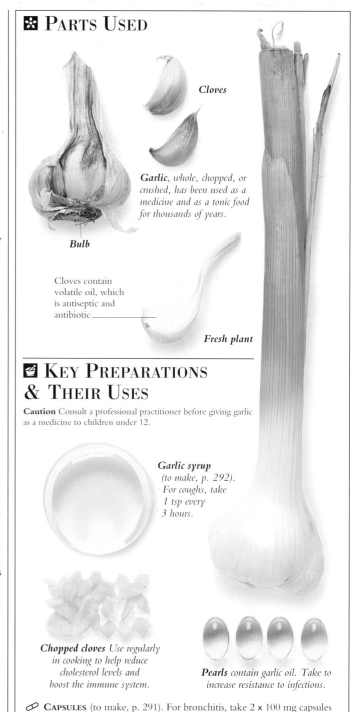

Cloves

Garlic, whole, chopped, or crushed, has been used as a medicine and as a tonic food for thousands of years.

Bulb

Cloves contain volatile oil, which is antiseptic and antibiotic

Fresh plant

✍ KEY PREPARATIONS & THEIR USES

Caution Consult a professional practitioner before giving garlic as a medicine to children under 12.

Garlic syrup (to make, p. 292). For coughs, take 1 tsp every 3 hours.

***Chopped cloves** Use regularly in cooking to help reduce cholesterol levels and boost the immune system.*

***Pearls** contain garlic oil. Take to increase resistance to infections.*

- ✑ **CAPSULES** (to make, p. 291). For bronchitis, take 2 x 100 mg capsules 3 times a day.
- ✑ **TABLETS** Take for high blood pressure and bronchitis.

SELF-HELP USES

- **Acne & boils**, p. 305.
- **Athlete's foot**, p. 304.
- **Colds & flu**, p. 311.
- **Cold sores**, p. 304.
- **Coughs & bronchitis**, p. 310.
- **Digestive infections**, p. 305.
- **Earache**, p. 312.
- **Fungal infections**, p. 314.
- **High blood pressure**, p. 301.
- **Old age tonic**, p. 319.
- **Tonsillitis**, p. 311.
- **Urinary infections**, p. 314.

Aloe vera syn. *A. barbadensis* (Liliaceae)

ALOE VERA, ALOES

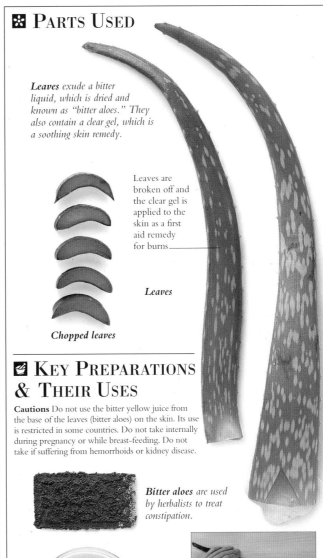

ALOE VERA
A perennial with succulent leaves 2 ft (60 cm) long and a spike of yellow or orange flowers.

NATIVE TO AFRICA, aloe vera is commonly cultivated as a potted plant and has two distinct types of medicinal use. The clear gel contained in the leaf is a remarkably effective healer of wounds and burns, speeding up the rate of healing and reducing the risk of infection. The yellow sap from the base of the leaf when dried is known as "bitter aloes." It is a strong laxative, useful for short-term constipation.

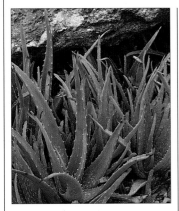

Aloe vera has prickly, gray-green, succulent leaves that yield effective medicinal substances.

HABITAT & CULTIVATION

Native to eastern and southern Africa, aloe vera grows wild in the tropics and is cultivated extensively worldwide. (The plants grown as potted plants have a low anthraquinone content.) Aloe vera is propagated by breaking off small rooted plantlets. To collect the gel and bitter liquid, the leaves are cut and drained as required.

RELATED SPECIES

Cape aloes (*A. ferox*) is used in herbal medicine as an irritant laxative. Many other *Aloe* species are also useful medicinally.

KEY CONSTITUENTS

- Anthraquinones (aloin, aloe-emodin)
- Resins
- Tannins
- Polysaccharides
- Aloectin B

KEY ACTIONS

- Heals wounds
- Emollient
- Stimulates secretions of bile
- Laxative

RESEARCH

- **Healing properties** Extensive research since the 1930s in the US and Russia has shown that the clear gel has a dramatic ability to heal wounds, ulcers, and burns, putting a protective coat on the affected area and speeding up the rate of healing. This action is in part due to the presence of aloectin B, which stimulates the immune system.

TRADITIONAL & CURRENT USES

- **Beauty treatment** Aloe vera has a long history as a skin lotion – Cleopatra is said to have attributed her beauty to it.
- **Western remedy** In the West, aloe vera first became popular in the 1950s when its ability to heal burns, in particular radiation burns, was discovered.
- **First aid** Aloe vera is an excellent first aid remedy to keep in the home for burns, scrapes, scalds, and sunburn. A leaf broken off releases soothing gel, which may be applied to the affected part.
- **Skin conditions** The gel is useful for almost any skin condition that needs soothing and astringing, and will help varicose veins to some degree.
- **Ulcers** The protective and healing effect of aloe vera also works internally, and the gel can be used for peptic ulcers and irritable bowel syndrome.
- **Laxative** The bitter yellow liquid in the leaves (bitter aloes) contains anthraquinones, which are strongly laxative. They cause

PARTS USED

Leaves exude a bitter liquid, which is dried and known as "bitter aloes." They also contain a clear gel, which is a soothing skin remedy.

Leaves are broken off and the clear gel is applied to the skin as a first aid remedy for burns

Leaves

Chopped leaves

KEY PREPARATIONS & THEIR USES

Cautions Do not use the bitter yellow juice from the base of the leaves (bitter aloes) on the skin. Its use is restricted in some countries. Do not take internally during pregnancy or while breast-feeding. Do not take if suffering from hemorrhoids or kidney disease.

Bitter aloes are used by herbalists to treat constipation.

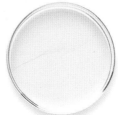

Juice is made commercially from the gel. For peptic ulcers, take 50 ml 3 times a day.

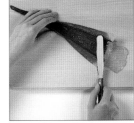

Leaves Break off a leaf and split open to collect the gel. For burns and eczema, apply liberally twice a day.

TINCTURE made from bitter aloes (see p. 291). To stimulate the appetite, take 1–3 ml with water before meals.

the colon to contract, generally producing a bowel movement 8–12 hours after consumption. At low doses, the bitter properties of the herb stimulate the digestion. At higher doses, bitter aloes are laxative and purgative.

SELF-HELP USES

- **Minor burns & sunburn**, p. 303.
- **Stretch marks**, p. 317.
- **Warts**, p. 304.
- **Weeping skin**, p. 303.
- **Wounds**, p. 304.

Alpinia officinarum (Zingiberaceae)
GALANGAL (HINDI), GAO LIANG (CHINESE)

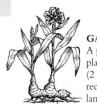

GALANGAL
A perennial aromatic plant growing to 6 ft (2 m) with white, red-lipped flowers and lance-shaped leaves.

LIKE OTHER MEMBERS OF THE ginger family, galangal is warming and comforting to the digestion. It has a pleasantly aromatic and mildly spicy taste, and is suitable for all conditions where the central areas of the body need greater warmth. Galangal was introduced into Europe in about the 9th century. The mystic Hildegard of Bingen regarded it literally as the "spice of life," given by God to ward off ill health.

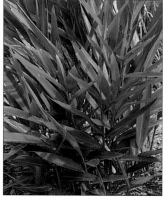

***Galangal** is an important spice in Thai cooking and is reportedly fed to Arabian horses to "fire them up" in parts of Asia.*

HABITAT & CULTIVATION

Native to grassland areas of southern China, and Southeast Asia in general, galangal is now cultivated as a spice and as a medicine throughout much of tropical Asia. It is propagated by dividing and replanting the rhizomes in spring, and it requires well-drained soil and a shady position. The rhizomes are harvested from 4- to 6-year-old plants at the end of the growing season and may be used fresh or dried.

RELATED SPECIES

Greater galangal, also known as Siamese ginger (*A. galanga*), though a close relative of galangal, has a much inferior taste and volatile oil content. It appears to have an antiulcer action. Two other *Alpinia* species, *cao dou cou* (*A. katsumadai*) and *yi zhi ren* (*A. oxyphylla*), are used in a broadly similar way to galangal in traditional Chinese medicine.

KEY CONSTITUENTS

- Volatile oil (about 1%) containing alpha-pinene, cineole, linalool
- Sesquiterpene lactones (galangol, galangin)

KEY ACTIONS

- Warming digestive tonic
- Stimulant
- Carminative
- Prevents vomiting
- Antifungal

RESEARCH

- **Antibacterial** In Chinese research trials, a decoction of galangal had an antibacterial action against a number of pathogens, including anthrax.
- **Antifungal** Research published in 1988 indicates that galangal is distinctly effective against *Candida albicans*.

TRADITIONAL & CURRENT USES

- **Chinese medicine** In traditional Chinese herbal medicine, galangal is a warming herb used for abdominal pain, vomiting, and hiccups, as well as for diarrhea due to internal cold. When used for hiccups, it is combined with codonopsis (*Codonopsis pilosula*, p. 84) and *fu ling* (*Poria cocos*, p. 253).
- **Indian tradition** In India and southwestern Asia, galangal is considered stomachic, anti-inflammatory, expectorant, and a nervine tonic. It is used in the treatment of hiccups, dyspepsia, stomach pain, rheumatoid arthritis, and intermittent fever.
- **Western herbalism** Galangal was introduced into Europe by Arabian physicians well over a

PARTS USED

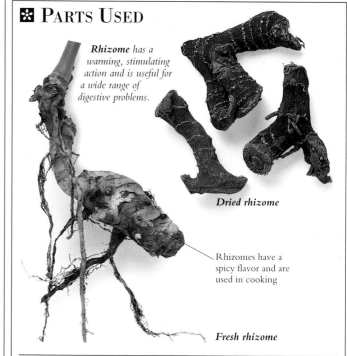

Rhizome has a warming, stimulating action and is useful for a wide range of digestive problems.

Dried rhizome

Rhizomes have a spicy flavor and are used in cooking

Fresh rhizome

KEY PREPARATIONS & THEIR USES

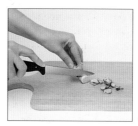

***Chopping root for a decoction** (to make, p. 290). For motion sickness, slowly sip up to a cupful.*

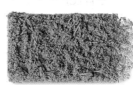

***Powder** For nausea, take a 250 mg capsule (to make, p. 291) twice a day.*

***Tincture** (to make, p. 291) is suitable for long-term use. To improve the digestion, take 20 drops diluted with 100 ml hot water 3 times a day.*

thousand years ago. In line with the Chinese and Indian herbal traditions, it is mainly used in the West for gas, indigestion, vomiting, and stomach pain. An infusion can be used to alleviate painful canker sores and sore gums. Galangal has long been recommended as a treatment for seasickness, which is not surprising given the well-established ability of its relative ginger (*Zingiber officinale*, p. 153) to relieve motion sickness.

- **Candidiasis** Galangal can be used with other antifungal herbs as part of a regimen to treat intestinal candidiasis.
- **Dosage** At a moderate dosage, galangal is a warming and gently stimulating herb for a weakened digestive system, but at a higher dosage it can be an irritant.

SELF-HELP USE

- **Nausea & motion sickness**, p. 306.

Ammi visnaga, syn. Daucus visnaga (Umbelliferae)

VISNAGA, KHELLA

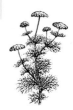

VISNAGA
An erect annual growing to 3 ft (1m) with leaves divided into wisps and clusters of small white flowers.

VISNAGA, WITH ITS AROMATIC, bitter scent and flavor, has greater medicinal than culinary value. It is an effective muscle relaxant and has been used for many centuries to alleviate the excruciating pain of kidney stones. Scientific research has confirmed the validity of this traditional use. Visnaga contains khellin, from which particularly safe pharmaceutical drugs for the treatment of asthma have been derived.

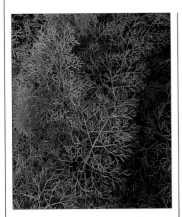

Visnaga is a member of the carrot family and has the characteristic delicate, wispy leaves.

HABITAT & CULTIVATION

Native to North Africa, visnaga grows wild in the Middle East and around the Mediterranean. It is naturalized in Australia and South America. Grown from seed, visnaga is widely cultivated. The tiny fruits containing the seeds are picked in late summer before they have fully ripened.

RELATED SPECIES

Bishop's Weed (*A. majus*, p. 164) is a close relative. This plant has been used to treat asthma but is mainly taken as a diuretic and to treat psoriasis.

KEY CONSTITUENTS

- Khellin (1%)
- Visnagin
- Khellol glycoside
- Volatile oil (0.2%)
- Flavonoids
- Sterols

KEY ACTIONS

- Antispasmodic
- Antiasthmatic
- Relaxant

RESEARCH

■ **Strong antispasmodic**
Research by a pharmacologist working in Egypt in 1946 revealed that visnaga (in particular its constituents khellin and visnagin) has a powerful antispasmodic action on the smaller bronchial muscles, on the coronary arteries that supply blood to the heart, and on the urinary tubules. Visnaga's ability to relax the small bronchi lasts for up to 6 hours, and the plant has practically no side effects.
■ **Khellin** Intal, an asthma drug widely used in conventional medicine, is derived chemically from khellin.

TRADITIONAL & CURRENT USES

■ **Kidney stones** Visnaga is a traditional Egyptian remedy for kidney stones. It was mentioned in the Ebers papyrus of Egypt (*c.* 1500 BC) and is still used there to relieve kidney stones. By relaxing the muscles of the ureter, visnaga reduces the pain caused by the trapped stone and helps ease the stone down into the bladder.
■ **Asthma remedy** Following research into its antispasmodic properties, visnaga is now given for asthma and is safe even for children to take. Although it does not always relieve acute asthma attacks, it does help to prevent their recurrence.
■ **Other respiratory conditions** Visnaga is an effective remedy for various respiratory problems, including bronchitis, emphysema, and whooping cough.
■ **Circulatory herb** By relaxing the coronary arteries, visnaga

PARTS USED

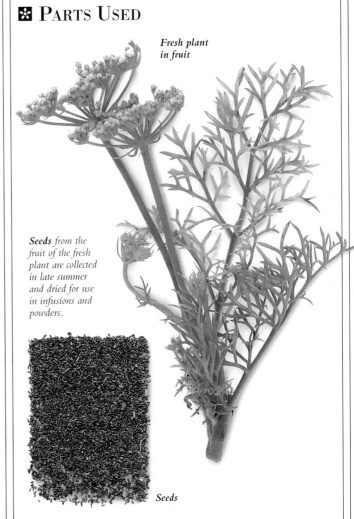

Fresh plant in fruit

Seeds from the fruit of the fresh plant are collected in late summer and dried for use in infusions and powders.

Seeds

KEY PREPARATIONS & THEIR USES

Caution Take only under professional supervision. Long-term use produces symptoms such as nausea, headaches, and insomnia. Subject to legal restrictions in some countries.

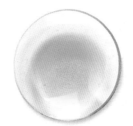

Infusion alleviates asthma, bronchitis, and kidney stones.

Powder is prescribed by doctors and medical herbalists to relieve angina.

helps to improve the blood supply to the heart muscle and thereby eases angina. Visnaga does not, however, reduce blood pressure.
■ **Dental hygiene** In Andalusia in Spain, the largest and best-

quality visnaga were employed to clean the teeth. The high value given to the herb in general was reflected in the saying: "Oro, plata, visnaga, o nada!" (Gold, silver, visnaga, or nothing!)

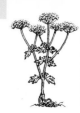

CHINESE ANGELICA
A sturdy, erect perennial growing to 6 ft (2 m), with large, bright green leaves and hollow stems.

Angelica sinensis syn. *A. polymorpha* (Umbelliferae)

CHINESE ANGELICA, DANG GUI (CHINESE)

IN THE CHINESE HERBAL TRADITION, Chinese angelica is the main tonic herb for conditions suffered by women. It is taken by millions of women around the world on a daily basis as an invigorating tonic, helping to regulate menstruation and tonify the blood. It has a sweet, pungent aroma that is very distinctive, and in China it is often used in cooking, which is the best way to take it as a blood tonic.

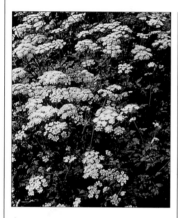

Chinese angelica has attractive clusters of white flowers in summer.

HABITAT & CULTIVATION

Chinese angelica is native to China and Japan, where it is now cultivated. The best rhizomes are in Gansu province in China. Seed is sown in spring, and the rhizomes are lifted in autumn.

RELATED SPECIES

American angelica (*A. atropurpurea*) has similar properties, although it is less aromatic. European angelica (*A. archangelica*, p. 166) is a warming tonic herb for the digestion and circulation, but does not have the same tonic action as Chinese angelica.

KEY CONSTITUENTS

- Coumarins
- Volatile oil (butylidine phthalide, ligustilide, sesquiterpenes, carvacrol)
- Vitamin B$_{12}$
- Beta-sitosterol

KEY ACTIONS

- Tonic
- Blood tonic
- Antispasmodic

- Sedative
- Promotes menstrual flow

RESEARCH

- **Gynecology** Research in China from the 1970s has shown that the herb regulates uterine contractions, which may explain its benefit for menstrual pain.
- **Whole plant** Research shows that the whole plant, including the rhizome, strengthens liver function. The whole rhizome has an antibiotic effect.

TRADITIONAL & CURRENT USES

- **Blood tonic** Famous in China as a tonic, Chinese angelica is taken for "deficient blood" conditions, anemia, and for the symptoms of anemia due to blood loss – a pale complexion, palpitations, and lowered vitality.
- **Women's health** Chinese angelica regulates the menstrual cycle, relieves menstrual pains and cramps, and is an ideal tonic for women with heavy menstrual bleeding who risk becoming anemic. However, as it stimulates menstrual bleeding, other tonic herbs, such as nettle (*Urtica dioica*, p. 145), are best taken during menstruation if the flow is heavy. It is also a uterine tonic and helps infertility.
- **Circulation** Chinese angelica is a "warming" herb, improving the circulation to the abdomen, and to the hands and feet. It strengthens the digestion and is also useful in the treatment of abscesses and boils.

SELF-HELP USES

- **Aiding conception**, p. 316.
- **Menstrual problems**, p. 315.

⚜ PARTS USED

Rhizome is valued for its medicinal properties and is often used in cooking.

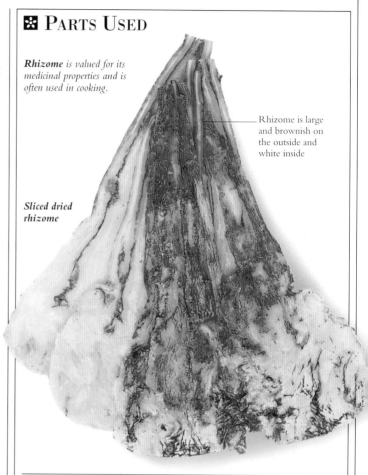

Rhizome is large and brownish on the outside and white inside

Sliced dried rhizome

⚗ KEY PREPARATIONS & THEIR USES

Caution Do not take during pregnancy.

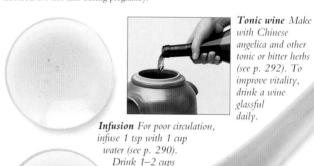

Tonic wine Make with Chinese angelica and other tonic or bitter herbs (see p. 292). To improve vitality, drink a wine glassful daily.

Infusion For poor circulation, infuse 1 tsp with 1 cup water (see p. 290). Drink 1–2 cups a day.

Tincture (to make, p. 291). For menstrual pain, take ½ tsp with water up to 4 times a day.

Chopped rhizome is commonly added to soups in China.

DECOCTION (to make, p. 290). For anemia, take 1 cup 2–3 times a day.

TABLETS Take as a general woman's tonic.

Apium graveolens (Umbelliferae)

CELERY, SMALLAGE

MORE FAMILIAR AS A VEGETABLE than as a medicine, celery stems and seeds have long been taken for urinary, rheumatic, and arthritic problems. Celery is a good cleansing, diuretic herb, and the seeds are used specifically for arthritic complaints where there is an accumulation of waste products. The seeds also have a reputation as a carminative with a mild tranquilizing effect. The stems are less significant medicinally.

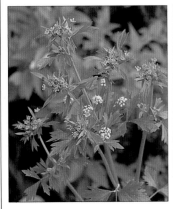

Celery is an important medicinal herb as well as a vegetable.

HABITAT & CULTIVATION

Native to Britain and other European countries, celery is often found growing wild along the English and Welsh coasts, and in marshlands. Widely grown as a vegetable, cultivated celery is less fragrant than the wild variety. It is propagated from seed in spring and harvested from midsummer to autumn.

RELATED SPECIES

Celeriac (*A. graveolens* var. *rapaceum*) is a "turnip-rooted" variety of celery. A medicinal food, it has some of the same qualities as celery.

KEY CONSTITUENTS

- Volatile oil (1.5–3%) containing limonene (60–70%), phthalides, and beta-selinene
- Coumarins
- Furanocoumarins (bergapten)
- Flavonoids (apiin)

KEY ACTIONS

- Antirheumatic
- Carminative
- Antispasmodic
- Diuretic
- Lowers blood pressure
- Urinary antiseptic

RESEARCH

- **Essential oil** Research in Germany and China during the 1970s and 1980s has shown that the essential oil has a calming effect on the central nervous system. Some of its constituents have antispasmodic, sedative, and anticonvulsant actions. Studies undertaken in China have confirmed the oil's usefulness in treating high blood pressure.

TRADITIONAL & CURRENT USES

- **Ancient herb** Records show that celery has been cultivated for at least 3,000 years, notably in pharaonic Egypt, and it was known in China in the 5th century BC. Throughout history, celery has been used as a food, and at various times both the whole plant and the seeds have been taken medicinally.
- **Cleansing properties** Today, the seeds are used for treating rheumatic conditions and gout. They help the kidneys dispose of urates and other unwanted waste products, as well as working to reduce acidity in the body as a whole. The seeds are useful in arthritis, helping to detoxify the body and improve the circulation of blood to the muscles and joints.
- **Diuretic** Celery seeds have a mildly diuretic and significantly antiseptic action. They are an effective treatment for cystitis, helping to disinfect the bladder and urinary tubules.

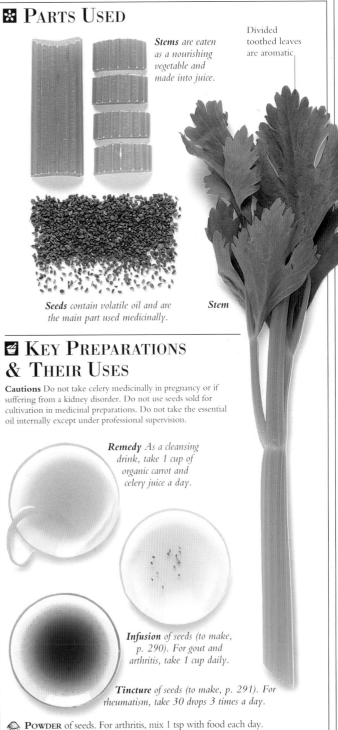

✿ PARTS USED

Stems are eaten as a nourishing vegetable and made into juice.

Divided toothed leaves are aromatic

Seeds contain volatile oil and are the main part used medicinally.

Stem

✍ KEY PREPARATIONS & THEIR USES

Cautions Do not take celery medicinally in pregnancy or if suffering from a kidney disorder. Do not use seeds sold for cultivation in medicinal preparations. Do not take the essential oil internally except under professional supervision.

Remedy As a cleansing drink, take 1 cup of organic carrot and celery juice a day.

Infusion of seeds (to make, p. 290). For gout and arthritis, take 1 cup daily.

Tincture of seeds (to make, p. 291). For rheumatism, take 30 drops 3 times a day.

🌿 **POWDER** of seeds. For arthritis, mix 1 tsp with food each day.

- **Nutritious drink** Celery and organic carrot juice make a nutritious, cleansing drink that is good for many chronic illnesses.
- **Other uses** Celery seeds are beneficial for chest problems such as asthma and bronchitis, and, when used in combination with other herbs, help to reduce blood pressure.

SELF-HELP USES

- **Arthritis**, p. 313.
- **Gout**, p. 313.

Arctium lappa (Compositae)

BURDOCK, NIU BANG ZI (CHINESE)

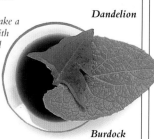

BURDOCK
A biennial with stems that grow to 5 ft (1.5 m), red-purple flower heads, and hooked bracts (burrs).

BURDOCK IS ONE OF THE foremost detoxifying herbs in both Western and Chinese herbal medicine. It is used to treat conditions caused by an "overload" of toxins, such as throat and other infections, boils and rashes, and chronic skin problems. The root and the seeds help to cleanse the body of waste products, and the root is thought to be particularly good at helping to eliminate heavy metals.

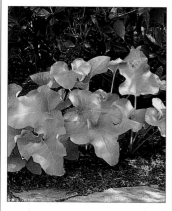

***Burdock** in its first year produces a rosette of large leaves.*

HABITAT & CULTIVATION

Native to Europe and Asia, burdock now grows in temperate regions throughout the world, including the US. Burdock is also cultivated in Europe and China and is propagated from seed in spring. The seeds are harvested in summer and the whole plant is dug up in midsummer.

RELATED SPECIES

A. minus and *A. tomentosum* are related species that are used in a similar way to burdock.

KEY CONSTITUENTS

- Bitter glycosides (arctiopicrin)
- Flavonoids (arctiin)
- Tannins
- Polyacetylenes
- Volatile oil
- Inulin (up to 45%)
- Sesquiterpenes

KEY ACTIONS

- Cleansing
- Mild diuretic
- Antibiotic
- Antiseptic

RESEARCH

- **Antibiotic** Studies in Germany (1967) and Japan (1986) showed that the polyacetylenes, especially in the fresh root, have an antibiotic effect.
- **Other research** Burdock has antibacterial and antifungal properties, and diuretic and hypoglycemic (lowering blood sugar levels) effects. It also appears to have an antitumor action. Arctiin is known to be a smooth muscle relaxant.

TRADITIONAL & CURRENT USES

- **History** Burdock was a traditional remedy for gout, fevers, and kidney stones. In the 17th century, Culpeper wrote, "The seed is much commended to break the stone and cause it to be expelled by urine."
- **Cleansing herb** Burdock is used in both Western and Chinese herbal medicine as a detoxifying herb. The seeds are used to remove toxins in fevers and infections such as mumps and measles, and the root helps the body to eliminate waste products in chronic skin and arthritic conditions.
- **Skin problems** Burdock's diuretic, antibiotic, and mildly bitter actions make it helpful for skin disorders, especially where toxicity is a key factor – for example, in acne, boils, abscesses, local skin infections, eczema, and psoriasis.
- **Combination remedies** Burdock is rarely used on its own in remedies. It is usually mixed with other herbs, such as dandelion (*Taraxacum officinale*, p. 140), to balance its strong cleansing action.

SELF-HELP USES

- **Acne & boils**, p. 305.
- **Skin rashes**, p. 303.

✽ PARTS USED

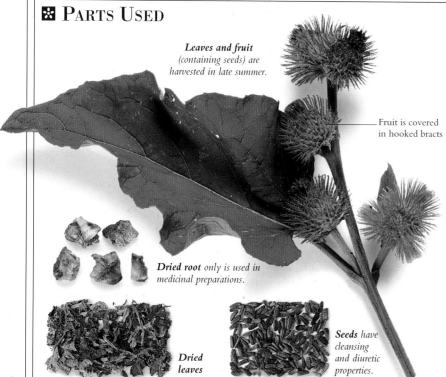

***Leaves and fruit** (containing seeds) are harvested in late summer.*

Fruit is covered in hooked bracts

***Dried root** only is used in medicinal preparations.*

Dried leaves

***Seeds** have cleansing and diuretic properties.*

✍ KEY PREPARATIONS & THEIR USES

***Remedy** For pimples, make a decoction (see p. 290) with 2 tsp burdock root and 5 tsp dandelion root. Drink 1 cup twice a day.*

Dandelion

Burdock

***Tincture** of root (to make, p. 291). For arthritis and skin disorders, take 20 drops diluted with water 2–3 times a day for up to 4 weeks.*

🥄 **DECOCTION** of root (to make, p. 290) is an alternative to tincture for arthritis and skin disorders. Drink 35 ml once a day for up to 4 weeks.

🫖 **INFUSION** of seeds (to make, p. 290). Use as a wash for acne and boils.

🥣 **POULTICE** of leaves (to make, p. 294). Apply to abscesses and boils.

Artemisia absinthium (Compositae)

WORMWOOD

WORMWOOD
A perennial reaching 3 ft (1 m), with gray-green stems and feathery leaves, both covered in fine hairs.

ONE OF THE TRULY BITTER PLANTS – *absinthium* means "without sweetness" – wormwood has a strong tonic effect on the digestive system, especially on the stomach and gallbladder. It is taken in small doses and sipped, the intensely bitter taste playing an important part in its therapeutic effect. In the past, wormwood was one of the main flavorings of vermouth (whose name derives from the German for wormwood).

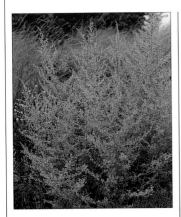

***Wormwood** is strongly aromatic and was used to flavor many alcoholic drinks.*

HABITAT & CULTIVATION

Wormwood is a wayside plant, native to Europe. It now grows wild in central Asia and in eastern parts of the US. It is also cultivated in temperate regions worldwide. Wormwood is propagated from seed in spring or by dividing the roots in autumn. The aerial parts are harvested in late summer.

RELATED SPECIES

Artemisia species with a medicinal use include: *A. abrotanum* (p. 170); *A. annua* (p. 64); *A. anomala; A. capillaris,* and *A. cina* (p. 170); *A. vulgaris* and *A. dracunculus* (p. 171).

KEY CONSTITUENTS

- Volatile oil containing sesquiterpene lactones (artabsin, anabsinthin); thujone; azulenes
- Flavonoids
- Phenolic acids
- Lignans

KEY ACTIONS

- Aromatic bitter
- Stimulates secretion of bile
- Anti-inflammatory
- Eliminates worms
- Eases stomach pain
- Mild antidepressant

RESEARCH

- **Bitter herb** Research into wormwood, mostly during the 1970s, has established that a range of the constituents within the plant contributes to its medicinal activity. Many are very bitter, affecting the bitter taste receptors on the tongue, which sets off a reflex action, stimulating stomach and other digestive secretions.
- **Other research** The azulenes are anti-inflammatory. The sesquiterpene lactones have an antitumor effect and are strongly insecticidal. Thujone is a stimulant to the brain. It is safe in small doses but toxic in excess.

TRADITIONAL & CURRENT USES

- **Absinthe** Wormwood is the source of *absinthe*, an addictive and toxic drink favored in 19th-century France. *Absinthe*, now banned, was flavored with essential oil of wormwood, which, due to its thujone content, is toxic in excess.
- **Digestive stimulant** Wormwood is an extremely useful medicine for those with weak and underactive digestions. It increases stomach acid and bile production and therefore improves digestion and the absorption of nutrients, making it helpful for many conditions, including anemia. Wormwood also eases gas and bloating, and if the tincture is taken regularly, it slowly strengthens the digestion and helps the body return to full vitality after a prolonged illness.
- **Worms** As its name suggests, wormwood is a traditional remedy for eliminating worms. It is moderately effective.
- **Traditional insect repellent** Wormwood is a good insecticide and insect repellent.
- **Other uses** The anti-inflammatory action of wormwood makes it useful for infections and it has occasionally been given as an antidepressant.

SELF-HELP USES

- **Anemia**, p. 301.
- **High fever**, p. 311.

✿ PARTS USED

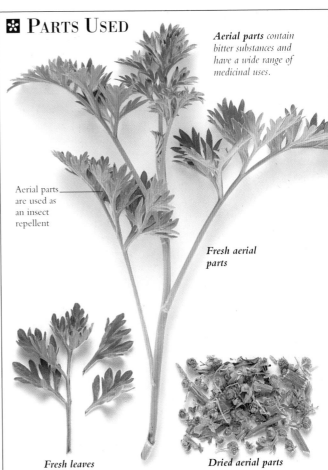

***Aerial parts** contain bitter substances and have a wide range of medicinal uses.*

Aerial parts are used as an insect repellent

Fresh aerial parts

Fresh leaves

Dried aerial parts

✍ KEY PREPARATIONS & THEIR USES

Cautions Take only under professional supervision. Take only in small doses, generally for no more than 4–5 weeks at a time. Do not take during pregnancy.

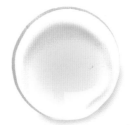

***Infusion** made from wormwood and other herbs, is used as a digestive remedy.*

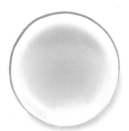

***Tincture** is used to treat digestive problems such as anemia.*

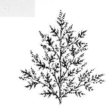

Artemisia annua (Compositae)

QING HAO, CHINESE WORMWOOD

UNTIL RECENTLY, QING HAO was regarded as just another *Artemisia*. It had one significant difference, though: its use in traditional Chinese medicine for treating malaria. Research has now vindicated this traditional use, revealing that *qing hao* prevents and cures malaria and is relatively free from side effects. Extracts of *qing hao* are currently being used in the tropics as an affordable and effective antimalarial.

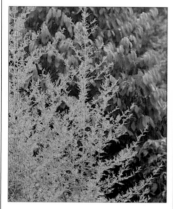

Qing hao *has bright green, saw-toothed leaves. It is used widely around the world as an effective antimalarial.*

HABITAT & CULTIVATION

Qing hao grows in grasslands and in open areas in Vietnam, Japan, China, Russia, and Korea. It is widely naturalized in the US. The herb is propagated from seed in spring or by dividing the rootstock in autumn. It is harvested in summer before the flowers bloom.

RELATED SPECIES

The related *A. apiacea* is used interchangeably with *qing hao* in China and is employed as a general tonic in Vietnam. Many other *Artemisia* species are used medicinally: *A. abrotanum* (p. 170); *A. absinthium* (p. 63); *A. capillaris* and *A. cina* (p. 170); *A. dracunculus* and *A. vulgaris* (p. 171).

KEY CONSTITUENTS

- Volatile oil (abrotamine, beta-bourbonene)
- Sesquiterpene lactone (artemisinin)
- Vitamin A

KEY ACTIONS

- Bitter
- Reduces fever
- Antimalarial
- Antibiotic

RESEARCH

- **Chinese research** *Qing hao* was extensively researched in China, especially in Guangzhou, in the 1980s. Studies revealed that it has an antibiotic effect against many fungal skin conditions and leptospirosis (Weil's disease). In addition, the plant has a direct effect against the malaria parasite *Plasmodium*, a protozoon introduced into the body by infected mosquitoes.
- **Artemisinin** Recent research has focused on the isolated compound artemisinin, which has proved to be a dramatically effective antimalarial. Recent clinical trials in Thailand have shown artemisinin to be 90% effective and to be more successful than the standard drug, chloroquine.

TRADITIONAL & CURRENT USES

- **History** The first mention of *qing hao* was in a Chinese text of 168 BC. Traditionally, it was seen as an herb that helped "to clear and relieve summer heat."
- **Cooling properties** *Qing hao* has a cool, bitter taste and is used for conditions brought on by heat, especially with symptoms such as fever, headaches, dizziness, and a tight-chested sensation. It treats chronic fevers, night fevers, and morning chills, and is a traditional remedy for nosebleeds associated with heat.

PARTS USED

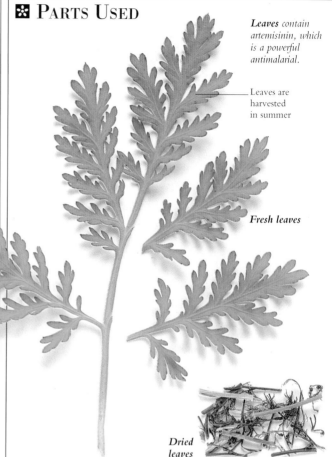

Leaves contain artemisinin, which is a powerful antimalarial.

Leaves are harvested in summer

Fresh leaves

Dried leaves

KEY PREPARATIONS & THEIR USES

Cautions Only take *qing hao* under professional supervision. Do not take during pregnancy.

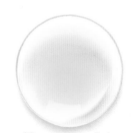

Tincture is prescribed to prevent malaria. It is also used to treat the illness itself.

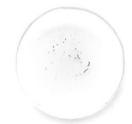

Infusion is strongly bitter. Herbalists use it to treat headaches and fever.

TABLETS containing artemisinin, which is extracted from the herb, are taken for malaria throughout the tropics.

- **Antimalarial** *Qing hao* has been used to treat the fevers and chills of malaria for thousands of years, and artemisinin is now used in many countries as an antimalarial. Artemisinin reduces the risks of developing malaria and aids a quick recovery. It is particularly helpful in treating drug-resistant strains of malaria. The whole plant may also be used to treat malaria and acts as a preventive, reducing the chances of infection.

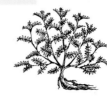

ASTRAGALUS
A perennial growing to 16 in (40 cm) with hairy stems and leaves divided into 12–18 pairs of leaflets.

Astragalus membranaceus (Leguminosae)

ASTRAGALUS, MILK VETCH, HUANG QI (CHINESE)

DESPITE THE FACT THAT astragalus is one of the most popular tonic herbs in China, it is not well known in the West. In China the root, known as *huang qi*, has been used for thousands of years. It has a sweet taste and is a warming tonic particularly suited to young, physically active people, increasing stamina and endurance, and improving resistance to the cold. It is often combined with other herbs as a blood tonic.

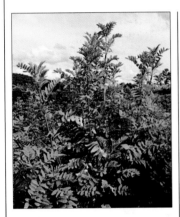

Astragalus is a typical member of the pea family and is closely related to licorice.

HABITAT & CULTIVATION

Astragalus is native to Mongolia and northern and eastern China. It is grown from seed in spring or autumn and thrives in sandy, well-drained soil, with plenty of sun. The root of 4-year-old plants is harvested in autumn.

KEY CONSTITUENTS

- Asparagine
- Calcyosin
- Formononetin
- Astragalosides
- Kumatakenin
- Sterols

KEY ACTIONS

- Adaptogenic
- Immune stimulant
- Diuretic
- Vasodilator
- Antiviral

RESEARCH

- **Chinese investigations**
Research in China indicates that astragalus is diuretic and that it lowers blood pressure and increases endurance.

- **Western research** Recent American research has focused on the ability of astragalus to restore normal immune function in cancer patients. Clinical evidence suggests that, as with a number of other herbs, cancer patients undergoing chemotherapy or radiotherapy recover faster and live longer if given astragalus concurrently.

TRADITIONAL & CURRENT USES

- **Tonic & endurance remedy** Astragalus is a classic energy tonic, perhaps even superior to ginseng (*Panax ginseng*, p. 116) for young people. In China it is believed to warm and tone the *wei qi* (a protective energy that circulates just beneath the skin), helping the body to adapt to external influences, especially to the cold. Astragalus raises immune resistance and manifestly improves physical endurance.

- **Control of fluids** Though a vasodilator (encouraging blood to flow to the surface), astragalus is used for excessive sweating, including night sweats. It is also helpful in both relieving fluid retention and reducing thirstiness. It encourages the system to function correctly.

- **Immune stimulant** Not an herb for acute illness, astragalus is nonetheless a very useful medicine for viral infections such as the common cold.

- **Other uses** Astragalus treats prolapsed organs, especially the uterus, and it is beneficial for uterine bleeding. It is often combined with Chinese angelica (*Angelica sinensis*, p. 60) as a blood tonic to treat anemia.

PARTS USED

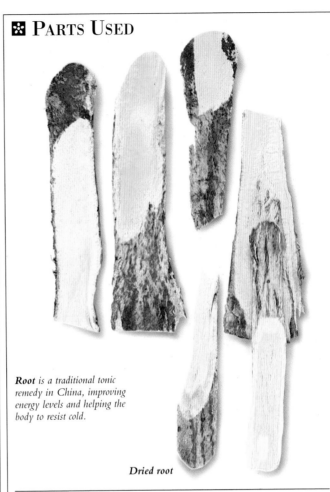

Root is a traditional tonic remedy in China, improving energy levels and helping the body to resist cold.

Dried root

KEY PREPARATIONS & THEIR USES

Caution Do not take astragalus if suffering from skin disorders.

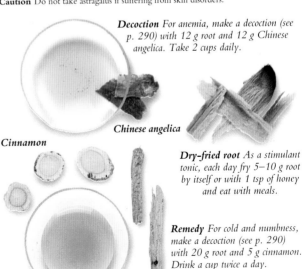

Decoction For anemia, make a decoction (see p. 290) with 12 g root and 12 g Chinese angelica. Take 2 cups daily.

Chinese angelica

Cinnamon

Dry-fried root As a stimulant tonic, each day fry 5–10 g root by itself or with 1 tsp of honey and eat with meals.

Remedy For cold and numbness, make a decoction (see p. 290) with 20 g root and 5 g cinnamon. Drink a cup twice a day.

Astragalus

TINCTURE (to make, p. 291). For night sweats, take 1 tsp with water 1–2 times daily.

Atropa belladonna (Solanaceae)
DEADLY NIGHTSHADE, BELLADONNA

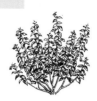

A perennial with large leaves and black berries, growing to 5 ft (1.5 m).

ALTHOUGH DEADLY NIGHTSHADE conjures up images of poison and death, like many plants it is an important and beneficial remedy when used correctly. Some of its constituents are employed in conventional medicine – for example, to dilate the pupils for eye examinations and as an anesthetic. In herbal medicine, deadly nightshade is mainly prescribed to relieve intestinal colic and to treat peptic ulcers.

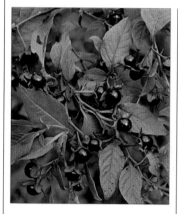

Deadly nightshade *produces unmistakable cherry-sized, glossy black berries in autumn.*

HABITAT & CULTIVATION
Deadly nightshade is native to Europe, western Asia, and northern Africa, and is now cultivated worldwide. It thrives in chalky soils, in woods, and on wasteground. The leaves are harvested in summer, and the root is collected from the first year onward in autumn.

RELATED SPECIES
Many of the *Solanaceae* family are powerful medicines, including eggplant (*Solanum melongena*, p. 268), tobacco (*Nicotiana tabacum*, p. 237), and henbane (*Hyoscyamus niger,* p. 219).

KEY CONSTITUENTS
- Tropane alkaloids (up to 0.6%), including hyoscyamine and atropine
- Flavonoids
- Coumarins
- Volatile bases (nicotine)

KEY ACTIONS
- Smooth muscle antispasmodic
- Narcotic

- Reduces sweating
- Sedative

RESEARCH
- **Tropane alkaloids** The tropane alkaloids inhibit the parasympathetic nervous system, which controls involuntary body activities. This reduces saliva; gastric, intestinal, and bronchial secretions; as well as the activity of the urinary tubules, bladder, and intestines. Tropane alkaloids also increase heart rate and dilate the pupils.

TRADITIONAL & CURRENT USES
- **Folklore** Deadly nightshade was believed to help witches to fly. Its other name "belladonna" (beautiful woman) is thought to refer to its use by Italian women to dilate the pupils of their eyes.
- **Relaxant** Deadly nightshade is prescribed to relax distended organs, especially the stomach and intestines, relieving intestinal colic and pain. It helps peptic ulcers, and it relaxes spasms of the urinary tubules.
- **Parkinson's disease** The herb can be used to treat the symptoms of Parkinson's disease, reducing tremors and rigidity, and improving speech and mobility.
- **Anesthetic** The smooth muscle relaxant properties of deadly nightshade make it useful in conventional medicine as an anesthetic, particularly when digestive or bronchial secretions need to be kept to a minimum.
- **Caution** The therapeutic dose of the plant is very close to the toxic amount. Excessive dosage can result in respiratory paralysis, coma, and death.

PARTS USED

Leaves are harvested in early summer. They have a weaker action than the root and are more commonly used.

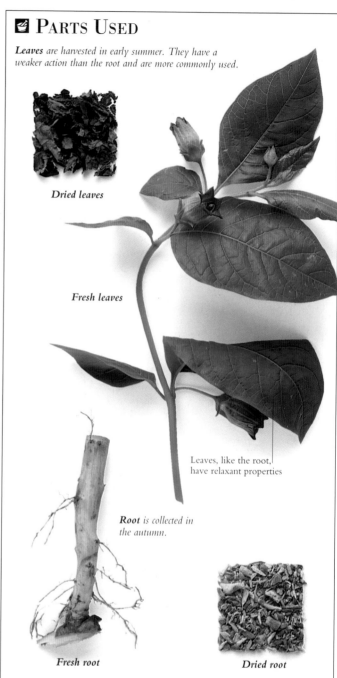

Dried leaves

Fresh leaves

Leaves, like the root, have relaxant properties

Root *is collected in the autumn.*

Fresh root

Dried root

KEY PREPARATIONS & THEIR USES

Caution Take only if prescribed by a medical herbalist or doctor. Deadly nightshade can be fatal if taken in the wrong dosage.

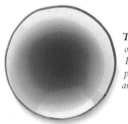

Tincture, made from the leaves or the root, is a strong relaxant. It is prescribed by herbal practitioners to relieve colic and to treat Parkinson's disease.

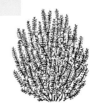

BUCHU
A bushy shrub growing to 6 ft (2 m), with stemless, slightly leathery leaves dotted with oil glands.

Barosma betulina (Rutaceae)

BUCHU

A TRADITIONAL SOUTH AFRICAN remedy, buchu is taken as a stimulant, a diuretic, and to relieve digestive complaints. In Western herbal medicine, it is valued as a urinary antiseptic and diuretic, and is used specifically to treat cystitis and other infections of the urinary tract. Buchu has a strongly distinctive aroma and taste, reminiscent of black currant, but is described by some as a mixture between rosemary and peppermint.

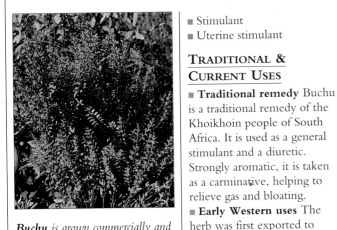

Buchu is grown commercially and used to enhance the black currant flavor of cassis.

HABITAT & CULTIVATION

Buchu is native to South Africa, where is it widely cultivated on hillsides. It is also grown in parts of South America. The herb is grown from cuttings in late summer and requires well-drained soil and plenty of sun. The leaves are harvested when the plant is flowering or fruiting in summer.

RELATED SPECIES

Two closely related species, *B. crenulata* and *B. serratifolia*, are used in a similar way to buchu but contain less volatile oil and are not as effective.

KEY CONSTITUENTS

- Volatile oil (1.5-2.5%), including pulegone, menthone, diosphenol
- Sulfur compounds
- Flavonoids (diosmin, rutin)
- Mucilage

KEY ACTIONS

- Urinary antiseptic
- Diuretic
- Stimulant
- Uterine stimulant

TRADITIONAL & CURRENT USES

- **Traditional remedy** Buchu is a traditional remedy of the Khoikhoin people of South Africa. It is used as a general stimulant and a diuretic. Strongly aromatic, it is taken as a carminative, helping to relieve gas and bloating.
- **Early Western uses** The herb was first exported to Britain in 1790 and became an official medicine in 1821, being listed in the *British Pharmacopoeia* as an effective remedy for "cystitis, urethritis, nephritis and catarrh of the bladder."
- **Modern urinary treatment** Broadly speaking, buchu is used today in Western herbal medicine for the same type of urinary complaints as in the 19th century. It is commonly prescribed for urinary tract infections, often proving effective in curing acute cystitis when combined with other herbs such as cornsilk (*Zea mays*, p. 152) and juniper (*Juniperus communis*, p. 223). Taken regularly, it can help to prevent recurrent attacks of chronic cystitis or urethritis. In addition, it is also taken for prostatitis and irritable bladder, often in combination with herbs such as uva-ursi (*Arctostaphylos uva-ursi*, p. 168) and cornsilk. The active constituent, diosphenol, has a diuretic action and may partly account for the herb's antiseptic effect on the urinary system.
- **Gynecological uses** Buchu infusion or tincture is useful in

PARTS USED

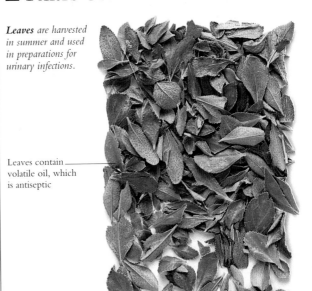

Leaves are harvested in summer and used in preparations for urinary infections.

Leaves contain volatile oil, which is antiseptic

Dried leaves

KEY PREPARATIONS & THEIR USES

Caution Do not take during pregnancy or while breast-feeding.

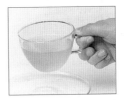

Infusion (to make, p. 290). For prostatitis, drink a cup twice a day.

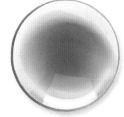

Tincture (to make, p. 291). For chronic urinary infections, take 40 drops with water 3 times a day.

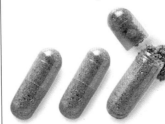

Capsules (to make, p. 291). For cystitis, take a 500 mg capsule twice daily.

treatments for cystitis and urethritis, especially when they are related to a preexisiting candida problem, such as yeast infections. The infusion is usually preferable to the tincture, particularly when the onset of infection is sudden. The infusion is also used as a douche for leucorrhea (white vaginal discharge) and occasionally for yeast infections. The herb is a

uterine stimulant and contains pulegone, which is also present in large quantities in pennyroyal (*Mentha pulegium*, p. 233). Pulegone is an abortifacient and a powerful emmanagogue (stimulates menstrual flow). Buchu should not, therefore, be taken during pregnancy.

SELF-HELP USE

- **Urinary infections**, p. 314.

BUPLEURUM CHINENSE

KEY MEDICINAL PLANTS

Bupleurum chinense syn. *B. scorzoneraefolium* (*Umbelliferae*)

BUPLEURUM, HARE'S EAR ROOT, CHAI HU (CHINESE)

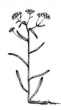

BUPLEURUM
A perennial growing up to 3 ft (1 m) high, with sickle-shaped leaves and clusters of small yellow flowers.

FIRST MENTIONED IN TEXTS from the 1st century BC, bupleurum is one of China's "harmony" herbs, balancing different organs and energies within the body. It is used as a tonic, strengthening the action of the digestive tract, improving liver function, and helping to push blood to the surface of the body. Recent research in Japan has confirmed tradititional use, showing that bupleurum protects the liver.

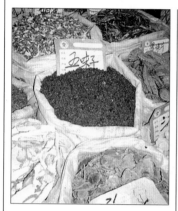

***Bupleurum** is commonly on sale in medicinal herb shops in China. It is widely taken as a liver tonic.*

HABITAT & CULTIVATION

Bupleurum grows in China and is cultivated throughout the central and eastern parts of that country. It is also found in other parts of Asia and in Europe. Bupleurum is propagated from seed in spring or by root division in autumn and requires well-drained soil and plenty of sun. The root is unearthed in spring and autumn.

KEY CONSTITUENTS

■ Bupleurumol
■ Triterpenoid saponins – saikosides (saikosaponins)
■ Flavonoids (rutin)

KEY ACTIONS

■ Protects liver
■ Anti-inflammatory
■ Tonic
■ Antiviral

RESEARCH

■ **Saikosides** Research in Japan from the 1960s onward into the *Bupleurum* genus has revealed that the saikosides are potent

medicines. They appear to protect the liver from toxicity and strengthen liver function, even in people suffering from immune system disorders. Following this discovery, clinical trials during the 1980s in Japan demonstrated that bupleurum is effective when used in the treatment of hepatitis and other chronic liver problems.
■ **Anti-inflammatory** The saikosides stimulate the body's production of corticosteroids and increase their anti-inflammatory effect.

TRADITIONAL & CURRENT USES

■ **Ancient Chinese remedy** Bupleurum has been taken in China for over 2,000 years as a liver tonic. It is traditionally believed to strengthen liver *qi* and to have a tonic action on the spleen and stomach. In Chinese medicine, bupleurum is used to treat "disharmony" between the liver and the spleen, a condition that manifests itself in problems of the digestive system such as abdominal pain, bloating, nausea, and indigestion.
■ **Liver problems** In common with milk thistle (*Carduus marianus*, p. 71) and members of the *Glycyrrhiza* genus – for example, licorice (*G. glabra*, p. 99) and *gan cao* (*G. uralensis*, p. 215) – bupleurum is an excellent remedy for a poorly functioning or weakened liver. Its anti-inflammatory action may contribute to its overall use in the treatment of liver disease.
■ **Fever** In China, bupleurum is

✠ PARTS USED

Roots *are harvested in the autumn, when they contain the most nutrients. They are a Chinese tonic, valuable for the liver.*

Sliced dried root

☑ KEY PREPARATIONS & THEIR USES

Caution Do not exceed the dose. Can occasionally cause nausea or vomiting.

Bupleurum

Licorice

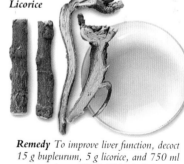

Decoction *(to make, p. 291). To stimulate sweating, thus reducing fever, drink a cup 3 times a day.*

Remedy *To improve liver function, decoct 15 g bupleurum, 5 g licorice, and 750 ml water. (see p. 290). Take in 3 doses during a 24-hour period.*

taken to reduce fever, especially in instances when it is accompanied by a bitter taste in the mouth, irritability, and either vomiting and abdominal pain, or dizziness and vertigo.
■ **Modern Japanese remedy** The traditional uses of bupleurum and scientific research accord so well that

many Japanese doctors practicing conventional Western medicine now use extracts of bupleurum root to treat patients with liver problems.
■ **Other uses** Bupleurum is sometimes useful in the treatment of hemorrhoids and of prolapsed tissue in the pelvis, such as a prolapse of the uterus.

68

Calendula officinalis (Compositae)
CALENDULA, POT MARIGOLD

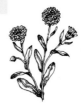

CALENDULA
An annual growing to 2 ft (60 cm), with vivid orange flower heads similar in structure to daisies.

CALENDULA IS ONE OF THE MOST well known and versatile herbs in Western herbal medicine. The bright orange petals are an excellent remedy for red and inflamed skin, their antiseptic and healing properties helping to prevent the spread of infection and speed up the rate of repair. Calendula is also a cleansing and detoxifying herb, and the infusion and tincture are used to treat chronic infections.

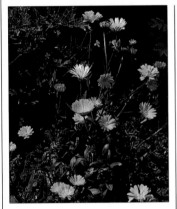

Calendula's colorful flowers were thought to lift the spirits and encourage cheerfulness.

HABITAT & CULTIVATION
Calendula, native to southern Europe, is cultivated in temperate regions around the world. Easily propagated from seed, it flourishes in almost all soils. The flowers are harvested as they open in early summer and are dried in the shade.

RELATED SPECIES
C. arvense, a wild species, seems to have similar therapeutic properties to calendula.

KEY CONSTITUENTS
- Triterpenes
- Resins
- Bitter glycosides
- Volatile oil
- Sterols
- Flavonoids
- Mucilage
- Carotones

KEY ACTIONS
- Anti-inflammatory
- Relieves muscle spasms
- Astringent
- Prevents hemorrhaging

- Heals wounds
- Antiseptic
- Detoxifying
- Mildly estrogenic

TRADITIONAL & CURRENT USES

Therapeutic properties Calendula is antiseptic. Some constituents are antifungal (particularly the resins), antibacterial, and antiviral. The herb also astringes the capillaries, an action that explains its effectiveness for cuts, wounds, varicose veins, and various inflammatory conditions.

Skin remedy Calendula is above all a remedy for the skin, providing effective treatment for most minor skin problems. It is used for cuts, scrapes, and wounds; for red and inflamed skin, including minor burns and sunburn; for acne and many rashes; and for fungal conditions such as ringworm, athlete's foot, and thrush. It is very helpful for diaper rash and cradle cap, and soothes nipples that are sore from breast-feeding.

Digestive disorders Taken internally, calendula infusion or tincture helps inflammatory problems of the digestive system such as gastritis, peptic ulcers, regional ileitis, and colitis.

Detoxifying Calendula has long been considered a detoxifying herb, and helps to treat the toxicity that underlies many fevers and infections, and systemic skin disorders, such as eczema and acne. The herb is also considered cleansing for the liver and gallbladder and can be used to treat problems affecting these organs.

PARTS USED

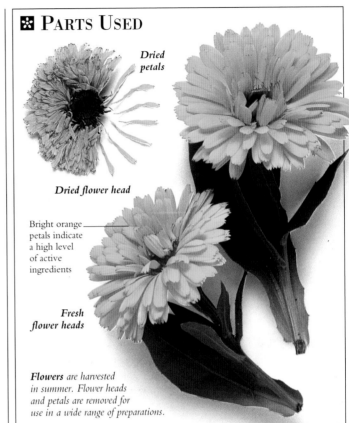

Dried petals

Dried flower head

Bright orange petals indicate a high level of active ingredients

Fresh flower heads

Flowers are harvested in summer. Flower heads and petals are removed for use in a wide range of preparations.

KEY PREPARATIONS & THEIR USES

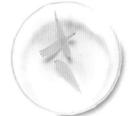

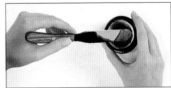

Cream is easy to make (see p. 295). Apply to cuts and scrapes.

Infusion (to make, p. 290). For chronic fungal infections, such as ringworm or oral thrush, drink 1 cup 3 times a day.

Ointment (to make, p. 294). For minor burns, apply up to 3 times a day.

INFUSED OIL (to make, p. 293). For inflamed dry skin, rub into the area 2–3 times a day.

TINCTURE (to make, p. 291). For eczema, take 30 drops with water 3 times a day.

Gynecological uses
Calendula has a mild estrogenic action and is often used to help reduce menstrual pain and regulate menstrual bleeding. The infusion makes an effective douche for yeast infections.

SELF-HELP USES
- **Acne & boils**, p. 305.

Capsicum frutescens (Solanaceae)
CAYENNE, CHILI

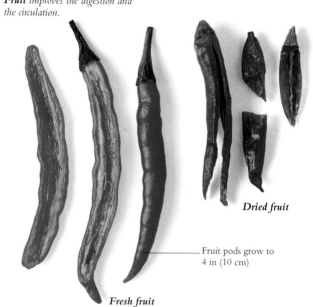

CAYENNE
A perennial, spiky shrub growing to 3 ft (1 m), with scarlet-red conical fruits filled with white seeds.

ORIGINALLY FROM THE TROPICAL regions of the Americas, cayenne was first introduced to the West in the 16th century. In cookery, it is renowned for its hot, burning taste, and it is not surprising to learn that, medicinally, it is a powerful warming stimulant. It acts on the circulation and the digestion, and is used to treat a wide range of complaints from arthritis and chilblains to colic and diarrhea.

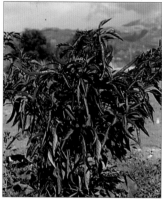

Cayenne is so popular in Mexico where it originated that it is even used to flavor ice cream.

HABITAT & CULTIVATION

Cayenne is native to the tropical Americas and is now cultivated throughout the tropics, especially in Africa and India. It is grown from seed in early spring and flourishes in hot, moist conditions. The fruit is harvested when ripe in summer and is dried in the shade.

RELATED SPECIES

Many closely related species and varieties of *C. frutescens* exist, all with different grades of pungency. Paprika, or Hungarian pepper (one of the mildest peppers), and the large green and red peppers that are eaten as vegetables are both varieties of *C. annuum* and are important medicinal foods.

KEY CONSTITUENTS

- Capsaicin (0.1–1.5%)
- Carotenoids
- Flavonoids
- Volatile oil
- Steroidal saponins (capsicidins – in seeds only)

KEY ACTIONS

- Stimulant
- Tonic
- Carminative
- Relieves muscle spasms
- Antiseptic
- Increases sweating
- Increases blood flow to the skin
- Analgesic

TRADITIONAL & CURRENT USES

- **Active constituents** Capsaicin is known to be the constituent responsible for stimulating the circulation and altering temperature regulation. Applied to the skin, capsaicin desensitizes nerve endings and it has been used in the past as a local analgesic. The capsicidins, found in the seeds, are thought to have antibiotic properties.
- **Warming stimulant** The herb's heating qualities make it a valuable remedy for poor circulation and related conditions. In particular, it improves blood flow to the hands and feet and to the central organs.
- **External uses** Applied locally to the skin, cayenne is mildly analgesic. It is also rubefacient, increasing blood flow to the affected part, and this helps to stimulate the circulation in "cold" rheumatic and arthritic conditions, aiding the removal of waste products and increasing the flow of nutrients to the tissues. Cayenne is also applied to unbroken chilblains, and powder placed inside the socks is a traditional remedy for those prone to permanently cold feet.
- **Internal uses** Cayenne is taken to relieve gas and colic, and to stimulate secretion of the digestive juices, thereby aiding digestion. It helps to prevent infections from establishing themselves in the digestive system and will counter infection if present. A pinch of cayenne is excellent in gargles for sore throats. Finally, extraordinary as it may seem, cayenne is useful for some types of diarrhea.

❖ PARTS USED

Fruit improves the digestion and the circulation.

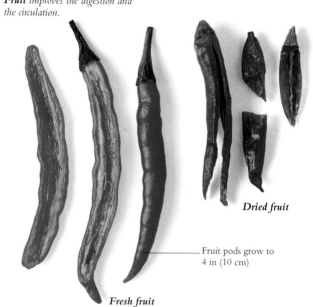

Dried fruit

Fruit pods grow to 4 in (10 cm)

Fresh fruit

🖐 KEY PREPARATIONS & THEIR USES

Cautions Do not exceed the stated dose. Do not take the seeds on their own. Do not take if suffering from peptic ulceration or acid indigestion. Do not take medicinal doses in pregnancy or if breast-feeding. Avoid touching the eyes or cuts after handling cayenne.

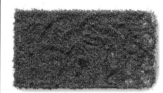

Powder For sore throats, add a pinch to 25 ml lemon juice. Dilute with hot water, add honey, and use as a gargle.

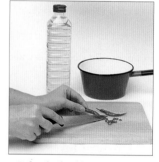

Infused oil Add 100 g chopped cayenne to 500 ml oil and simmer (see p. 293). Gently massage into rheumatic limbs.

Tincture (to make, p. 291). For arthritis, combine 20 drops with 100 ml of willow bark tincture. Take 1 tsp with water twice a day.

⊘ **TABLETS** are convenient for long-term use. Take for poor circulation.
☁ **OINTMENT** (to make, p. 294). Apply to chilblains (only if the skin is unbroken).

SELF-HELP USES

- **High fever**, p. 311
- **Poor circulation**, p. 302.

Carduus marianus syn. *Silybum marianum* (Compositae)

MILK THISTLE, MARY THISTLE

MILK THISTLE
A spiny biennial
growing to 5 ft
(1.5 m), with white-
veined leaves and
purple flower heads.

MILK THISTLE HAS BEEN USED in Europe as a remedy
for depression and liver problems for hundreds, if not
thousands, of years. Recent research has confirmed
traditional herbal knowledge, proving that the herb
has a remarkable ability to protect the liver from
damage resulting from alcoholic and other types of
poisoning. Today, milk thistle is widely used in the
West for treating a range of liver conditions.

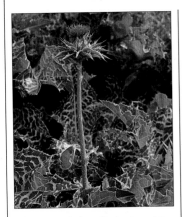

*Milk thistle has distinctive white
markings on its leaves caused,
according to tradition, by the
Virgin Mary's milk.*

HABITAT & CULTIVATION

Native to the Mediterranean,
milk thistle grows wild
throughout Europe and is widely
naturalized in California and
Australia. It thrives in open areas.
Also cultivated as an ornamental
plant, it prefers a sunny position
and self-seeds readily. The
flower heads are picked in full
bloom in early summer. Seeds
are collected in late summer.

OTHER SPECIES

There are other herbs with a less
effective though beneficial effect
on the liver, such as holy thistle
(*Cnicus benedictus*, p. 196). Other
herbs, including globe artichoke
(*Cynara scolymus*, p. 196),
protect liver function against
toxins but they are not as
effective as milk thistle.

KEY CONSTITUENTS

- Flavonlignans (1–4%)
  (silymarin)
- Bitter principles
- Polyacetylenes

KEY ACTIONS

- Protects the liver
- Stimulates secretion of bile
- Increases breast-milk production
- Antidepressant

RESEARCH

- **Silymarin** German research
from the 1970s onward has
focused on silymarin, a substance
contained in the seeds. This
exerts a highly protective effect
on the liver, maintaining its
function and preventing damage
from compounds that are
normally highly toxic. It has
been shown that severe liver
breakdown, resulting from
ingesting carbon tetrachloride
or death cap mushrooms, may
be prevented if silymarin is taken
immediately before, or within
48 hours. In Germany, silymarin
has been used successfully to
treat hepatitis and liver cirrhosis.

TRADITIONAL & CURRENT USES

- **Traditional uses** Milk thistle
flower heads, boiled and eaten
like artichokes, were useful as
a spring tonic after the winter
months when people had been
deprived of fresh vegetables.
They were also taken to increase
breast-milk production, and
were considered excellent for
melancholia (depression), which
was traditionally associated with
the liver. Gerard stated in his
Herball of 1597, "My opinion is
that this [milk thistle] is the best
remedy that grows against all
melancholy diseases."
- **Liver disorders** Today, milk
thistle is the main remedy used
in Western herbal medicine to
protect the liver and its many

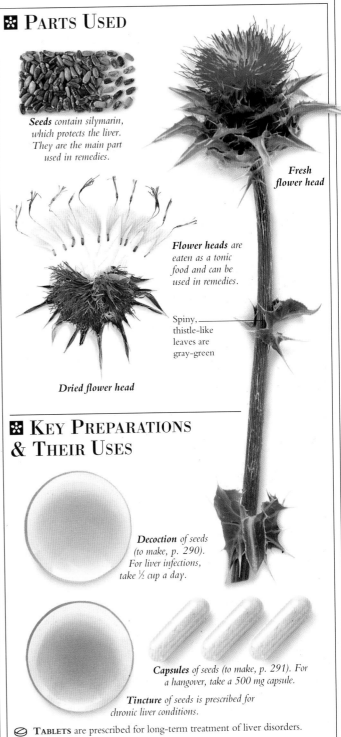

☸ PARTS USED

*Seeds contain silymarin,
which protects the liver.
They are the main part
used in remedies.*

*Fresh
flower head*

*Flower heads are
eaten as a tonic
food and can be
used in remedies.*

*Spiny,
thistle-like
leaves are
gray-green*

Dried flower head

☸ KEY PREPARATIONS & THEIR USES

*Decoction of seeds
(to make, p. 290).
For liver infections,
take ½ cup a day.*

*Capsules of seeds (to make, p. 291). For
a hangover, take a 500 mg capsule.*

*Tincture of seeds is prescribed for
chronic liver conditions.*

◎ **TABLETS** are prescribed for long-term treatment of liver disorders.

metabolic activities, and help
renew its cells. The herb is used
in the treatment of hepatitis and
jaundice, as well as in conditions
where the liver is under stress –
whether from infection, excess
alcohol, or from chemotherapy

prescribed to treat diseases such
as cancer. In this last instance,
milk thistle can help to limit
damage done to the liver by
chemotherapy and speed up
recovery from side effects once
the treatment is completed.

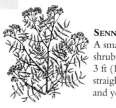

SENNA
A small perennial shrub growing to 3 ft (1 m), with a straight, woody stem and yellow flowers.

Cassia senna syn. *Senna alexandrina* (Leguminosae)
SENNA, ALEXANDRIAN SENNA

ALMOST EVERYONE WILL HAVE TAKEN a preparation containing senna at some time in their lives. Senna is probably one of the best-known herbal medicines, not least because it is still widely used in conventional medicine. It is a very efficient laxative and is a particularly useful remedy for the occasional bout of constipation. It has a slightly bitter, nauseating taste, and is therefore generally mixed with other herbs.

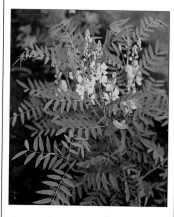

Senna shrubs have pairs of lance-shaped leaflets arranged on either side of a central stem.

- Naphthalene glycosides
- Mucilage
- Flavonoids
- Volatile oil

KEY ACTIONS
- Stimulant
- Laxative
- Cathartic

RESEARCH
■ **Sennosides** Extensive research during the last 50 years has led to a clear understanding of senna's action. The sennosides irritate the lining of the large intestine, causing the muscles to contract strongly, resulting in a bowel movement about 10 hours after the dose is taken. They also stop fluid from being absorbed from the large bowel, helping to keep the stool soft.

TRADITIONAL & CURRENT USES
■ **Early records** The herb was first used medicinally by Arabian physicians in the 9th century AD.
■ **Constipation** Senna has always been specifically used for constipation. It is particularly appropriate when a soft stool is required – for example, in cases of anal fissure. Senna is a good short-term laxative but should not be taken for more than 10 days since this leads to weakening of the large bowel muscles.
■ **Cathartic** As a cathartic (very strong laxative), senna can cause griping and colic, and is therefore normally taken with aromatic, carminative herbs that relax the intestinal muscles.

SELF-HELP USE
■ **Constipation**, p. 307.

HABITAT & CULTIVATION
Senna is native to tropical Africa and is now cultivated throughout that continent. It is grown from seed in spring or from cuttings in early summer and requires plenty of sun. The leaves may be picked before, or while, the plant is in flower and the pods are collected when they are ripe in autumn.

RELATED SPECIES
There are over 400 species of *Cassia*. Tinnevelly senna (*C. angustifolia*) is grown in the Indian subcontinent and has the same therapeutic properties as *C. senna*. In Ayurvedic medicine, it is used for skin problems, jaundice, bronchitis, and anemia, as well as for constipation. *Jue ming zi* (*C. obtusifolia*) is used in traditional Chinese medicine for "liver fire" patterns, and for constipation and atherosclerosis.

KEY CONSTITUENTS
■ Anthraquinone glycosides (sennosides)

☒ PARTS USED

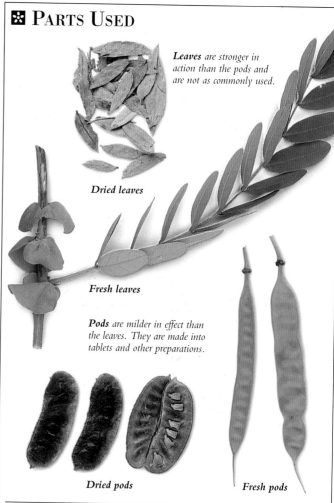

Leaves are stronger in action than the pods and are not as commonly used.

Dried leaves

Fresh leaves

Pods are milder in effect than the leaves. They are made into tablets and other preparations.

Dried pods

Fresh pods

☒ KEY PREPARATIONS & THEIR USES

Cautions Do not give to children under 12. Do not take for more than 10 days at a time. Do not take if suffering from colitis. Do not take during pregnancy.

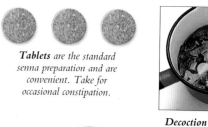

Tablets are the standard senna preparation and are convenient. Take for occasional constipation.

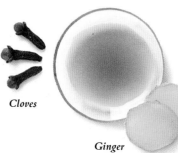

Cloves

Ginger

Decoction For constipation, steep 3–6 senna pods and 1 g fresh ginger in 1 cup freshly boiled water for 6–12 hours. Strain and drink.

Infusion For mild constipation, infuse 1–2 senna pods, 1 g fresh ginger, and 1–2 cloves in 1 cup freshly boiled water for 15 minutes. Strain and drink.

TINCTURE is prescribed by herbalists to treat short-term constipation.

Caulophyllum thalictroides (Berberidaceae)

BLUE COHOSH, SQUAW ROOT, PAPOOSE ROOT

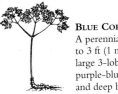

BLUE COHOSH
A perennial growing
to 3 ft (1 m), with
large 3-lobed leaves,
purple-blue flowers,
and deep blue berries.

BLUE COHOSH IS A traditional Native American herb,
still found growing in the woods of eastern North
America. It was used extensively by various tribes to
facilitate childbirth – hence its common name "squaw
root." Blue cohosh is still considered to be a woman's
herb and is currently mainly used in Western herbal
medicine to treat a range of gynecological conditions,
although it is also useful for arthritis.

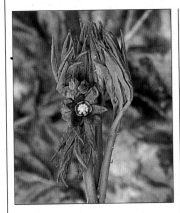

*Blue cohosh has a striking
appearance. It has 3 purple-blue
stems that divide into leaves at the
top, surrounding a single flower.*

HABITAT & CULTIVATION
Blue cohosh grows wild in
much of eastern North America,
from Manitoba to Alabama, and
prefers woodland valleys, north-
facing slopes, and damp banks.
It is mainly gathered from the
wild, but it can be cultivated, in
which case it is propagated from
seed sown when ripe or by root
division in autumn. The root and
rhizome are harvested in autumn.

RELATED SPECIES
C. robustum, a related Russian
species, is thought to have
similar properties. It is known
to have fungicidal constituents.

KEY CONSTITUENTS
- Alkaloids (caulophylline,
  laburnine, magnoflorine)
- Steroidal saponins
  (caulosapogenin)
- Resin

KEY ACTIONS
- Antispasmodic
- Diuretic

- Promotes menstrual flow
- Uterine tonic
- Antirheumatic
- Increases sweating
- Anti-inflammatory

RESEARCH
- **Steroidal saponins** A poorly
researched plant, blue cohosh
deserves further investigation. Its
consistent reputation as an herb
for facilitating childbirth and for
gynecological conditions maybe
due in part to the steroidal
saponins, which are known
to stimulate the uterus.

TRADITIONAL & CURRENT USES
- **Traditional woman's herb**
"Cohosh" is an Algonquin
name, and blue cohosh was
a popular medicinal herb with
a large number of Native
American tribes. It was primarily
considered a "woman's herb"
helping to improve contractions
during labor, rectify delayed or
irregular menstruation, and
alleviate heavy bleeding and
pain during menstruation.
- **Other traditional uses**
The root was taken by Native
Americans as a contraceptive
and was used by both sexes to
treat genitourinary conditions.
- **Modern remedy** The
European settlers in North
America learned of blue
cohosh's value from Native
peoples, and the herb was
included in the *Pharmacopoeia
of the United States* until 1905.
Current medicinal uses of
blue cohosh are not radically
different from its traditional
uses. It is still considered an
herb that is particularly suited

⬛ PARTS USED

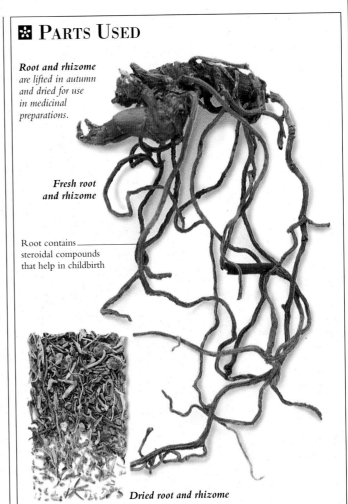

Root and rhizome
are lifted in autumn
and dried for use
in medicinal
preparations.

*Fresh root
and rhizome*

Root contains
steroidal compounds
that help in childbirth

Dried root and rhizome

☛ KEY PREPARATIONS & THEIR USES

Cautions Take only under professional supervision. Do not take during pregnancy. The
plant can cause contact dermatitis.

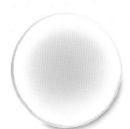

*Decoction is prescribed
by herbalists to relieve
menstrual pain and
to treat arthritis.*

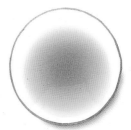

*Tincture is given during
labor to relieve the pain
of childbirth and to
speed delivery.*

to women and is chiefly
employed as a uterine tonic,
bringing relief from uterine
and ovarian pain and helping
to improve menstrual blood
flow. It should not be taken
during pregnancy since it is

a uterine stimulant, but
it is useful during labor.
- **Anti-inflammatory** Blue
cohosh can reduce inflammation,
and is sometimes used in
treatments for arthritic and
rheumatic conditions.

Centella asiatica syn. *Hydrocotyle asiatica* (Umbelliferae)

GOTU KOLA (HINDI), INDIAN PENNYWORT

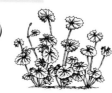

GOTU KOLA
A perennial, herbaceous creeper growing to 20 in (50 cm), with fan-shaped leaves.

GOTU KOLA IS AN ANCIENT Ayurvedic remedy that is now used extensively in the West. It is a useful tonic and cleansing herb for skin problems and digestive disorders. In India, it is used to treat a variety of conditions, including leprosy, but it is valued chiefly as a revitalizing herb that strengthens nervous function and memory. It has a bittersweet, acrid taste, and in India it is sometimes used in salads and as a vegetable.

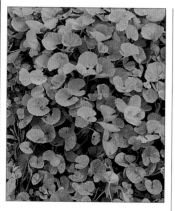

***Gotu kola** is found growing wild throughout India.*

HABITAT & CULTIVATION

Gotu kola is native to India and the southern US. It also grows in tropical and subtropical parts of Australia, southern Africa, and South America. It prefers marshy areas and riverbanks. Although usually gathered wild, gotu kola can be cultivated from seed in spring. The aerial parts are harvested throughout the year.

RELATED SPECIES

Marsh pennywort (*Hydrocotyle vulgaris*) is a related European species, but, unlike gotu kola, it does not have any known therapeutic uses.

KEY CONSTITUENTS

- Triterpenoid saponins (asiaticocide, brahmoside, thankuniside)
- Alkaloids (hydrocotyline)
- Bitter principles (vellarin)

KEY ACTIONS

- Tonic
- Antirheumatic
- Mild diuretic
- Sedative
- Peripheral vasodilator

RESEARCH

- **Fertility** Research in the mid-1990s suggests that asiaticocide and thankuniside may reduce fertility, a finding that contrasts with one of the herb's traditional uses – in India it is taken to improve fertility.
- **Other research** Gotu kola is known to thin the blood, and, in large dosages, it helps to lower blood sugar levels.

TRADITIONAL & CURRENT USES

- **Leprosy & skin disorders** Gotu kola has been used for thousands of years in India and still has a central place in Ayurvedic medicine. It is used specifically to treat leprosy, skin ulcers, and other skin problems.
- **Tonic herb** The herb has a longstanding reputation in India as a "rejuvenator," helping concentration and memory. It is also taken for fertility and as a tonic for poor digestion and rheumatism.
- **Other Indian uses** Fresh leaves are given to children for dysentery. The plant is also thought helpful for fevers, abdominal disorders, asthma, and bronchitis. An oil extract is used to promote hair growth.
- **Western uses** Despite its reputation as a tonic herb, Gotu kola is used mainly for skin problems and wounds. It is now also considered to have an anti-inflammatory effect and is given for rheumatism, rheumatoid arthritis, and poor venous circulation.

SELF-HELP USE

- **Eczema**, p. 300.

❖ PARTS USED

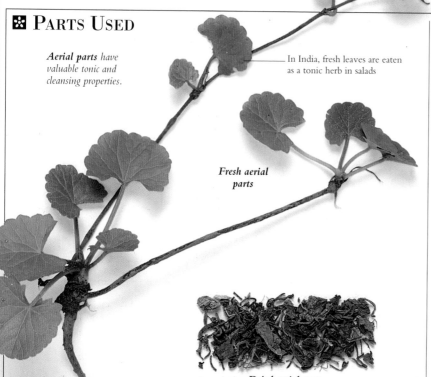

***Aerial parts** have valuable tonic and cleansing properties.*

In India, fresh leaves are eaten as a tonic herb in salads

Fresh aerial parts

Dried aerial parts

🥣 KEY PREPARATIONS & THEIR USES

Cautions Can occasionally cause sensitivity to sunlight. Restricted herb in some countries.

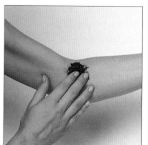

***Powder** is an important Ayurvedic remedy. Take 1–2 g a day with water as a general tonic.*

***Paste** made from powder. Mix 2 tsp powder with 25 ml water and apply to patches of eczema.*

***Infusion** (to make, p. 290). For rheumatism, take 35 ml twice a day.*

➤ **TINCTURE** (to make, p. 291). For poor memory and concentration, take 30 drops with water 3 times a day.

Chamaelirium luteum syn. *Helonias dioica* (Liliaceae)

HELONIAS, FALSE UNICORN ROOT, BLAZING STAR

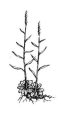

HELONIAS
An herbaceous perennial growing to 3 ft (1 m), with long green leaves and green-white flowers.

A NATIVE NORTH AMERICAN plant, helonias is used specifically for female reproductive disorders, and it has a central place in American and British herbal medicine. It is a valuable remedy for menstrual problems and ovarian cysts, and can also be very beneficial during menopause. The herb also helps to treat digestive problems. Despite its therapeutic usefulness, helonias has been poorly investigated.

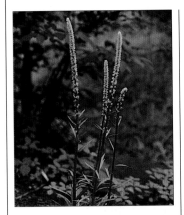

Helonias is called "fairywand" in some countries because of the appearance of its flowers.

HABITAT & CULTIVATION

Native to North America, helonias grows in low, moist, well-drained ground east of the Mississippi River. It is generally harvested from the wild and is rarely cultivated. It can, however, be propagated from seed that is sown in autumn. Helonias flowers in early summer and the root is dug up in autumn.

KEY CONSTITUENTS

- Steroidal saponins (up to 9%)
- Glycosides (chamaelirin, helonin)

KEY ACTIONS

- Uterine & ovarian tonic
- Promotes menstrual flow
- Diuretic

RESEARCH

- **Lack of investigation** The experience of Western herbalists shows helonias to be a valuable medicine for menstrual and uterine problems. The presence of steroidal saponins, which stimulate the uterus, indicates

that claims for helonias's helping gynecological problems could well be substantiated. However, virtually no research has taken place. One can only wonder why herbs such as ginseng (*Panax ginseng*, p. 116), which also contain steroidal saponins, have been extensively researched and helonias has not. Could it be because the former mainly affect the male rather than the female reproductive system? Helonias is an herb that urgently needs to be researched.

TRADITIONAL & CURRENT USES

- **Traditional remedy** Helonias is a traditional Native North American remedy. There is some confusion about its use since a number of other herbs have shared the same name or had similar names. It is thought that helonias was used by Native Americans mainly as a woman's herb, but it may also have been the remedy taken by the Arkansas people for wounds and ulcers. The root was listed as a uterine tonic and a diuretic in the *US National Formulary* from 1916 to 1947.
- **Modern gynecological herb** Today, helonias is valued by Western medical herbalists as a key remedy for conditions affecting the uterus and the ovaries. It seems to have a "normalizing" effect on the female reproductive system, encouraging a regular menstrual cycle, and it is given to women with irregular or absent periods. Helonias also encourages the ovaries to release their hormones at the right point in the month.

PARTS USED

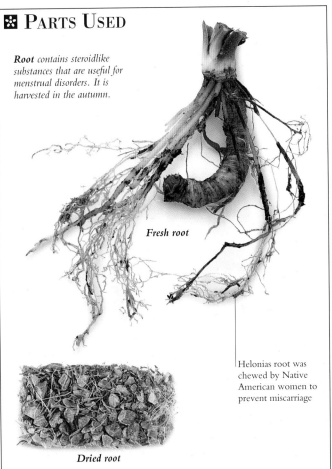

Root contains steroidlike substances that are useful for menstrual disorders. It is harvested in the autumn.

Fresh root

Helonias root was chewed by Native American women to prevent miscarriage

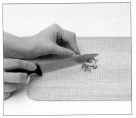

Dried root

KEY PREPARATIONS & THEIR USES

Caution Do not exceed the dose or take during pregnancy.

Chopping root for decoction (to make, p. 290). For menopausal problems, take ½ cup twice a day.

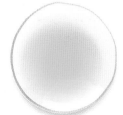

Tincture (to make, p. 291) is recommended for long-term use as a uterine tonic. Take 10 drops 3 times a day.

Tablets Take tablets, which often contain other herbs, for menopausal symptoms.

It can take some months, however, for the herb to have a significant effect on the cycle. In addition, helonias is used to treat endometriosis, uterine infections, ovarian cysts, and menopausal symptoms.

- **Additional uses** Helonias is a tonic for digestive and genitourinary conditions.

SELF-HELP USES

- **Decreased estrogen & progesterone levels**, p. 316.

75

Chamomilla recutita syn. *Matricaria recutita* (Compositae)

GERMAN CHAMOMILE

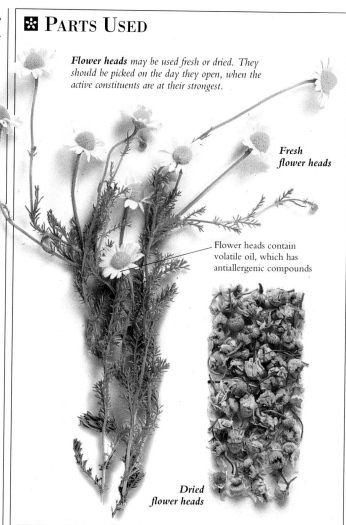

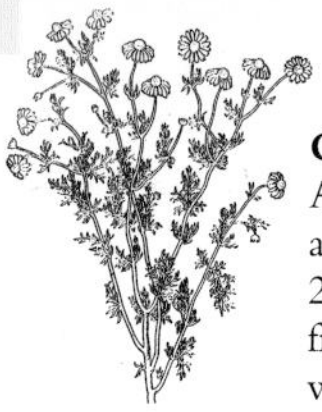

GERMAN CHAMOMILE
A sweetly aromatic annual growing to 2 ft (60 cm), with finely cut leaves and white flower heads.

GERMAN CHAMOMILE'S AROMATIC, slightly bitter taste, reminiscent of apples, is familiar to herbal tea drinkers. The herb's varied medicinal uses, however, are not as well known. It is an excellent herb for many digestive disorders and for nervous tension and irritability. Externally, it is used for sore skin and eczema. Roman chamomile (*Chamaemelum nobile*, p. 184) is a close relative, used in a similar way.

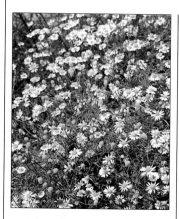

***German chamomile** is a valuable herb to cultivate for home use.*

HABITAT & CULTIVATION

German chamomile grows wild and is cultivated in much of Europe and other temperate regions. The seeds are sown in spring or autumn and the flower heads are picked in full bloom, in summer.

KEY CONSTITUENTS

- Volatile oil (proazulenes, farnesine, alpha-bisabolol, spiroether)
- Flavonoids (anthemidin, luteolin, rutin)
- Bitter glycosides (anthemic acid)
- Coumarins
- Tannins

KEY ACTIONS

- Anti-inflammatory
- Antispasmodic
- Relaxant
- Carminative
- Mild bitter
- Antiallergenic

RESEARCH

- **Trials in Germany** A cream made from German chamomile was tested in 1987 for its ability to heal wounds and produced very positive results. In 1993, a trial using German chamomile and 4 other herbs showed them to be most effective at easing infantile colic.

TRADITIONAL & CURRENT USES

- **Digestive problems** German chamomile has been taken for digestive problems since at least the 1st century AD. Gentle and efficacious, it is very suitable for children. The herb is valuable for pain, indigestion, acidity, gas, gastritis, bloating, and colic. It is also used for hiatus hernia, peptic ulcer, Crohn's disease, and irritable bowel syndrome.
- **Tension** German chamomile, which contains spiroether, a very strong antispasmodic, relaxes tense, aching muscles and eases menstrual pain. It also relieves irritability and promotes sleep, especially in children.
- **Irritation** German chamomile is useful for hay fever and asthma. The proazulenes in the herb produce chamazulene on steam distillation, which is markedly antiallergenic. Externally, it can be applied to sore, itchy skin and eczema. It also relieves eyestrain.

SELF-HELP USES

- **Bites & stings**, p. 303.
- **Colic**, p.318.
- **Congestion**, p. 312.
- **Eczema**, p. 300.
- **Indigestion**, p. 307.
- **Insomnia**, p. 309.
- **Mild asthma**, p. 301.
- **Morning sickness**, p. 317.
- **Sore & tired eyes**, p. 310.
- **Sore nipples**, p. 315.
- **Stomachache**, p. 305.

�֍ PARTS USED

***Flower heads** may be used fresh or dried. They should be picked on the day they open, when the active constituents are at their strongest.*

Fresh flower heads

Flower heads contain volatile oil, which has antiallergenic compounds

Dried flower heads

✍ KEY PREPARATIONS & THEIR USES

Cautions The fresh plant can cause dermatitis. Do not take the essential oil internally except under professional supervision. Do not use the oil externally during pregnancy.

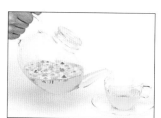

***Cream** (to make, p. 295). Rub onto sore or itchy skin.*

***Making infusion** with flower heads (see p. 290). For a good night's sleep, drink a cup last thing at night.*

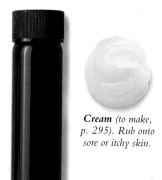

***Essential oil** For diaper rash, combine 5 drops with 20 ml carrier oil and apply.*

 INFUSION To relax fractious and overtired children, infuse 4 tsp dried herb in 500 ml water (see p. 290) and strain into a bath.

 OINTMENT (to make, p. 294). Rub onto sore or inflamed skin.

 TINCTURE (to make, p. 291). For irritable bowel syndrome, take 1 tsp diluted with 100 ml water 3 times a day.

Chrysanthemum × morifolium (Compositae)

JU HUA (CHINESE), CHRYSANTHEMUM FLOWERS

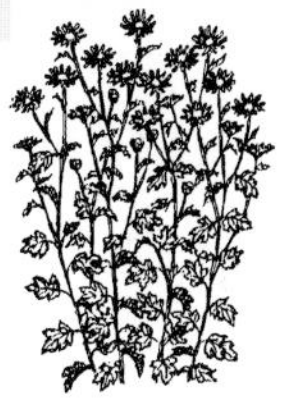

JU HUA
A perennial growing to about 5 ft (1.5 m), with flower heads composed of yellow ray florets.

JU HUA IS KNOWN in the West as florists' chrysanthemum and is valued for its ornamental qualities. In China, however, it is a popular medicinal herb and is also commonly drunk as a refreshing tisane. *Ju hua* is used to improve vision and soothe sore eyes, to relieve headaches and to counter infections such as colds and flu. Furthermore, research has demonstrated that it is a valuable remedy for high blood pressure.

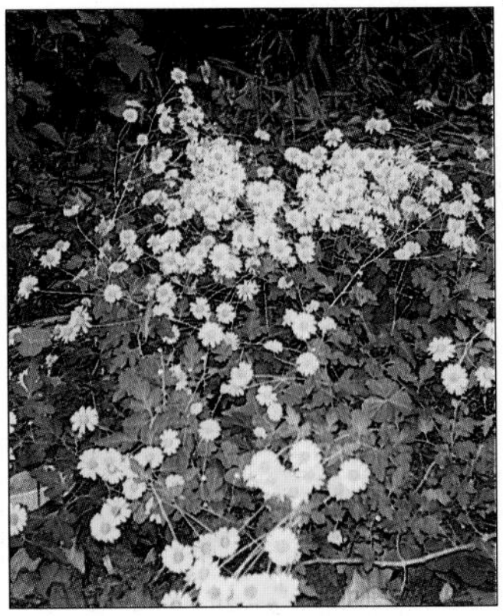

***Ju hua** flowers are colorful and have been used medicinally in China since the 1st century AD.*

HABITAT & CULTIVATION

Ju hua is native to China. Today, it is mostly cultivated, and is propagated from cuttings in spring or early summer. The flower heads are gathered in autumn when fully open. They are usually dried in the sun, which can take a long time.

RELATED SPECIES

Wild chrysanthemum, *ye hu hua* (*C. indicum*), has a similar use in Chinese herbal medicine. There are many other closely related species with an established therapeutic value, for example, tansy (*C. vulgare*) and feverfew (*Tanacetum parthenium*, p. 139).

KEY CONSTITUENTS

- Alkaloids, including stachydrine
- Volatile oil
- Sesquiterpene lactones
- Flavonoids, including apigenin
- Betaine & choline
- Vitamin B_1

KEY ACTIONS

- Increases sweating
- Antiseptic
- Lowers blood pressure
- Cooling
- Reduces fever

RESEARCH

- **Blood pressure** A number of Chinese and Japanese clinical trials during the 1970s showed that *ju hua* is most effective at lowering blood pressure and relieving associated symptoms, such as headaches, dizziness, and insomnia. In these trials, *ju hua* was mixed with *jin yin hua* (*Lonicera* spp., p. 228).
- **Other research** *Ju hua* has proved to be helpful in the treatment of angina and to have an antibiotic effect against a range of pathogens.

TRADITIONAL & CURRENT USES

- **Longstanding remedy** *Ju hua* has been taken in China as a medicine and as a beverage for thousands of years. It was first categorized in the *Divine Husbandman's Classic (Shen'nong Bencaojing)*, written in the 1st century AD.
- **Eye problems** In China, the infused flower heads are popular as a remedy for red, sore eyes, especially after long periods of close work, such as reading or working at a computer. The warm flower heads are placed on closed eyes and then replaced when cool. *Ju hua* infusion is taken as a remedy to improve the eyesight.
- **Cooling & antiseptic** *Ju hua* infusion is used to reduce fever, to counter infection, and to detoxify the body. It relieves mild fevers and tension headaches, soothes a dry mouth or throat, and treats bad breath.
- **Skin complaints** The fresh leaves make an antiseptic poultice for acne, pimples, boils, and sores.
- **High blood pressure** Symptoms often associated with high blood pressure, such as dizziness, headaches, and tinnitus, are treated with *ju hua*.
- **Convulsions** *Ju hua* is given mixed with other herbs to children suffering from convulsions.

SELF-HELP USE

- **Sore & tired eyes**, p. 310.

PARTS USED

***Flower heads** are gathered in late autumn. In China, they are steamed before drying to reduce bitterness.*

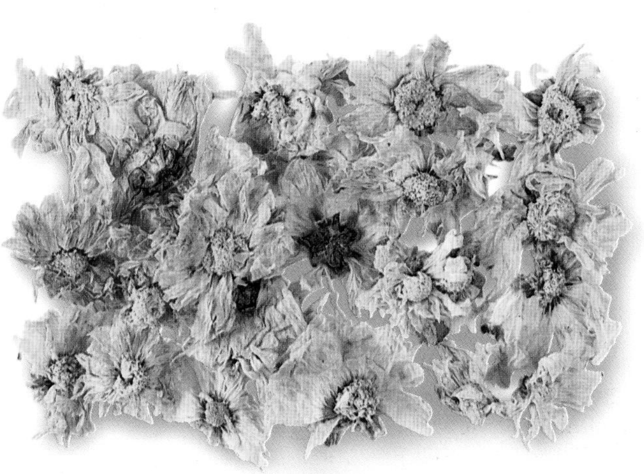

Dried flower heads

KEY PREPARATIONS & THEIR USES

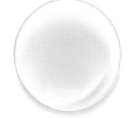

***Infusion** of flower heads (p. 290). For tension headaches, drink 1 cup at hourly intervals.*

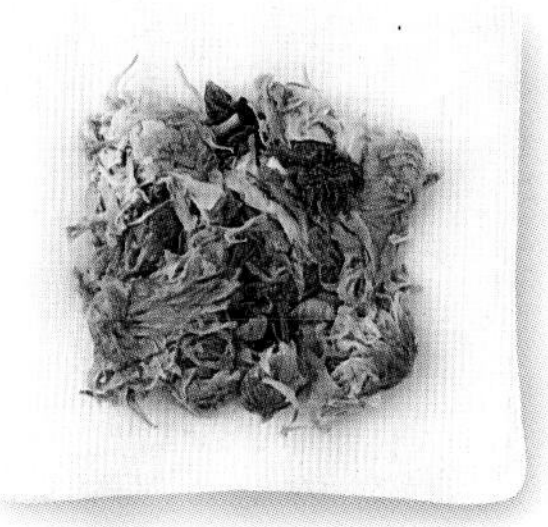

***Poultice** (to make, p. 294). For eyestrain, steep flower heads in hot water for 10 minutes and place them on closed eyes.*

***Powdered leaves** For acne, mix 1 tsp with 2–3 tsp water and apply to pimples.*

POULTICE of fresh leaves (to make, p. 294). For boils and pimples, apply directly to the skin.

KEY MEDICINAL PLANTS

Cimicifuga racemosa (Ranunculaceae)
BLACK COHOSH, BLACK SNAKEROOT, SQUAWROOT

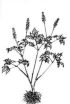

BLACK COHOSH
An herbaceous perennial growing to 8 ft (2.5 m) high, with creamy white flower spikes.

THE ROOT OF BLACK COHOSH is a Native American remedy. It has long been used for women's complaints, especially painful periods and problems associated with menopause, and was used by the Penobscot people for kidney troubles. It also benefits rheumatic problems, including rheumatoid arthritis and nerve conditions such as tinnitus (ringing in the ears). The root has a bitter, acrid taste and a disagreeable odor.

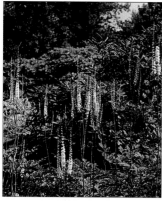

***Black cohosh** was used by Native Americans to treat gynecological problems and complaints such as rheumatism and headaches.*

HABITAT & CULTIVATION

Black cohosh is native to Canada and the eastern states of the US, growing as far south as Florida. It prefers shady spots in woods and shrubby areas. The herb is now grown in Europe and can be found in the wild, having self-seeded from cultivated plants. It is grown from seed, and the root is harvested in autumn.

RELATED SPECIES

A number of *Cimicifuga* species are used in traditional Chinese medicine, including *sheng ma* (*C. dahurica*) and *C. foetida*. They are thought to "clear heat" and relieve toxicity and are used to treat asthma, headaches, and measles, among other conditions.

KEY CONSTITUENTS

- Triterpene glycosides (actein, cimicifugoside)
- Isoflavones (formononetin)
- Isoferulic acid

- Salicylic acid
- Tannins
- Resin

KEY ACTIONS

- Promotes menstrual flow
- Antirheumatic
- Expectorant
- Sedative

RESEARCH

- **Menopause herb** Research has confirmed the validity of traditional knowledge. The results of a German trial, published in 1995, revealed that black cohosh in combination with St. John's wort (*Hypericum perforatum*, p. 104) was 78% effective at treating hot flashes and other menopausal problems.
- **Estrogenic properties** Black cohosh has a well-established estrogenic action and is thought to reduce levels of pituitary luteinizing hormone, thereby decreasing the ovaries' production of progesterone.

TRADITIONAL & CURRENT USES

- **Gynecological uses** Black cohosh has long been used by Native Americans for female problems, for which reason it was also known as "squawroot." It is used today for menstrual pain and problems where progesterone production is too high, and for menopausal symptoms, especially hot flashes, debility, and depression.
- **Inflammation** Black cohosh is useful for inflammatory arthritis, especially when it is associated with menopause, and it is also an effective remedy for rheumatic problems, including

rheumatoid arthritis.
- **Sedative properties** The sedative action of black cohosh makes it valuable for treating a variety of conditions, including high blood pressure and tinnitus (ringing in the ears). It is also

valuable for whooping cough and asthma.

SELF-HELP USES

- **Arthritis**, p. 313.
- **Decreased estrogen & progesterone levels**, p. 316.

✣ PARTS USED

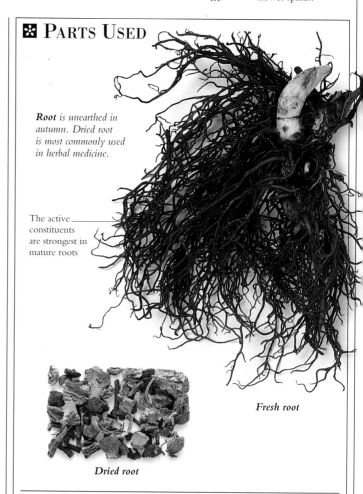

***Root** is unearthed in autumn. Dried root is most commonly used in herbal medicine.*

The active constituents are strongest in mature roots

Fresh root

Dried root

⚘ KEY PREPARATIONS & THEIR USES

Cautions Do not take in pregnancy or if breast-feeding. Restricted in some countries.

Decoction (to make, p. 290). For rheumatism, take ½ cup twice a day.

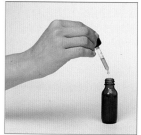

Tincture (to make, p. 291). To relieve menstrual pain, add 40 drops to 100 ml water and take 3 times a day.

◯ **TABLETS** are made from the powdered herb. Take for menopausal symptoms such as mood swings and hot flashes.

CINCHONA
An evergreen tree reaching 80 ft (25m), with reddish bark and leaves that grow to 20 in (50 cm).

Cinchona spp. *(Rubiaceae)*
CINCHONA, PERUVIAN BARK

CINCHONA IS BEST KNOWN as the source of quinine, which for centuries was the most widely taken anti-malarial remedy in the world. It was first documented in Peru by a Jesuit missionary in 1633. As well as being a remedy for malaria, the herb is also used for fevers and digestive problems. Various *Cinchona* species are used medicinally, including *C. calisaya*, *C. ledgeriana*, and *C. officinalis*.

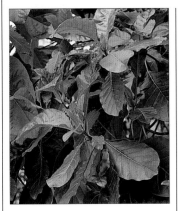

Cinchona bark has a bitter taste, and it, or its constituent quinine, is used to flavor tonic water.

HABITAT & CULTIVATION

Native to mountainous tropical regions of South America, especially Peru, cinchona is now also grown in India, Java, and parts of Africa, and is cultivated intensively on tree farms. The trees are propagated from cuttings in late spring, and the bark of the trunk, branches, and root are removed from 6- to 8-year-old trees, and then dried in the sun. The annual production of cinchona bark has been estimated at about 8,000 tons (8,200 tonnes) a year.

KEY CONSTITUENTS

- Alkaloids (up to 15%), mainly quinoline alkaloids (quinine, quinidine), and also indole alkaloids (cinchonamine)
- Bitter triterpenic glycosides (quinovin)
- Tannins
- Quinic acid

KEY ACTIONS

- Bitter
- Reduces fever

- Antimalarial
- Tonic
- Stimulates the appetite
- Antispasmodic
- Astringent
- Antibacterial

RESEARCH

- **Pharmacology** Cinchona has been thoroughly researched, and its pharmacological actions are well established.
- **Quinine** Quinine is both strongly antimalarial and antibacterial. Like the other alkaloids, it is antispasmodic.
- **Bitter** The bitter constituents in cinchona, including the alkaloids and quinovin, produce a reflex stimulation of the digestion as a whole, increasing stomach secretions.
- **Quinidine** A cardiac depressant, quinidine is known to reduce heart rate and improve irregularity of heartbeat.

TRADITIONAL & CURRENT USES

- **Traditional remedy** The indigenous people of Peru have taken cinchona for many centuries, and it is still a well-used remedy for fevers, digestive problems, and infections.
- **Antimalarial** Cinchona, and in particular quinine, were the principal remedies for malaria until World War I. From the 1960s on, resistance of the malarial parasite to the synthetic drug chloroquine led to quinine's use once again in preventing and treating malaria. Quinine is also used to treat other acute feverish conditions.
- **Digestive stimulant** As a bitter tonic, cinchona stimulates

saliva, digestive secretions, and the appetite, and improves weak digestive function.
- **Gargle** Cinchona is useful as a gargle for sore, infected throats.
- **Muscle spasms** The herb is used in herbal medicine for

✦ PARTS USED

Bark of the trunk, branches, and root contains alkaloids, especially quinine. The bark of the trunk is most commonly used medicinally.

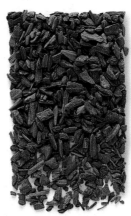

Dried bark

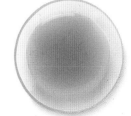

Fresh bark

⚘ KEY PREPARATIONS & THEIR USES

Cautions Take only under professional supervision. Do not take during pregnancy. Excessive use causes "cinchonism," which in extreme cases leads to coma and death. Restricted in some countries.

Powder is used to treat malaria.

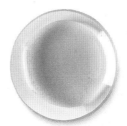

Decoction is a well-known remedy for fevers. It is also used as a gargle for sore throats.

Tincture is strongly bitter and is prescribed to improve the digestion.

cramps, especially night cramps. It also relieves arthritis.
- **Indian remedy** In India, cinchona is used to treat sciatica and dysentery, as well as problems associated with *kapha* (*see* pp. 35).

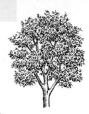

Cinnamomum verum syn. *C. zeylanicum* (Lauraceae)

CINNAMON, DALCINI (HINDI)

CINNAMON TREE
An evergreen tree, growing to 25–60 ft (8–18 m), with soft, reddish brown bark and yellow flowers.

AS WELL AS BEING ONE OF the world's most important spices, cinnamon is an ancient herbal medicine, first written about in the Jewish religious text, the Torah. Cinnamon has a long history of use in India and was first used medicinally in Egypt and parts of Europe from about 500 BC. Traditionally, the herb was taken for colds, flu, and digestive problems, and it is still used in much the same way today.

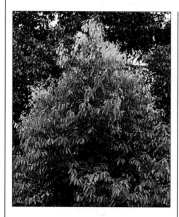

Cinnamon is now widely cultivated as a spice and a medicine, but, traditionally, only bark from wild trees was used medicinally.

HABITAT & CULTIVATION

Cinnamon is native to Sri Lanka and India, growing in tropical forests to an altitude of 1,500 ft (500 m). It is extensively cultivated throughout the tropical regions of the world, especially in the Philippines and West Indies. Cinnamon is propagated from cuttings, and every second year, during the rainy season, the young trees are cut back to just above ground level. The bark is harvested from the many stump shoots and left for 24 hours to ferment. The outer bark is then scraped away, revealing the inner bark.

RELATED SPECIES

Cassia (*rou gui* – *C. cassia*) is a very close relative with similar constituents and therapeutic properties. It is native to China and Japan, and is widely used in Chinese herbal medicine in much the same way as cinnamon. It is valued as a strong *yang* tonic (*see* p. 38).

KEY CONSTITUENTS

- Volatile oil up to 4% (cinnamaldehyde 65–75%, eugenol 4–10%)
- Tannins (condensed)
- Coumarins
- Mucilage

KEY ACTIONS

- Warming stimulant
- Carminative
- Antispasmodic
- Antiseptic
- Antiviral

RESEARCH

- **Japanese research** In the 1980s, Japanese research into the constituent cinnamaldehyde showed it to be sedative and analgesic. It is also thought to reduce blood pressure and fevers.
- **Bark extracts** Extracts of the bark have antibacterial and anti-fungal actions.

TRADITIONAL & CURRENT USES

- **Therapeutic properties** Cinnamon's medicinal value is largely due to its volatile oil, which has antiviral and stimulating properties.
- **Ancient warming remedy** In both India and Europe, cinnamon has been traditionally taken as a warming herb for "cold" conditions, often in combination with ginger (*Zingiber officinale*, p. 153). The herb stimulates the circulation, especially to the fingers and toes. Cinnamon is also a traditional remedy for digestive problems, such as nausea, vomiting, and diarrhea, as well as for aching muscles and other symptoms of viral conditions such as colds.

✵ PARTS USED

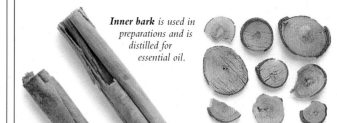

Inner bark is used in preparations and is distilled for essential oil.

Twigs of closely related C. cassia are widely used in Chinese medicine to relieve "cold" conditions.

📜 KEY PREPARATIONS & THEIR USES

Cautions Cinnamon can be toxic if taken in excess. Do not take the essential oil internally except under professional supervision. Do not take as a medicine during pregnancy.

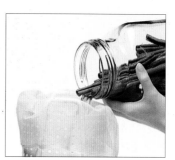

Tincture To make, infuse the herb in alcohol (see p. 291). For flatulence, take 20 drops with water up to 4 times a day.

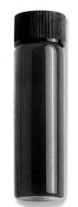

Essential oil For wasp stings, dab on oil as often as required.

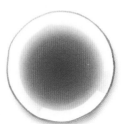

Infusion (to make p. 290) For colds and flu, drink ½ cup 2–3 times a day.

Powder is used mainly in India. For a weak digestion, take ¼ tsp 2–3 times a day with water.

- **Convalescence** Cinnamon is a supportive and strengthening herb for weak digestions. It is used specifically in the treatment of debility and in convalescence.
- **Gynecological remedy** The herb has a slight emmenagogic action – stimulating the uterus and encouraging menstrual bleeding. In India, it is taken after childbirth as a contraceptive.

SELF-HELP USE

- **Colds**, p. 311.

Citrus limon (Rutaceae)

LEMON

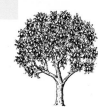

LEMON TREE
A small evergreen tree growing to about 22 ft (7 m), with light green toothed leaves.

LEMON IS ONE OF THE most important and versatile natural medicines for home use. A familiar food as well as a remedy, it has a high vitamin C content that helps to improve resistance to infection, making it effective against colds and flu. It is taken as a preventive for many conditions, including stomach infections, circulatory problems, and arteriosclerosis (thickening of the arterial walls).

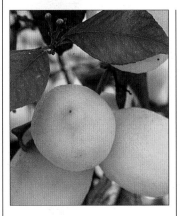

Lemons *were a remedy for scurvy (caused by lack of vitamin C) long before vitamin C was identified.*

HABITAT & CULTIVATION

Thought to be native to India, lemon trees were first grown in Europe in the 2nd century AD and are now cultivated in Mediterranean and subtropical climates worldwide. Propagated from seed in spring, they prefer well-drained soil and plenty of sun. The fruit is best harvested in winter when the vitamin C content is at its highest.

KEY CONSTITUENTS

- Volatile oil (about 2.5% of the peel), limonene (up to 70%), alpha-terpinene, alpha-pinene, beta-pinene, citral
- Coumarins
- Bioflavonoids
- Vitamins A, B_1, B_2, B_3, and C (40–50 mg per 100 g of fruit)
- Mucilage

KEY ACTIONS

- Antiseptic
- Antirheumatic
- Antibacterial
- Antioxidant
- Reduces fever

TRADITIONAL & CURRENT USES

- **Valuable medicine** Spanish popular medicine ascribes so many medicinal uses to lemon that whole books have been written about it.
- **Established properties** Despite its acid content, once digested, lemon has an alkaline effect within the body, making it useful in rheumatic conditions where acidity is a contributory factor. The volatile oil is antiseptic and antibacterial. The bioflavonoids strengthen the inner lining of blood vessels, especially veins and capillaries, and help counter varicose veins and easy bruising.
- **Preventive** Lemon is a valuable preventive medicine. Its antiseptic and cleansing actions make it valuable for those prone to arteriosclerosis, and to infections and fevers (especially of the stomach, liver, and intestines). Its ability to strengthen blood vessel walls helps to prevent circulatory disorders and bleeding gums. Lemon is also useful as a general tonic for many chronic illnesses. Above all, it is a food that helps to maintain general good health.
- **Strengthening vein walls** The whole fruit, especially the pith, treats arteriosclerosis, weak capillaries, and varicose veins.
- **Juice** Lemon juice is good for colds, flu, and chest infections. It also acts as a tonic for the liver and pancreas, improves the appetite and helps to ease stomach acidity, ulcers, arthritis, gout, and rheumatism. As a gargle, lemon juice relieves sore throats, gingivitis, and canker sores. Externally lemon juice can be applied directly to acne, athlete's foot, chilblains, stings, ringworm, sunburn, and warts.

SELF-HELP USES

- **Acne & boils**, p. 305.
- **Arthritis**, p. 313.
- **Bites & stings**, p. 303.
- **Chilblains**, p. 302.
- **Colds & flu**, p. 311.
- **Cold sores**, p. 304.
- **Sore throats**, p. 311.
- **Weak digestion**, p 306.

❖ PARTS USED

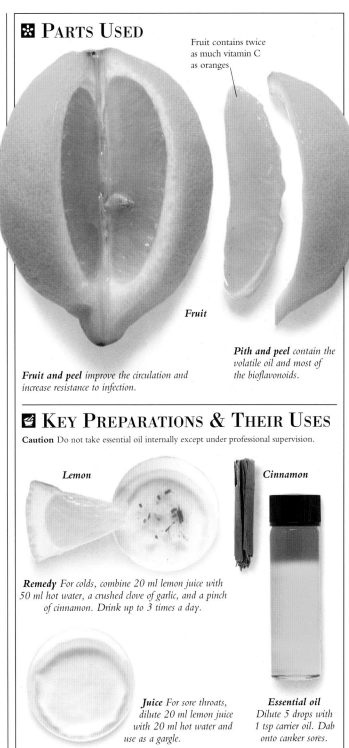

Fruit contains twice as much vitamin C as oranges

Fruit

Fruit and peel *improve the circulation and increase resistance to infection.*

Pith and peel *contain the volatile oil and most of the bioflavonoids.*

⬛ KEY PREPARATIONS & THEIR USES

Caution Do not take essential oil internally except under professional supervision.

Lemon

Cinnamon

Remedy *For colds, combine 20 ml lemon juice with 50 ml hot water, a crushed clove of garlic, and a pinch of cinnamon. Drink up to 3 times a day.*

Juice *For sore throats, dilute 20 ml lemon juice with 20 ml hot water and use as a gargle.*

Essential oil *Dilute 5 drops with 1 tsp carrier oil. Dab onto canker sores.*

Codonopsis pilosula (Campanulaceae)
CODONOPSIS, DANG SHEN (CHINESE)

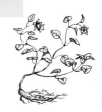

CODONOPSIS
A twining perennial growing to 5 ft (1.5 m), with oval leaves and green to purple flowers.

CODONOPSIS HAS A CENTRAL PLACE in Chinese herbal medicine as a gentle tonic that increases energy levels and helps the body adapt to stress. Research has confirmed this use. Codonopsis is thought to be similar in action to ginseng, but it is milder and has a shorter-lasting effect. It is given to those who find ginseng too strong a tonic and is used interchangeably with ginseng in Chinese herbal formulas.

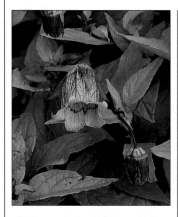

Codonopsis *bears solitary bell-shaped flowers with purple markings in summer.*

HABITAT & CULTIVATION
Codonopsis is native to northeastern China and grows throughout much of the region, especially in the Shanxi and Szechuan provinces. It is propagated from seed in spring or autumn. The root is harvested in autumn once the aerial parts have died down.

KEY CONSTITUENTS
- Triterpenoid saponins
- Sterins
- Alkaloid (perlolyrin)
- Alkenyl & alkenyl glycosides
- Polysaccharides
- Tangshenoside I

KEY ACTIONS
- Adaptogenic
- Stimulant
- Tonic

RESEARCH
- **Blood remedy** Laboratory experiments have demonstrated that codonopsis increases hemoglobin and red blood cell levels, and lowers blood pressure.

- **Stamina** Other research has confirmed the ability of codonopsis to help increase endurance to stress and to maintain alertness.

TRADITIONAL & CURRENT USES
- **Tonic herb** In Chinese herbal medicine, codonopsis is considered to tone the *qi* (vital force – *see* pp. 22–23), lungs, and spleen. It improves vitality and helps to balance metabolic function. It is a gentle tonic remedy that helps to revive the system as a whole.
- **Primary uses** Codonopsis is taken in particular for tired limbs, general fatigue, and for digestive problems such as appetite loss, vomiting, and diarrhea. It is thought to nourish the *yin* (*see* pp. 38–39) of the stomach without making it too "wet," and at the same time to tone the spleen without making it too "dry." It is beneficial in any chronic illness where "spleen *qi* deficiency" is a contributory factor.
- **False-fire** Perhaps most interestingly, codonopsis is given as a tonic to people who are stressed and have "false-fire" symptoms, including tense neck muscles, headaches, irritability, and high blood pressure, and who find the tonic action of ginseng (*Panax ginseng*, p. 116) too strong. Codonopsis is reputedly more successful in reducing levels of adrenaline, and therefore stress, than ginseng.
- **Breast-feeding tonic** The herb is taken regularly by nursing mothers in China to increase milk production and as a tonic to "build strong blood."
- **Respiratory problems** Codonopsis clears excessive mucus from the lungs and is useful for respiratory problems, including shortness of breath and asthma.

❖ PARTS USED

Root is used in cooking or dried for use in tinctures and decoctions.

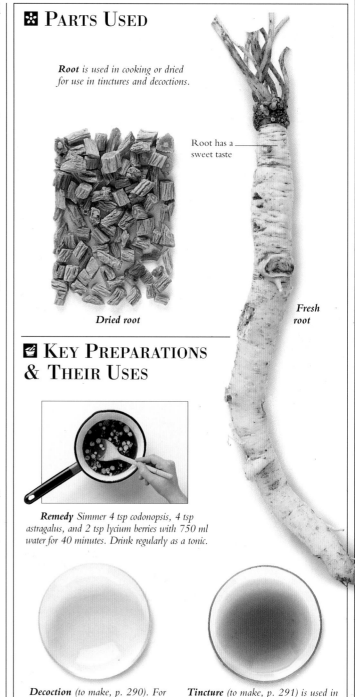

Root has a sweet taste

Dried root

Fresh root

☙ KEY PREPARATIONS & THEIR USES

Remedy *Simmer 4 tsp codonopsis, 4 tsp astragalus, and 2 tsp lycium berries with 750 ml water for 40 minutes. Drink regularly as a tonic.*

Decoction *(to make, p. 290). For fatigue, drink ½ cup twice a day.*

Tincture *(to make, p. 291) is used in the West but not in Chinese herbal medicine. As a tonic, take ½ tsp with water 3 times a day.*

SELF-HELP USES
- **Loss of appetite & vomiting**, p. 306.
- **Nervous exhaustion, muscle tension & headaches**, p. 308.
- **Stress or convalescence**, p. 319.

Coleus forskohlii syn. *Plectranthus barbatus* (Labiatae)

COLEUS

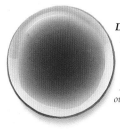

COLEUS
An aromatic perennial with tuberlike roots and an erect stem reaching 2 ft (60 cm).

NATIVE TO INDIA, COLEUS is used in Indian folk medicine rather than within the Ayurvedic tradition, and is a traditional digestive remedy. It shot to fame in Western medical circles when one of its constituents, forskolin, was first isolated in the 1970s. Research by an Indian/German company showed that forskolin was a powerful medicine for various conditions, including heart failure, glaucoma, and bronchial asthma.

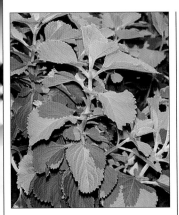

Coleus is strongly aromatic and the leaves have a distinctive camphorlike scent.

HABITAT & CULTIVATION

Native to India, coleus grows on the dry slopes of the Indian plains and in the foothills of the Himalayas. It is also found in subtropical or warm temperate areas, including Nepal, Sri Lanka, Myanmar (Burma), and parts of eastern Africa. Coleus was popular as an ornamental plant in the 19th century and today is cultivated on a large scale in Gujarat, India, for use in pickles – approximately 980 tons (1,000 tonnes) are harvested yearly. The plant is propagated by stem cuttings or root division in spring or summer. It flourishes in well-drained soil in sun or partial shade. Both root and leaves are harvested in autumn.

RELATED SPECIES

Six other species of *Coleus* have been investigated but only *C. forskohlii* contains forskolin. Indian borage (*C. amboinicus*) is used traditionally within Ayurvedic and Unani Tibb herbal medicine to help reduce inflammation and is prescribed for bronchitis and asthma.

KEY CONSTITUENTS

- Volatile oil
- Diterpenes (forskolin)

KEY ACTIONS

- Lowers blood pressure
- Antispasmodic
- Dilates the bronchioles (small airways of the lungs)
- Dilates the blood vessels
- Heart tonic

RESEARCH

- **Forskolin** The active constituent forskolin was first isolated in the 1970s. It has important therapeutic benefits, which include lowering high blood pressure, relaxing smooth muscle, increasing the release of hormones from the thyroid gland, stimulating digestive secretions, and reducing pressure within the eye.
- **Whole herb** Research into coleus has focused on the action of forskolin in isolation, and the herb as a whole has not been researched.

TRADITIONAL & CURRENT USES

- **Traditional uses** Coleus is a traditional herb in India for a wide range of digestive problems. It is given to relieve gas, bloating, and abdominal discomfort.
- **Circulatory remedy** An important heart and circulatory tonic, coleus is used to treat congestive heart failure and poor coronary blood flow. It also improves circulation of blood to the brain.
- **Respiratory problems** Its antispasmodic action makes coleus valuable for respiratory complaints, including asthma and bronchitis.
- **Glaucoma** Coleus is used topically in treatments to relieve glaucoma (excess pressure within the eye, which, if untreated, can result in loss of vision).
- **Potential use** Judging by the therapeutic effects of the constituent forskolin, coleus may be of use in combination with other herbs, such as hawthorn (*Crataegus oxyacantha*, p. 86), in helping to reduce high blood pressure.

✿ PARTS USED

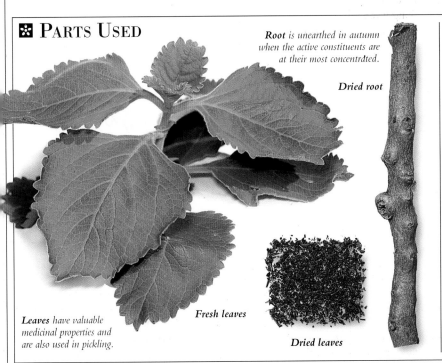

Root is unearthed in autumn when the active constituents are at their most concentrated.

Dried root

Leaves *have valuable medicinal properties and are also used in pickling.*

Fresh leaves

Dried leaves

☛ KEY PREPARATIONS & THEIR USES

Caution Do not take for circulatory problems or glaucoma without professional advice.

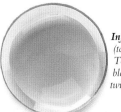

Decoction *of root. For bronchial asthma, make a decoction with 15 g root and 500 ml water (see p. 291). Drink in small doses over 2 days.*

Infusion *of leaves (to make, p. 290). To relieve gas and bloating, drink 1 cup twice a day.*

KEY MEDICINAL PLANTS

Commiphora molmol syn. *C. myrrha* (Burseraceae)

MYRRH

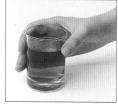

MYRRH
A spiny, deciduous tree growing to 15 ft (5 m), with yellow-red flowers and pointed fruit.

MYRRH HAS BEEN USED IN perfumes, incense, and embalming, and, as a symbol of suffering, was one of the three gifts believed to have been offered to the infant Jesus by the Magi. Myrrh is also one of the oldest known medicines and was widely used by the ancient Egyptians. It is an excellent remedy for mouth and throat problems, with a drying, slightly bitter taste, and it is also useful for skin problems.

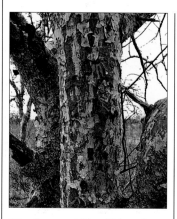

***Myrrh** trees yield a thick, yellow resin which has a distinct, aromatic odor. It is used in mouthwashes.*

HABITAT & CULTIVATION

Native to northeastern Africa, especially Somalia, myrrh is now also found in Ethiopia, Saudi Arabia, India, Iran, and Thailand. It grows in thickets and likes well-drained soil in the sun.

Myrrh is propagated from seed in spring or from cuttings at the end of the growing season. The resin is collected from cut branches and is dried for use.

RELATED SPECIES

A number of closely related *Commiphora* species are used interchangeably with myrrh. Guggulu (*C. mukul*) is known to contain phytosterols, which have a hormonal action. Myrrh and guggulu are so similar that myrrh probably also contains these constituents, which would explain myrrh's use in traditional Indian medicine for menstrual problems and as an aphrodisiac.

KEY CONSTITUENTS

- Gum (30–60%), acidic polysaccharides
- Resin (25–40%)
- Volatile oil (3–8%), including heerabolene, eugenol and many furanosesquiterpenes

KEY ACTIONS

- Stimulant
- Antiseptic
- Anti-inflammatory
- Astringent
- Expectorant
- Antispasmodic
- Carminative

TRADITIONAL & CURRENT USES

- **Therapeutic properties** The medicinal actions of myrrh have not been well researched, although its astringent, antiseptic, and antimicrobial actions have been confirmed. Myrrh is not soluble in water and is therefore normally taken in the form of a powder or a tincture, rather than as an infusion. It is not easily absorbed by the intestines and so is generally used in external treatments or gargles rather than in internal remedies.
- **Ayurvedic remedy** In Ayurvedic medicine, myrrh is considered to be tonic and aphrodisiac and to cleanse the blood. It also has a reputation for improving the intellect.

Myrrh is widely used throughout India and the Middle East for the treatment of mouth, gum, throat, and digestive problems, as well as for irregular and painful menstruation.

- **Mouth & gum remedy** Myrrh is one of the most effective herbal medicines in the world for sore throats, canker sores, and gingivitis (gum infections). The diluted tincture is used as a mouthwash and is effective as a gargle, helping to counter infection and inflammation and tighten the affected tissue.
- **External uses** Externally, myrrh's astringent and antiseptic actions make it a useful treatment for acne and boils, as well as for mild inflammatory skin problems. The herb's drying and slightly anesthetizing effect has led to its use in Germany as a treatment for pressure sores caused by prosthetic limbs.

SELF-HELP USES

- **Acne & boils**, p. 305.
- **Canker sores**, p. 306.
- **Gum problems**, p. 306.
- **Oral thrush**, p. 314.
- **Sore throats**, p. 311.

❖ PARTS USED

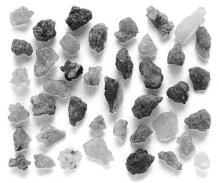

Dried gum resin

Gum resin *oozes from fissures or cuts in the bark of the tree and dries into yellow-red solid pieces.*

☘ KEY PREPARATIONS & THEIR USES

Cautions Do not use in pregnancy. Do not take the essential oil internally.

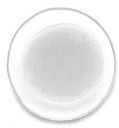

Tincture *(to make, p. 291). For canker sores, carefully dab on a little every hour.*

Powder *Rub a little onto sore gums 3 times daily.*

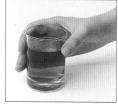

Essential oil *For congested sinuses, dilute 3 drops in 1 tsp carrier oil and massage gently (see p. 296).*

Mouthwash *Dilute 1 tsp (to make, p. 291) with 100 ml water and use as mouthwash for sore throats.*

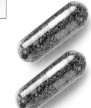

Capsules *(to make, p. 291). For bronchial congestion, take a 300 mg capsule twice a day.*

Corydalis·yanhusuo syn. *C. soldida* (Papaveraceae)

CORYDALIS, YAN HU SUO (CHINESE)

CORYDALIS
A small herbaceous plant growing to 8 in (20 cm) with narrow leaves and pink flowers.

CORYDALIS IS AN IMPORTANT Chinese remedy used at least since the 8th century to help "invigorate the blood" and relieve almost any painful condition. It is particularly used for menstrual cramps, and for chest and abdominal pain. Research in China has confirmed the validity of corydalis's traditional use, revealing that it contains powerful alkaloids that are responsible for its analgesic effect.

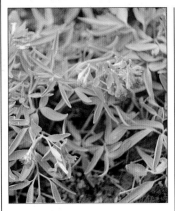

Corydalis is commonly prescribed by the Chinese in formulations for menstrual pain.

HABITAT & CULTIVATION

Native to Siberia, northern China, and Japan, corydalis is commonly cultivated in eastern and northeastern parts of China. It is propagated from seed in early spring or autumn, and the rhizome is harvested in late spring and early summer when the aerial parts have withered.

RELATED SPECIES

C. cava, a related species from southern Europe, has been shown to provide relief from involuntary tremors and ataxia (shaky movements). *C. gariana*, native to the Himalayas, is used in India as a detoxifying and tonic herb for skin problems and genitourinary infections. Fumitory (*Fumaria officinalis*, p. 211), used to treat skin problems, is also closely related.

KEY CONSTITUENTS

- Alkaloids (including corydalis L, corydaline, tetrahydropalmatine [THP], and protopine)
- Protoberberine-type alkaloid (leonticine)

KEY ACTIONS

- Analgesic
- Antispasmodic
- Sedative

RESEARCH

- **Analgesic properties**
Research in China from the 1950s onward has shown that corydalis has useful pain-relieving properties. The powdered rhizome has one-hundredth of the analgesic potency of morphine – an alkaloid derived from opium poppy (*Papaver somniferum*, p. 242). Morphine is highly concentrated and the strongest analgesic in medical use. Although this research shows corydalis to be much weaker in its effect than morphine, it nonetheless indicates the value of corydalis in pain relief.
- **Alkaloids** The strongest analgesic alkaloid in corydalis is corydaline. Tetrahydropalmatine (THP), another alkaloid, is analgesic and sedative and has been shown to work, at least in part, by blocking the dopamine receptors in the central nervous system. This constituent is also known to stimulate secretion of the adrenocorticotrophic hormone (ACTH) by the anterior pituitary gland, which controls aspects of stress.
- **Menstrual pain** Clinical trials in China have shown corydalis to be very effective in relieving menstrual pain.

TRADITIONAL & CURRENT USES

- **Pain relief** Corydalis is specifically taken to treat pain and is used in Chinese herbal medicine to relieve pain resulting from almost any cause. It is rarely taken on its own, being combined with various other herbs as appropriate.
- **Menstrual pain** Corydalis is most commonly used to relieve menstrual pain.
- **Abdominal conditions** Many types of abdominal pain, whether in the lower abdomen, as in appendicitis, or in the upper abdomen, as in peptic ulcer, are treated with corydalis.
- **Injuries** In Chinese medical theory, and in other herbal traditions, pain is often thought to stem from obstruction of normal blood flow. As corydalis is thought to "invigorate the blood," it is considered to be especially useful as a treatment for the pain that results from a traumatic injury.

✺ PARTS USED

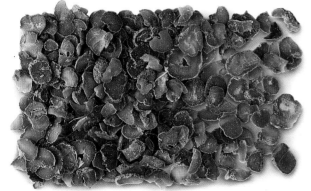

Dried rhizome

Rhizome contains powerful alkaloids that research shows help alleviate pain. It is unearthed in autumn, then dried and chopped.

✐ KEY PREPARATIONS & THEIR USES

Caution Do not take during pregnancy.

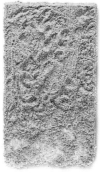

Powder *To ease pain, take 2 g of powder with food twice a day.*

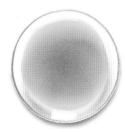

Decoction *Make a decoction with 10 g corydalis, 3 g cinnamon, and 500 ml water (see p. 290). For menstrual pain, take 100 ml twice a day.*

➴ **TINCTURE** (to make, p. 291). For abdominal pain, take up to 1 tsp with water twice a day.

HAWTHORN
A deciduous, thorny tree with small leaves, white flowers, and red berries, growing to 25 ft (8 m).

KEY MEDICINAL PLANTS

Crataegus oxyacantha & C. monogyna (Rosaceae)
HAWTHORN

HAWTHORN IS AN EXTREMELY valuable medicinal herb. It was known in the Middle Ages as a symbol of hope and taken for many ailments. Today it is used mainly for heart and circulatory disorders, in particular for angina. Western herbalists consider it literally to be a "food for the heart," increasing blood flow to the heart muscles and restoring normal heartbeat. Recent research has confirmed the validity of these uses.

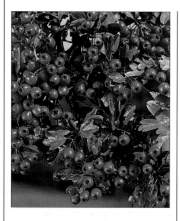

Hawthorn has bright red berries in autumn. They are used in remedies to treat a variety of circulatory disorders.

HABITAT & CULTIVATION

Hawthorn trees grow in pastures and along hedges throughout most of the temperate regions of the northern hemisphere. The seeds take 18 months to germinate, but the trees are usually cultivated from cuttings. The flowering tops are harvested in late spring and the berries are gathered in late summer to early autumn.

KEY CONSTITUENTS

- Bioflavonoids (rutin, quercitin)
- Triterpenoids
- Oligomeric procyanidin
- Amines (trimethylamine – in flowers only)
- Polyphenols
- Coumarins
- Tannins

KEY ACTIONS

- Cardiotonic
- Dilates blood vessels
- Relaxant
- Antioxidant

RESEARCH

■ **Bioflavonoids** Hawthorn has been fairly well researched. Its main medicinal benefit is due to its bioflavonoid content. These constituents relax and dilate the arteries, especially the coronary arteries. This increases the flow of blood to the heart muscles and reduces symptoms of angina. The bioflavonoids are also strongly antioxidant, helping to prevent or reduce degeneration of the blood vessels.
■ **Cardiac herb** A number of trials have confirmed hawthorn's value in treating chronic heart failure, notably a 1994 trial in Germany that showed hawthorn improved heartbeat rate and lowered blood pressure.

TRADITIONAL & CURRENT USES

■ **Historical uses** Hawthorn was traditionally used in Europe for kidney and bladder stones, and as a diuretic. The 16th- and 18th-century herbals of Gerard, Culpeper, and K'Eogh all list these uses. Its current use for circulatory and cardiac problems stems from an Irish physician who started using it successfully on his patients for such conditions toward the end of the 19th century.
■ **Heart remedy** Hawthorn is used today to treat angina and coronary artery disease. It is also useful for mild congestive heart failure and irregular heartbeat. It works well but may take some months to produce notable results. Like many herbs, hawthorn works in tune with the body's own physiological processes, and it

takes time for change to occur.
■ **Blood pressure** Not only is hawthorn a valuable remedy for high blood pressure but it also raises low blood pressure. Herbalists using hawthorn have found that it restores blood pressure to normal.

■ **Poor memory** Combined with ginkgo (*Ginkgo biloba*, p. 98), hawthorn is used to enhance poor memory. It works by improving the circulation of blood within the head, thereby increasing the amount of oxygen to the brain.

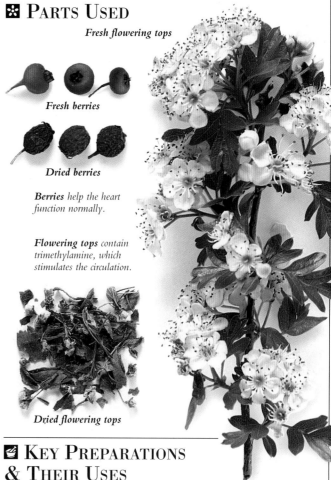

✵ PARTS USED

Fresh flowering tops

Fresh berries

Dried berries

Berries help the heart function normally.

Flowering tops contain trimethylamine, which stimulates the circulation.

Dried flowering tops

🍵 KEY PREPARATIONS & THEIR USES

Caution Take only under professional supervision.

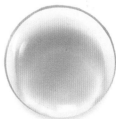
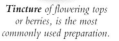

Tincture of flowering tops or berries, is the most commonly used preparation.

Decoction of flowering tops is valuable for circulatory disorders.

Tablets containing powdered flowering tops are convenient for long-term use.

INFUSION made from the flowers or leaves helps to restore blood pressure levels to normal.

Crataeva nurvula (*Capparaceae*)

VARUNA, BARUN (HINDI) THREE-LEAVED CAPER

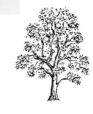

VARUNA
A large, deciduous tree growing to 50 ft (15 m) high, with smooth bark and pale yellow flowers.

THE BARK OF THE VARUNA TREE is an important herb for problems affecting the kidneys and bladder, especially kidney and bladder stones. In Ayurvedic medicine, it has been used for around 3,000 years to treat these problems, and, as is the case with so many herbs, recent scientific research is confirming the appropriateness of its traditional usage, demonstrating that it prevents the formation of kidney stones.

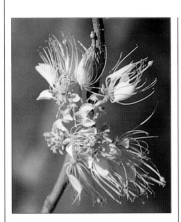

Varuna is frequently cultivated in the vicinity of temples in central India and Bangladesh.

HABITAT & CULTIVATION

Varuna grows throughout India and is often found along river-banks. Grown from seed in spring, the leaves are harvested in spring and the bark is collected throughout the year.

KEY CONSTITUENTS

- Saponins
- Flavonoids
- Plant sterols
- Glucosilinates

KEY ACTIONS

- Diuretic
- Inhibits the formation of stones

RESEARCH

■ **Bladder & kidney stones**
Clinical research in India from the 1980s onward indicates that varuna increases bladder tone and inhibits the formation of bladder stones. It reduces the production within the body of oxalates, substances that can precipitate in the kidneys and bladder to form stones. Varuna also seems to reduce the rate at which stone-forming constituents within the urine are deposited in the kidneys.

■ **Urinary system** Indian research in the 1980s and 1990s points to varuna being valuable in the treatment of urinary tract infections and bladder problems caused by an enlarged prostate gland. In one clinical trial 85% of patients with chronic urinary tract infections were symptom-free after undergoing 4 weeks' treatment with varuna.

TRADITIONAL & CURRENT USES

■ **Ancient urinary remedy**
Texts dating back to the 8th century BC document varuna's use in Ayurvedic medicine for kidney and bladder problems. From around AD 1100, varuna became the main Indian herbal medicine for kidney stones.

■ **Other traditional uses**
Traditionally, varuna bark is considered useful in Ayurveda (*see* p. 35) for weakened conditions of *vata* (air) and *kapha* (earth), and is used to treat many conditions, including asthma, bronchitis, and skin diseases. The bark is also used to treat fevers, gastritis, and vomiting, as well as snakebite. The fresh leaves, bruised and mixed with vinegar, relieve sore and inflamed joints.

■ **Kidney stones** Today, varuna is beginning to be used in the West, as well as in India, in the prevention and treatment of kidney stones. It is given to people who are prone to develop kidney stones, reducing the tendency to stone formation.

◆ PARTS USED

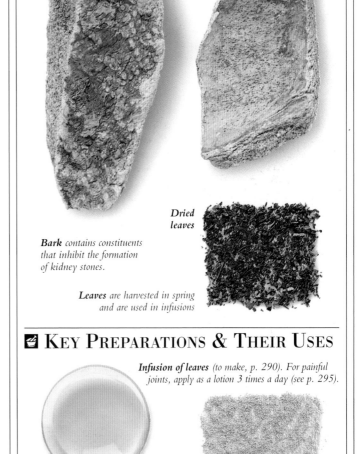

Dried bark

Dried leaves

Bark *contains constituents that inhibit the formation of kidney stones.*

Leaves *are harvested in spring and are used in infusions*

◆ KEY PREPARATIONS & THEIR USES

Infusion of leaves *(to make, p. 290). For painful joints, apply as a lotion 3 times a day (see p. 295).*

Powdered bark *is used in Ayurveda. For urinary infections, take 15 g with water daily.*

Decoction *of bark (to make, p. 290) is the most common preparation. To prevent kidney stone formation, take 1 cup 3 times a day.*

It is also prescribed for people who already have small stones. Varuna improves smooth muscle tone and encourages the removal of stones in the urine.

■ **Urinary tract remedy**
Combined with antiseptic and immune-stimulating herbs, varuna is very useful for urinary tract infections, including cystitis. It is also sometimes effective for bladder conditions involving poor muscle tone, some cases of incontinence, and urinary problems associated with prostate enlargement.

Curcuma longa syn. *C. domestica* (Zingiberaceae)
TURMERIC, HALDI (HINDI), JIANG HUANG (CHINESE)

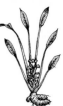

ALTHOUGH TURMERIC'S BRIGHT yellow color and spicy taste are familiar to lovers of Indian food, its medicinal value is not as well known. During the last two decades, turmeric's ancient use as a treatment for digestive and liver problems has been largely confirmed by scientific research. The herb has also been shown to inhibit blood-clotting, relieve inflammatory conditions, and help to lower cholesterol levels.

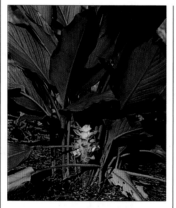

Turmeric is a valuable remedy for arthritic and skin conditions.

HABITAT & CULTIVATION

Turmeric is native to India and southern Asia, and is cultivated throughout southern and eastern Asia. It is propagated by cuttings from the root, and needs well-drained soil and a humid climate. The rhizome is unearthed in winter.

KEY CONSTITUENTS

- Volatile oil (3–5%), including zingiberen and turmerone
- Curcumin
- Bitter principles
- Resin

KEY ACTIONS

- Stimulates secretion of bile
- Anti-inflammatory
- Eases stomach pain
- Antioxidant
- Antibacterial

RESEARCH

- **New interest in turmeric**
Despite its longstanding use in India and China, the therapeutic actions of turmeric were not researched until recent decades when there was an upsurge of interest in foods and medicines that lower cholesterol levels or have antioxidant properties (neutralize harmful free radicals). Research since the early 1970s, mainly in India, has confirmed turmeric's traditional actions and revealed potential new uses for it.
- **Anti-inflammatory** Turmeric is a powerful anti-inflammatory. It has an even stronger action than hydrocortisone, according to research studies conducted between 1971 and 1991.
- **Curcumin** When applied to the skin and exposed to sunlight, turmeric is strongly antibacterial. Curcumin is the constituent responsible for this action. Curcumin is also more strongly antioxidant than vitamin E.
- **Cholesterol** Chinese clinical trials in 1987 indicate that turmeric lowers cholesterol levels.
- **Cancer** Turmeric may be a valuable preventive remedy for those at risk of developing cancer, but more research is needed.
- **Other actions** Research has shown that turmeric has an anti-coagulant action, keeping the blood thin. It also increases bile production and flow, and has a protective action on the stomach and liver.

TRADITIONAL & CURRENT USES

- **Traditional remedy**
Turmeric improves the action of the liver and is a traditional remedy for jaundice in both Ayurvedic and Chinese herbal medicine. It is also an ancient herb for digestive problems such as gastritis and acidity, helping to increase mucus production and protect the stomach. The herb also alleviates nausea.
- **Arthritis & allergies** Even though turmeric does not relieve pain, its anti-inflammatory action makes it useful for arthritis, and other inflammatory conditions such as asthma and eczema.
- **Circulatory disorders** Due to its anti-inflammatory, blood-thinning, and cholesterol-lowering properties, turmeric is now used to reduce the risk of strokes and heart attacks.
- **Skin conditions** Applied to the skin, turmeric is useful in treating a number of conditions, including psoriasis, and fungal infections such as athlete's foot.

SELF-HELP USES

- **Athlete's foot**, p. 304.
- **Nausea & motion sickness**, p. 306.

⚙ PARTS USED

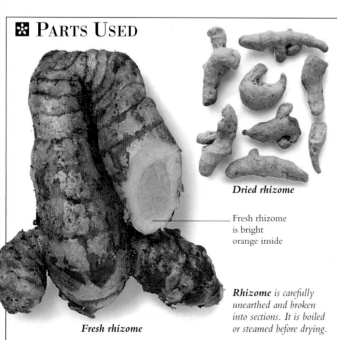

Fresh rhizome

Fresh rhizome is bright orange inside

Dried rhizome

Rhizome is carefully unearthed and broken into sections. It is boiled or steamed before drying.

✍ KEY PREPARATIONS & THEIR USES

Cautions Turmeric occasionally causes skin rashes. Those taking turmeric medicinally should avoid overexposure to the sun since the herb can increase sensitivity to sunlight.

Decoction (to make, p. 290). For gastritis, take ½ cup 3 times a day.

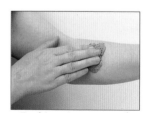

Poultice using a paste made with powder. For psoriasis, mix 1 tsp with a little water and apply 3 times a day.

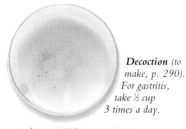

Powder is the most common preparation in Ayurvedic medicine. For gastritis, take 1 tsp with water 3 times a day.

✒ TINCTURE (to make, p. 291). For eczema, take 1 tsp diluted with 100 ml of water 3 times a day.

Dioscorea villosa (Dioscoreaceae)
WILD YAM

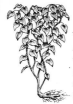

WILD YAM
A deciduous perennial vine, climbing to 20 ft (6 m) with heart-shaped leaves and tiny green flowers.

WILD YAM IS THE PLANT SOURCE of a steroidlike substance, diosgenin, which was the starting point in the creation of the first contraceptive pill. There is no suggestion that the plant was used as a contraceptive in the past, although it has traditionally been taken in Central America to relieve menstrual, ovarian, and labor pains. The herb is also valuable for digestive problems, arthritis, and muscle cramps.

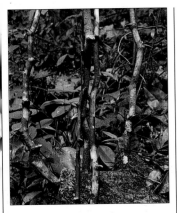

Wild yam can be found growing wild in damp woodlands in North America.

HABITAT & CULTIVATION

Wild yam is native to North and Central America and has now become naturalized in tropical, semitropical, and temperate climates around the world. The plant is propagated from seed in spring, from sections of tubers, or by root division in spring or autumn. It thrives in sunny conditions and rich soil. The root and tuber of wild yam are harvested in autumn.

RELATED SPECIES

Many yam species have a hormonal action. *Shan yao* (*Dioscorea opposita*, p. 200) is an important tonic for the spleen and stomach in traditional Chinese medicine and is taken for appetite loss and wheezing.

KEY CONSTITUENTS

- Steroidal saponins (mainly dioscin)
- Phytosterols (beta-sitosterol)
- Alkaloids
- Tannins
- Starch

KEY ACTIONS

- Antispasmodic
- Anti-inflammatory
- Antirheumatic
- Increases sweating
- Diuretic

RESEARCH

■ Synthesis of hormones
Diosgenin, a breakdown product of dioscin, was first identified by Japanese scientists in 1936. This discovery paved the way for the synthesis of progesterone (one of the main female sex hormones) and of corticosteroid hormones such as cortisone.

■ Anti-inflammatory The discovery that wild yam contains large amounts of dioscin, which has an anti-inflammatory action, supports its use in treating rheumatic conditions.

TRADITIONAL & CURRENT USES

■ Traditional uses Both the Maya and the Aztec peoples used wild yam medicinally – possibly to relieve pain. The plant is also known as colic root and rheumatism root in North America, indicating its use by European settlers for these conditions.

■ Gynecological problems
In North and Central America, wild yam is a traditional relaxing remedy for painful menstruation, ovarian pain, and labor.

■ Arthritis & rheumatism
The herb's combination of anti-inflammatory and antispasmodic actions makes it extremely useful in treatments for arthritis and rheumatism. It reduces inflammation and pain, and

✻ PARTS USED

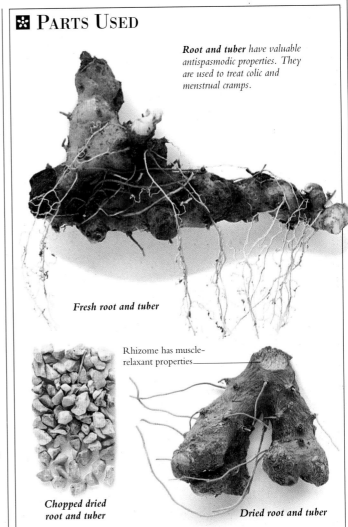

Root and tuber have valuable antispasmodic properties. They are used to treat colic and menstrual cramps.

Fresh root and tuber

Rhizome has muscle-relaxant properties

Chopped dried root and tuber

Dried root and tuber

❧ KEY PREPARATIONS & THEIR USES

Caution Do not take during pregnancy.

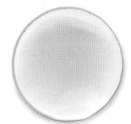

Decoction (to make, p. 290). For irritable bowel syndrome, take ½ cup twice a day.

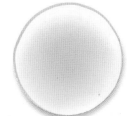

Tincture (to make, p. 291). For arthritis, take ½ tsp with water twice a day.

relaxes stiff muscles in the affected area.

■ Muscle spasms & pain Wild yam helps to relieve cramps, muscle tension, and colic.

■ Digestive problems The herb can be an effective treatment for digestive problems, including gallbladder inflammation, irritable bowel syndrome, and diverticulitis.

SELF-HELP USE

- **Menstrual pain**, p. 315.

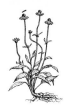

ECHINACEA
A perennial growing to 20 in (50 cm), with daisylike purple flowers and leaves covered in coarse hair.

Echinacea angustifolia & E. purpurea (Compositae)
ECHINACEA, PURPLE CONEFLOWER

NATIVE TO NORTH AMERICA, echinacea is one of the world's most important medicinal herbs. Research shows that it has the ability to raise the body's resistance to bacterial and viral infections by stimulating the immune system. Echinacea is also antibiotic and helps to relieve allergies, and it has been used for centuries to clear skin infections. Both *E. angustifolia* and *E. purpurea* are cultivated for therapeutic purposes.

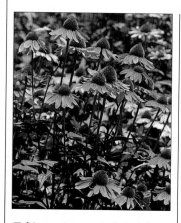

Echinacea's name is derived from the Greek word for hedgehog and was inspired by the appearance of the flower's central cone.

- Anti-inflammatory
- Antibiotic
- Detoxifying
- Increases sweating
- Heals wounds
- Antiallergenic

HABITAT & CULTIVATION

Native to central parts of the US, echinacea, particularly *E. purpurea*, which is easier to grow, is now commercially cultivated in Europe and the US. Grown from seed in spring or by root division in winter, it thrives best in rich, sandy soil. The flowers are gathered in full bloom, and the roots of 4-year-old plants are lifted in autumn.

RELATED SPECIES

E. pallida is also used medicinally.

KEY CONSTITUENTS

- Alkamides (mostly isobutylamides with olefinic and acetylenic bonds)
- Caffeic acid esters (mainly echinacoside and cynarin)
- Polysaccharides
- Volatile oil (humulene)
- Echinolone
- Betaine

KEY ACTIONS

- Immune stimulant

RESEARCH

- **Immune system** Echinacea's effect is not yet fully understood, but it is known that a number of constituents stimulate the immune system to counter both bacterial and viral infections. The polysaccharides have an anti-hyaluronidase action, inhibiting the ability of viruses to enter and take over cells, while the alkamides are antibacterial and antifungal. Echinacea also has a general stimulating effect on the body's immune defenses and is currently being investigated as a treatment for HIV and AIDS.

TRADITIONAL & CURRENT USES

- **Native American medicine** The Comanche used echinacea as a remedy for toothache and sore throats and the Sioux took it for rabies, snakebite, and septic conditions.
- **Western uses** Echinacea is the most important immune stimulant in Western herbal medicine. It is used for infections of all kinds and is particularly helpful for chronic infections, such as postviral fatigue syndrome (ME). It is also good for chilblains, colds, flu, skin disorders, and respiratory problems, and is very effective as a gargle for throat infections.
- **Allergies** The herb is a helpful remedy for treating allergies, such as asthma.

❖ PARTS USED

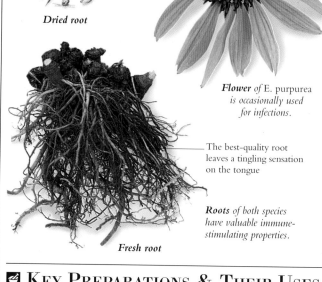

Dried root

Flower of E. purpurea *is occasionally used for infections.*

The best-quality root leaves a tingling sensation on the tongue

Roots of both species have valuable immune-stimulating properties.

Fresh root

KEY PREPARATIONS & THEIR USES

Caution High doses can cause nausea.

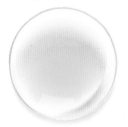

Tincture of root (to make, p. 291). For chronic infections, take ½ tsp in water 3 times a day.

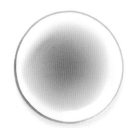

Decoction of root (to make, p. 290). To treat throat infections, gargle with 50 ml 3 times a day.

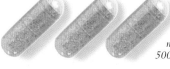

Capsules of powdered root (to make, p. 291). For colds, take a 500 mg capsule 3 times a day.

⊘ **TABLETS** Take as an immune-stimulant for infections.

SELF-HELP USES

Eletteria cardamomum (Zingiberaceae)
CARDAMOM, ELACI (HINDI)

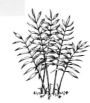

CARDAMOM
A perennial growing to 15 ft (5 m), with mauve-marked, white flowers and very long, lance-shaped leaves.

CARDAMOM IS ONE OF THE oldest spices in the world and was used extensively in ancient Egypt to make perfumes. Its medicinal uses, however, are less well known. Cardamom has been employed in Ayurvedic medicine for thousands of years and is an excellent remedy for many digestive problems, helping to soothe indigestion and gas. It has an aromatic, pungent taste and combines well with other herbs.

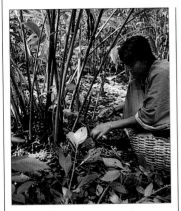

Cardamom seedpods are harvested by hand. Each pod contains up to 20 aromatic, dark red-brown seeds.

HABITAT & CULTIVATION

Cardamom is native to southern India and Sri Lanka, where it grows abundantly in forests at 2,500–5,000 ft (800–1,500 m) above sea level. It is also widely cultivated in India, southern Asia, Indonesia, and Guatemala. Cardamom is propagated from seed in autumn or by root division in spring and summer, and needs a shady position and rich and moist but well-drained soil. The seedpods are harvested just before they start to open in dry weather during the autumn and are dried whole in the sun.

KEY CONSTITUENTS

- Volatile oil (borneol, camphor, pinene, humulene, caryophyllene, carvone, eucalyptole, terpinene, sabinene)

KEY ACTIONS

- Eases stomach pain
- Carminative
- Aromatic

- Warming digestive stimulant
- Antispasmodic

RESEARCH

- **Volatile oil** Research in the 1960s showed that the volatile oil has a strong antispasmodic action, confirming the herb's effectiveness in relieving gas and treating colic and cramps.

TRADITIONAL & CURRENT USES

- **Ancient herb** Cardamom has been highly valued both as a spice and a medicine and was known in Greece in the 4th century BC.
- **Digestive problems** Throughout history, cardamom has been used for the relief of digestive problems, especially indigestion, gas, and cramps. It has a pleasant taste and is often used in digestive remedies, its delicate flavor helping to counteract the taste of less palatable herbs.
- **Current Indian uses** Cardamom is used in India for many conditions, including asthma, bronchitis, kidney stones, anorexia, debility, and weakened *vata* (see p. 35).
- **Chinese remedy** In China, the herb is taken for urinary incontinence and as a tonic.
- **Bad breath** Cardamom is an effective treatment for bad breath, and when taken with garlic helps to reduce garlic's strong smell.
- **Aphrodisiac** The herb has a long-lasting reputation as an aphrodisiac.

SELF-HELP USE

- **Gas & bloating**, p. 306

PARTS USED

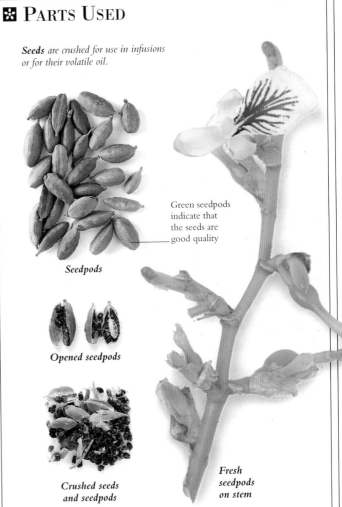

Seeds are crushed for use in infusions or for their volatile oil.

Green seedpods indicate that the seeds are good quality

Seedpods

Opened seedpods

Crushed seeds and seedpods

Fresh seedpods on stem

KEY PREPARATIONS & THEIR USES

Caution Do not take the essential oil internally.

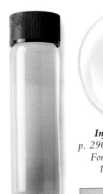

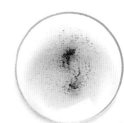

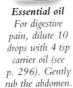

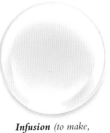

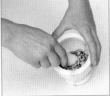

Infusion (to make, p. 290) is a pleasant drink. For indigestion, drink 1 cup after meals.

Tincture (to make, p. 291) improves the appetite. For poor appetite, combine 5 drops with 15 drops gentian tincture and take 3 times a day.

Essential oil For digestive pain, dilute 10 drops with 4 tsp carrier oil (see p. 296). Gently rub the abdomen.

Crush cardamom seeds using a mortar and pestle just before you are about to use them.

Eleutherococcus senticosus (Araliaceae)
SIBERIAN GINSENG

SIBERIAN GINSENG
A deciduous, hardy shrub, growing to 10 ft (3 m). It has 3–7 toothed leaflets on each stem.

SIBERIAN GINSENG IS A POWERFUL tonic herb with an impressive range of health benefits. Unlike many herbs with a medicinal use, it is more useful for maintaining good health rather than treating ill health. Research has shown that Siberian ginseng stimulates resistance to stress and it is now widely used as a tonic during times of stress and pressure. It has a similar effect to *Panax ginseng* (p. 116) but is more stimulating.

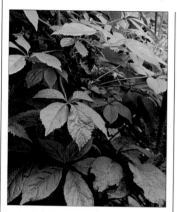

Siberian ginseng can help those exposed to toxic chemicals and radiation and was given to people folowing the nuclear disaster at Chernobyl in 1986.

HABITAT & CULTIVATION
Siberian ginseng is native to eastern Russia, China, Korea, and Japan. It can be grown from seed, but it is a difficult plant to germinate. The root is lifted in autumn and dried.

RELATED SPECIES
Wu jia pi (Acanthopanacis gracilistylus) is a very close relative of Siberian ginseng, used in Chinese herbal medicine to treat "cold, damp" conditions.

KEY CONSTITUENTS
- Eleutherosides (0.6–0.9%)
- Phenylpropanoids
- Lignans
- Coumarins
- Sugars
- Polysaccharides
- Triterpenoid saponins
- Glycans

KEY ACTIONS
- Adaptogenic
- Tonic
- Stimulant
- Protects the immune system

RESEARCH
- **Russian studies** There has been much research into Siberian ginseng in Russia since the 1950s, although the exact method by which it stimulates stamina and resistance to stress is not yet understood.
- **Tonic herb** Siberian ginseng seems to have a general tonic effect on the body, in particular on the adrenal glands, helping the body to withstand heat, cold, infection, other physical stresses, and radiation. It has even been given to astronauts to counter the effects of weightlessness.
- **Stamina** Athletes have experienced as much as a 9% improvement in stamina when taking Siberian ginseng.

TRADITIONAL & CURRENT USES
- **Enhancing resilience** Siberian ginseng is given to improve mental resilience, for example, during exams, and to reduce the effects of physical stress, for example during athletic training.
- **Exhaustion remedy** Siberian ginseng is most effective in the treatment of prolonged exhaustion and debility, resulting from overwork and long-term stress. The herb also stimulates immune resistance and can be taken in convalescence to aid recovery from chronic illness. As a general tonic, Siberian ginseng helps both to prevent infection and to maintain well-being. It is also used in treatments for impotence.

SELF-HELP USES
- **Insomnia**, p. 309.
- **Stress**, p. 308.

⊞ PARTS USED

Root is unearthed in autumn, dried whole, and then chopped up for use in medicinal preparations.

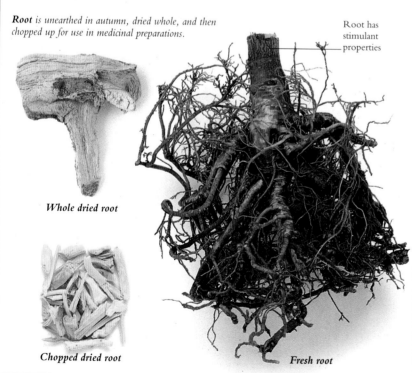

Root has stimulant properties

Whole dried root

Chopped dried root

Fresh root

☟ KEY PREPARATIONS & THEIR USES

Cautions Do not take for more than 6 weeks at a time. Do not take during illness without professional advice. Avoid caffeine when taking Siberian ginseng. Side effects are rare, but more likely if the standard dose is exceeded.

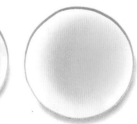

Decoction (to make, p. 290). Take 35 ml twice a day as a general tonic.

Tincture (to make, p. 291). During busy periods, take ½ tsp with water 3 times a day.

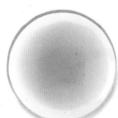

Capsules Make with powder (see p. 291) and for long-term stress take a 1 g capsule daily.

⊘ **TABLETS** are a convenient way of taking Siberian ginseng. Use before exams or other stressful events.

Ephedra sinica (Ephedraceae)

EPHEDRA, MA HUANG (CHINESE), DESERT TEA

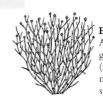

EPHEDRA
An evergreen shrub growing to 20 in (50 cm) with long, narrow, sprawling stems and tiny leaves.

EPHEDRA IS A STRONGLY STIMULANT, acrid-tasting herb that has a central place in Chinese and other herbal traditions. According to legend, the bodyguards of Genghis Khan, threatened with beheading if they fell asleep on sentry duty, used to take a tea containing ephedra to stay alert. Today, ephedra is used in the West and in China for problems ranging from chills and fevers to asthma and hay fever.

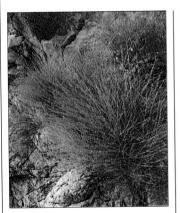

Ephedra was found in a Middle Eastern neolithic grave, indicating that it may have been used as a medicine 60,000 years ago.

HABITAT & CULTIVATION

Native to northern China and Inner Mongolia, ephedra often grows in desert areas. It is propagated from seed in autumn or by root division in autumn or spring and needs well-drained soil. The stems are gathered throughout the year and dried.

RELATED SPECIES

Other *Ephedra* species with similar medicinal properties to ephedra grow throughout the northern hemisphere. In North America, related species were used to treat fevers and relieve kidney pain, while in India, *Ephedra* species were taken for asthma, hay fever, and rheumatism.

KEY CONSTITUENTS

- Protoalkaloids (ephedrine, pseudoephedrine)
- Tannins
- Saponin
- Flavone
- Volatile oil

KEY ACTIONS

Western herbal medicine:
- Increases sweating
- Dilates the bronchioles (small airways in the lungs)
- Diuretic
- Stimulant
- Raises blood pressure

Chinese herbal medicine:
- Disperses cold
- Helps problems caused by "external cold"
- Aids movement of lung *qi*

RESEARCH

- **Active constituents** Most of the active constituents mimic the effect of adrenaline within the body, increasing alertness. Ephedrine, extracted originally from ephedra, was first synthesized in 1927 and was used as a decongestant and anti-asthmatic. It is still commonly used in conventional medicine for its decongestant properties.
- **Whole herb** The whole plant contains many compounds – some active, some inert – which in combination seem to act synergistically. The whole plant can be used at a much lower dosage than isolated constituents and it has significant therapeutic effects – including dilating the bronchial airways and increasing blood flow to the skin. Unlike ephedrine, the whole plant rarely gives rise to side effects.

TRADITIONAL & CURRENT USES

- **Historical uses** Traditionally, Zen monks used ephedra to promote calm concentration during meditation.
- **Chinese herb** In China, ephedra is popular for chills and

PARTS USED

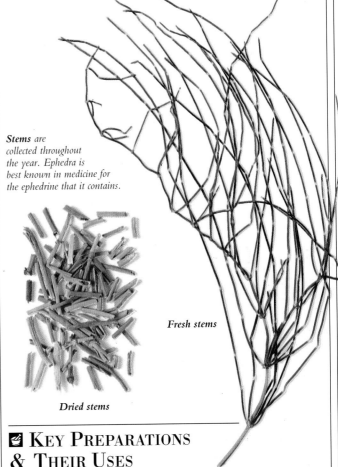

Stems are collected throughout the year. Ephedra is best known in medicine for the ephedrine that it contains.

Fresh stems

Dried stems

KEY PREPARATIONS & THEIR USES

Cautions Take only under professional supervision. Do not take if suffering from angina, glaucoma, high blood pressure, enlarged prostate gland, or overactive thyroid gland. Ephedra occasionally causes side effects, including headaches, tremors, and insomnia. Restricted herb in some countries.

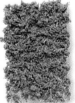

Decoction is prescribed by herbalists for asthma.

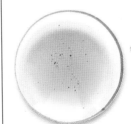

Powder is used by the Chinese to treat kidney energy deficiency.

Tincture is used in treatments to alleviate the aches and pains of rheumatism.

fevers, coughs, and wheezing, and in combination with rehmannia (*Rehmannia glutinosa*, p. 123) is given to treat kidney *yin* deficiency (*see* pp. 38–39).
- **Current Western uses** Ephedra is used principally in current Western herbal medicine as a treatment for asthma and hay fever, and for the acute onset of colds and flu. It also helps to raise blood pressure, cool fevers, and alleviate rheumatism.

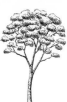

EUCALYPTUS
An evergreen tree
growing to 300 ft
(100 m), with a
blue-gray trunk and
green leaves.

Eucalyptus globulus (Myrtaceae)
EUCALYPTUS, BLUE GUM

EUCALYPTUS, A TRADITIONAL Aboriginal remedy,
is a powerful antiseptic used all over the world for
relieving coughs and colds, sore throats, and other
infections. It is warming and stimulating and, for
many people, its scent conjures up days spent in bed
during a childhood illness, with eucalyptus and other
oils rubbed on the chest. Eucalpytus is a common
ingredient in many over-the-counter cold remedies.

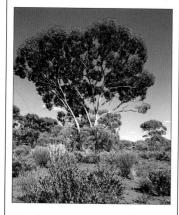

Eucalyptus *was first introduced
to the West from Australia in
the 19th century.*

HABITAT & CULTIVATION

Native to Australia, eucalyptus
is cultivated on plantations in
tropical, subtropical, and
temperate areas of the world.
Planting can cause ecological
problems because the trees
absorb huge quantities of water
and prevent the growth of
native plants. This can be
beneficial, however, for drying
up marshy areas and so reducing
the risk of malaria. The leaves
are harvested as required and
are dried or distilled for oil.

RELATED SPECIES

Many other *Eucalyptus* species
contain valuable essential oils,
including *E. smithii* (p. 205).

KEY CONSTITUENTS

- Volatile oil (cineole, up to
  80%)
- Flavonoids
- Tannins
- Resin

KEY ACTIONS

- Antiseptic

- Expectorant
- Stimulates local blood flow

RESEARCH

- **Essential oil** Extensive
research into eucalyptus essential
oil during the last 50 years has
shown it to have a marked
antiseptic action and the ability
to dilate the bronchioles (small
airways) of the lungs. The
action of the essential oil as a
whole is stronger than that of
its main constituent, cineole.

TRADITIONAL & CURRENT USES

- **Infections** Eucalyptus is a
traditional Aboriginal remedy
for infections and fevers. It
is now used throughout the
world for these ailments.
- **Antiseptic** The herb is an
antiseptic and is very helpful
for colds, flu, and sore throats.
- **Expectorant** Eucalyptus is a
strong expectorant, suitable for
chest infections, including
bronchitis and pneumonia.
- **Warming** The diluted essential
oil, applied to the skin as a chest
or sinus rub, has a warming and
slightly anesthetic effect, helping
to relieve respiratory infections.
The same effect takes place
when the infusion or tincture
is used as a gargle.
- **Pain relief** Diluted essential
oil applied to the affected area
can help to relieve rheumatic
joints characterized by aching
pains and stiffness, as well as
neuralgia, and some bacterial
skin infections.

SELF-HELP USES

- **Congestion**, p. 312.
- **Coughs & bronchitis**, p. 310.

✺ PARTS USED

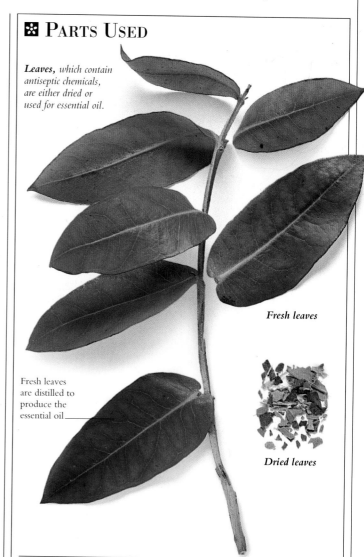

Leaves, *which contain
antiseptic chemicals,
are either dried or
used for essential oil.*

Fresh leaves

Fresh leaves
are distilled to
produce the
essential oil

Dried leaves

☙ KEY PREPARATIONS & THEIR USES

Caution Do not take the essential oil internally except under professional supervision.

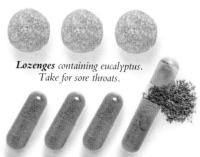

Lozenges *containing eucalyptus.
Take for sore throats.*

Capsules *(to make, p. 291). For bronchitis,
take a 200 mg capsule 3 times a day.*

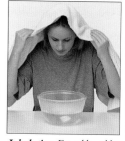

Inhalation *For colds, add
10 drops essential oil to
boiling water (p. 296).*

- **ESSENTIAL OIL** (to use, p. 296). Use 5 drops diluted with 10 ml carrier
oil as a chest or sinus rub.
- **INFUSION** (to make, p. 290). Drink 1 cup 3 times a day for bronchitis.
- **TINCTURE** (to make, p. 291). For chest coughs, add ½ tsp tincture to
100 ml water and take twice a day.

Eugenia carophyllata syn. *Syzgium aromaticum* (Myrtaceae)

CLOVE

CLOVE TREE
An evergreen, pyramid-shaped tree growing to 50 ft (15 m). The tree is strongly aromatic.

CLOVES, THE DRIED FLOWER BUDS of the clove tree, are best known as a spice but are also highly valued as an herbal medicine, particularly in India and Southeast Asia. Native to the Molucca Islands, cloves were one of the earliest spices to be traded and were imported into Alexandria in AD 176. The cloves contain the best essential oil, but the stems and leaves of the tree can also be distilled for their oil.

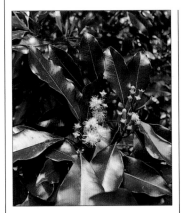

Cloves *are pink when unripe, but later turn brown when they are dried outside in the sun.*

HABITAT & CULTIVATION

Originally from the Molucca Islands (Indonesia) and the southern Phillipines, cloves are now grown extensively in Tanzania and Madagascar and, to a lesser extent, in the West Indies and Brazil. The tree is grown from seed in spring or from semiripe cuttings in summer. Twice a year, the unopened flower buds are picked and then sun-dried.

KEY CONSTITUENTS

- Volatile oil containing eugenol (up to 85%), acetyl eugenol, methyl salicylate, pinene, vanillin
- Gum
- Tannins

KEY ACTIONS

- Antiseptic
- Carminative
- Stimulant
- Analgesic
- Prevents vomiting
- Antispasmodic
- Eliminates parasites

RESEARCH

- **Volatile oil** Argentinian research in 1994 showed clove's volatile oil to be strongly antibacterial. Eugenol (a phenol) is the largest and most important component of the volatile oil. It is strongly anesthetic and antiseptic, and therefore useful in pain relief for toothache and as an antiseptic for many conditions.
- **Acetyl eugenol** Acetyl eugenol, another component of the volatile oil, has been shown to be strongly antispasmodic.

TRADITIONAL & CURRENT USES

- **Ancient all-purpose remedy** Cloves have been used in Southeast Asia for thousands of years and were regarded as a panacea for almost all ills.
- **Antiseptic** The antiseptic property of cloves makes them useful for treating certain viral conditions. In tropical Asia, they have often been given to treat infections such as malaria, cholera, and tuberculosis, and parasites such as scabies.
- **Antispasmodic** Digestive discomfort, such as gas, colic, and abdominal bloating, can be relieved with cloves. Their antispasmodic property also eases coughs and, applied topically, relieves muscle spasms.
- **Mind & body stimulant** Cloves are a stimulant, both to the mind (improving memory) and to the body as a whole, and have been used as an aphrodisiac both in India and in the West. The herb has also been used to prepare for childbirth. It helps stimulate and strengthen uterine

PARTS USED

Flower buds are picked unopened and dried for use in infusions or powders and for oil extraction.

Fresh flower buds

Leaves and stems are occasionally used for oil extraction

Dried flower buds (cloves)

KEY PREPARATIONS & THEIR USES

Cautions External use can cause dermatitis. Do not take essential oil internally except under professional supervision.

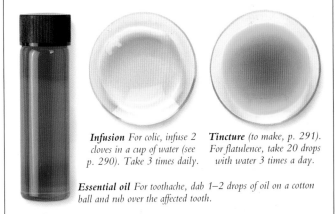

Infusion *For colic, infuse 2 cloves in a cup of water (see p. 290). Take 3 times daily.*

Tincture *(to make, p. 291). For flatulence, take 20 drops with water 3 times a day.*

Essential oil *For toothache, dab 1–2 drops of oil on a cotton ball and rub over the affected tooth.*

muscle contractions in labor.
- **Additional uses** Besides all their other uses, cloves can be used to treat acne, skin ulcers, sores, and styes. They also make a potent mosquito and moth repellent. Oranges studded with cloves were used in the Moluccas as insect repellents.
- **Western herbalism** Despite the bewildering variety of their therapeutic uses, cloves are

underrated in the West. They are used regularly only in mouthwashes and for their local anesthetic effect – for example, in relieving toothache.

SELF-HELP USES

Filipendula ulmaria (Rosaceae)

MEADOWSWEET, QUEEN OF THE MEADOW

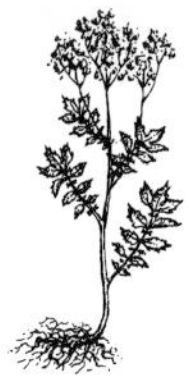

MEADOWSWEET A perennial reaching 5 ft (1.5 m), with toothed leaves and clusters of creamy, scented flowers.

IN MEDIEVAL TIMES, MEADOWSWEET was a favorite strewing herb – Gerard wrote in his *Herball* (1597) that "the smell thereof makes the heart merry and joyful and delighteth the senses." Salicylic acid isolated from the plant was first synthesized in the 1890s and used to make aspirin. Nowadays, meadowsweet is taken for gastric problems and inflammatory conditions, such as arthritis.

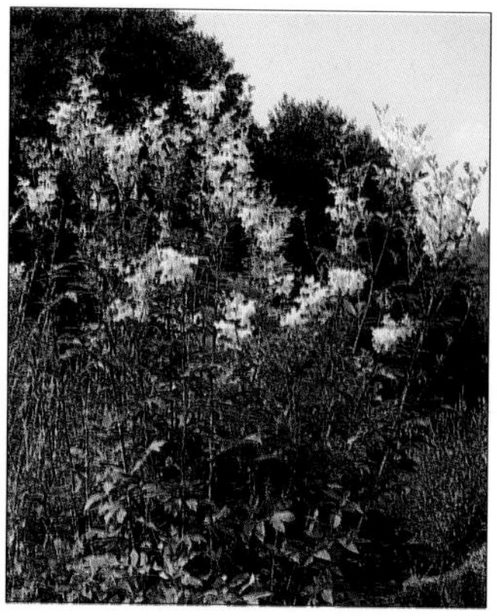

***Meadowsweet** was known as "meadwort" in the Middle Ages, because it was used to flavor mead.*

HABITAT & CULTIVATION

Native to Europe, meadowsweet grows easily in damp places, preferring ditches and the banks of streams and rivers. It seeds itself freely, but can also be propagated by root division in autumn or spring. Leaves and flowering tops are harvested in summer when the flowers open.

KEY CONSTITUENTS

- Flavonol glycosides (approximately 1%), mainly glycosides of quercetin
- Phenolic glycosides (salicylates)
- Volatile oil (salicylaldehyde)
- Polyphenols (tannins)

KEY ACTIONS

- Anti-inflammatory
- Antirheumatic
- Astringent
- Diuretic
- Eases stomach pain

RESEARCH

■ **Salicylates** The salicylates are aspirin-like substances, which help to reduce inflammation and relieve pain – for example, in arthritic conditions.

■ **Protective combination** Unlike aspirin, which at high doses causes gastric ulceration, the combination of salicylates, tannins, and other constituents in meadowsweet acts to protect the inner lining of the stomach and intestines, while providing the anti-inflammatory benefit of the salicylates. Meadowsweet illustrates well the fact that herbal medicines cannot be understood by simply considering their active constituents in isolation.

TRADITIONAL & CURRENT USES

■ **Early European uses** Meadowsweet was one of the most sacred herbs of the Druids, although whether it was used as a medicine is not known. It has been a longstanding folk remedy in much of Europe. Nicholas Culpeper wrote in 1652 that "it helpeth speedily those that are troubled with the cholic being boiled in wine; and stayeth the flux on the belly."

■ **Neutralizing acid** The herb is a remedy for acid indigestion, helping to heal and to reduce acidity. Its ability to reduce acid levels throughout the body is not established, but its effectiveness in painful arthritic and rheumatic problems is probably not due entirely to its anti-inflammatory action. It would seem that reducing acidity within the stomach can help to reduce acid levels in the body as a whole, thereby helping joint problems (which are associated with acidity).

PARTS USED

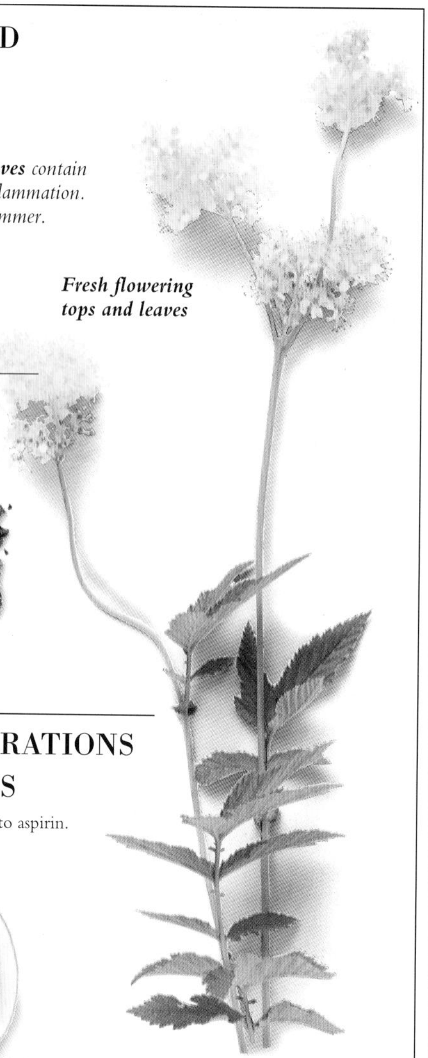

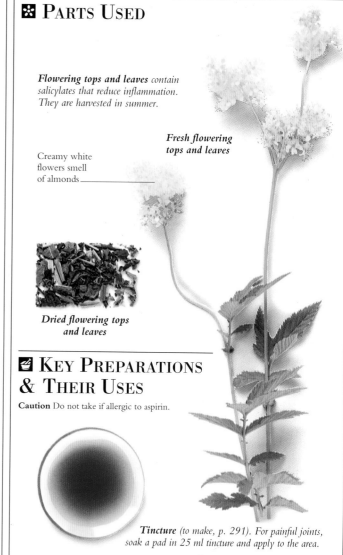

***Flowering tops and leaves** contain salicylates that reduce inflammation. They are harvested in summer.*

Fresh flowering tops and leaves

Creamy white flowers smell of almonds

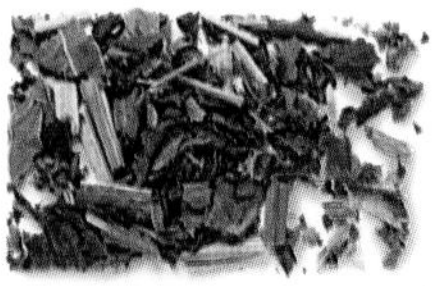

Dried flowering tops and leaves

KEY PREPARATIONS & THEIR USES

Caution Do not take if allergic to aspirin.

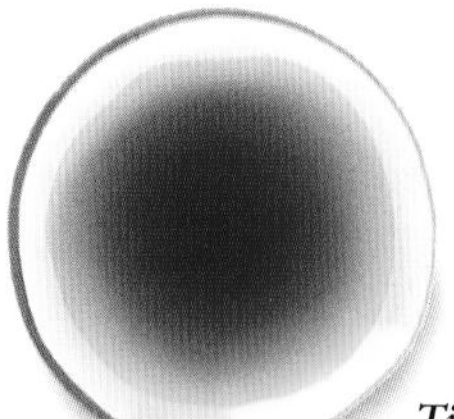

***Tincture** (to make, p. 291). For painful joints, soak a pad in 25 ml tincture and apply to the area.*

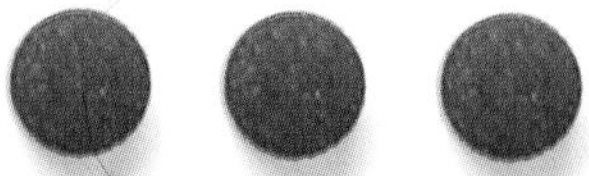

***Tablets** are convenient. Take for rheumatic aches.*

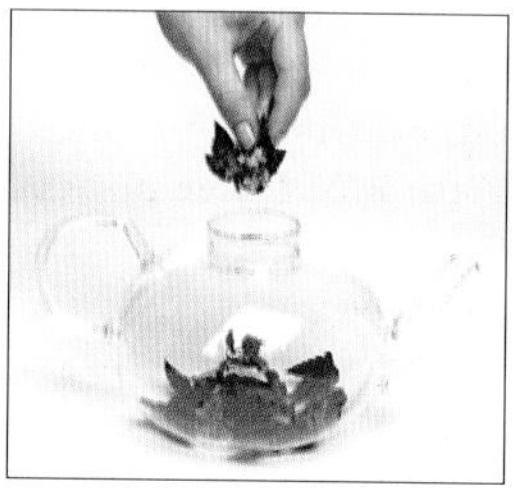

***Infusion** Make by adding freshly boiled water to the herb (see p. 290). For indigestion, take 100 ml every 2 hours.*

DECOCTION (to make, p. 290). For diarrhea, take 1 cup 2–3 times a day.

POWDER For acidity, take ½ tsp mixed with a little water 3 times a day.

Meadowsweet is also occasionally used for cystitis.

■ **Digestive remedy** Meadowsweet is a safe remedy for diarrhea, even in children, and is used with other herbs for irritable bowel syndrome.

SELF-HELP USES

- **Acidity with gastritis**, p. 307.
- **Arthritis associated with acid indigestion or a peptic ulcer**, p. 313.
- **Heartburn**, p. 317.

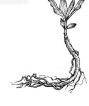

GENTIAN
An erect perennial growing to 4 ft (1.2 m) with star-shaped yellow flowers and oval leaves.

Gentiana lutea (Gentianaceae)

GENTIAN

GENTIAN IS A POWERFUL BITTER, and the herb is an essential ingredient of traditional aperitifs and bitters such as Angostura bitters. The customary aperitif about half an hour before a meal is more than a social nicety – the bitter constituents stimulate gastric juices and prime the stomach, enabling it to cope effectively with a heavy meal. Medicinally, gentian strengthens a weak or underactive digestive system.

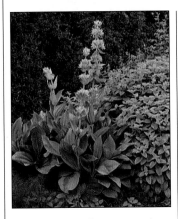

Gentian is a tall, attractive plant and has been cultivated in gardens at least since the time of the 16th-century herbalist Gerard.

HABITAT & CULTIVATION

This largest member of the diverse gentian family is native to the Alps and other mountainous regions of central and southern Europe from Spain to the Balkans, flourishing at altitudes of 2,300–8,000 ft (700–2,400 m). The large root crowns can be split, or, alternatively, the plant can be readily grown from seed. It needs a loamy soil and a sheltered position. The root is dug up in early autumn and dried as quickly as possible.

RELATED SPECIES

Many gentian species are bitter-tasting plants, and a number are used in herbal medicine as a result – for example, Japanese gentian (*G. scabra*) and qin jiao (*G. macrophylla*, p. 214).

KEY CONSTITUENTS

■ Bitter principles (gentiopicroside, amarogentin)
■ Gentianose

■ Inulin
■ Pectin
■ Phenolic acids

KEY ACTIONS

■ Bitter
■ Digestive stimulant
■ Eases stomach pain

RESEARCH

■ **Amarogentin** Although present in much smaller quantities than gentiopicroside, amarogentin is the constituent largely responsible for the bitterness of gentian. It is 3,000 times more bitter than gentiopicroside, and, tasted at dilutions of 1:50,000, it is possibly the most bitter substance on the planet.

TRADITIONAL & CURRENT USES

■ **Origin of the name** Gentius, king of Illyria in the 2nd century BC, reputedly discovered the virtues of the plant. The name gentian attests to its use in classical times.
■ **Action of bitter principles** There are 4 main taste receptors on the tongue – sweet, sour, salt, and bitter. It has been shown that the bitter principles in gentian stimulate the bitter taste receptors on the tongue, causing an increase in the production of saliva and gastric secretions. This in turn stimulates the appetite and improves the action of the digestive system in general.
■ **Digestive stimulant** By stimulating the action of the stomach, many symptoms associated with a weak digestion such as gas, indigestion, and poor appetite are relieved.

PARTS USED

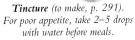

Fresh root

Root *is harvested in autumn for use in remedies to improve the digestion.*

Root contains bitter principles

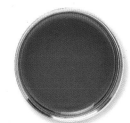

Dried chopped root

KEY PREPARATIONS & THEIR USES

Caution Do not take if suffering from acid indigestion and peptic ulcer.

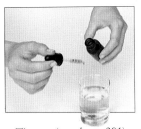

Tincture *(to make, p. 291). For poor appetite, take 2–5 drops with water before meals.*

Decoction *(to make, p. 290). For anemia and weakened digestion, take 25 ml 3–5 times a day.*

Stomach and other secretions are improved, which in turn helps to increase the absorption of nutrients. The herb also acts as a stimulant on the gallbladder and liver, encouraging them to function more efficiently. Gentian is therefore useful in almost any condition where the digestive system needs to be toned up. It is often taken as a digestive tonic in old age.
■ **Nutrient absorption** By improving digestive function, gentian increases the absorption of nutrients across the gut wall. It aids the absorption of a wide range of nutrients, including iron and vitamin B_{12}, and is therefore useful for iron-deficiency anemia (usually resulting from blood loss). It is often added to prescriptions for women with heavy menstrual bleeding.

SELF-HELP USES

■ **Anemia**, p. 301.
■ **Fever**, p. 311.
■ **Gas & bloating**, p. 306.
■ **Weakened digestion**, p. 319.

KEY MEDICINAL PLANTS

Ginkgo biloba (Ginkgoaceae)
GINKGO, MAIDENHAIR TREE, BAI GUO (CHINESE)

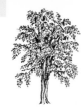

GINKGO
A deciduous tree with one or several main trunks and spreading branches. It grows to 100 ft (30 m).

GINKGO IS THOUGHT TO BE the oldest tree on the planet, first growing about 190 million years ago. Though it has long been used as a medicine in its native China, its therapeutic actions have only recently been researched. The leaves (and their extract) are used to treat poor circulation to the brain and to maintain a plentiful blood flow to the central nervous system. Ginkgo is also valuable for asthma.

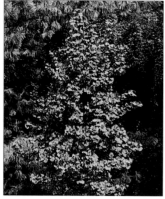

***Ginkgo trees** are widely cultivated for their leaves, which are an excellent herbal remedy for poor memory and dementia.*

HABITAT & CULTIVATION
Native to China and possibly to Japan, ginkgo trees are grown on large plantations in China, France, and South Carolina. They produce green to yellow fan-shaped leaves with radiating veins, and round fruits about 1 in (3 cm) across that contain a single seed. The leaves and fruit are harvested in autumn.

KEY CONSTITUENTS
- Flavonoids
- Ginkgolides
- Bilobalides

KEY ACTIONS
- Circulatory stimulant & tonic
- Antiasthmatic
- Antispasmodic
- Antiallergenic
- Anti-inflammatory

RESEARCH
- **Circulation** Extensive research since the 1960s has established the importance of ginkgo in improving poor cerebral circulation, aiding memory and concentration, and helping in cases of dementia.
- **Anti-inflammatory action** Ginkgo's ability to reduce inflammation may make it valuable in the future for conditions as varied as auto-immune problems, multiple sclerosis, and organ transplants.
- **Platelet activating factor** Research into ginkgo has led to the understanding of a new branch of human physiology. Ginkgo inhibits platelet activating factor (PAF), a substance released by a range of blood cells. PAF causes the blood to become stickier and therefore more likely to produce blood clots, and it also makes various inflammatory and allergenic changes take place.

TRADITIONAL & CURRENT USES
- **Chinese herbal medicine** Ginkgo seeds are used to relieve wheezing and to lessen phlegm. They are also given to treat vaginal discharge, a weak bladder, and incontinence. The leaves are traditionally used for treating asthma.
- **Western herbal medicine** Western interest in ginkgo has concentrated on the remarkable ability of the leaves to improve the circulation, especially poor circulation to the brain, and the herb's antiallergenic and anti-inflammatory actions, which make it a particularly useful remedy for the treatment of asthma. Ginkgo is the best selling herbal medicine in France and Germany, where

❖ PARTS USED

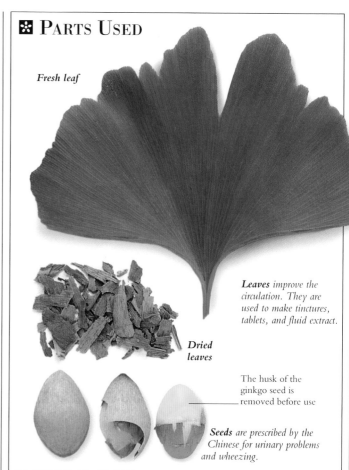

Fresh leaf

***Leaves** improve the circulation. They are used to make tinctures, tablets, and fluid extract.*

Dried leaves

The husk of the ginkgo seed is removed before use

***Seeds** are prescribed by the Chinese for urinary problems and wheezing.*

✍ KEY PREPARATIONS & THEIR USES

Cautions Do not exceed the dose. May cause toxic reactions if taken to excess. Restricted herb in some countries.

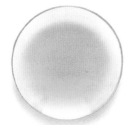

***Tincture** of leaves (to make, p. 291). For poor circulation, take 1 tsp 2–3 times a day with water.*

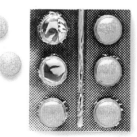

***Tablets** Take for poor circulation and memory loss.*

DECOCTION of the seeds is used by herbalists to treat wheezing.

FLUID EXTRACT An extract from the fresh leaves is prescribed by medical herbalists for asthma.

it is taken daily by millions of people from middle age onward to maintain and improve cerebral circulation and the memory and to reduce the possibility of a stroke. It is probably one of the most useful herbs for the treatment of senile dementia.

SELF-HELP USES
- **Failing memory**, p. 319.
- **High blood pressure & arteriosclerosis**, p. 301.

LICORICE
A woody-stemmed perennial growing to 6 ft (2 m), with dark leaves and cream to mauve flowers.

Glycyrrhiza glabra (*Leguminosae*)
LICORICE

WITH A CONSTITUENT – glycyrrhizic acid – that is 50 times sweeter than sugar, it is not surprising that licorice is mainly thought of as a candy. Yet it is also one of the most valuable of all herbal medicines, a powerful anti-inflammatory that is effective in conditions as varied as arthritis and canker sores. It is among the most used herbs in European medicine and has been taken medicinally for several thousand years.

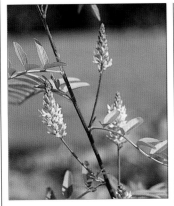

Licorice has pealike cream flowers in summer. It is cultivated commercially for its roots.

HABITAT & CULTIVATION

Growing wild in southeastern Europe and southwestern Asia, licorice is now extensively cultivated. It is propagated by dividing the roots in spring. The root of 3–4-year-old plants is unearthed in late autumn.

RELATED SPECIES

Various *Glycyrrhiza* species are used medicinally in a similar way to licorice. See *gan cao* (*G. uralensis*, p. 215).

KEY CONSTITUENTS

- Triterpene saponins (glycyrrhizin, up to 6%)
- Flavonoids (isoflavones: liquiritin, isoliquiritin, formononetin)
- Polysaccharides
- Sterols
- Coumarins
- Asparagin

KEY ACTIONS

- Anti-inflammatory
- Expectorant
- Demulcent
- Adrenal agent
- Mild laxative

RESEARCH

- **Adrenal agent** Research shows that on being broken down in the gut, glycyrrhizin has an anti-inflammatory and antiarthritic action similar to hydrocortisone and other corticosteroid hormones. It stimulates the production of hormones by the adrenal glands and reduces the breakdown of steroids by the liver and kidneys.
- **Glycyrrhizin** Research in Japan in 1985 showed that glycyrrhizin was effective in the treatment of chronic hepatitis and liver cirrhosis.
- **Protective mucus** Licorice as a whole reduces stomach secretions but produces a thick protective mucus for the lining of the stomach, making it a useful remedy in inflammatory stomach conditions.
- **Isoflavones** The isoflavones are known to be estrogenic.

TRADITIONAL & CURRENT USES

- **Traditional uses** Licorice has long been valued for its medicinal uses. It was taken in ancient Greece for asthma, chest problems, and canker sores.
- **Soothing herb** Inflammatory conditions of the digestive system, such as canker sores, gastritis, peptic ulceration, and excessive acid problems, benefit from licorice's demulcent and healing properties, as do many chest complaints, arthritis, inflamed joints, and some skin problems. Licorice is also soothing for inflamed eyes.

✿ PARTS USED

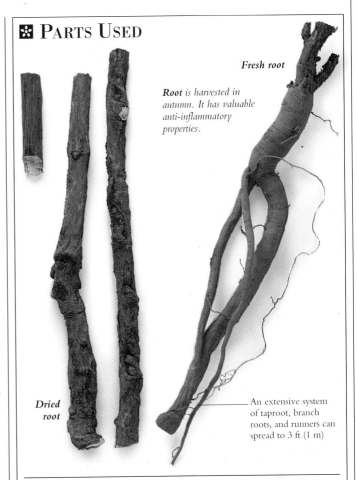

Fresh root

Root is harvested in autumn. It has valuable anti-inflammatory properties.

Dried root

An extensive system of taproot, branch roots, and runners can spread to 3 ft (1 m)

🍵 KEY PREPARATIONS & THEIR USES

Caution Do not take if anemic, suffering from high blood pressure, or in pregnancy.

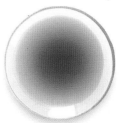

Tincture (to make, p. 291). For gastritis, add ½ tsp to 100 ml water and take twice a day.

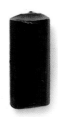

Dried juice stick Chew for indigestion.

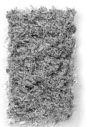

Powder Gently rub onto canker sores.

🥣 **DECOCTION** For constipation, make a decoction (see p. 290) with 1 part licorice and 3 parts dandelion root. Drink 1 cup twice a day.

💧 **FLUID EXTRACT** is prescribed for peptic ulcers.

- **Adrenal stimulation** Licorice stimulates the adrenal glands, helping in Addison's disease where the adrenal glands cease to function normally.
- **Constipation** Licorice is useful as a gentle laxative.

SELF-HELP USES

- **Canker sores**, p. 306.
- **Constipation**, p. 307.
- **Coughs & bronchitis**, p. 310.
- **Loss of appetite & vomiting**, p. 306.
- **Oral thrush**, p. 307.

Hamamelis virginiana (Hamamelidaceae)
WITCH HAZEL

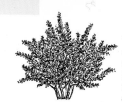

WITCH HAZEL
A small deciduous tree growing to 15 ft (5 m), with coarsely toothed, broadly oval leaves.

WITCH HAZEL WAS A traditional remedy of many Native North American people. They used poultices soaked in a decoction of bark to treat tumors and inflammations, especially of the eye, and took the herb internally for hemorrhaging and heavy menstrual bleeding. European settlers in the 18th century soon came to value witch hazel for its astringency, and its use spread to Europe and beyond.

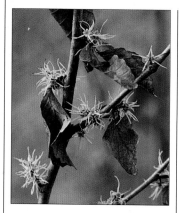

Witch hazel produces distinctive flowers in winter followed by brown fruit capsules that, when ripe, eject 2 seeds up to 12 ft (4 m) away from the tree.

HABITAT & CULTIVATION

Witch hazel is a woodland tree, indigenous to Canada and eastern parts of the US. Today it is commonly cultivated in Europe. The trees are grown from hardwood cuttings or from seed, both of which are planted in autumn. The leaves are gathered in summer and dried. The bark is harvested during the autumn and dried as quickly as possible in the shade.

OTHER SPECIES

European hazel (*Corylus avellana*) is a similar herb. It is used occasionally in European herbal medicine as an astringent to treat diarrhea. The oil is nutritious and can be used to treat threadworms in children.

KEY CONSTITUENTS

- Tannins (8–10%)
- Flavonoids
- Bitter principle
- Volatile oil (leaves only)

KEY ACTIONS

- Astringent
- Anti-inflammatory
- Stops external and internal bleeding

TRADITIONAL & CURRENT USES

■ **Established properties** Witch hazel contains large quantities of tannins. These have a drying, astringent effect, causing the tightening up of proteins in the skin and across the surface of abrasions. This creates a protective covering that increases resistance to inflammation and promotes healing of broken skin. Witch hazel also appears to help damaged blood vessels beneath the skin. It is thought that this effect may be due to the flavonoids as well as to the tannins. When witch hazel is distilled it retains its astringency, suggesting that astringent agents other than tannins are present.

■ **Skin problems** Witch hazel is a very useful herb for inflamed and tender skin conditions, such as eczema. It is mainly used where the skin has not been significantly broken and helps to protect the affected area and prevent infection.

■ **Damaged veins** Witch hazel is valuable for damaged facial veins, varicose veins, and hemorrhoids, and is an effective remedy for bruises. Due to its astringent properties, it helps to tighten distended veins and restore their normal structure.

■ **Other uses** A lotion can be applied to the skin for under-lying problems such as cysts or tumors. Witch hazel also makes

❋ PARTS USED

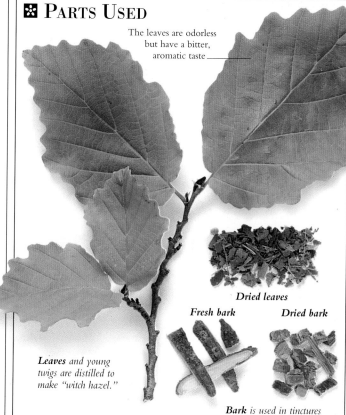

The leaves are odorless but have a bitter, aromatic taste

Dried leaves

Fresh bark

Dried bark

Leaves and young twigs are distilled to make "witch hazel."

Bark is used in tinctures and ointments.

✎ KEY PREPARATIONS & THEIR USES

Caution Take only under professional supervision.

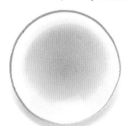

Tincture of bark (to make, p. 291). Dilute 20 ml in 400 ml cold water and sponge onto varicose veins.

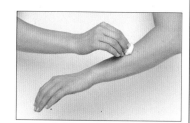

Distilled witch hazel Dab onto insect stings, sore skin, and broken veins.

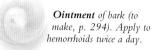

Ointment of bark (to make, p. 294). Apply to hemorrhoids twice a day.

⛵ **INFUSION** of the leaves (to make, p. 290). Use as a lotion for broken veins and cysts.

an effective eyewash for inflammation of the eyes. Less commonly, it is taken internally to alleviate diarrhea, helping to tighten up the mucous membranes of the intestines, and for bleeding of any kind.

SELF-HELP USES

- **Bruises**, p. 304.
- **Cleansing wounds**, p. 304.
- **Eczema**, p. 300.
- **Hemorrhoids**, p. 302.
- **Varicose veins**, p. 303.
- **Weeping skin**, p. 302.

Harpagophytum procumbens (Pedaliaceae)

DEVIL'S CLAW

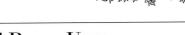

DEVIL'S CLAW
A trailing perennial, reaching 5 ft (1.5 m) in length, with fleshy lobed leaves and barbed, woody fruit.

THE COLORFUL NAME of this African plant is derived from the appearance of its tough, barbed fruit. The medicinal properties of devil's claw were first discovered by various southern African peoples, who used a decoction of the tuber to treat digestive problems and arthritis. The herb is now widely available in pharmacies and health food stores in the West as a remedy for arthritis and rheumatism.

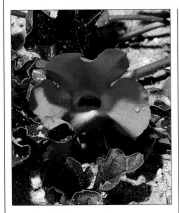

Devil's claw, found growing in the Transvaal, has bright purple flowers in spring.

HABITAT & CULTIVATION

Devil's claw is native to southern and eastern Africa, and is found most commonly on the veldt of the Transvaal. It thrives in clay or sandy soils, preferring roadsides and wasteground, especially places where natural vegetation has been cleared. Propagated from seed in spring, the young tubers are unearthed in autumn and cut into pieces about ¾ in (2 cm) long. Care is taken not to mix the tubers, which contain the active constituents, with the roots, since this can render the herb ineffective.

RELATED SPECIES

Two related species, both growing in Africa, are used medicinally in a more or less similar way to devil's claw.

KEY CONSTITUENTS

- Iridoid glycosides (harpagoside)
- Sugars (stachyose)
- Phytosterols
- Flavonoids
- Harpagoquinone

KEY ACTIONS

- Anti-inflammatory
- Analgesic
- Digestive stimulant

RESEARCH

- **Anti-inflammatory** French research (1992) indicated that devil's claw is anti-inflammatory, but opinion is divided on its effectiveness in practice.
- **Pain relief** There is some evidence to confirm devil claw's use as an analgesic, since it seems to be effective in easing the symptoms of joint pain.
- **Bitter** The strongly bitter action of devil's claw stimulates and tones the digestive system. Many arthritic conditions are associated with poor digestion and absorption of food, and the stimulant effect of this herb on the stomach and gallbladder contributes to its overall therapeutic value as an anti-arthritic remedy.

TRADITIONAL & CURRENT USES

- **African traditional remedy** Devil's claw is used by various peoples in southern Africa, including the Khoikhoin and the Bantu. Traditionally it has been used as a tonic, especially for digestive problems; for arthritis and rheumatism; to reduce fevers; and as an ointment for sores, ulcers, and boils.
- **Western uses** Current Western use of devil's claw is broadly in line with its traditional application. It is commonly available over the counter in tablet form for arthritic and rheumatic conditions and can bring relief from pain arising from a range of joint and muscular problems, including gout, back pain, fibrositis, and rheumatoid arthritis.

❊ PARTS USED

Tuber is harvested in autumn and used in a variety of antiarthritic preparations.

Sliced dried tuber

Chopped dried tuber

🖾 KEY PREPARATIONS & THEIR USES

Cautions Do not take if suffering from a stomach or duodenal ulcer. Do not take during pregnancy.

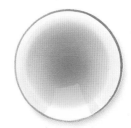

Decoction *(to make, p. 290). For rheumatism, simmer 1 tsp root in 1 cup water for 15 minutes. Take in small doses over 1–2 days.*

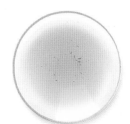

Tincture *(to make, p. 291). For arthritis associated with poor digestion, take 30 drops with water twice daily.*

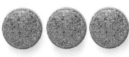

Tablets *Take for arthritis and rheumatism.*

SELF-HELP USES

- **Arthritis & inflamed joints**, p. 313.
- **Back pain due to joint inflammation**, p. 313.

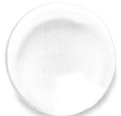

HOPS
A tall, climbing perennial growing up to 22 ft (7 m). Hop plants are either male or female.

Humulus lupulus (Cannabaceae)
HOPS

THE BITTER TASTE OF HOPS, which is well known to beer drinkers, largely accounts for this herb's ability to strengthen and stimulate the digestion. Hops are also sedative and make a valuable remedy for sleeplessness and excitability. When the plant was first used to brew beer in England in the 16th century, it aroused great opposition: a petition to Parliament described it as "a wicked weed" that would "endanger the people."

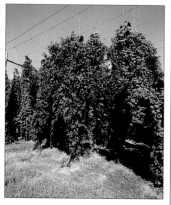

Hops have been cultivated for brewing beer since at least the 11th century. The bines (stems) are trained up raised wire runners.

HABITAT & CULTIVATION

Indigenous to Europe and Asia, hops flourish there on dumps and along roadsides. They are grown commercially throughout northern Europe. Flowers of the female plant (strobiles) are picked in early autumn and dried at a low temperature.

RELATED SPECIES

Hops are related to marijuana (*Cannabis sativa*, p. 180).

KEY CONSTITUENTS

- Bitter principles (lupulin containing humulon, lupulon, and valerianic acid)

- Volatile oil (1%), humulene
- Flavonoids
- Polyphenolic tannins
- Estrogenic substances
- Asparagin

KEY ACTIONS

- Sedative
- Soporific
- Antispasmodic
- Aromatic bitter

RESEARCH

- **Bitter principles** The bitter principles as a whole strongly stimulate the digestive system, increasing gastric and other secretions. A number of constituents, such as valerianic acid, are sedative, though it is not yet fully understood how they work. Lupulon and humulon are antiseptic.
- **Other research** The herb relaxes smooth muscle and is believed to have an estrogenic effect. Some isolated constituents are thought to depress central nervous activity.

TRADITIONAL & CURRENT USES

- **Historical uses** Hops feature only occasionally in early herbals, and the health benefits ascribed to them are similar to our understanding today.
- **Sedative** The herb is used mostly for its sedative effect. A sachet placed inside a bed pillow releases an aroma that calms the mind. Hops help to reduce irritability and restlessness and promote a good night's sleep.
- **Tension** Blended with other herbs, hops are good for stress, anxiety, tension, and headaches, though they should not be used if depression is a factor. The antispasmodic action also makes them useful for certain types of asthma and for menstrual pain.
- **Aid to digestion** Hops are beneficial for the digestion, increasing stomach secretions and relaxing spasms and colic.

SELF-HELP USE

- **Insomnia**, p. 309.

❖ PARTS USED

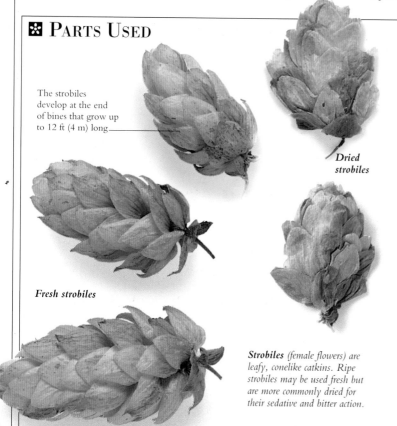

The strobiles develop at the end of bines that grow up to 12 ft (4 m) long

Dried strobiles

Fresh strobiles

Strobiles (female flowers) are leafy, conelike catkins. Ripe strobiles may be used fresh but are more commonly dried for their sedative and bitter action.

☙ KEY PREPARATIONS & THEIR USES

Caution Do not take if suffering from depression.

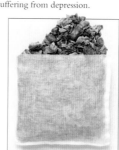

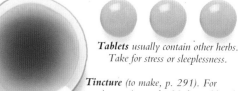

Infusion (to make, p. 290). For insomnia, drink 1 cup at night.

Sachet Make a sachet with 100 g dried herb. Put inside a pillow to aid sleep.

Tablets usually contain other herbs. Take for stress or sleeplessness.

Tincture (to make, p. 291). For excessive anxiety, take 20 drops diluted in a glass of water 3 times a day. For digestive headaches, take 10 drops with water up to 5 times a day.

CAPSULES (to make, p. 291). To stimulate the appetite, take a 500 mg capsule 3 times a day before meals.

Hydrastis canadensis (Ranunculaceae)

GOLDENSEAL

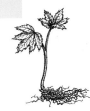

GOLDENSEAL
A small herbaceous perennial, with a thick yellow root and an erect stem growing to 1 ft (30 cm).

GOLDENSEAL IS A NORTH AMERICAN remedy, prized during the 19th century as a cure-all. The Cherokee and other Native Americans used it, mixed with bear fat as an insect repellent, and they also made it into a lotion for wounds, ulcers, and sore, inflamed eyes. It was given internally for stomach and liver problems. Today it is employed as an astringent, antibacterial remedy for the mucous membranes of the body.

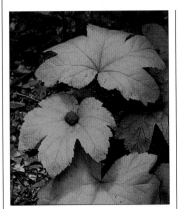

Goldenseal is an unusual-looking plant with a single, red, inedible fruit.

HABITAT & CULTIVATION

Goldenseal grows wild in moist mountainous woodland areas of North America and prefers soil that is well covered with dead leaves. Due to excessive harvesting, goldenseal is now rare in its natural habitat and has to be cultivated, but to flourish, it requires an environment very similar to its native habitat. It is propagated by root division. Rhizomes from 3-year-old plants are dug up in the autumn and dried in the open air on cloth.

KEY CONSTITUENTS

- Isoquinoline alkaloids (hydrastine, berberine, canadine)
- Volatile oil
- Resin

KEY ACTIONS

- Tonic
- Mild laxative
- Anti-inflammatory
- Antibacterial
- Bitter
- Uterine stimulant
- Stops internal bleeding
- Astringent

RESEARCH

- **Alkaloids** For an herb with such a tremendous medicinal reputation, there has been very little research into its pharmacology, but it is known that goldenseal's medicinal actions are due largely to the isoqinoline alkaloids.
- **Hydrastine** Research in Canada in the late 1960s showed that hydrastine constricts the blood vessels and stimulates the autonomic nervous system.
- **Berberine** Berberine is bitter, antibacterial, and amebicidal. It also has a sedative action on the central nervous system.
- **Canadine** Research shows that this alkaloid stimulates the muscles of the uterus.

TRADITIONAL & CURRENT USES

- **Mucous membranes** Most authorities agree that goldenseal is a potent remedy for disorders affecting mucous membranes of the body, notably of the eye, ear, nose and throat, the stomach and intestines, and the vagina.
- **Countering infection** As a dilute infusion, goldenseal can be used as an eyewash and as a mouthwash for infected gums. It is an extremely effective wash or douche for yeast infections and other vaginal infections generally. The infusion is also valued as a remedy for psoriasis.
- **Digestive problems** Taken internally, goldenseal increases digestive secretions, astringes the mucous membranes that line the gut, and checks inflammation. It should not be taken for extended periods of time since it reduces the gut's capacity to absorb some nutrients, notably B vitamins.
- **Gynecological uses** Goldenseal helps to reduce heavy menstrual bleeding and is used by herbal practitioners and midwives to help stop bleeding following childbirth (postpartum hemorrhage). Goldenseal should not be taken during pregnancy.

☙ PARTS USED

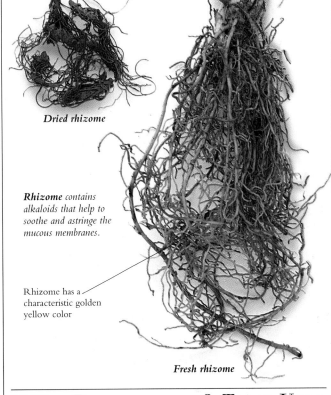

Dried rhizome

Rhizome contains alkaloids that help to soothe and astringe the mucous membranes.

Rhizome has a characteristic golden yellow color

Fresh rhizome

☙ KEY PREPARATIONS & THEIR USES

Cautions Toxic if taken to excess. Do not take if suffering from high blood pressure. Do not take during pregnancy or while breast-feeding.

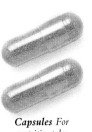

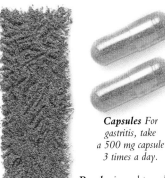

Capsules For gastritis, take a 500 mg capsule 3 times a day.

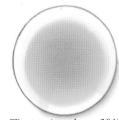

Tincture (to make, p. 291). For excess mucus, take 20 drops with water 3 times a day.

Powder is used to make capsules (see p. 291).

DECOCTION (to make, p. 290). For sore throats, gargle with 50 ml 3–4 times a day.

INFUSION of powder (to make, p. 290). For yeast infections, apply 150 ml.

Hypericum perforatum (Guttiferae)
St. John's Wort, Y Fendigedig (Welsh)

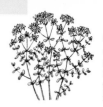

St. John's Wort
An erect perennial growing to 32 in (80 cm) with bright yellow flowers in a flat-topped cluster.

St. John's wort flowers at the time of the summer solstice, and in medieval Europe it was considered to have powerful magical properties that enabled it to repel evil. Medicinally, it was used to treat emotional and nervous complaints. In the 19th century the herb fell into disuse, but recent research has brought it back into prominence as an extremely valuable remedy for nervous problems.

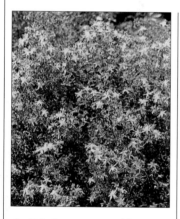

St. John's wort *was a folk remedy for insanity in the Middle Ages.*

HABITAT & CULTIVATION
Native to Britain and Europe, St. John's wort now grows wild throughout much of the world. It is found in meadows, on banks, and by roadsides, and prefers sunny positions and chalky soils. It can be grown from seed in spring or by dividing the rootstock in autumn. The flowering tops are harvested in midsummer.

RELATED SPECIES
A number of *Hypericum* species contain hypericin, but in smaller quantities than St. John's wort.

KEY CONSTITUENTS
- Volatile oil (carophyllene)
- Hypericin & pseudohypericin
- Flavonoids

KEY ACTIONS
- Antidepressant
- Antispasmodic
- Stimulates bile flow
- Astringent
- Sedative
- Relieves pain
- Antiviral

RESEARCH
- **Depression** In a recent research study in Austria, 67% of patients with mild to moderate depression improved when given an extract of St. John's wort. This confirmed findings of earlier trials that showed the herb to be good for depression.
- **Hypericin** The red color of the oil is due to products of hypericin. This constituent is antidepressant and so strongly antiviral that it is being researched for use in treating HIV and AIDS.
- **Whole herb** Research shows that the whole herb is effective against many viral infections.

TRADITIONAL & CURRENT USES
- **Nervous complaints** St. John's wort is one of the most valuable European medicinal plants for nervous problems. Herbalists have long used it as a tonic for anxiety, tension, insomnia, and depression – particularly that associated with menopause.
- **Menopause** The herb is especially helpful for menopausal problems, alleviating the symptoms of hormonal change and treating decreased vitality.
- **Tonic properties** St. John's wort is a valuable tonic for the liver and gallbladder.
- **Infused oil** The red oil is an excellent antiseptic. Externally, it is used for wounds and burns and to relieve cramp and nerve pain. Internally, the oil may be taken for peptic ulcers and gastric inflammation. Its antiviral, anti-inflammatory, and healing powers work just as well within the body as externally.

✱ PARTS USED

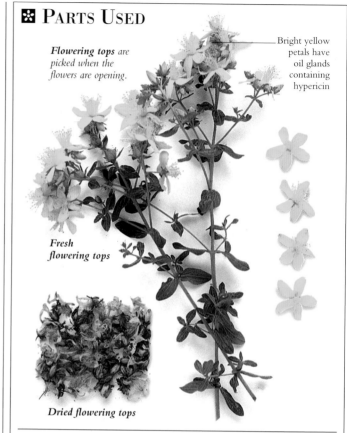

Flowering tops are picked when the flowers are opening.

Bright yellow petals have oil glands containing hypericin

Fresh flowering tops

Dried flowering tops

✍ KEY PREPARATIONS & THEIR USES

Cautions Can cause sensitivity to sunlight. Restricted herb in some countries.

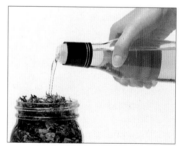

Infused oil is made by steeping the herb in oil for 6 weeks (see p. 293). Dab onto minor wounds and burns.

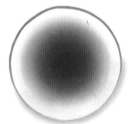

Cream *(to make, p. 295). For cramps or neuralgia, rub onto the affected part.*

Tincture *(to make, p. 291). For depression, take ½ tsp with water 3 times a day.*

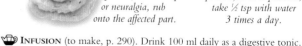

INFUSION (to make, p. 290). Drink 100 ml daily as a digestive tonic.

SELF-HELP USES
- **Anxiety, depression, & tension**, p. 308.
- **Back pain**, p. 313.
- **Bites & stings**, p. 303.
- **Cold sores, chickenpox & shingles**, p. 304.
- **Depression & decreased vitality due to menopause**, p. 316.
- **Neuralgia**, p. 308.
- **Stiff & aching joints**, p. 313.
- **Tired & aching muscles**, p. 312.

Inula helenium (Compositae)

ELECAMPANE

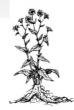

PRIZED BY THE ROMANS as a medicine and as a food, this herb derives its botanical name from Helen of Troy, who, according to legend, was holding elecampane in her hand when she set off with Paris to live with him in Troy. The root has long been considered to be a gently warming and tonic herb, and is particularly useful for chronic bronchitis and other respiratory problems.

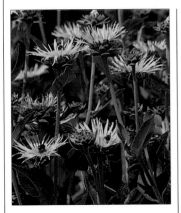

"Elecampane will the spirits sustain," is a medieval saying. It reflects the herb's tonic properties.

HABITAT & CULTIVATION

Native to southeastern Europe and western Asia, elecampane now grows in many temperate regions, including parts of the US. It is also cultivated. Propagated from seed in spring or by root division, it prefers moist, well-drained ground. The root is unearthed in the autumn, cut up, and then dried at a high temperature.

RELATED SPECIES

Xuan fu hua (*I. japonica*, p. 221) grows in China and Japan. Other relatives used medicinally include sunflower (*Helianthus annuus*), common fleabane (*Pulicaria dysenterica*), and echinacea (*Echinacea* spp, p. 90).

KEY CONSTITUENTS

- Inulin (up to 44%)
- Volatile oil (up to 4%), containing alantol and sesquiterpene lactones (including alantolactone)
- Triterpene saponins (dammaranedienol)

- Sterols
- Polyacetylenes

KEY ACTIONS

- Expectorant
- Soothes coughing
- Increases sweating
- Mildly bitter
- Eliminates worms
- Antiseptic

RESEARCH

- **Inulin** Inulin was first isolated from elecampane in 1804 and took its name from the herb. It has mucilaginous qualities that help soothe the bronchial linings.
- **Alantolactone** This constituent is thought to be anti-inflammatory. It also reduces mucous secretions and stimulates the immune system.
- **Whole herb** As a whole, the herb has a stimulant, expectorant effect, encouraging the coughing up of mucus from the lungs. The volatile oil is known to be partly responsible for this and also for the herb's antiseptic properties.

TRADITIONAL & CURRENT USES

- **Chest infections** Elecampane has long been valued as a tonic herb for the respiratory system. Its warming effect on the lungs, combined with its ability to gently stimulate the coughing up and clearing of mucus from the chest, makes it a safe remedy for young and old. Elecampane can be used in almost all chesty conditions, and is very useful when the patient is debilitated.
- **Chronic chest complaints** Elecampane's attributes have led to its specific use for chronic bronchitis and bronchial asthma.

✴ PARTS USED

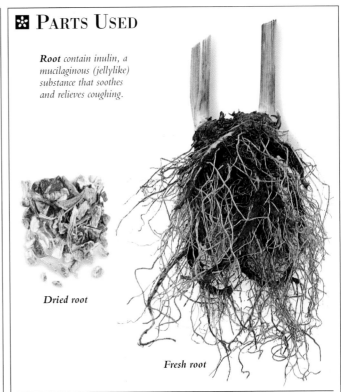

Root contain inulin, a mucilaginous (jellylike) substance that soothes and relieves coughing.

Dried root

Fresh root

✍ KEY PREPARATIONS & THEIR USES

Cautions Can cause skin reactions. Do not take internally in pregnancy or if breast-feeding.

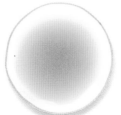

Decoction (to make, p. 290) For irritable coughs, take ½ cup 2–3 times a day.

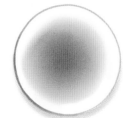

Tincture (to make, p. 291). For bronchitis, mix 50 ml with 50 ml thyme tincture. Take 1 tsp 3 times a day.

☞ **SYRUP** For coughs, make an infusion (see p. 290) and simmer until it has reduced to half the volume, before adding the sugar or honey (to make, p. 292). Take 1–2 tsp every 2 hours.

It is particularly useful because it both soothes the bronchial tube linings and is an expectorant. In addition, the herb is mildly bitter, helping recovery by improving digestion and the absorption of nutrients.

- **Digestive problems** Elecampane has been taken traditionally as a tonic herb for the digestion. It stimulates the appetite and relieves dyspepsia. It is a useful remedy for the treatment of worms.
- **Infection** In the past, elecampane was used in the treatment of tuberculosis. It combines well with other antiseptic herbs and is used for infections such as flu and tonsillitis. Its restorative, tonic action complements its ability to counter infection.

SELF-HELP USE

- **Coughs & bronchitis**, p. 310.

Jateorhiza palmata syn. *J. calumba* (Menispermaceae)

CALUMBA

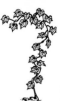

CALUMBA
A twining perennial growing to 50 ft (15 m) with large palmlike leaves and green-white flowers.

A PROFOUNDLY BITTER HERB, the root of the calumba vine is an East African herbal remedy traditionally used as a digestive tonic, and to treat a variety of digestive infections, including dysentery. It stimulates the appetite and digestive activity, making it a valuable herbal medicine in the treatment of anorexia nervosa. Calumba has a soft, slippery texture and, as might be expected, a strongly bitter taste.

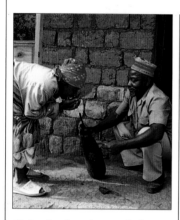

Calumba decoction, made from the root, is a traditional East African cure for digestive problems.

HABITAT & CULTIVATION

Calumba is a creeping vine, native to the rainforests of East Africa, especially Mozambique and Madagascar. It grows to a great height, often reaching the tops of trees. Calumba is cultivated in other tropical regions and also in Europe. It is grown from seed planted in spring and trained along supports. The root is dug up in dry weather in early spring.

KEY CONSTITUENTS

- Isoquinoline alkaloids (palmatine, columbamine, jatrorrhizine)
- Bitter principles (furanoditerpenol, palmanin)
- Volatile oil (up to 1% – mostly thymol)
- Mucilage

KEY ACTIONS

- Bitter
- Eases stomach pain
- Tonic
- Reduces fever
- Expels worms

RESEARCH

■ **Isoquinoline alkaloids**
Research in Singapore in 1986 indicated that 2 of the isquinoline alkaloids, palmatine and jatrorrhizine, reduce blood pressure. In addition, palmatine is a uterine stimulant, while jatrorrhizine is sedative and antifungal. The isoquinoline alkaloids are similar in action to those present in barberry (*Berberis vulgaris*, p. 175) and goldenseal (*Hydrastis canadensis*, p. 103).

TRADITIONAL & CURRENT USES

■ **Bitter properties** Calumba's bitter properties are due to its bitter principles and, to a lesser extent, its isoquinoline alkaloids. These stimulate specific taste receptors on the tongue that in turn stimulate secretion of digestive juices. One of the bitterest of all plants, calumba has much in common with gentian (*Gentiana lutea*, p. 97), although it owes its bitterness to a different range of constituents. Unlike many bitter herbs, calumba contains very little volatile oil and no tannins (which give astringency) and is therefore always classed as a "pure bitter."
■ **Digestive problems** By making the stomach more acidic (and therefore hostile to pathogens), calumba helps to prevent digestive infections. It increases the level of digestive secretions, thereby improving the breakdown and absorption of food. Calumba also relieves indigestion when this results from deficient digestive

secretions – in particular, reduced stomach acid levels.
■ **Loss of appetite** The pure bitter action of calumba makes it an extremely good remedy, not only for a weakened or under-active digestion but also for poor appetite. Calumba is used specifically to treat loss of appetite and anorexia nervosa.
■ **Chronic illness** As with other bitter herbs, calumba is useful in the treatment of many chronic illnesses. Taken regularly before meals (preferably in tincture form), it tones the digestion and

improves the absorption of nutrients. It is particularly helpful in the treatment of chronic fatigue syndrome, which is often associated with deficient stomach acid production.
■ **Other uses** Calumba is given to treat dysentery, being used traditionally for this purpose in East Africa, and to expel worms. Although this herb should generally be avoided during pregnancy, small doses have been prescribed to relieve morning sickness.

✿ PARTS USED

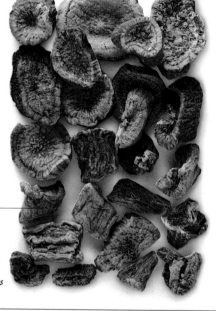

Root of the calumba vine is harvested in dry weather and dried.

The bitter constituents in the root stimulate the appetite

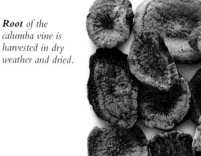

Dried root slices

☙ KEY PREPARATIONS & THEIR USES

Caution Do not take during pregnancy.

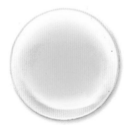

Decoction is best with other herbs. For indigestion, make a decoction (see p. 290) with 5 g calumba, 10 g sweet flag, and 750 ml water. Take ½ cup twice daily.

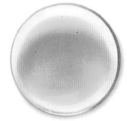

Tincture (to make, see p. 291) is a strong digestive stimulant and tonic. For a weak digestion, take 20 drops with water 2–3 times a day before meals.

Lavandula officinalis syn. *L. angustifolia (Labiatae)*

LAVENDER

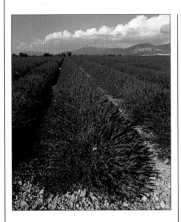

LAVENDER
A perennial shrub growing to 3 ft (1 m), with spikes of violet-blue flowers extending above the foliage.

LAVENDER IS AN IMPORTANT relaxing herb, but it is better known for its sweet-scented aroma than for its medicinal properties. It became popular as a medicine during the late Middle Ages, and in 1620 it was one of the medicinal herbs taken to the New World by the Pilgrims. It was described by the herbalist John Parkinson (1640) as being of "especiall good use for all griefes and paines of the head and brain."

Lavender is widely cultivated for perfume and medicinal use.

HABITAT & CULTIVATION

Native to France and the western Mediterranean, lavender is cultivated worldwide for its volatile oil, and is grown as a garden plant as far north as Norway. It is propagated from seed or cuttings and needs a sunny position. The flowers are picked in the morning in midsummer and are dried or are distilled to produce essential oil.

RELATED SPECIES

Spike lavender (*L. spica*) yields more oil than *L. officinalis*, but of an inferior quality. *L. stoechas* is used as an antiseptic wash for wounds, ulcers, and sores in Spain and Portugal. Its oil is also inferior to that of *L. officinalis*.

KEY CONSTITUENTS

- Volatile oil (up to 3%) containing over 40 constituents, including linalyl acetate (30–60%), cineole (10%), linalool, nerol, borneol
- Flavonoids
- Tannins
- Coumarins

KEY ACTIONS

- Carminative
- Relieves muscle spasms
- Antidepressant
- Antiseptic & antibacterial
- Stimulates blood flow

RESEARCH

- **Lavender oil** Research into the essential oil has been under way for many decades, and it is understood to have a very low toxicity and significant antiseptic and antibacterial actions. It reduces pain and nervous excitability.
- **Flowers** Lavender flowers, as a whole, are also known to be antibacterial and antiseptic. They calm the nerves, reduce muscle tension, and relieve cramps and gas. Applied externally, they are insecticidal and rubefacient (irritant and stimulating to the local circulation).

TRADITIONAL & CURRENT USES

- **Nervous system** Lavender is well known for its soothing and calming effect, and is combined with other sedative herbs to relieve sleeplessness, irritability, headaches, and migraine. It also helps to alleviate depression.
- **Digestion** Like many herbs with a significant volatile oil content, lavender soothes indigestion and colic, and relieves gas and bloating.
- **Asthma** Lavender's relaxing effect makes it helpful for some types of asthma, especially where excessive nervousness is a feature.
- **Essential oil** The oil is an invaluable first aid remedy. It is strongly antiseptic, helping to heal burns, wounds, and sores.

✦ PARTS USED

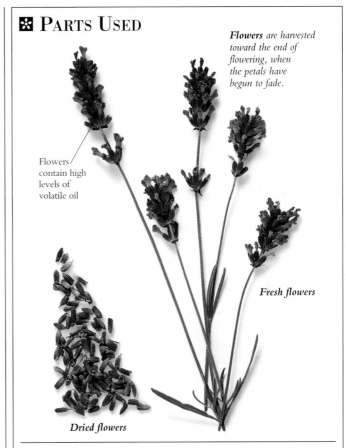

Flowers are harvested toward the end of flowering, when the petals have begun to fade.

Flowers contain high levels of volatile oil

Fresh flowers

Dried flowers

☕ KEY PREPARATIONS & THEIR USES

Caution Do not take the essential oil internally except under professional supervision.

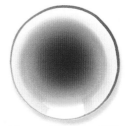

Tincture (to make, p. 291) For insomnia, take ½–1 tsp with water at night.

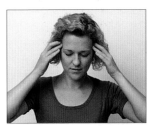

Massage oil For headaches, combine 20 drops with 20 ml carrier oil and apply (see p. 296).

🗴 **ESSENTIAL OIL** Apply undiluted to insect stings.

🥣 **INFUSION** (to make, p. 290) is a calming remedy for digestive problems. For indigestion, take ½ cup twice a day.

Rubbed on insect stings, it relieves pain and inflammation, and it can be used to treat scabies and head lice. Massaging a few drops on the temples eases headaches, and 5 drops added to a bath at night relieves muscle tension, tones the nervous system, and encourages a good night's sleep.

SELF-HELP USES

- **Back pain**, p. 313.
- **Bites & stings**, p. 303.
- **Burns & sunburn**, p. 309.
- **Earache**, p. 312.
- **Headaches & migraine**, p. 309.
- **Insomnia**, p. 309.
- **Neuralgia**, p. 308.
- **Stiff & aching joints**, p. 313.

Lobelia inflata (Campanulaceae)

LOBELIA, INDIAN TOBACCO

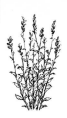

LOBELIA
An annual growing to 20 in (50 cm), with lance-shaped leaves and pale blue flowers.

LOBELIA IS A POWERFUL ANTISPASMODIC, used for respiratory and muscle disorders. In common with other *Lobelia* species, it was a traditional Native American remedy for many conditions. It was used as a "puke weed" to induce vomiting, as a remedy for worms and venereal disease, and as an expectorant. Lobelia was also smoked as a substitute for tobacco and was reputed to share some of its magical qualities.

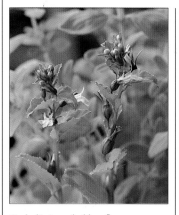

Lobelia's *pale blue flowers were believed to have magical properties and were used to ward off ghosts.*

HABITAT & CULTIVATION

An indigenous American plant, lobelia is found in much of North America, especially in eastern parts of the US. It grows by roadsides and in neglected areas and prefers acid soil. The aerial parts are harvested in early autumn, when the seed capsules are most numerous, and are carefully dried.

RELATED SPECIES

At least 4 other *Lobelia* species were used traditionally by Native Americans. One species, great lobelia (*L. siphilitica*), as its Latin name suggests, was credited by Native Americans and European settlers as having the power to cure syphilis. Chinese lobelia (*ban bian lian, L. chinensis*) is used in Chinese herbal medicine as a diuretic and for snake bite.

KEY CONSTITUENTS

- Piperidine alkaloids (principally lobeline, but many others present)
- Carboxylic acids

KEY ACTIONS

- Respiratory stimulant
- Antispasmodic
- Expectorant
- Induces vomiting
- Increases sweating

RESEARCH

- **Antispasmodic** The whole leaf, as opposed to isolated constituents, is known to be strongly antispasmodic.
- **Piperidine alkaloids** The piperidine alkaloids, especially lobeline, have similar chemical effects to nicotine (*Nicotiana tabacum*, p. 237).
- **Lobeline** It has been shown that lobeline stimulates the respiratory center within the brain stem, producing stronger and deeper breathing, which helps explain why lobelia is useful for respiratory complaints.

TRADITIONAL & CURRENT USES

- **Native American remedy** Lobelia was a traditional Native American remedy and its use was later championed by the American herbalist Samuel Thomson (1769–1843), who made the herb the mainstay of his controversial therapeutic system (*see* p. 48). He mainly used it to induce vomiting.
- **Respiratory problems** A powerful antispasmodic and respiratory stimulant, lobelia is valuable for asthma, especially bronchial asthma, and chronic bronchitis. It relaxes the muscles of the smaller bronchial tubes, thus opening the airways, stimulating breathing, and promoting the coughing up of phlegm. In the Anglo-American

PARTS USED

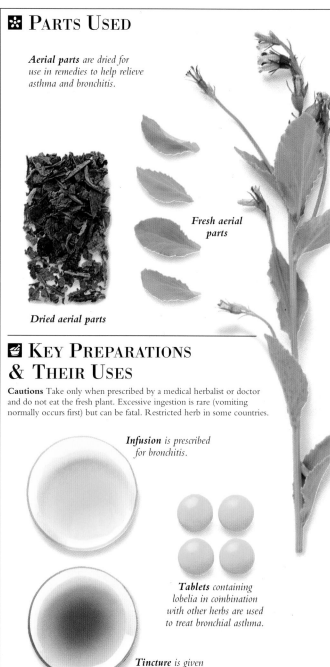

Aerial parts are dried for use in remedies to help relieve asthma and bronchitis.

Fresh aerial parts

Dried aerial parts

KEY PREPARATIONS & THEIR USES

Cautions Take only when prescribed by a medical herbalist or doctor and do not eat the fresh plant. Excessive ingestion is rare (vomiting normally occurs first) but can be fatal. Restricted herb in some countries.

Infusion is prescribed for bronchitis.

Tablets containing lobelia in combination with other herbs are used to treat bronchial asthma.

Tincture is given to relieve asthma.

herbal tradition, lobelia has always been combined with cayenne (*Capsicum frutescens*, p. 70), its hot stimulant action helping to push blood into areas that lobelia has relaxed.
- **Relaxant** Lobelia is often most effective when the infusion or diluted tincture is applied externally. It relaxes muscles, particularly smooth muscle, which makes it useful for sprains, and back problems where muscle tension is a key factor. Combined with cayenne, lobelia has been used as a chest and sinus rub.
- **Tobacco addiction** Due to its chemical similarity to nicotine, lobelia is employed by herbalists to help patients give up smoking.

Lycium chinense (Solanaceae)
LYCIUM, CHINESE WOLFBERRY

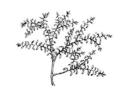

LYCIUM
A deciduous shrub growing to 12 ft (4 m), with bright green leaves and scarlet berries.

LYCIUM IS A MAJOR CHINESE TONIC HERB, first mentioned in the *Divine Husbandman's Classic (Shen'nong Bencaojing)*, written in the 1st century AD. Traditionally it is believed to promote long life – a Chinese herbalist said to have lived for 252 years ascribed his longevity to tonic herbs, including lycium. Today both the berries and the root have a wide range of medicinal uses.

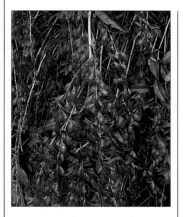

Lycium produces berries that are a blood tonic. In China, they are eaten raw and used in cooking.

HABITAT & CULTIVATION
Lycium grows throughout much of China and Tibet, and is cultivated extensively across central and northern China. It is grown from seed in autumn. The root can be unearthed at any time of the year but is most commonly harvested in spring. The berries are picked in late summer or early autumn.

KEY CONSTITUENTS
- Betaine
- Beta-sitosterol
Berries only:
- Physalien
- Carotene
- Vitamins B_1, B_{12}, and C
Root only:
- Cinnamic acid
- Psyllic acid

KEY ACTIONS
Berries:
- Tonic
- Protect the liver
Root:
- Reduces fever
- Lowers blood pressure

RESEARCH
- **Fruit** The berries protect the liver from damage caused by exposure to toxins.
- **Root** The root is known to stimulate the parasympathetic nervous system, which controls involuntary bodily functions. It also relaxes the artery muscles, thereby lowering blood pressure. Chinese research has shown the root to have a notable ability to reduce fever, and in one clinical trial it had a significant effect in reducing fever in malaria.

TRADITIONAL & CURRENT USES
- **Blood tonic** In China, lycium berries are taken as a blood tonic. They improve the circulation and absorption of nutrients by the cells and help with many symptoms, including dizziness, tinnitus, blurred vision, and wasting conditions.
- **Liver & eye tonic** The berries are a liver and kidney tonic. In Chinese medicine, the liver is associated with the eyes, and lycium berries are considered excellent for failing eyesight.
- **Cooling properties** Lycium root is used in China to "cool the blood," helping to reduce fever, sweating, irritability, and thirst. These cooling qualities also help to stop nosebleeds, reduce vomiting of blood, and soothe coughs and wheezing, whenever they are due to "patterns of excess heat."
- **Blood pressure** As a result of recent research, lycium root is beginning to be used in China to treat people suffering from high blood pressure.

✥ PARTS USED

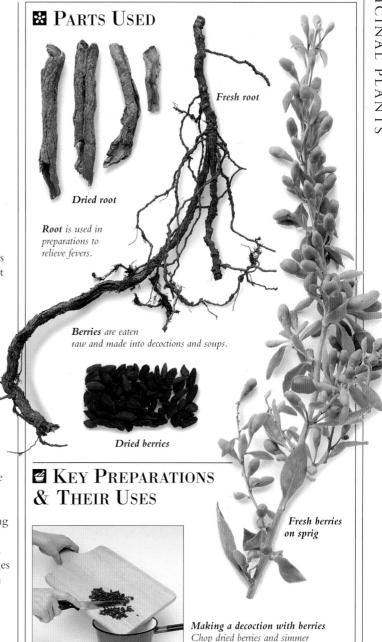

Fresh root

Dried root

Root *is used in preparations to relieve fevers.*

Berries *are eaten raw and made into decoctions and soups.*

Dried berries

Fresh berries on sprig

☙ KEY PREPARATIONS & THEIR USES

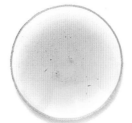

Making a decoction with berries
Chop dried berries and simmer (see p. 290). For poor eyesight, take 100 ml daily.

Decoction of the root (to make, p. 290). For fevers, take 100 ml daily.

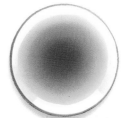

Tincture of the root (to make, p. 291). For coughs and wheezing, take 3 ml diluted with water 3 times a day.

Melaleuca alternifolia (Myrtaceae)

TEA TREE

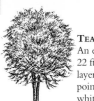

TEA TREE
An evergreen reaching
22 ft (7 m), with
layers of papery bark,
pointed leaves, and
white flower spikes.

TEA TREE, AND IN PARTICULAR its essential oil, is one of the most important natural antiseptics. Useful for stings, burns, wounds, and skin infections of all kinds, the herb merits a place in every medicine chest. Tea tree is native to Australia and is a traditional remedy of the Aborigines. Its therapeutic properties were first researched during the 1920s and it is now widely used in Europe, North America, and Australia.

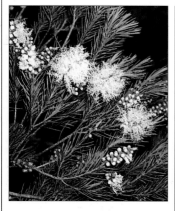

Tea tree *provides one of the most effective natural antiseptics.*

HABITAT & CULTIVATION

Tea tree is native to Australia, flourishing in moist soils in northern New South Wales and Queensland. It is now cultivated extensively, especially in New South Wales. Tea tree is grown from cuttings in summer. The leaves and small branches are picked throughout the year and distilled to produce essential oil.

RELATED SPECIES

Other *Melaleuca* species that provide valuable essential oils include cajuput (*M. leucadendron*, p. 232), broad-leaved paperbark tree (*M. viridiflora*), and *M. linariifolia*, the essential oil of which is very similar to tea tree.

KEY CONSTITUENTS

- Volatile oil (percentages are variable), terpinen-4-ol (40%), gamma-terpinene (24%), alpha-terpinene (10%), cineol (5%)

KEY ACTIONS

- Antiseptic
- Antibacterial
- Antifungal

- Antiviral
- Immune stimulant

RESEARCH

Antiseptic properties

Tea tree essential oil was first researched in 1923 in Australia. Since the 1960s it has been intensively investigated, and its antiseptic properties are well established. Clinical trials, mainly in Australia, have shown that it is effective at treating a broad range of infectious conditions, notably fungal and skin problems such as vaginal yeast infections, acne, and warts.

Active constituents One of the most important constituents is known to be terpinen-4-ol, which is significantly antiseptic and well tolerated by the skin. The oil also contains cineol, which can irritate the skin. The cineol content varies – poor-quality oil has more than 10%; in some cases up to 65%.

TRADITIONAL & CURRENT USES

Traditional remedy Tea tree is a traditional Aboriginal remedy. The leaves are crushed, and either inhaled or used in infusions for coughs, colds, and skin infections.

Skin problems Tea tree oil or cream can be applied to skin infections such as athlete's foot and ringworm, as well as to corns, warts, acne and boils, infected burns, scrapes, wounds, insect bites and stings, and other skin conditions.

Chronic infections Tea tree may be taken internally to treat infections, notably cystitis, glandular fever, and postviral

PARTS USED

Leaves have high levels of an antiseptic volatile oil and are used in preparations for skin problems and infections.

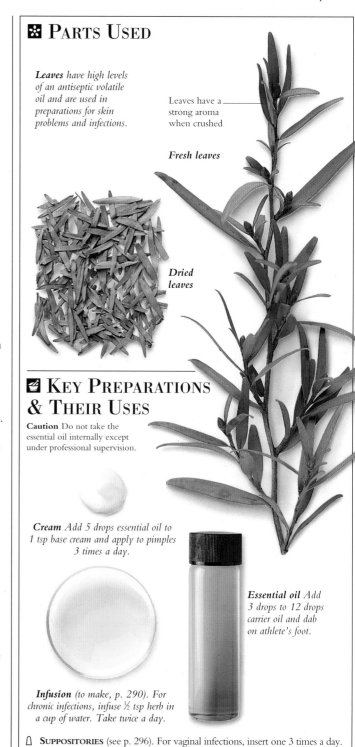

Leaves have a strong aroma when crushed

Fresh leaves

Dried leaves

KEY PREPARATIONS & THEIR USES

Caution Do not take the essential oil internally except under professional supervision.

Cream *Add 5 drops essential oil to 1 tsp base cream and apply to pimples 3 times a day.*

Essential oil *Add 3 drops to 12 drops carrier oil and dab on athlete's foot.*

Infusion *(to make, p. 290). For chronic infections, infuse ½ tsp herb in a cup of water. Take twice a day.*

SUPPOSITORIES (see p. 296). For vaginal infections, insert one 3 times a day.

fatigue syndrome (ME).

Oral infections The herb is effective in mouthwashes, countering oral infection and gum disease, and it can also be used as a gargle for sore throats.

Vaginal infections Tea tree is

an excellent remedy for a range of vaginal yeast infections.

SELF-HELP USES

- **Acne & boils**, p. 305.
- **Athlete's foot**, p. 304.
- **Vaginal infections**, p. 314.

Melissa officinalis (Labiatae)

LEMON BALM, BALM

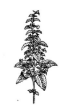

LEMON BALM
A perennial growing to 5 ft (1.5 m), with tiny white flowers and deeply veined, toothed leaves.

IN WRITING THAT "Balm is sovereign for the brain, strengthening the memory and powerfully chasing away melancholy," John Evelyn (1620–1706) neatly summarized lemon balm's long tradition as a tonic remedy that raises the spirits and comforts the heart. Today, this sweet-smelling herb is still widely valued for its calming properties, and new research shows that it can help significantly in the treatment of cold sores.

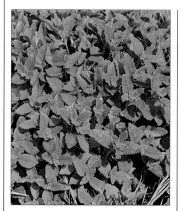

Lemon balm's botanical name, Melissa, *comes from the Greek for bee and refers to the great attraction the plant holds for bees.*

HABITAT & CULTIVATION

A native of southern Europe, western Asia, and northern Africa, lemon balm now grows throughout the world. The plant is propagated from seed or cuttings in spring. The aerial parts are picked from early summer onward and are best harvested just before the flowers open, when the concentration of volatile oil is at its highest.

KEY CONSTITUENTS

- Volatile oil up to 0.2% (citral, caryophyllene oxide, linalool, and citronellal)
- Flavonoids
- Triterpenes
- Polyphenols
- Tannins

KEY ACTIONS

- Relaxant
- Antispasmodic
- Increases sweating
- Carminative
- Antiviral
- Nerve tonic

RESEARCH

- **Volatile oil** German research has shown that the volatile oil, and in particular citral and citronellal, calm the central nervous system. The oil is also strongly antispasmodic.
- **Polyphenols** Polyphenols are antiviral. In particular, they combat the herpes simplex virus, which produces cold sores. In one research study, the average healing time of cold sores was halved to about 5 days and the time between outbreaks doubled.
- **Thyroid** Lemon balm inhibits thyroid function.

TRADITIONAL & CURRENT USES

- **Traditional uses** This herb has always been taken to lift the spirits. Taken regularly, it was believed to encourage longevity. Other traditional uses include healing wounds, relieving palpitations and relaxing the heart, and treating toothache.
- **Modern relaxing tonic** Lemon balm is a relaxing tonic for anxiety, mild depression, restlessness, and irritability. It reduces feelings of nervousness and panic and will often quiet a racing heart, being a valuable remedy for palpitations of a nervous origin. Lemon balm is also useful when overanxiety is causing digestive problems such as indigestion, acidity, nausea, bloating, and colicky pains.
- **Cold sores** Lemon balm relieves cold sores and reduces the chances of further outbreaks.
- **Hormonal herb** Following the discovery of its antithyroid effect, the herb is given to people with an overactive thyroid.

✢ PARTS USED

Aerial parts are used in a variety of preparations as a calming remedy.

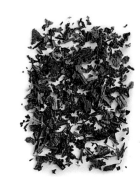

Dried aerial parts

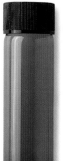

Leaves produce a lemon scent when crushed

Fresh aerial parts

✍ KEY PREPARATIONS & THEIR USES

Caution Do not take the essential oil internally except under professional supervision.

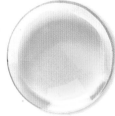

Essential oil *For shingles, add 5 drops to 1 tsp olive oil and massage the painful area gently (see p. 296).*

Infusion *(to make, p. 290). For nervous headaches, drink a cup 3 times a day.*

Tincture *(to make, p. 291). For anxiety and mild depression, take ½ tsp with water 3 times a day.*

🥄 **LOTION** For cold sores, make an infusion (see p. 290) and apply regularly (see p. 295).

🍶 **JUICE** Apply as needed to cuts and scrapes.

🥣 **OINTMENT** (to make, p. 294). Apply to insect stings.

- **Other uses** Lemon balm is a first-aid remedy for cuts and insect stings and is good for fevers.

SELF-HELP USES

- **Anxiety, depression & tension**, p. 308.
- **Cold sores, chicken pox & shingles**, p. 304.
- **Flu with muscle aches & pains**, p. 311.
- **Nausea due to emotional problems**, p. 306.
- **Stomachache**, p. 305.

Mentha × piperita (Labiatae)
PEPPERMINT

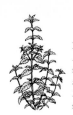

PEPPERMINT
A strongly aromatic, square-stemmed annual, growing to 32 in (80 cm), with serrated leaves.

PEPPERMINT'S ORIGIN IS A MYSTERY, but it has been in existence for a long time – dried leaves were found in Egyptian pyramids dating from about 1000 BC. It was highly valued by the Greeks and Romans but only became popular in Western Europe in the 18th century. Peppermint's chief therapeutic value lies in its ability to relieve gas, flatulence, bloating, and colic, although it has many other applications.

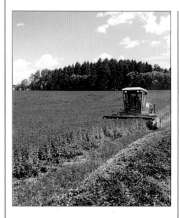

***Peppermint** is cultivated in many parts of the world for its oil.*

HABITAT & CULTIVATION
Peppermint is grown commercially and in gardens throughout Europe, Asia, and North America. It is propagated from seed in spring and is harvested just before it flowers in summer, in dry sunny weather.

RELATED SPECIES
Peppermint is a hybrid of watermint (*M. aquatica*) and spearmint (*M. spicata*), which have similar, though milder, therapeutic properties.

KEY CONSTITUENTS
- Volatile oil (up to 1.5%), including menthol (35–55%), menthone (10–40%)
- Flavonoids (luteolin, menthoside)
- Phenolic acids
- Triterpenes

KEY ACTIONS
- Carminative
- Relieves muscle spasms
- Increases sweating
- Stimulates secretion of bile
- Antiseptic

RESEARCH
- **Volatile oil** Research has shown that the volatile oil is strongly antibacterial. Menthol (a constituent of the oil) is antiseptic, antifungal, cooling, and anesthetic to the skin, although it is also an irritant.
- **Whole herb** The whole plant has an antispasmodic effect on the digestive system. Clinical trials in Denmark and Britain during the 1990s have confirmed its value in the treatment of irritable bowel syndrome.

TRADITIONAL & CURRENT USES
- **Digestive problems** Peppermint is excellent for the digestive system, increasing the flow of digestive juices and bile and relaxing the muscles of the gut. It reduces colic, cramps, and gas, and helps to soothe an irritated bowel. In soothing the lining and muscles of the colon, it helps diarrhea and relieves a spastic colon (often the cause of constipation).
- **Pain relief** Applied to the skin, peppermint relieves pain and reduces sensitivity. It also relieves headaches and migraines linked to digestive weakness.
- **Infection** Diluted oil is used as an inhalant and chest rub for respiratory infections. The whole herb is important for digestive infections.

SELF-HELP USES
- **Digestive headaches**, p. 309.
- **Eczema**, p. 300.
- **Gas & bloating**, p. 306.
- **Nausea with headache**, p. 306.
- **Neuralgia**, p. 308.

✦ PARTS USED

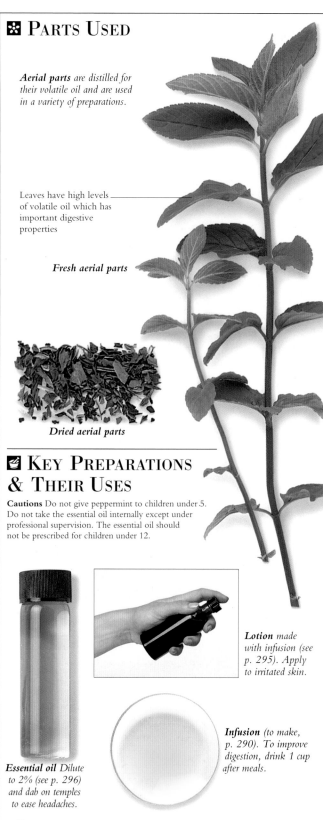

***Aerial parts** are distilled for their volatile oil and are used in a variety of preparations.*

Leaves have high levels of volatile oil which has important digestive properties

Fresh aerial parts

Dried aerial parts

✍ KEY PREPARATIONS & THEIR USES

Cautions Do not give peppermint to children under 5. Do not take the essential oil internally except under professional supervision. The essential oil should not be prescribed for children under 12.

***Lotion** made with infusion (see p. 295). Apply to irritated skin.*

***Infusion** (to make, p. 290). To improve digestion, drink 1 cup after meals.*

***Essential oil** Dilute to 2% (see p. 296) and dab on temples to ease headaches.*

✦ **TINCTURE** mixed with other herbs is prescribed mainly for digestive problems.

✦ **CAPSULES** are prescribed for irritable bowel syndrome.

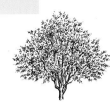

NUTMEG & MACE
An evergreen tree growing to 40 ft (12 m), with aromatic leaves and clusters of small yellow flowers.

Myristica fragrans (Myristicaceae)
NUTMEG & MACE, ROU DOU KOU (CHINESE)

NUTMEG AND MACE BOTH COME from the nutmeg tree and have very similar medicinal properties. They are infrequently used in the West because of their toxity at high dosages, but nonetheless are important medicines, employed principally to stimulate the digestion and to treat infections of the digestive tract. Nutmeg has also long been valued as an aphrodisiac and as a remedy for eczema and rheumatism.

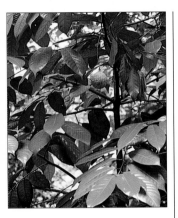

Nutmeg and mace *are cultivated commercially in the tropics.*

HABITAT & CULTIVATION
Native to the Molucca Islands of Indonesia, nutmeg trees are now widely cultivated. They are propagated from seed, sown when ripe. The tree yields fruit after about 8 years, and can continue to fruit for over 60 years. The fruit is picked when ripe and the nutmeg and mace are separated and dried.

KEY CONSTITUENTS
Nutmeg:
- Volatile oil (up to 15%), including alpha-pinene, beta-pinene, alpha-terpinene, beta-terpinene, myristicin, elincin, safrole
- Fixed oil ("nutmeg butter"), myristine, butyrin

Mace:
- Volatile oil (similar to nutmeg but with a higher concentration of myristicin)

KEY ACTIONS
Nutmeg:
- Carminative
- Relieves muscle spasms
- Prevents vomiting

- Stimulant

Mace:
- Stimulant
- Carminative

TRADITIONAL & CURRENT USES
- **Digestive problems** Nutmeg essential oil has an anesthetic and stimulating effect on the stomach and intestines, increasing appetite and reducing nausea, vomiting and diarrhea. It is a helpful remedy for many digestive problems, especially gastroenteritis.
- **Chinese medicine** In China, nutmeg is used specifically for diarrhea, helping to bind and warm the intestines and relieve abdominal pain and distension due to "cold."
- **Aphrodisiac** In India, nutmeg has a long reputation as an aphrodisiac. It is believed to increase sexual stamina.
- **External uses** Ointments based on the fixed oil (nutmeg butter) are used to treat rheumatic conditions. They have a counterirritant effect, stimulating blood flow to the area. In India, nutmeg is ground into a paste and applied directly to areas of eczema and ringworm.
- **Safety** Low medicinal doses and culinary amounts of nutmeg and mace are safe. In excess, however, the herbs are strongly stimulant, hallucinogenic, and toxic. The consumption of just 2 whole nutmegs has been known to cause death. Myristicin is the constituent most responsible for this toxicity, and it is also hallucinogenic. In addition, safrole in isolation and at a high dosage is carcinogenic.

PARTS USED

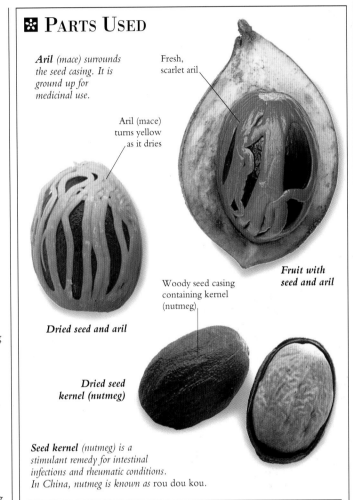

Aril *(mace) surrounds the seed casing. It is ground up for medicinal use.*

Fresh, scarlet aril

Aril (mace) turns yellow as it dries

Dried seed and aril

Woody seed casing containing kernel (nutmeg)

Fruit with seed and aril

Dried seed kernel (nutmeg)

Seed kernel *(nutmeg) is a stimulant remedy for intestinal infections and rheumatic conditions. In China, nutmeg is known as* rou dou kou.

KEY PREPARATIONS & THEIR USES

Cautions Take the essential oil internally only under professional supervision. Do not take more than 3 g of either herb a day. Do not use during pregnancy.

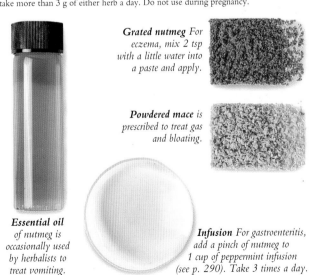

Grated nutmeg *For eczema, mix 2 tsp with a little water into a paste and apply.*

Powdered mace *is prescribed to treat gas and bloating.*

Essential oil *of nutmeg is occasionally used by herbalists to treat vomiting.*

Infusion *For gastroenteritis, add a pinch of nutmeg to 1 cup of peppermint infusion (see p. 290). Take 3 times a day.*

OINTMENT made from fixed oil (nutmeg butter). For rheumatic conditions, apply several times a day.

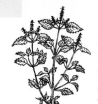

HOLY BASIL
An aromatic annual growing to about 28 in (70 cm), with small purple-red or white flowers.

Ocimum sanctum (Labiatae)
HOLY BASIL, TULSI (HINDI)

HOLY BASIL, LIKE SWEET (culinary) basil, comes from India, where it is revered as the herb sacred to the goddess *Lakshmi*, wife of *Vishnu*, the god who preserves life. *Tulsi* means "matchless," and the herb has very important medicinal properties – notably its ability to reduce blood sugar levels. In Indian herbal medicine, holy basil has a wide range of uses, relieving fevers, bronchitis, asthma, stress, and canker sores.

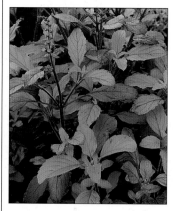

Holy basil is so called because it is often planted around temples and courtyards in India.

HABITAT & CULTIVATION

Holy basil is indigenous to India and other tropical regions of Asia. It is also grown extensively in Central and South America, mainly for its medicinal properties. The herb can be grown from seed and is often cultivated as a pot plant. It is harvested before the flowers open, in early summer.

RELATED SPECIES

Sweet basil (*O. basilicum*, p. 238) is a close relative.

KEY CONSTITUENTS

- Volatile oil (1%), including eugenol (70–80%), methyl chavicol, methyl eugenol, caryophyllene
- Flavonoids (apigenin, luteolin)
- Triterpene: ursolic acid

KEY ACTIONS

- Lowers blood sugar levels
- Antispasmodic
- Analgesic
- Lowers blood pressure
- Reduces fever

- Adaptogenic
- Anti-inflammatory

RESEARCH

- **Diabetes** Research into holy basil's ability to reduce blood sugar levels, and thus help diabetes, has been going on for some decades. It has now been established as a useful medicine for some types of diabetes.
- **Indian research** Research in India has shown that the plant helps lower blood pressure and has anti-inflammatory, analgesic, and fever-reducing properties. In addition, the herb appears to inhibit sperm production.

TRADITIONAL & CURRENT USES

- **Traditional use** Holy basil has always been considered to be a tonic, invigorating herb, useful for improving vitality.
- **Ayurvedic remedy** In Ayurvedic medicine, holy basil is chiefly employed for fevers. A classic Indian recipe mixes holy basil, black pepper (*Piper nigrum*, p. 248), ginger (*Zingiber officinale*, p. 153), and honey in a remedy that prevents infection and controls high fever.
- **Heart & stress** Holy basil is thought to have an affinity with the heart, protecting it from stress and lowering blood pressure and cholesterol levels. It has a reputation for reducing stress and is regarded as adaptogenic – helping the body to adapt to new demands and stresses.
- **Diabetic remedy** The herb's ability to help stabilize blood sugar levels makes it useful in the treatment of diabetes.
- **Respiratory problems** Holy

PARTS USED

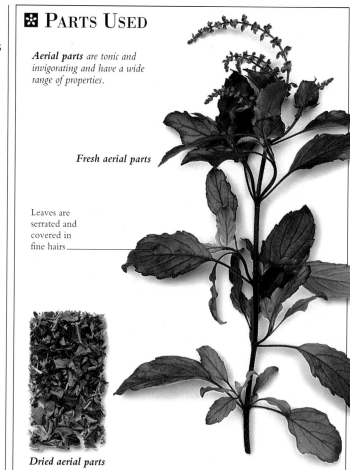

Aerial parts are tonic and invigorating and have a wide range of properties.

Fresh aerial parts

Leaves are serrated and covered in fine hairs

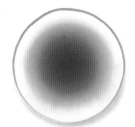

Dried aerial parts

KEY PREPARATIONS & THEIR USES

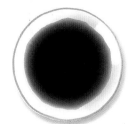

Juice For skin infections, apply 10 ml to the affected part twice a day.

Decoction (to make, p. 290) is used for fevers and as a tonic. Take 1 cup daily as a general tonic.

Powder For canker sores, rub powder gently into painful areas several times a day.

basil is a valuable herb for respiratory infections, especially colds, coughs, bronchitis, and pleurisy. It is also useful in the treatment of asthma.

- **Other uses** Juice is extracted and applied to insect stings, ringworm, and skin diseases. It is also used as ear drops for ear infections. Juice or powdered herb helps canker sores to heal.

SELF-HELP USE

- **Bites & stings**, p. 303.

Paeonia lactiflora syn. *P. albiflora* (Paeoniaceae)
WHITE PEONY, BAI SHAO YAO (CHINESE)

WHITE PEONY
An upright perennial, growing to 6 ft (2 m), with large, white flowers and divided, dark green leaves.

WHITE PEONY'S HISTORY of medicinal use in China stretches back for at least 1,500 years. It is known most widely as one of the herbs used to make "four things soup," a female tonic, and it is also a remedy for gynecological problems and for cramps, pain, and dizziness. Traditionally, it is considered that women who take the herb on a regular basis become as radiant as the flower itself.

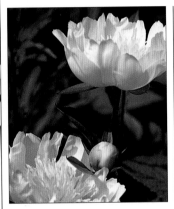

***White peony** is cultivated in China both for its beautiful fragrant flowers and for its root, which has tonic properties.*

HABITAT & CULTIVATION

White peony root is grown throughout northeastern China and Inner Mongolia. It is propagated from seed in spring, or from root cuttings taken in winter. The root of 4- or 5-year-old plants is harvested in spring or autumn.

RELATED SPECIES

Mu dan pi (*P. suffruticosa*) and the wild form of white peony, *chi shao yao* (*P. rubrae*), are both used medicinally in China and have similar properties to white peony. Peony (*Paeonia officinalis*, p. 241) a common European plant, is also closely related.

KEY CONSTITUENTS

- Monoterpenoid glycosides (paeoniflorin, albiflorin)
- Benzoic acid
- Pentagalloyl glucose

KEY ACTIONS

- Antispasmodic
- Tonic

- Astringent
- Analgesic

RESEARCH

- **Paenoiflorin** Paenoiflorin is significantly antispasmodic, relaxing intestinal tissue as well as the muscles of the uterus. In Chinese experiments during the 1980s it was shown to counter oxytocin, the hormone that induces contraction of the uterus. Paenoiflorin is thought to be mildly hypotensive, lowering blood pressure and increasing blood flow to the heart through the coronary arteries. It also exhibits mild anti-inflammatory and fever reducing properties.
- **Cold sores** Pentagalloyl glucose may have an antiviral effect against the cold sore virus herpes simplex.

TRADITIONAL & CURRENT USES

- **Four things soup** White peony is regarded primarily as a woman's herb. Together with rehmannia (*Rehmannia glutinosa*, p. 123), *chuan xiong* (*Ligusticum wallachii*), and Chinese angelica (*Angelica sinensis*, p. 60) it is an ingredient in "four things soup," the most widely used female tonic in China.
- **Gynecological remedy** White peony helps menstrual disorders, including heavy bleeding between periods, and is specifically used to treat menstrual pain and cramps. It is a blood and *yin* tonic (*see* pp. 38–39) and will help "blood deficiency" states, as well as hot flashes and night sweats resulting from *yin* deficiency.

✵ PARTS USED

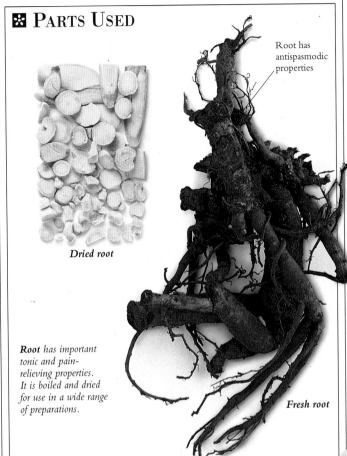

Dried root

Root *has important tonic and pain-relieving properties. It is boiled and dried for use in a wide range of preparations.*

Root has antispasmodic properties

Fresh root

☙ KEY PREPARATIONS & THEIR USES

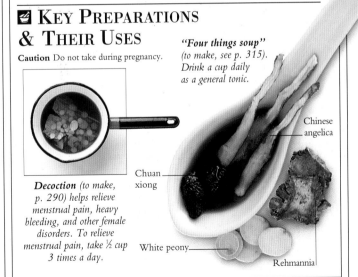

Caution Do not take during pregnancy.

"Four things soup" (to make, see p. 315). Drink a cup daily as a general tonic.

***Decoction** (to make, p. 290) helps relieve menstrual pain, heavy bleeding, and other female disorders. To relieve menstrual pain, take ½ cup 3 times a day.*

Chinese angelica

Chuan xiong

White peony

Rehmannia

- **Antispasmodic** White peony is prescribed for cramping abdominal pain, especially in dysentery, for muscle cramps, and numb hands and feet. It also treats headaches, ringing in the ear, dizziness, and blurred vision.

SELF-HELP USES

- **Heavy menstrual bleeding**, p. 315.
- **Hot flashes & night sweats**, p. 316.
- **Menstrual pain**, p. 315.

Panax ginseng (Araliaceae)

GINSENG, REN SHEN (CHINESE)

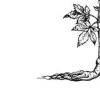

GINSENG
A perennial growing to 3 ft (1 m), with oval, toothed leaves and a cluster of small green-yellow flowers.

GINSENG IS THE MOST FAMOUS Chinese herb of all. It has been valued for its remarkable therapeutic benefits for about 7,000 years and was so revered that wars were fought for control of the forests in which it thrived. An Arabian physician brought ginseng back to Europe in the 9th century, yet its ability to improve stamina and resistance to stress became common knowledge in the West only in the 18th century.

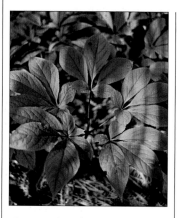

Ginseng has always been valued as a tonic in old age.

HABITAT & CULTIVATION

Ginseng is native to northeastern China, eastern Russia, and North Korea, but is now extremely rare in the wild. Ginseng cultivation requires great skill. It is propagated from seed in spring and requires rich, moist, but well-drained soil. The plant takes at least 4 years to mature. The root is then normally harvested in autumn, washed, and steamed before being dried.

RELATED SPECIES

San qi (P. notoginseng, p. 241), *P. pseudoginseng,* and American ginseng *(P. quinquefolium,* p. 241) all have significant benefits.

KEY CONSTITUENTS

- Triterpenoid saponins (0.7–3%), ginsenosides – at least 25 have been identified
- Acetylenic compounds
- Panaxans
- Sesquiterpenes

KEY ACTIONS

- Adaptogenic
- Tonic

RESEARCH

- **Adaptogenic** Ginseng has been researched in detail over the past 20–30 years in China, Japan, Korea, Russia, and many other countries. Its remarkable "adaptogenic" quality (helping the body to adapt to stress, fatigue, and cold) has been confirmed. Trials show that ginseng significantly improves the body's capacity to cope with hunger, extremes of temperature, and mental and emotional stress. Furthermore, ginseng produces a sedative effect when the body requires sleep. The ginsenosides that are responsible for this action are similar in structure to the body's own stress hormones.
- **Other research** Ginseng also increases immune function and resistance to infection, and supports liver function.

TRADITIONAL & CURRENT USES

- **Therapeutic actions** As an adaptogenic, ginseng's action varies. It has a stimulating effect on young people with strong *qi* (vital force, *see* pp. 38–39), but is tonic, restorative, and even sedative for those weakened by illness or old age.
- **Chinese remedy** In China, ginseng is best known as a stimulant, tonic herb for athletes and those subject to physical stress, and as a male aphrodisiac. It is also a tonic for old age, and is traditionally taken by people in northern and central China from late middle age onward, helping them to endure the long hard winters.
- **Western tonic** In the West, ginseng is viewed not so much as a medicine, but as a life-enhancing tonic. It is useful for those coping with stressful events, such as taking exams. Ginseng is often abused in the West and should not be taken for more than 6 weeks.

✤ PARTS USED

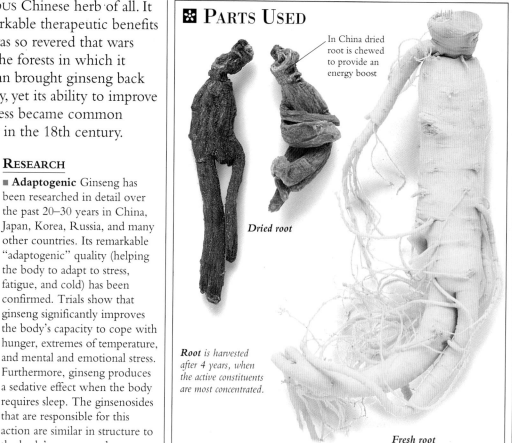

In China dried root is chewed to provide an energy boost

Dried root

Root is harvested after 4 years, when the active constituents are most concentrated.

Fresh root

☙ KEY PREPARATIONS & THEIR USES

Cautions Do not exceed the dose (can cause insomnia and high blood pressure). Do not take for more than 6 weeks. Avoid caffeine while taking ginseng. Do not take if pregnant.

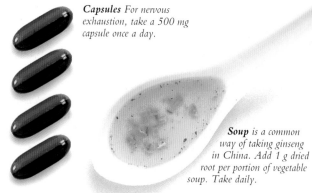

Capsules For nervous exhaustion, take a 500 mg capsule once a day.

Soup is a common way of taking ginseng in China. Add 1 g dried root per portion of vegetable soup. Take daily.

TABLETS are a convenient way of taking ginseng. Take for short-term stressful events, such as moving a household.

SELF-HELP USES

- **Impotence and premature ejaculation**, p. 316.
- **Maintaining vitality**, p. 319.
- **Poor sleep and nervous exhaustion**, p. 309.
- **Short-term stress**, p. 308.

Passiflora incarnata (Passifloraceae)

PASSIONFLOWER, PASSIFLORA, MAYPOP

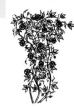

PASSIONFLOWER
A climbing vine growing to 28 ft (9 m), with 3-lobed leaves, ornate flowers, and egg-shaped fruit.

PASSIONFLOWER'S NAME COMES from its beautiful flowers, thought to represent Christ's crucifixion – 5 stamens for the 5 wounds, 3 styles for the 3 nails, and white and purple-blue colors for purity and heaven. The herb has valuable sedative and tranquilizing properties, and has a long use as a medicine in Central and North American herbal traditions, being taken in Mexico for insomnia, epilepsy, and hysteria.

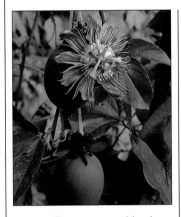

Passionflower was used by the Algonquin people of North America as an herbal tranquilizer.

HABITAT & CULTIVATION

Native to southern US (Virginia, Texas, and Tennessee) and to Central and South America, passionflower is now extensively cultivated in Europe, notably in Italy, as well as in North America. It is propagated from seed in spring and needs plenty of sun. The aerial parts are gathered when the plant is flowering or in fruit.

RELATED SPECIES

There are approximately 400 *Passiflora* species, some of which are popular garden plants. A number have a similar sedative action to passionflower. *P. quadrangularis* has been found to contain serotonin, one of the main chemical messengers within the brain.

KEY CONSTITUENTS

- Flavonoids (apigenin)
- Maltol
- Cyanogenic glycosides (gynocardin)
- Indole alkaloids (harman)

KEY ACTIONS

- Sedative
- Antispasmodic
- Tranquilizing

RESEARCH

Tranquilizing properties
Passionflower has been fairly well researched but its mode of action on the central nervous system is poorly understood. The aerial parts have established sedative, tranquilizing, and sleep-inducing properties, but the constituents that cause these actions have not been identified.

Indole alkaloids Research has not yet conclusively established that passionflower contains indole alkaloids.

TRADITIONAL & CURRENT USES

Insomnia Passionflower is best known as a remedy for insomnia and disturbed sleep patterns, and is useful for short-term bouts of sleeplessness.

Gentle sedative This herb is widely acknowledged as a good medicine for anxiety, tension, irritability, and insomnia. Its gentle sedative properties produce a relaxing effect, reducing nervous overactivity and panic, and making it a mild and nonaddictive herbal tranquilizer, comparable in some ways to valerian (*Valeriana officinalis*, p. 146). Occasionally, it is prescribed for convulsions.

Pain relief Passionflower has valuable painkilling properties and is given for toothache, period pain, and headaches.

Tranquilizing effects Its ability to reduce anxiety makes passionflower valuable for many

✲ PARTS USED

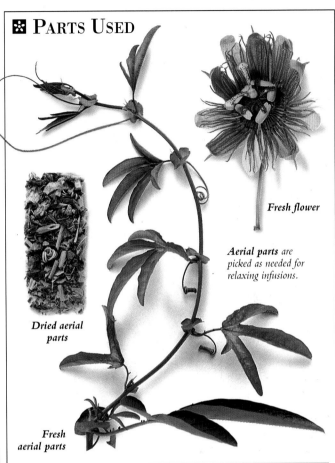

Fresh flower

Aerial parts are picked as needed for relaxing infusions.

Dried aerial parts

Fresh aerial parts

✍ KEY PREPARATIONS & THEIR USES

Cautions Passionflower can cause drowsiness. Do not take high doses in pregnancy.

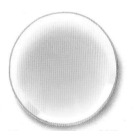

Tincture *(to make, p. 291) is a useful sedative for an overactive mind. Take 1 tsp with water daily.*

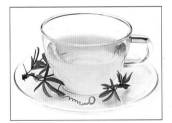

Infusion *(to make, p. 290). For occasional sleeplessness, drink up to 2 cups during the evening.*

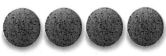

Tablets *are a common over-the-counter remedy for insomnia and stress.*

nervous states, and it is used to treat conditions as diverse as asthma, palpitations, high blood pressure, and muscle cramps. In each case, its antispasmodic and tranquilizing properties are the key to its usefulness, reducing the overactivity responsible for the disorder.

SELF-HELP USES

- **Insomnia**, p. 309.
- **Sleeplessness due to backache**, p. 313.

Persea americana (Lauraceae)

AVOCADO

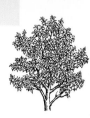

AVOCADO TREE
An evergreen tree, growing to 70 ft (20 m), with dark green, leathery leaves and white flowers.

MANY PARTS OF THE avocado tree have a use in herbal medicine. The leaves and bark are effective remedies for digestive problems and coughs. As well as being extremely nutritious, the fruit has a wide range of medicinal uses. Native peoples of Guatemala, for example, use the pulp to stimulate hair growth, the rind to expel worms, and the seeds to treat diarrhea. The fruit pulp is used as a baby food in West Africa.

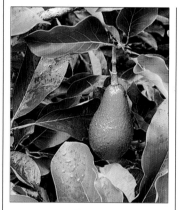

***Avocado** is very nutritious and makes an excellent baby food.*

HABITAT & CULTIVATION

Indigenous to Central America, avocado is widely cultivated for its fruit in tropical and subtropical areas, including Israel, Spain, and South Africa. It is propagated from seed. The leaves are harvested as needed, and the unripe fruit is picked when fully grown.

RELATED SPECIES

Other *Persea* species have similar fruits to avocado and are used in a similar way.

KEY CONSTITUENTS

Leaves & bark:
■ Volatile oil (methylchavicol, alpha-pinene)
■ Flavonoids
■ Tannins
Fruit pulp:
■ Unsaturated fats
■ Protein (about 25%)
■ Sesquiterpenes
■ Vitamins A, B₁, B₂

KEY ACTIONS

Leaves & bark:
■ Astringent

■ Carminative
■ Relieve coughs
■ Promote menstrual flow
Fruit pulp:
■ Emollient
■ Carminative
Rind:
■ Eliminates worms

RESEARCH

■ **Cholesterol** Research shows that the fruit helps to lower cholesterol levels.
■ **Poisons** Livestock that have grazed on avocado leaves, fruit, or bark have been observed to suffer fewer toxic effects from snakebite and other poisons.

TRADITIONAL & CURRENT USES

■ **Leaves & bark** Avocado leaves and the bark of young stems stimulate menstruation and can induce abortion. Being astringent and carminative, the leaves are taken for diarrhea, gas, and bloating, and are considered valuable for relieving coughs, for liver obstructions, and for clearing high uric acid levels, which cause gout.
■ **Fruit** The rind of the fruit is used as a remedy to expel worms. The mashed fruit pulp is a nourishing food and is considered to have aphrodisiac properties. Used externally, the pulp is cooling and soothing to the skin. It is applied to suppurating wounds and to the scalp to stimulate hair growth.
■ **Oil** The expressed oil of the avocado seed nourishes and maintains skin tone. It softens rough, dry, or flaking skin and, massaged into the scalp, improves hair growth.

✤ PARTS USED

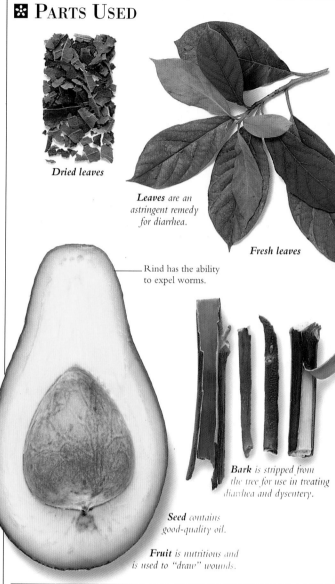

Dried leaves

Leaves *are an astringent remedy for diarrhea.*

Fresh leaves

Rind has the ability to expel worms.

Bark *is stripped from the tree for use in treating diarrhea and dysentery.*

Seed *contains good-quality oil.*

Fruit *is nutritious and is used to "draw" wounds.*

☙ KEY PREPARATIONS & THEIR USES

Caution The leaves and bark should not be used during pregnancy.

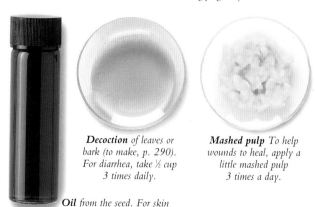

***Decoction** of leaves or bark (to make, p. 290). For diarrhea, take ½ cup 3 times daily.*

***Mashed pulp** To help wounds to heal, apply a little mashed pulp 3 times a day.*

Oil *from the seed. For skin blemishes, rub a little oil on the area daily.*

Piper methysticum (Piperaceae)

KAVA KAVA

KAVA KAVA An evergreen shrub climbing to 10 ft (3 m), with fleshy stems and heart-shaped leaves.

KAVA KAVA IS AN HERB with major ritual and cultural significance among the peoples of the Pacific Islands, who use it for social ceremonies and to communicate with their gods. Kava kava's calming and stimulating qualities in large doses produce intoxication and euphoria, and the herb has a longstanding reputation as an aphrodisiac. It has a hot, aromatic, and bitter taste, and leaves the mouth feeling slightly numbed.

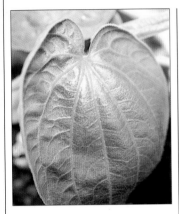

Kava kava has huge tapering leaves, growing to 10 in (25 cm) across. Its root is used medicinally to relieve pain.

HABITAT & CULTIVATION

Kava kava is an indigenous Polynesian vine and grows throughout the Pacific Islands as far east as Hawaii. It is cultivated commercially in the US and Australia. Kava kava is propagated from runners in late winter or early spring and is usually grown on frames. It needs well-drained stony soil and a shady position. The root is harvested at any time of year.

RELATED SPECIES

The closely related *P. sanctum* is native to Mexico. It is similar to kava kava in many ways; for example, it also contains kava lactones and is traditionally taken as a stimulant. Other related species include matico, betel, cubeb, and pepper (*P. angustifolia*, *P. betle*, *P. cubeba*, and *P. nigrum*, pp. 247–248).

KEY CONSTITUENTS

- Resin – containing kava lactones, including kawain
- Piperidine alkaloid (pipermethysticine)

KEY ACTIONS

- Stimulant
- Tonic
- Reduces anxiety
- Urinary antiseptic
- Analgesic
- Induces sleep

RESEARCH

- **Lactones** The kava lactones have a depressant effect on the central nervous system and are antispasmodic. Research shows that kawain, in particular, is sedative. The kava lactones also have an anesthetic effect on the lining of the urinary tubules and the bladder.
- **Relieving anxiety** The results of a clinical trial in Germany published in 1990 revealed that kawain is as effective as benzodiazepene in helping to relieve anxiety.

TRADITIONAL & CURRENT USES

- **Traditional aphrodisiac** Kava kava is valued in the South Sea Islands as a calming and stimulating intoxicant. Taken in large quantities it produces a euphoric state, which is probably why it has long been considered an aphrodisiac.
- **Narcotic** Experience in the Pacific Islands and among the Aborigines in Australia has shown that if taken to excess kava kava has a narcotic effect, inducing stupor.
- **Antiseptic** Kava kava has an antiseptic action and in the past it was used specifically to treat venereal disease, especially gonorrhea. Although kava kava is no longer generally employed in this way, it is a valuable urinary antiseptic, helping to counter urinary infections and to settle an irritable bladder.
- **Pain relief** With its tonic, strengthening, and mildly analgesic properties, kava kava is a good remedy for chronic pain, helping to reduce sensitivity and to relax muscles that are tensed in response to pain.
- **Arthritic conditions** Kava kava's analgesic and cleansing diuretic effect often makes it beneficial for treating rheumatic and arthritic problems such as gout. The herb helps to bring relief from pain and to remove waste products from the affected joint.
- **Relaxing remedy** Kava kava is a safe and proven remedy for anxiety that does not cause drowsiness or affect the user's ability to operate machinery. It may be taken long term to help relieve chronic stress, and its combination of anxiety-relieving and muscle-relaxant properties makes it of value for treating muscle tension as well as emotional stress.
- **External uses** The herb makes a useful analgesic mouthwash for toothache and canker sores.

❊ PARTS USED

Root relieves pain and counters urinary tract infections.

Traditionally the root is chewed and fermented with saliva

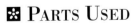

Dried root

☙ KEY PREPARATIONS & THEIR USES

Cautions Do not exceed the recommended dose. Do not take for more than 4 weeks. Do not take during pregnancy.

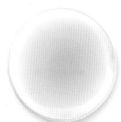

Infusion (to make, p. 290). To alleviate urinary infections, drink ½ cup twice a day.

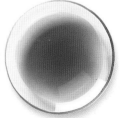

Tincture (to make, p. 291) is a soothing and relaxing tonic. For stress, take 30 drops with water 3 times a day.

Plantago spp. *(Plantaginaceae)*
PSYLLIUM, ISPAGHULA (HINDI), FLEA SEED

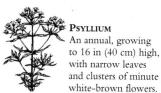

PSYLLIUM
An annual, growing to 16 in (40 cm) high, with narrow leaves and clusters of minute white-brown flowers.

PRODUCED BY SEVERAL *Plantago* species – *P. ovata*, *P. psyllium*, and *P. indica* – psyllium has been used as a safe and effective laxative for thousands of years in Europe, North Africa, and Asia. Given their small size and brown color, psyllium husks and seeds have been mistaken for fleas, hence their folk name flea seed. Bland-tasting, they swell when moistened and have a jellylike consistency in the mouth.

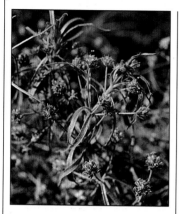

Psyllium is widely cultivated for its husks and seeds, which are used as a remedy for bowel problems.

HABITAT & CULTIVATION
The 3 species that produce psyllium grow variously throughout southern Europe, North Africa, and Asia, especially in India, and are extensively cultivated. They are propagated from seed in spring and require plenty of sun. The seeds are harvested when ripe in late summer and early autumn.

RELATED SPECIES
Common plantain (*P. major*, p. 249) is prescribed for diarrhea and irritable bowel syndrome. *Che qian zi* (*P. asiatica*) is used in China as a diuretic, for diarrhea, and for bronchial congestion. The powdered husk is given to women in the later stages of pregnancy to encourage normal presentation of the fetus (head-down position in the uterus).

KEY CONSTITUENTS
- Mucilage (arabinoxylan)
- Fixed oil (2.5%) – mainly linoleic, oleic, and palmitic fatty acids
- Starch

KEY ACTIONS
- Demulcent
- Bulk laxative
- Antidiarrheal

RESEARCH
- **Regulating bowel function** Clinical trials in the US, Germany, and Scandinavia during the 1980s have shown that psyllium has both a laxative and an antidiarrheal action. As with so many herbs, it helps to restore normal function of a body organ.

TRADITIONAL & CURRENT USES
- **Laxative** Psyllium is a well-known laxative. It is prescribed in conventional as well as herbal medicine for constipation, especially when the condition is resulting from an overtensed or overrelaxed bowel. Both husks and seeds contain high levels of fiber (the mucilage) and expand, becoming highly gelatinous when soaked in water. By maintaining a high water content within the large bowel, they increase the bulk of the stool, easing its passage.
- **Other bowel problems** Contrary to expectation, psyllium is a useful remedy for diarrhea. The herb is also an effective treatment for many other bowel problems, including irritable bowel syndrome, ulcerative colitis, and Crohn's disease (regional ileitis). In India, psyllium is commonly used to treat dysentery.
- **Hemorrhoid relief** Psyllium is valuable for hemorrhoids, helping to soften the stool and to reduce irritation of the distended vein.
- **Detoxifying herb** The jellylike mucilage produced when psyllium is soaked in water has the ability to absorb toxins within the large bowel. Psyllium is commonly taken to reduce autotoxicity (the toxins are expelled from the body with the husks and seeds in the feces).
- **Digestive ailments** The soothing, protective effect imparted by the mucilage-rich husks and seeds benefits the whole gastrointestinal tract. Psyllium is taken for stomach and duodenal ulcers, and for acid indigestion.
- **Urinary infections** The demulcent action of psyllium extends to the urinary tract. In India, an infusion of the seeds (the only time this preparation is used) is given for urethritis.
- **External uses** When psyllium husks are soaked in an infusion of calendula (*Calendula officinalis*, p. 69) they make an effective poultice for external use, drawing out infection from boils, abscesses, and whitlows (pus-filled swellings on the fingertips).

SELF-HELP USES
- **Chronic diarrhea & irritable bowel syndrome**, p. 307.
- **Constipation**, p. 317.
- **Difficult passage of the stool & hemorrhoids**, p. 302.

✤ PARTS USED

Seeds should be soaked in water before they are used.

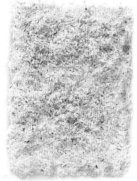

Husks are generally powdered for use in a variety of preparations.

� KEY PREPARATIONS & THEIR USES

Caution Do not exceed the stated dose. Always take with plenty of water.

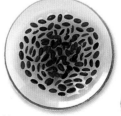

Cold maceration For constipation, soak 20 g of seeds in 200 ml water for 10 hours. Take the whole dose at night.

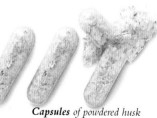

Capsules of powdered husk (p. 291). For hemorrhoids, take a 200 mg capsule 3 times a day.

POULTICE For boils, mix 5 g of powdered husks with sufficient infusion of calendula to make a thick paste. Apply (see p. 294) 3 times a day.

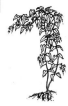

HE SHOU WU
A perennial climber, growing to 30 ft (10 m), with red stems and white or pink flowers.

Polygonum multiflorum (Polygonaceae)
HE SHOU WU (CHINESE), FLOWERY KNOTWEED

A CHINESE TONIC HERB with a bittersweet taste, *he shou wu* is thought to concentrate *qi* (vital energy) in its root, so that taking this herb gives vitality to the body. It has always been considered a rejuvenating herb, helping to prevent aging and encouraging longevity. Traditionally, much folklore is attached to *he shou wu*, and large old roots are thought to have remarkable powers.

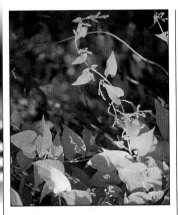

He shou wu is one of the oldest Chinese tonic herbs. It helps to lower blood cholesterol levels.

HABITAT & CULTIVATION

He shou wu is native to central and southern China and is cultivated throughout that region. It is propagated from seed, or by root division in spring, or from cuttings in summer. The plant requires well-fertilized soil and plenty of protection from winter weather. The roots of 3- to 4-year-old plants are unearthed and dried in the autumn. Older, larger roots are prized for their therapeutic properties but are generally not available commercially.

RELATED SPECIES

Bistort (*P. bistorta*, p. 251), one of the most strongly astringent of all herbs, and knotgrass (*P. aviculare*, p. 251) are used in European herbal medicine. They do not have the same tonic therapeutic properties as *P. multiflorum*. In Chinese herbal medicine, *P. cuspidatum* is used to treat amenorrhea (absence of periods).

KEY CONSTITUENTS

- Chrysophanic acid
- Anthraquinones (emodin, rhein)
- Lecithin

KEY ACTIONS

- Mildly sedative
- Nourishes the blood
- Tonic

RESEARCH

- **Cholesterol levels** In animal experiments in China, *he shou wu* was shown to reduce raised blood cholesterol levels significantly. Also, in a clinical trial, over 80% of patients with high blood cholesterol who had been taking decoctions of the root showed an improvement.
- **Blood sugar levels** Chinese research has revealed that *he shou wu* helps to increase the levels of sugar in the blood.
- **Countering infection** In China, experiments have demonstrated that *he shou wu* has the ability to counter the tuberculosis bacillus, and it is thought that it may be helpful in the treatment of malaria.

TRADITIONAL & CURRENT USES

- **Popular Chinese tonic** Although *he shou wu* is not the earliest tonic herb listed in Chinese herbal medicine (it is first mentioned in AD 713), it has certainly become one of the most important and widely used. It is taken regularly by millions of people throughout the East for its rejuvenating and toning properties and to increase fertility in both men and women.

✿ PARTS USED

Root is highly valued in Chinese medicine for its tonic properties. It is unearthed in the autumn.

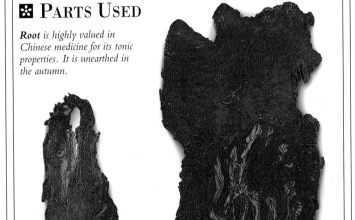

Dried root

☘ KEY PREPARATIONS & THEIR USES

Caution Only the prepared root from Chinese herbal supplierss should be used.

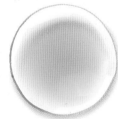

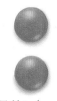

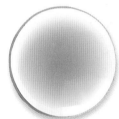

Decoction (to make, p. 290). As a general tonic, take the decoction over 2 days.

Tablets, known as shou wu pian, are taken in China for their rejuvenating properties.

Tincture (to make, p. 291). To reduce blood cholesterol levels, take 1 tsp twice a day with water.

❧ **POWDER** may be added to food for its tonic effect. Take 5 g a day.

- **Liver & kidney remedy** In Chinese herbal medicine, *he shou wu's* most important use is as a tonic for the liver and kidneys. By strengthening liver and kidney function, it helps to cleanse the blood, enabling the *qi* to circulate freely around the whole body.
- **Nerve & blood tonic** *He shou wu* is given in Chinese herbal medicine to people with symptoms, such as dizziness, weakness, numbness, and blurred vision, which indicate inefficient nerves and "blood deficiency."

- **Premature aging** *He shou wu* is prescribed in China for people showing signs of premature aging, including graying of the hair. This use suggests that the herb supports the body, helping it function in a balanced, healthy way.
- **Malaria** The herb is prescribed in the treatment of chronic malaria; when it is often combined with ginseng (*Panax ginseng*, p. 116), Chinese angelica (*Angelica sinensis*, p. 60), and green tangerine peel (*Citrus reticulata*).

Prunella vulgaris (Labiatae)

SELF-HEAL, XU KU CAO (CHINESE)

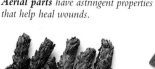

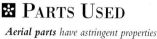

SELF-HEAL
A creeping perennial, growing to 20 in (50 cm), with pointed oval leaves and violet-blue or pink flowers.

A NATIVE EUROPEAN PLANT, self-heal has a long history as a wound healer and general tonic. Self-heal flowers, *xu ku cao*, are a remedy in Chinese herbal medicine. Unusually, the herb's application in China bears no relation to its traditional European usage. In China, the flowers are used for fevers and "liver weakness." Self-heal is little used in contemporary European herbal medicine and merits further investigation.

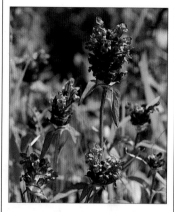

Self-heal's *throat-shaped flowers inspired its use for throat problems under the Doctrine of Signatures theory (see p. 16).*

HABITAT & CULTIVATION

Native to Europe and Asia, self-heal can be found in temperate regions worldwide. It is a wayside plant, growing in meadows and by roadsides, and thrives in sunny areas. Self-heal spreads by self-seeding or via its roots. It germinates easily and can be grown from seed in spring or by root division. The aerial parts are picked in midsummer when the plant is in bloom.

RELATED SPECIES

P. grandiflora, a closely related species, is thought to have similar properties.

KEY CONSTITUENTS

- Pentacyclic triterpenes (based on ursolic, betulinic, and oleanolic acids)
- Tannins
- Caffeic acid
- Vitamins B$_1$, C, K

KEY ACTIONS

- Heals wounds

- Astringent
- Stops internal bleeding
- Gently lowers blood pressure

RESEARCH

- **Blood pressure** Studies in China indicate that self-heal has a mildly dilating effect on the blood vessels, helping to lower blood pressure.
- **Countering infection** Chinese research shows the herb to have a moderately strong antibiotic action against a broad range of pathogens, including the *Shigella* species and *E. coli*, strains of which can cause enteritis and urinary infections.

TRADITIONAL & CURRENT USES

- **Traditional uses** Self-heal has been used as a wound herb for centuries. It staunches bleeding and accelerates the rate of repair. John Gerard wrote: "there is not a better wounde herbe in the world than that of selfe-heale" (1597). The Irish herbalist K'Eogh stated that self-heal "heals all internal and external wounds, removes obstructions of the liver and gall, and is therefore good for jaundice" (1735).
- **Modern European remedy** Not used in European herbal medicine on the same scale as in the past, self-heal is mainly employed as a wound herb. It is also sometimes taken to reduce internal bleeding, and as a gargle to treat sore throats. Externally, self-heal is applied topically to treat leucorrhea (vaginal discharge) and hemorrhoids. It has been considered by some practitioners to be a tonic.

✱ PARTS USED

Aerial parts *have astringent properties that help heal wounds.*

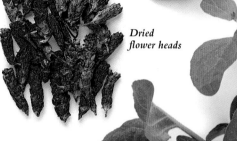

Dried flower heads

Dried aerial parts

Fresh aerial parts

🌿 KEY PREPARATIONS & THEIR USES

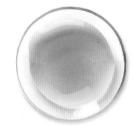

Infusion *(to make, p. 290). For sore throats, gargle 3 times a day.*

Tincture *(to make, p. 291). For bleeding gums, add 1 tsp to 20 ml of water and use as a mouthwash.*

Ointment *(to make, p. 294). Apply to cuts and scrapes, hemorrhoids, and varicose veins.*

📄 **POULTICE** *(to make, p. 294). Apply to sprains and minor wounds.*

- **Chinese treatment** In China, self-heal is taken on its own or with *ju hua* (*Chrysanthemum x morifolium*, p. 77) for fevers, headaches, dizziness, and vertigo, and to soothe and calm inflamed and sore eyes. It is thought to cool "liver fire" resulting from liver weakness, and is prescribed for infected and enlarged glands, especially the lymph nodes of the neck. In light of recent research, it is now sometimes used for high blood pressure.

Rehmannia glutinosa (Scrophulariaceae)

REHMANNIA, DI HUANG (CHINESE)

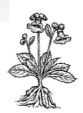

REHMANNIA
A perennial, reaching 1–2 ft (30–60 cm), with large sticky leaves and purple flowers.

AN IMPORTANT CHINESE TONIC HERB, rehmannia has figured extensively in many traditional herbal formulas and has an ancient history; it was referred to by Ge Hong, the 4th-century AD Chinese physician and alchemist. It is a "longevity" herb and has a marked tonic action on the liver and kidneys. Research has confirmed its traditional use, showing that it protects the liver and is useful for hepatitis.

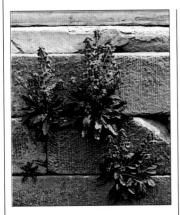

Rehmannia's appearance gave rise to its Western folkname "Chinese foxglove."

HABITAT & CULTIVATION

Rehmannia grows wild on sunny mountain slopes in northern and northeastern parts of China, especially in Henan province. It can be cultivated, in which case it is propagated from seed sown in autumn or spring. The root is harvested in autumn after the plant has flowered.

RELATED SPECIES

R. lutea is used in Chinese herbal medicine as a diuretic.

KEY CONSTITUENTS

- Phytosterols (B-sitosterol, stigmasterol)
- Sugars (mannitol)
- Rehmannin

KEY ACTIONS

- Tonic
- Kidney tonic
- Lowers blood pressure
- Protects the liver

RESEARCH

- **Liver remedy** Chinese research has shown rehmannia

to be a very important liver-protective herb, preventing poisoning and liver damage. Clinical trials in China have demonstrated that it is effective in treating hepatitis. ·
- **Other research** Trials have indicated that rehmannia lowers blood pressure and blood cholesterol levels. In addition, its ability to reduce fevers may make it useful for rheumatoid arthritis.

TRADITIONAL & CURRENT USES

- **Raw & prepared root** In Chinese herbal medicine, the root (*di huang*) is known as *sheng di huang* when it is eaten raw and *shu di huang* when it has been cooked in wine. The former is the most commonly taken remedy. Both are *yin* tonics (*see p. 38*), but have different therapeutic indications.
- **Sheng di huang** The raw root "cools the blood" and is given to help lower fever in acute and chronic illnesses. Its cooling nature is reflected in its use for problems such as thirst and a red tongue that arise from "heat patterns." *Sheng di huang* is useful for treating people with impaired liver function and is used specifically to treat hepatitis and other liver conditions.
- **Shu di huang** This preparation is used specifically for blood loss and "blood deficiency" states such as irregular and heavy menstrual bleeding. It is warming rather than cooling, and is considered to be a prime kidney tonic.
- **Blood pressure** Rehmannia is used to treat high blood pressure. Interestingly, while

PARTS USED

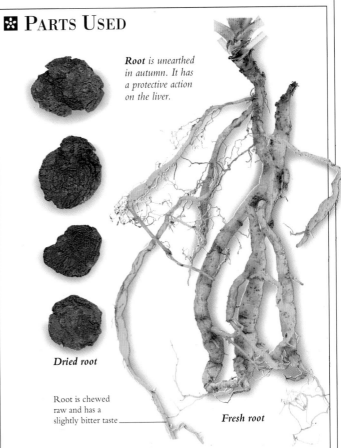

Root is unearthed in autumn. It has a protective action on the liver.

Dried root

Root is chewed raw and has a slightly bitter taste

Fresh root

KEY PREPARATIONS & THEIR USES

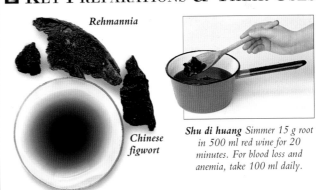

Rehmannia

Chinese figwort

Shu di huang *Simmer 15 g root in 500 ml red wine for 20 minutes. For blood loss and anemia, take 100 ml daily.*

Remedy *Decoct 15 g rehmannia and 10 g Chinese figwort (see p. 290). For fevers, take 1 cup 2–3 times daily.*

sheng di huang appears to raise blood pressure, *shu di huang* has the opposite effect.
- **Longevity** Rehmannia is a traditional and valuable tonic for old age. It is considered to help prevent senility.
- **Chinese formulas** The herb is an ingredient of many famous herbal formulas, most notably

"the pill of eight ingredients," which contemporary Chinese herbalists consider to "warm and invigorate the *yang* of the loins."

SELF-HELP USES

- **Heavy menstrual bleeding**, p. 315.
- **Weakened liver & metabolism**, p. 319.

Rheum palmatum (*Polygonaceae*)

CHINESE RHUBARB, DA HUANG (CHINESE)

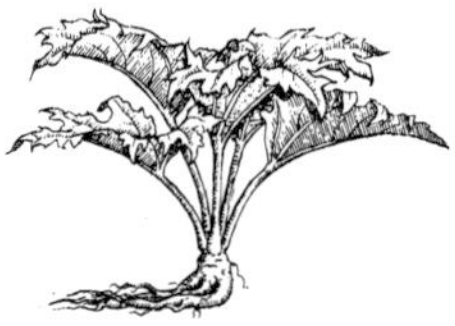

CHINESE RHUBARB A thick-rhizomed perennial growing to 10 ft (3 m), with large palm-shaped leaves and small flowers.

CHINESE RHUBARB HAS LONG been prized as the most useful purge in herbal medicine, safe even for young children due to its gentle action. It has been used in China for over 2,000 years and is an extremely effective treatment for many digestive problems. Paradoxically, it is a laxative when taken in large doses but has a constipating effect in small measures. The rhizome has an astringent, unpleasant taste.

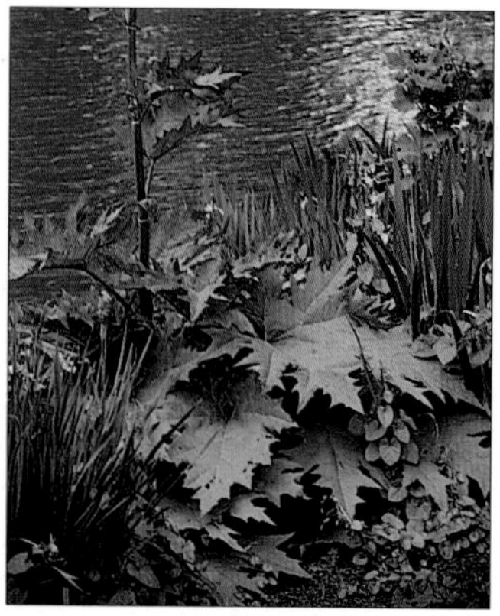

Chinese rhubarb *grows best close to water. In summer it produces clusters of red flowers.*

HABITAT & CULTIVATION

Native to China and Tibet, where the best-quality rhubarb is still found, Chinese rhubarb now also grows in the West. It is found in the wild and is widely cultivated. It is grown from seed in spring or by root division in spring or autumn and requires a sunny position and well-drained soil. The rhizomes of 6–10-year-old plants are dug up in the autumn after the stem and leaves have turned yellow.

RELATED SPECIES

R. tanguticum and *R. officinale* have similar uses to *R. palmatum*. These 3 species are considered to be superior in action to other rhubarbs. The familiar, edible rhubarb is *R. rhaponticum*.

KEY CONSTITUENTS

- Anthraquinones (about 3–5%), rhein, aloe-emodin, emodin
- Flavonoids (catechin)
- Phenolic acids
- Tannins (5–10%)
- Calcium oxalate

KEY ACTIONS

- Laxative
- Constipating
- Astringent
- Eases stomach pain
- Antibacterial

RESEARCH

- **Anthraquinones & tannins** Chinese rhubarb's medicinal value is largely due to the irritant, laxative, and purgative properties of the anthraquinones and in large doses the rhizome is strongly laxative. The high levels of tannins contained in the herb, however, counterbalance the laxative action, and it has been demonstrated that in small doses the tannins predominate, causing a constipating effect.
- **Antibacterial** Decoctions of the root have been shown to be effective against *Staphylococcus aureus*, an infectious bacterium that causes canker sores and folliculitis (an acne-type infection of the beard area).

TRADITIONAL & CURRENT USES

- **History** Chinese rhubarb was first mentioned in the 1st-century AD Chinese classic *Materia Medica* and has been grown in the West since 1732. It is one of the relatively few herbs still used today in conventional as well as herbal medicine, and is listed in the *British Pharmacopoeia* of 1988.
- **Constipation** Large doses of Chinese rhubarb are combined with carminative herbs and taken as a laxative, helping to clear the colon without causing excessive cramps. This is useful for treating constipation where the muscles of the large bowel are weak.
- **Diarrhea** Small doses of the root are astringent, relieving irritation of the inner lining of the gut, thus reducing diarrhea.
- **Other uses** The herb can be applied to burns, boils, and carbuncles. It is a tonic and mild appetite stimulant and is a useful mouthwash for canker sores.

SELF-HELP USE

- **Constipation**, p. 307.

PARTS USED

Rhizome is a mild appetite stimulant and helps to improve digestion

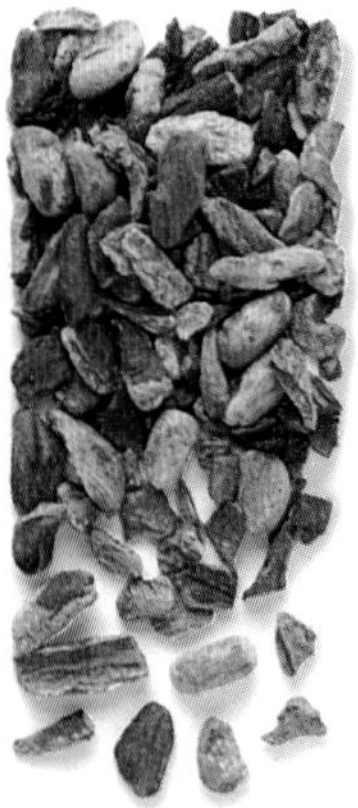

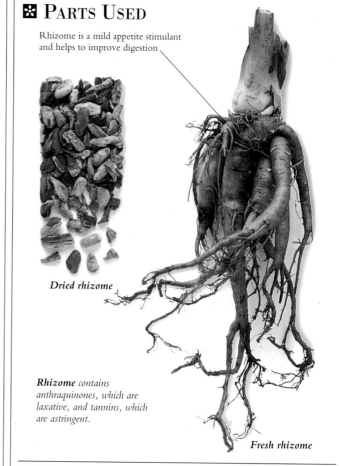

Dried rhizome

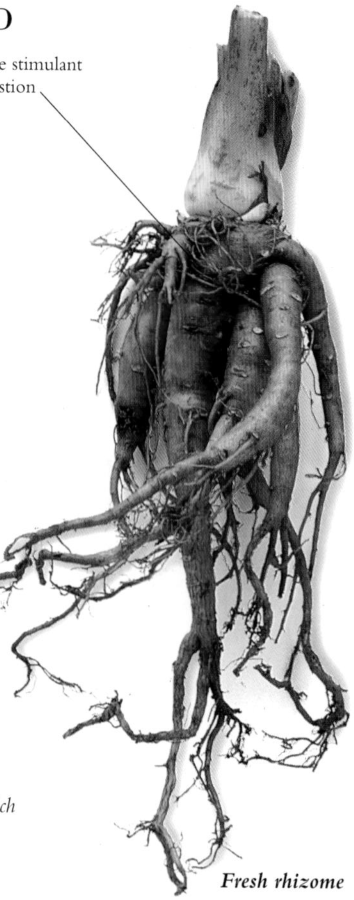

Rhizome *contains anthraquinones, which are laxative, and tannins, which are astringent.*

Fresh rhizome

KEY PREPARATIONS & THEIR USES

Cautions Do not take during pregnancy or while breast-feeding. Do not take during menstruation or if prone to gout or kidney stones.

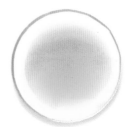

Decoction *(to make, p. 290). For an occasional bout of constipation, take 100 ml each evening.*

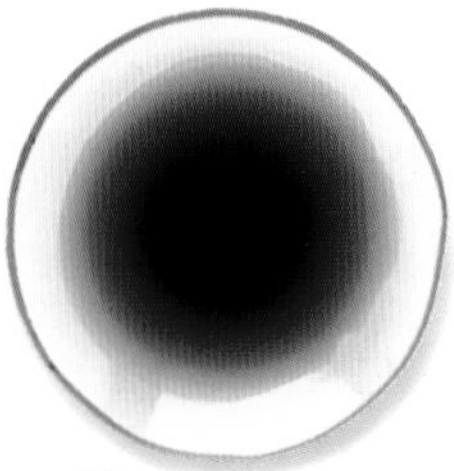

Tincture *(to make, p. 291). To stimulate the appetite, take 20 drops with water twice a day.*

TABLETS are one of the most convenient ways of taking the herb. Take for one-off bouts of constipation.

Rosmarinus officinalis (Labiatiae)
ROSEMARY

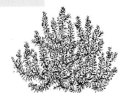

ROSEMARY
A strongly aromatic evergreen shrub growing to 7 ft (2 m), with narrow, dark green, pinelike leaves.

ROSEMARY IS A WELL-KNOWN and greatly valued herb that is native to southern Europe. It has been used since antiquity to improve and strengthen the memory. To this day it is burned in the homes of students in Greece who are about to take exams. Rosemary has a longstanding reputation as a tonic, invigorating herb, imparting a zest for life that is to some degree reflected in its distinctive aromatic taste.

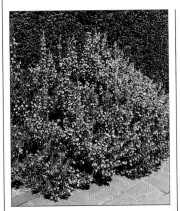

Rosemary was a symbol of fidelity between lovers, on account of its ability to improve the memory.

HABITAT & CULTIVATION

Native to the Mediterranean, rosemary grows freely in much of southern Europe and is cultivated throughout the world. It is propagated from seed or cuttings in spring and prefers a warm, moderately dry climate and a sheltered site. The branches are gathered during the summer after flowering and dried in the shade.

KEY CONSTITUENTS

- Volatile oil (1–2%) containing borneol, camphene, camphor, cineole
- Flavonoids (apigenin, diosmin)
- Tannins
- Rosmarinic acid
- Diterpenes (picrosalvin)
- Rosmaricine

KEY ACTIONS

- Tonic
- Stimulant
- Astringent
- Nervine
- Anti-inflammatory
- Carminative

RESEARCH

- **Rosmaricine** Research has shown that rosmaricine is a stimulant and mild analgesic.
- **Volatile oil** The oil content varies within the plant. It is analgesic and stimulant, especially when applied to the skin.
- **Other research** Rosemary's anti-inflammatory effect is due mainly to rosmarinic acid and flavonoids. The flavonoids also strengthen the capillaries. The herb, as a whole, has bitter and astringent properties.

TRADITIONAL & CURRENT USES

- **Circulatory stimulant** Rosemary has a central place in European herbal medicine. A warming herb, it stimulates circulation of blood to the head, improving concentration and memory. It also eases headaches and migraine, and encourages hair growth by improving blood flow to the scalp.
- **Nervous problems** Rosemary has been used to treat epilepsy and vertigo.
- **Poor circulation** Thought to raise low blood pressure, rosemary is valuable for fainting and weakness associated with deficient circulation.
- **Restorative** Rosemary aids recovery from long-term stress and chronic illness. It is thought to stimulate the adrenal glands and is used specifically for debility, especially when accompanied by poor circulation and digestion.
- **Uplifting** Rosemary is often prescribed for people who, though not actually ill, are stressed and "failing to thrive." It is valued as an herb that raises

PARTS USED

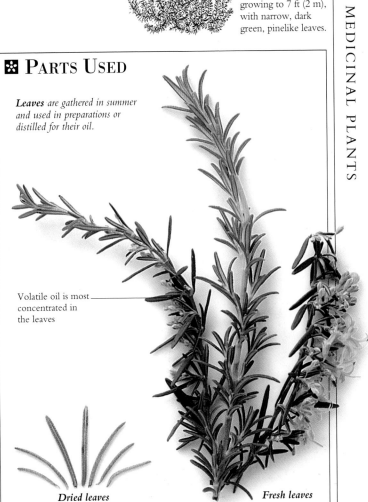

Leaves are gathered in summer and used in preparations or distilled for their oil.

Volatile oil is most concentrated in the leaves

Dried leaves

Fresh leaves

KEY PREPARATIONS & THEIR USES

Caution Do not take the essential oil internally except under professional supervision.

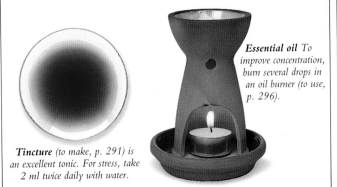

Tincture (to make, p. 291) is an excellent tonic. For stress, take 2 ml twice daily with water.

Essential oil *To improve concentration, burn several drops in an oil burner (to use, p. 296).*

INFUSION (to make, p. 290). To relieve headaches, take 50 ml every 3 hours. The infusion, rubbed into the scalp, improves hair growth.

the spirits, and is useful for mild to moderate depression.
- **Other uses** Applied as a lotion or diluted essential oil, rosemary eases aching, rheumatic muscles. Add the infusion or essential oil to bathwater for a reviving soak.

SELF-HELP USES

- **Migraine**, p. 309.
- **Premenstrual tension**, p. 315.
- **Sore throats**, p. 311.
- **Tired & aching muscles**, p. 312.

Rumex crispus (Polygonaceae)
YELLOW DOCK, CURLED DOCK

YELLOW DOCK
A perennial growing from 1–5 ft (30 cm–1.5 m), with lance-shaped leaves up to 10 in (25 cm) long.

IN COMMON WITH OTHER SPECIES of dock, this herb has valuable cleansing properties and is useful for skin problems. It is not as famous a laxative as Chinese rhubarb (*Rheum palmatum*, p. 124), but its gentle, less intense effect on the bowel makes it particularly useful for mild constipation. The root has a slightly bitter taste and is the only part used medicinally. In the past, the leaves were eaten as a spring tonic.

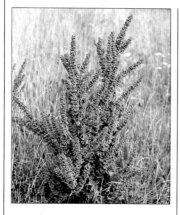

Yellow dock has spikes of small, red, woody fruits in autumn.

HABITAT & CULTIVATION
Native to Europe and Africa, yellow dock is commonly found growing wild in many regions of the world. It thrives on dumps, roadsides, and in ditches. The root is dug up in autumn, chopped, and dried.

RELATED SPECIES
Many other docks have a similar action – for example, broad-leaved dock (*R. obtusifolius*). Certain sorrels, such as sheep's sorrel (*R. acetosella*, p. 262), are also used similarly to yellow dock. The *Rumex* family has long been used as a purge: Nicholas Culpeper (1616–1654) described monk's rhubarb (*R. alpinus*) as "purging choler and flegm downwards very gently and safely without danger."

KEY CONSTITUENTS
- Anthraquinones (up to 4%), nepodin, emodin, chrysaphanol
- Tannins
- Oxalates
- Volatile oil

KEY ACTIONS
- Mild laxative
- Stimulates bile flow
- Cleansing

RESEARCH
- **Anthraquinones** Yellow dock has not been well researched, but its laxative, cleansing properties are known to be largely due to the anthraquinones. These constituents have a laxative, and, at high doses, a purgative effect on the colon. This action is similar, but milder, to that of Chinese rhubarb.
- **Oxalates** The leaves of yellow dock were a traditional spring tonic, but research shows that they contain large amounts of oxalates, which in high doses can cause kidney stones and gout. (The level of oxalates in the root, however, is safe.)

TRADITIONAL & CURRENT USES
- **Laxative effect** The herb's gentle laxative action makes it an important remedy in mild cases of constipation. This action is enhanced if the fiber content of the diet is increased. By stimulating the colon, feces are eliminated more efficiently, reducing reabsorption of toxins.
- **Bile stimulant** Yellow dock is thought to improve the flow of bile, which further contributes to its detoxifying action. (Waste products are removed through the bile ducts.)
- **Cleansing herb** Generally combined with other cleansing herbs such as burdock (*Arctium lappa*, p. 62) and dandelion (*Taraxacum officinale*, p. 140), yellow dock is used to treat a wide range of conditions resulting from high levels of toxins in the body. These include skin conditions such as acne, boils, eczema, and psoriasis, as well as fungal infections, sluggish digestion and constipation, and arthritic and rheumatic problems, especially osteoarthritis.

▣ PARTS USED

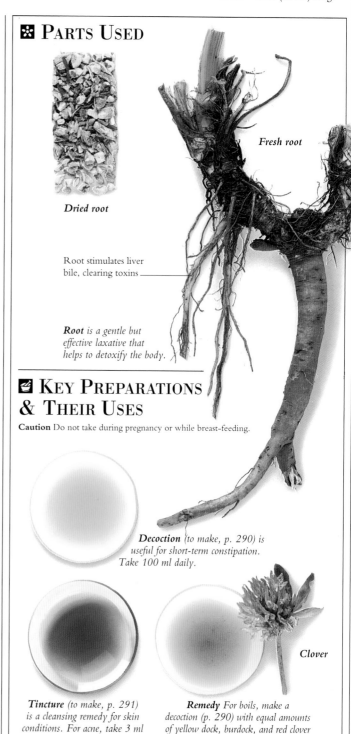

Dried root

Fresh root

Root stimulates liver bile, clearing toxins

Root is a gentle but effective laxative that helps to detoxify the body.

▣ KEY PREPARATIONS & THEIR USES

Caution Do not take during pregnancy or while breast-feeding.

Decoction (to make, p. 290) is useful for short-term constipation. Take 100 ml daily.

Clover

Tincture (to make, p. 291) is a cleansing remedy for skin conditions. For acne, take 3 ml with water twice a day.

Remedy For boils, make a decoction (p. 290) with equal amounts of yellow dock, burdock, and red clover root. Drink ½ cup daily.

SELF-HELP USES
- **Constipation**, p. 307.
- **Nettle rash**, p. 303.

Sabal serrulata syn. *Serenoa serrulata* (Palmaceae)

SAW PALMETTO

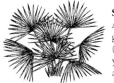

SAW PALMETTO
A small palm growing to 20 ft (6 m), with fans of yellow-green leaves and ivory flowers.

SAW PALMETTO BERRIES WERE EATEN by Native North Americans and also by animals. According to legend, on seeing the animals grow "sleek and fat," European settlers tried them and attributed medicinal properties to them. The fruit pulp was used as a tonic from the 19th century onward, and today it is used to help in debility, for urinary tract problems, and for reducing enlarged prostate glands.

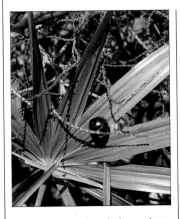

Saw palmetto has dark purple to black berries growing in the center of the leaf fans.

HABITAT & CULTIVATION

Saw palmetto is indigenous to North America and can be found growing in sand dunes along the Atlantic and Caribbean coasts from South Carolina to Texas. It is propagated from seed in spring and needs well-drained soil and plenty of sun. The berries are harvested when ripe in autumn, then dried, often with the seeds removed.

RELATED SPECIES

The Maya of Central America used the roots or leaves of *S. japa*, another small palm, as a remedy for dysentery and abdominal pain. The crushed roots of *S. adamsonii* were used by the Houma, who also lived in Central America, as an eye lotion.

KEY CONSTITUENTS

- Volatile oil (1–2%)
- Fixed oil
- Steroidal saponin
- Polysaccharides
- Tannins

KEY ACTIONS

- Tonic
- Diuretic
- Sedative
- Anabolic
- Estrogenic

RESEARCH

- **Need for treatment** There has been little research into saw palmetto, despite its potential as a treatment for enlarged prostate gland, and its anabolic action (*see below*). With the probable presence of steroidal constituents, and an apparent estrogenic action, saw palmetto is a plant that could have significant hormonal actions. It needs to be researched in depth.

TRADITIONAL & CURRENT USES

- **Anabolic action** Saw palmetto is a tonic and is one of the few Western remedies that is considered to be anabolic – it strengthens and builds body tissues and encourages weight gain. Fruit pulp or tincture is given to those suffering from wasting illnesses and for general debility and failure to thrive.
- **Hormonal disorders** Although it is generally considered to be a man's herb, given its probable estrogenic action saw palmetto is also a useful herbal remedy for women. It is prescribed for impotence, reduced or absent sex drive, and testicular atrophy in men, and in women has been given to stimulate breast enlargement.
- **Urinary remedy** Saw palmetto has been nicknamed the "plant catheter." This is because it has the ability to strengthen the neck of the bladder and to reduce enlarged prostate glands. It is used chiefly as a diuretic to improve urine flow and as a urinary antiseptic in cystitis. It combines well with horsetail (*Equisetum arvense*, p. 202) and hydrangea (*Hydrangea arborescens*, p. 219) in the treatment of prostate infection.

SELF-HELP USE

- **Impotence & premature ejaculation**, see p. 316.

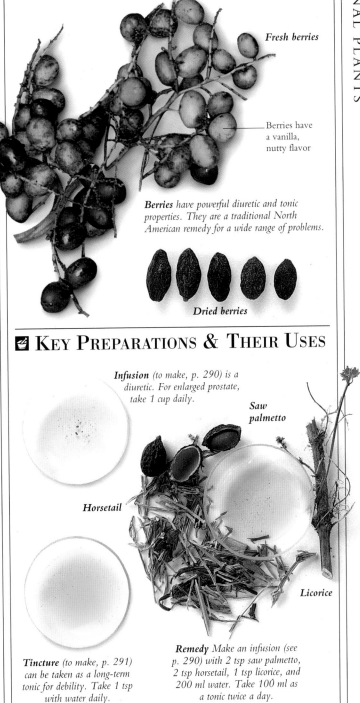

✤ PARTS USED

Fresh berries

Berries have a vanilla, nutty flavor

Berries have powerful diuretic and tonic properties. They are a traditional North American remedy for a wide range of problems.

Dried berries

☙ KEY PREPARATIONS & THEIR USES

Infusion (to make, p. 290) is a diuretic. For enlarged prostate, take 1 cup daily.

Saw palmetto

Horsetail

Licorice

Tincture (to make, p. 291) can be taken as a long-term tonic for debility. Take 1 tsp with water daily.

Remedy Make an infusion (see p. 290) with 2 tsp saw palmetto, 2 tsp horsetail, 1 tsp licorice, and 200 ml water. Take 100 ml as a tonic twice a day.

127

Salix alba (Salicaceae)
WHITE WILLOW

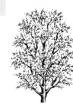

WHITE WILLOW
A deciduous tree growing to 80 ft (25 m), with green tapering leaves, and catkins in spring.

JUSTLY FAMOUS AS THE ORIGINAL source of salicylic acid (the forerunner of aspirin), white willow and closely related species have been used for thousands of years in Europe, Africa, Asia, and North America to relieve joint pain and manage fevers. Dioscorides, a Greek physician in the 1st century AD, suggested taking "willow leaves, mashed with a little pepper and drunk with wine" to relieve lower back pain.

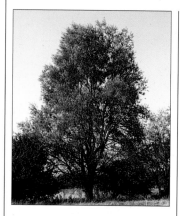

White willow *is used in Britain to make cricket bats. The bark has anti-inflammatory properties.*

HABITAT & CULTIVATION

Native to much of Europe, white willow is also found in North Africa and Asia, thriving in damp areas, such as on riverbanks. It is propagated from semiripe cuttings in summer or from hardwood cuttings in winter. The trees are frequently pollarded, and bark is stripped from branches of 2- to 5-year-old trees in spring.

RELATED SPECIES

Many *Salix* species – for example, crack willow (*S. fragilis*) – are used interchangeably with white willow. *S. acmophylla* is used in the Indian subcontinent as a remedy for fevers. In North American herbal medicine, black willow (*S. nigra*) is given as an anaphrodisiac (sexual depressant).

KEY CONSTITUENTS

- Phenolic glycosides (up to 11%) – salicylic acid
- Flavonoids
- Tannins (up to 20%)

KEY ACTIONS

- Anti-inflammatory
- Analgesic
- Reduces fever
- Antirheumatic
- Astringent

RESEARCH

- **Salicylic acid & aspirin**
There has been little research into white willow as a whole, but salicylic acid, its main active constituent, was first isolated in 1838. It was the forerunner of aspirin, a chemical drug first produced in 1899. Salicylic acid has many of the same analgesic and anti-inflammatory actions as aspirin. It inhibits prostaglandin production, relieves pain, and soothes fevers. Unlike aspirin, it does not thin the blood. Nor does it irritate the stomach lining – a common side effect of aspirin.

TRADITIONAL & CURRENT USES

- **Past uses** White willow is astringent and was formerly used to staunch internal bleeding. In his herbal (1652), Nicholas Culpeper advised that the burnt ashes of the bark be "mixed with vinegar, [to] take away warts, corns and superfluous flesh."
- **Joint remedy** White willow is an excellent remedy for arthritic and rheumatic pain affecting the back, and joints such as the knees and hips. In combination with other herbs and dietary changes, it relieves inflammation and swelling, and improves mobility in painful or creaky joints. Though aspirin-based conventional medicines are stronger acting, they can have unwanted side effects.

- **Fevers & pain** White willow is taken to manage high fevers. It may also be used to ease headaches and head pain.
- **Menopause** By reducing sweating, white willow helps hot flashes and night sweats.

PARTS USED

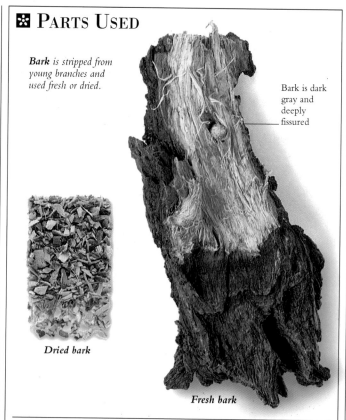

Bark *is stripped from young branches and used fresh or dried.*

Bark is dark gray and deeply fissured

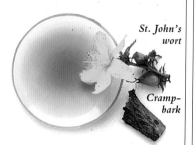

Dried bark

Fresh bark

KEY PREPARATIONS & THEIR USES

Caution Avoid if allergic to aspirin.

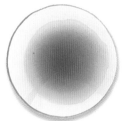

St. John's wort

Cramp-bark

Tincture *(to make, see p. 291). For rheumatism, take ½ tsp with water 3 times a day.*

Remedy *Make a decoction (see p. 290) with 10 g each of white willow, St. John's wort, and crampbark. For aching muscles, drink 1 cup twice a day.*

Tablets *usually also contain other herbs. Take for arthritis.*

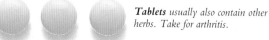 **DECOCTION** (to make, p. 290). For painful joints and aching rheumatic muscles, take ½ cup 3 times a day.

SELF-HELP USES

- **Arthritis & inflamed joints**, p. 313.
- **Back pain due to joint inflammation**, p. 313.
- **Hot flashes & night sweats**, p. 316.

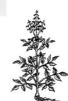

DAN SHEN
A hardy perennial growing to 32 in (80 cm), with toothed oval leaves and clusters of purple flowers.

Salvia miltiorrhiza (Labiatae)
DAN SHEN, RED SAGE

RECENT SCIENTIFIC RESEARCH has confirmed the validity of *dan shen's* traditional usage for heart and circulatory problems. *The Divine Husbandman's Classic (Shen'nong Bencaojing)*, the earliest of all Chinese herbal texts, listed *dan shen* as an herb that "invigorates the blood," and it is still used as a circulatory remedy. In particular, it is taken for menstrual pain and other conditions resulting from circulatory congestion.

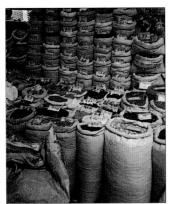

Dan shen is an important circulatory stimulant. It is sold in herbal markets across China for use in medicinal formulas.

HABITAT & CULTIVATION

Native to China, *dan shen* is now cultivated in northeastern China and Inner Mongolia. It requires moist sandy soil and is propagated by root division in spring. The root is harvested from late autumn through to early spring.

RELATED SPECIES

Sage (*S. officinalis*, p. 130) is a closely related species but is used for an entirely different range of medical problems. In Mexico, the related species *S. divinorum* is used as a hallucinogen.

KEY CONSTITUENTS

- Tanshinones
- Tanshinol
- Salviol
- Vitamin E
- Volatile oil

KEY ACTIONS

- Circulatory tonic
- Dilates the blood vessels
- Sedative
- Antibacterial

RESEARCH

- **Tanshinones** There has been extensive research into *dan shen* in China, and the tanshinones have been shown to have a profound effect on the coronary circulation, reducing the symptoms of angina and improving heart function.
- **Heart attack** The whole herb (rather than isolated constituents) has been used in China to assist patients who are recovering from a heart attack, and it appears to support heart function at this critical time. Clinical trials in China, however, have shown that *dan shen* is most effective when taken as a preventive, rather than as a remedy after the heart attack has taken place.
- **Other research** *Dan shen* is known to inhibit the action of tubercle bacillus.

TRADITIONAL & CURRENT USES

- **Circulatory stimulant** *Dan shen* has been esteemed by the Chinese for thousands of years as a circulatory stimulant. Like hawthorn (*Crataegus oxyacantha*, p. 86), it is a safe effective remedy for many circulatory problems. It particularly benefits the coronary circulation, opening up the arteries and improving blood flow to the heart, and is therefore helpful in treating coronary heart disease. Although it does not lower blood pressure, *dan shen* relaxes the blood vessels and improves circulation throughout the body.
- **Circulatory congestion** *Dan shen* is used traditionally to treat conditions caused by blood stagnation, primarily those affecting the lower abdomen, such as absent or painful menstrual periods and fibroids.
- **Sedative** The sedative action of *dan shen* helps calm the nerves, and it is therefore helpful in treating angina, a condition made worse by anxiety and worry. Palpitations, insomnia, and irritability also benefit from *dan shen's* sedative properties.
- **Cooling herb** *Dan shen* is a soothing remedy that is used to remove "excess heat," particularly in the heart and liver. It can also alleviate inflammatory skin problems, such as abscesses, boils, and sores.

SELF-HELP USE

- **Palpitations**, p. 302.

✿ PARTS USED

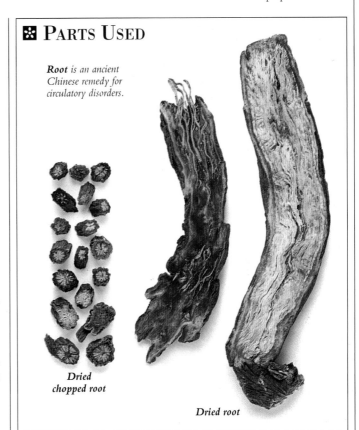

Root is an ancient Chinese remedy for circulatory disorders.

Dried chopped root

Dried root

☕ KEY PREPARATIONS & THEIR USES

Cautions For serious circulatory or heart problems, take only under professional supervision. The tincture may produce digestive and skin reactions. Avoid in pregnancy.

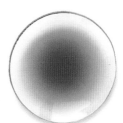

Tincture is used by herbalists to treat angina and other circulatory problems.

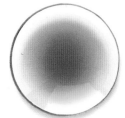

Decoction (to make, p. 290). For painful menstrual periods, take ½ cup up to 3 times a day.

SAGE
An evergreen growing
to 32 in (80 cm), with
square stems and hairy
gray-green or
purple leaves.

Salvia officinalis (Labiatae)
SAGE

SAGE'S BOTANICAL NAME is a clue to its medicinal importance: *Salvia* comes from *salvare*, meaning "to cure" in Latin. A medieval saying echoes this: "Why should a man die while sage grows in his garden?" Today, sage is an excellent remedy for sore throats, poor digestion, and irregular menstruation, and it is also taken as a gently stimulating tonic. It has a slightly warm but noticeably bitter and astringent taste.

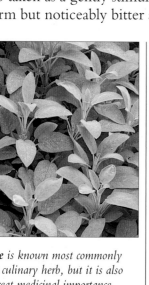

Sage is known most commonly as a culinary herb, but it is also of great medicinal importance.

HABITAT & CULTIVATION

Native to the Mediterranean, sage is cultivated all round the world, thriving in sunny conditions. It is grown from seed in spring and the plants are replaced after 3–4 years. The leaves are picked in summer.

RELATED SPECIES

In all, there are about 500 species of *Salvia*. Spanish sage (*S. lavandulifolia*) is the most familiar culinary variety and does not contain thujone. Two close relatives of *S. officinalis* are *dan shen* (*S. miltiorrhiza*, p. 129) and clary sage (*S. sclarea*, p. 263).

KEY CONSTITUENTS

- Volatile oil (thujone – about 50%)
- Diterpene bitters
- Flavonoids
- Phenolic acids
- Tannins

KEY ACTIONS

- Astringent
- Antiseptic
- Aromatic
- Carminative
- Estrogenic
- Reduces sweating
- Tonic

RESEARCH

- **Thujone** Research shows that thujone, contained in the volatile oil, is strongly antiseptic and carminative. It also has an estrogenic action that is partly responsible for sage's hormonal effect, especially in reducing breast-milk production. In excess, thujone is toxic.
- **Other research** Rosmarinic acid, a phenol, is known to be strongly anti-inflammatory, while the volatile oil, as a whole, relieves muscle spasms and is antimicrobial.

TRADITIONAL & CURRENT USES

- **Antiseptic & astringent** Sage's combination of antiseptic, relaxing, and astringent actions makes it ideal for almost all types of sore throat, and it is widely used in gargles. It is also used for canker sores and sore gums. Sage's astringency also makes it useful for mild diarrhea.
- **Tonic** Sage is a digestive tonic and stimulant. In Chinese medicine it is a *yin* tonic (*see* pp. 38–39) with a well-deserved reputation as a nerve tonic, helping both to calm and stimulate the nervous system.
- **Hormonal stimulant** Sage is a valuable remedy for irregular and light menstruation, encouraging a better flow of blood. Although its hormonal action is not completely understood, there is no doubt

that it reduces sweating, which, coupled with its tonic and estrogenic effects, makes it an excellent remedy for menopause, not only reducing hot flashes but helping the body to adapt to the hormonal changes involved.
- **Asthma remedy** Sage has traditionally been used to treat asthma, and the dried leaves are

still included in herbal smoking mixtures for this complaint.

SELF-HELP USES

- **Bites & stings**, p. 303.
- **Canker sores**, p. 306.
- **Diarrhea**, p. 307.
- **Hot flashes & night sweats**, p. 316.
- **Sore throats**, p. 311.

✻ PARTS USED

Leaves have valuable antiseptic and astringent properties.

Fresh leaves

Purple sage, *S. officinalis purpurascens*, is the preferred medicinal variety

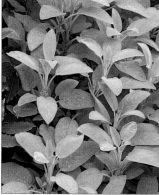

Dried leaves

✎ KEY PREPARATIONS & THEIR USES

Cautions Do not take therapeutic doses during pregnancy or if epileptic.

Infusion (to make, p. 290). Use as a gargle for sore throats up to 3 times a day.

Fresh sage leaves are a useful first aid remedy. Rub on stings and bites.

Tincture (to make, p. 291) is a digestive tonic. Take 2 ml with water twice a day.

Sambucus nigra (Caprifoliaceae)
ELDER

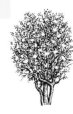

ELDER HAS MORE FOLKLORE attached to it than almost any other European plant, except perhaps mandrake (*Mandragora officinarum*, p. 230). Chopping elder branches was considered dangerous in rural England because it was believed that the tree was inhabited by the Elder Mother. To avoid her wrath, woodcutters would recite a placatory rhyme. Elder is a valuable remedy for flu, colds, and chesty conditions.

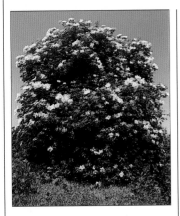

Elder was traditionally known as "Nature's medicine chest."

HABITAT & CULTIVATION

Native to Europe, elder thrives in woods, hedges, and on wasteground. It is now found in most temperate regions and is often cultivated. Elder is propagated from cuttings in spring. The flowering tops are harvested in late spring and the berries are picked in early autumn.

KEY CONSTITUENTS

Flowers:
- Flavonoids (up to 3%) – rutin
- Phenolic acids
- Triterpenes
- Sterols
- Volatile oil (up to 0.2%)
- Mucilage
- Tannins

Leaves:
- Cyanogenic glycosides

Berries:
- Flavonoids
- Anthocyanins
- Vitamins A and C

KEY ACTIONS

- Increases sweating
- Diuretic
- Anti-inflammatory

RESEARCH

- **Lack of research** Research indicates that the flowers reduce inflammation, but on the whole elder is a poorly researched herb. Its diaphoretic effect (increasing sweating) is well known but even this is not completely understood.

TRADITIONAL & CURRENT USES

- **Coughs & colds** Flowering tops are ideal for coughs, colds, and flu. The infusion is relaxing and produces a mild perspiration that helps to reduce fever.
- **Congestion & allergies** The flowering tops tone the mucous linings of the nose and throat, increasing their resistance to infection. They are prescribed for chronic congestion, allergies, ear infections, and candidiasis. Infusions of the flowering tops and other herbs can reduce the severity of hay fever attacks if taken for some months before the onset of the hay fever season.
- **Arthritis** By encouraging sweating and urine production, elder flowering tops promote the removal of waste products from the body and are of value in arthritic conditions.
- **Berries** Rich in vitamin C, elder berries have been taken for rheumatism and erysipelas (a skin infection). They are mildly laxative and also help diarrhea.

SELF-HELP USES

- **Allergic rhinitis, including hay fever**, p. 300.
- **Candidiasis**, p. 314.
- **Earache due to chronic congestion**, p. 312.
- **Flu**, p. 311.

✦ PARTS USED

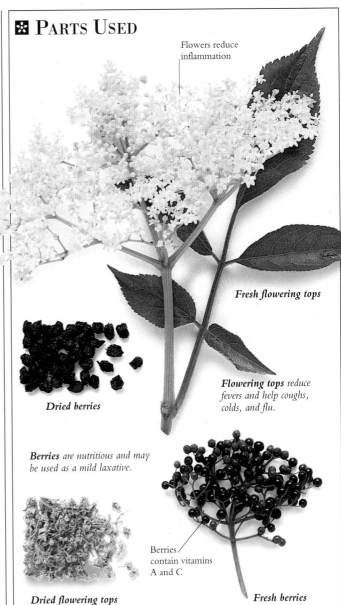

Flowers reduce inflammation

Fresh flowering tops

Dried berries

Flowering tops reduce fevers and help coughs, colds, and flu.

Berries are nutritious and may be used as a mild laxative.

Berries contain vitamins A and C

Dried flowering tops

Fresh berries

☙ KEY PREPARATIONS & THEIR USES

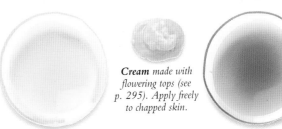

Cream made with flowering tops (see p. 295). Apply freely to chapped skin.

Infusion of flowering tops (to make, p. 290). For colds, drink 1 cup 3 times a day.

Tincture of flowering tops (to make, p. 291). For hay fever, take 1 tsp with water 3–4 times a day.

DECOCTION of berries (to make, p. 290). For rheumatic aches, take 100 ml 3 times a day.

Schisandra chinensis (Schisandraceae)

SCHISANDRA, WU WEI ZI (CHINESE)

SCHISANDRA
An aromatic, woody vine reaching up to 25 ft (8 m) with pink flowers and spikes of red berries.

SCHISANDRA RANKS ALONG WITH other Chinese tonic herbs as an excellent tonic and restorative. It helps in stressful times and increases zest for life. The berries tone the kidneys and sexual organs, protect the liver, strengthen nervous function, and cleanse the blood. The name *wu wei zi* means "5-flavored herb," since this herb reputedly tastes of the 5 main elemental energies (*see* p. 38). It has a sour, salty, and slightly warm taste.

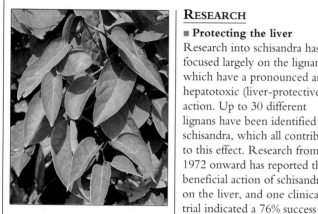

***Schisandra** is one of China's most important tonic herbs, widely taken as a sexual tonic.*

HABITAT & CULTIVATION

Schisandra is cultivated in northeastern China, especially in the provinces of Jilin, Lianoning, Heilongjiang, and Hebei. It is propagated from seed in spring. The fruit is harvested in autumn when it is fully ripe.

RELATED SPECIES

Though less therapeutically active than schisandra, the berries of the related *nan wu wei zi (S. sphenanthera)* are commonly used in Chinese medicine for acute coughs.

KEY CONSTITUENTS

- Lignans (schizandrin, deoxyschizandrin, gomisin)
- Phytosterols (beta-sitosterol, stigmasterol)
- Volatile oil
- Vitamins C and E

KEY ACTIONS

- Tonic
- Adaptogenic
- Protects liver

RESEARCH

■ Protecting the liver
Research into schisandra has focused largely on the lignans, which have a pronounced anti-hepatotoxic (liver-protective) action. Up to 30 different lignans have been identified in schisandra, which all contribute to this effect. Research from 1972 onward has reported the beneficial action of schisandra on the liver, and one clinical trial indicated a 76% success rate in treating patients with hepatitis, with no side effects being noted.
■ Nervous system Schisandra is known to stimulate the nervous system, increasing the speed of reflex nervous responses and improving mental clarity. The berries are thought to be potentially useful in the treatment of depression, and are known to help improve irritability and forgetfulness.
■ Uterus Schisandra stimulates the uterus, strengthening rhythmic contractions.
■ Adaptogenic herb Research has shown that in common with ginseng (*Panax ginseng*, p. 116), schisandra has adaptogenic properties, helping the body to adapt to stress.

TRADITIONAL & CURRENT USES

■ Tonic Schisandra is a major tonic herb and acts throughout the body, strengthening and toning many different organs.
■ Sexual stimulant Probably best known as a sexual tonic for both men and women, schisandra reputedly increases the secretion of sexual fluids

and, in men, it also improves sexual stamina.
■ Liver treatment herb
Schisandra has proven benefits for the liver, and is used in the treatment of hepatitis and poor liver function.
■ Sedative Although a stimulant, schisandra is used in Chinese medicine to "quiet the spirit and calm the heart." It is given for insomnia and dream-disturbed sleep, and is a fine example of how adaptogenic herbs often work in apparently contradictory ways to restore normal body function.
■ Mental & emotional remedy
In China, schisandra berries have traditionally been prescribed to treat mental illnesses such as neuroses. They are also given to improve concentration and coordination, and are a traditional remedy for forgetfulness and irritability. Schisandra's effectiveness for treating these problems has now been borne out by research.

■ Respiratory infections The herb is used in the treatment of respiratory infections such as chronic coughs, shortness of breath, and wheezing.
■ Balancing fluid levels
Schisandra is used to tone up and strengthen kidney function and to help the body to balance levels of fluid, making it helpful for treating night sweats, thirst, and urinary frequency.
■ Skin rashes Recently, Chinese herbalists have started to use schisandra to treat urticaria (hives) and other skin problems, including eczema. It is usually given for these conditions in the form of a medicinal wine.
■ Additional uses Schisandra is used for a wide variety of other physical disorders, including diarrhea and dysentery, as well as to help improve failing sight and hearing.

SELF-HELP USE

- **Low sex drive**, p. 316.

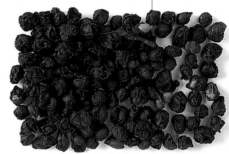

✣ PARTS USED

***Fruit** helps the body to cope with stress.*

Berries are chewed every day for 100 days as a tonic in China

Dried fruit

▨ KEY PREPARATIONS & THEIR USES

Caution Large doses can cause heartburn.

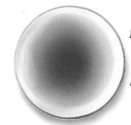

***Decoction** (to make, p. 291). For coughs and shortness of breath, decoct 5 g crushed berries with 100 ml water. Divide into 3 doses and drink during a 24-hour period.*

Scutellaria baicalensis syn. *S. macrantha* (Labiatae)
BAICAL SKULLCAP, HUANG QUIN

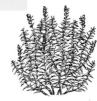

BAICAL SKULLCAP
A perennial growing to 1–4 ft (30–120 cm) high, with lance-shaped leaves and purplish-blue flowers.

IN 1973, 92 WOODEN TABLETS WERE discovered in a 2nd-century AD tomb in northwestern China. Among other herbs listed in prescriptions for decoctions, tinctures, pills, and ointments was Baical skullcap. The herb has had a central place in Chinese herbal medicine at least since that time and is one of the main remedies for "hot and damp" conditions, such as dysentery and diarrhea.

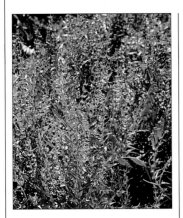

Baical skullcap is an important medicinal plant in China and is also cultivated as an ornamental.

HABITAT & CULTIVATION

Baical skullcap is found in China, Japan, Korea, Mongolia, and Russia. It thrives on sunny grassy slopes and in open areas between 350 ft (100 m) and 8,000 ft (2,000 m) above sea level. Baical skullcap is propagated from seed sown in autumn and the root of 3- to 4-year-old plants is harvested in autumn or spring.

RELATED SPECIES

Skullcap (*S. lateriflora*, p. 134) is a close relative. It is a Native North American remedy for anxiety or stress.

KEY CONSTITUENTS

- Flavonoids (about 12%)– baicalin, wogoniside
- Sterols
- Benzoic acid

KEY ACTIONS

- Sedative
- Antiallergenic
- Antibiotic
- Anti-inflammatory

RESEARCH

- **Flavonoids** Baical skullcap has been extensively researched in China, and it is clear that it has a marked anti-inflammatory and antiallergenic action. This is largely due to the flavonoids. In common with other herbs that have significant levels of flavonoids, such as hawthorn (*Crataegus oxyacantha*, p. 86), it is likely that Baical skullcap may help venous problems and fragile capillaries.
- **Verifying traditional uses** Clinical trials suggest that Baical skullcap's traditional use for high fevers and infections such as dysentery are justified.
- **Diabetes** The herb may be useful for problems arising from diabetes, including cataracts.

TRADITIONAL & CURRENT USES

- **Cold & bitter herb** In traditional Chinese medicine, Baical skullcap is "cold" and "bitter" (*see* p. 39). It is prescribed in China for hot and thirsty conditions such as high fevers, coughs with thick yellow phlegm, and gastrointestinal infections that cause diarrhea, such as dysentery. It is also given to people suffering from painful urinary conditions.
- **Anti-inflammatory** In the light of recent research, Baical skullcap is now used for allergic conditions such as asthma, hay fever, eczema, and nettle rash, although undoubtedly its anti-inflammatory action is most useful for digestive infections.
- **Circulatory remedy** Baical skullcap is a valuable remedy for the circulation. In combination with other herbs, it is used to treat high blood pressure, arteriosclerosis, varicose veins, and easy bruising.
- **Other uses** Applied to the skin, Baical skullcap treats sores, swelling, and boils. It appears to be useful for circulatory problems that arise from diabetes.

SELF-HELP USES

- **Allergic rhinitis**, p. 300.
- **Wheezing & shortness of breath**, p. 301.

❊ PARTS USED

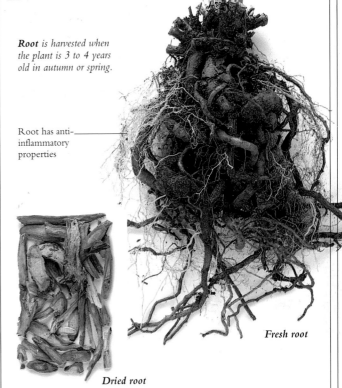

Root is harvested when the plant is 3 to 4 years old in autumn or spring.

Root has anti-inflammatory properties

Fresh root

Dried root

✍ KEY PREPARATIONS & THEIR USES

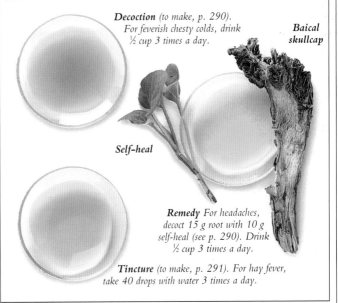

Decoction (to make, p. 290). For feverish chesty colds, drink ½ cup 3 times a day.

Baical skullcap

Self-heal

Remedy For headaches, decoct 15 g root with 10 g self-heal (see p. 290). Drink ½ cup 3 times a day.

Tincture (to make, p. 291). For hay fever, take 40 drops with water 3 times a day.

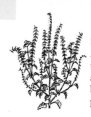

SKULLCAP
A perennial growing to 2 ft (60 cm), with an erect, many-branched stem and pink to blue flowers.

Scutellaria lateriflora (*Labiatae*)
SKULLCAP, VIRGINIA SKULLCAP, MAD DOG

A NATIVE AMERICAN HERB, skullcap was traditionally taken for menstrual problems. It was also used in purification ceremonies when menstrual taboos had been broken. Skullcap became well known in 19th-century America as a treatment for rabies, hence its folk name "mad dog." Today, it is mainly used as a tonic and sedative for the nerves in times of stress. It has a bitter slightly astringent taste.

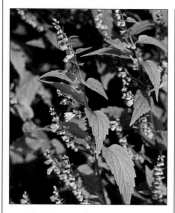

***Skullcap** is easy to recognize. It has pairs of pink to blue flowers and distinctive seed capsules.*

HABITAT & CULTIVATION
A native of North America, skullcap still grows wild in much of the US and Canada. It thrives in damp conditions, for example, on riverbanks, and needs plenty of sun. Skullcap can be propagated from seed or by root division in spring. The aerial parts of 3- to 4-year-old plants are harvested in summer, when in flower.

RELATED SPECIES
There are about 100 species of *Scutellaria*. In the past, European skullcap (*S. galericulata*) and lesser skullcap (*S. minor*) were used in a similar way to *S. lateriflora*, but today they are considered to have a less important therapeutic action. Baical skullcap (*S. baicalensis*, p. 133) is also closely related.

KEY CONSTITUENTS
- Flavonoids (scutellarin)
- Bitter iridoids (catalpol)
- Volatile oil
- Tannins

KEY ACTIONS
- Sedative
- Nervine tonic
- Antispasmodic
- Mild bitter

RESEARCH
- **Scutellaria species** Very little research has been carried out on this species of *Scutellaria*, despite its long use in North American and British herbal medicine. It is likely that it contains similar constituents to other *Scutellaria* species, notably Baical skullcap (*S. baicalensis*, p. 133), which has been well researched and is strongly anti-inflammatory.

TRADITIONAL & CURRENT USES
- **Native American cure** The Cherokee used skullcap to stimulate menstruation, relieve breast pain, and encourage expulsion of the placenta.
- **19th-century remedy** The Physiomedicalists (followers of a 19th-century Anglo-American school of herbal medicine) first discovered skullcap's use as a nervine. They recognized that it has a "deeper" action on the nervous system than any other herb and used it for hysteria, epilepsy, convulsions, and rabies, as well as for serious mental illnesses such as schizophrenia.
- **Current uses** Today, skullcap is taken mainly as a nerve tonic and for its restorative properties. It helps to support and nourish the nervous system, and calms and relieves stress and anxiety. Its antispasmodic action makes it useful for conditions where stress and worry cause muscular tension. Skullcap is often prescribed on its own or mixed with other sedative herbs, to treat insomnia and it is also given to relieve menstrual pain. Research into skullcap is sorely needed and may reveal more uses for this valuable herb.

✱ PARTS USED

***Aerial parts** are harvested in summer for use in a number of calming preparations.*

Seed capsules, when dry, look like skullcaps

Dried aerial parts

Fresh aerial parts

✍ KEY PREPARATIONS & THEIR USES

Infusion (to make, p. 290). For short-term relief of stress and anxiety, take 50 ml 3 times a day.

Capsules (to make, p. 291). For nervous exhaustion, take a 200 mg capsule twice daily.

Tincture (to make, p. 291). For nervous tension and headaches, take 3 ml with water twice a day.

TABLETS often contain other sedative herbs. Take for insomnia.

SELF-HELP USES
- **Anxiety, depression & tension**, p. 308.
- **Migraine**, p. 309.
- **Panic attacks & headaches**, p. 308.

Swertia chirata syn. *Ophelia chirata* (Gentianiaceae)
CHIRETTA, CHIRAYATA (HINDI)

CHIRETTA
An annual growing to about 3ft (1m) high, with smooth leaves and purple-tinged, pale green flowers.

NATIVE TO INDIA, CHIRETTA is a traditional Ayurvedic herb. It is a strongly bitter tonic and is used to treat *pitta* (fire) conditions. Chiretta is perhaps best known in India as the main ingredient in *mahasudarshana churna* – a remedy containing more than 50 herbs, that is prescribed for fevers, including malaria, as well as for liver problems, gallstones, indigestion, and nausea. Research has shown chiretta protects the liver.

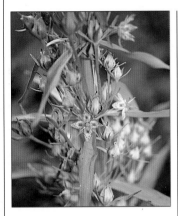

Chiretta can be found growing wild in pastureland on the lower slopes of the Himalayas.

HABITAT & CULTIVATION
Chiretta is native to northern India and Nepal and grows wild throughout that region at high altitudes. It can be cultivated and is propagated from seed sown in spring or autumn. Chiretta prefers well-drained soil and plenty of sun. The aerial parts are harvested in summer when the plant is in flower.

RELATED SPECIES
Other *Swertia* species also valued for their bitter properties include *S. japonica*, which is widely used in Japan. Chiretta is a member of the *Gentianaceae* family, many of which are strongly bitter and are used for digestive problems. *See* gentian (*Gentiana lutea*, p. 97) and centaury (*Erythrea centaurea*, p. 204).

KEY CONSTITUENTS
- Xanthones
- Iridoids (including amarogentin)
- Alkaloids
- Flavones

KEY ACTIONS
- Bitter
- Tonic
- Stimulates the appetite
- Eases stomach pain
- Reduces fever
- Antimalarial

RESEARCH
- **Bitter constituents** In common with other members of the *Gentianaceae* family, chiretta is known to contain appreciable quantities of highly bitter substances. These include iridoids, especially amarogentin, and alkaloids.
- **Liver-protective action** The constituent amarogentin has a protective action on the liver.
- **Other research** Research in India demonstrated that the xanthones are antimalarial and protect against tuberculosis.

TRADITIONAL & CURRENT USES
- **Therapeutic properties** Chiretta is a strongly bitter herb. It stimulates the bitter taste receptors on the tongue, which sets off a reflex action, stimulating the whole digestive tract.
- **Digestive remedy** Chiretta is an excellent remedy for a weak stomach, especially when this gives rise to nausea, indigestion, and bloating. The infusion, which should be taken in small doses, helps to improve the appetite and digestive function as a whole. The infusion may also be taken to expel worms.
- **Fevers** Like most bitters, chiretta reduces fevers, cooling the body and increasing blood flow to the liver. It is a useful remedy for malaria.

PARTS USED

Aerial parts are collected when the plant is in flower in summer. They contain strongly bitter substances and are useful for digestive problems.

Dried aerial parts

Leaves contain amaragentin, which gives them a bitter taste

Fresh aerial parts

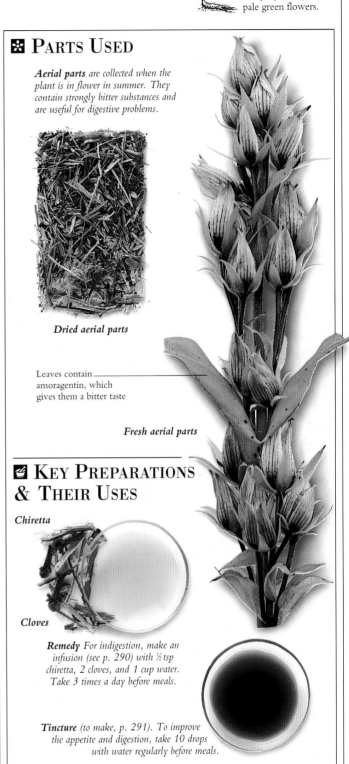

KEY PREPARATIONS & THEIR USES

Chiretta

Cloves

Remedy *For indigestion, make an infusion (see p. 290) with ½ tsp chiretta, 2 cloves, and 1 cup water. Take 3 times a day before meals.*

Tincture *(to make, p. 291). To improve the appetite and digestion, take 10 drops with water regularly before meals.*

- **Hiccups** In India chiretta is prescribed for hiccups. The infusion is taken with honey in small doses at frequent intervals.
- **Other uses** Recently chiretta has been used with other herbs to treat allergies, and its strong tonic properties make it very useful for treating debility and in convalescence.

SELF-HELP USES
- **Anemia**, p. 301.
- **Weak digestion**, p. 306.

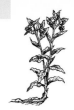

COMFREY
A perennial growing to 3 ft (1 m), with thick leaves and bell-like white to pink or mauve flowers.

Symphytum officinale (Boraginaceae)
COMFREY, KNITBONE

COMFREY'S NAMES TESTIFY TO its traditional use in mending broken bones. "Comfrey" is a corruption of *con firma*, meaning the bone is "made firm"; *symphytum* is derived from the Greek for "to unite"; and knitbone speaks for itself. Comfrey is also a wound herb. K'Eogh in his *Irish Herbal* (1735) wrote that it "heals all inward wounds and ruptures." Today, it is still highly regarded for its healing properties.

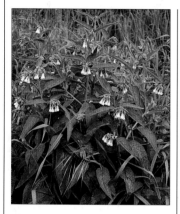

Comfrey was known to the Greek physician Dioscorides in the 1st century AD who wrote about it in his Materia Medica.

HABITAT & CULTIVATION

An indigenous European plant, comfrey grows in all temperate regions of the world, including western Asia, North America, and Australia. It thrives in moist, marshy places. It can be grown from seed in spring or by root division in autumn, and the leaves and flowering tops are harvested in summer. The root is unearthed in autumn.

KEY CONSTITUENTS

- Allantoin (up to 4.7%)
- Mucilage (about 29%)
- Triterpenoids
- Phenolic acids (rosmarinic acid)
- Asparagine
- Pyrrolizidine alkaloids (0.02–0.07%)
- Tannins

KEY ACTIONS

- Demulcent
- Astringent
- Anti-inflammatory
- Heals wounds & bones

RESEARCH

- **Allantoin** Comfrey contains allantoin, a cell-proliferant that helps repair damaged tissue.
- **Rosmarinic acid** The herb has a significant anti-inflammatory action, partly due to the presence of rosmarinic acid and other phenolic acids.
- **Pyrrolizidine alkaloids** Research shows that, as isolated substances, the pyrrolizidine alkaloids are highly toxic to the liver. It is still unclear whether they are toxic in the context of the whole plant, as they are only present in minute amounts, often being completely absent from samples of dried aerial parts. The highest concentration is in the root and, until its safety is confirmed (or denied), comfrey root should not be used internally. (The aerial parts are considered safe.)

The legitimate question mark over comfrey's safety as a medicine needs to be balanced by a deeper understanding of its therapeutic properties.

TRADITIONAL & CURRENT USES

- **Past uses** The herb has been used to treat stomach ulcers, irritable bowel syndrome, and a range of respiratory conditions, including bronchitis and pleurisy.
- **Injuries** Comfrey's ability to promote the healing of bruises, sprains, fractures, and broken bones has been known for thousands of years. It encourages ligaments and bones to knit together firmly. A comfrey compress applied immediately to a sprained ankle can significantly reduce the severity of the injury.

✵ PARTS USED

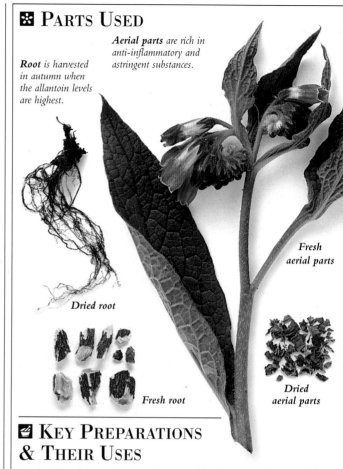

Root is harvested in autumn when the allantoin levels are highest.

Aerial parts are rich in anti-inflammatory and astringent substances.

Dried root

Fresh aerial parts

Fresh root

Dried aerial parts

🥄 KEY PREPARATIONS & THEIR USES

Cautions Do not use on dirty wounds, since rapid healing can trap dirt or pus. Take internally only under professional supervision. Restricted in some countries.

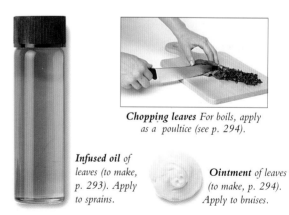

Chopping leaves For boils, apply as a poultice (see p. 294).

Infused oil of leaves (to make, p. 293). Apply to sprains.

Ointment of leaves (to make, p. 294). Apply to bruises.

TINCTURE of root (to make, p. 291). Apply undiluted to acne.

The combination of tannins and mucilage helps to soothe bruises and scrapes.
- **Skin problems** Comfrey oil or ointment is used to treat acne and boils and to relieve psoriasis. It is also valuable in the treatment of scars.

SELF-HELP USES

- **Acne & boils**, p. 305.
- **Fractures,** p. 312.
- **Fungal skin infections**, p. 304.
- **Healing wounds**, p. 304.
- **Inflamed skin rashes**, p. 303.
- **Stiff & aching joints**, p. 313.

Syzygium cumini (Myrtaceae)
JAMBUL, JAVA PLUM

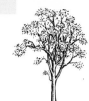

JAMBUL
An evergreen tree growing to 33 ft (10 m), with lance-shaped leaves and green-yellow flowers.

NATIVE TO PARTS OF southern Asia and Australia, jambul is a typical example of a medicinal plant that is both a food and a medicine. The fruit, when ripe, has the scent and taste of a ripe apricot and is eaten as a preserve. Both the seeds and the fruit have important carminative and astringent properties. The fresh seeds reduce blood sugar levels and are beneficial in treating conditions such as diabetes.

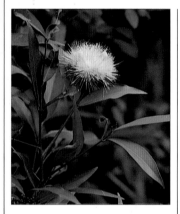

***Jambul** helps to lower blood sugar levels and is an important remedy for diabetes.*

HABITAT & CULTIVATION

A native of southern Asia and Australia, jambul can now also be found growing throughout tropical regions of India, Indonesia, and Africa. It is cultivated commercially for its fruit. Jambul is propagated from seed or from semiripe cuttings in summer and requires well-drained soil and plenty of sun. The fruit is harvested when ripe in autumn.

RELATED SPECIES

There are many other closely related species that are valued for their therapeutic properties. Cloves (*Eugenia caryophyllata*, p. 95) are taken for many digestive problems, helping to relieve gas and bloating, as well as for infections such as malaria. *E. chequeri* from Chile and *E. gerrodi* from South Africa are used to treat coughs and congestion. In Brazil, the leaves of *E. uniflora* are employed to help repel mosquitoes and other insects.

KEY CONSTITUENTS

- Phenols (methylxanthoxylin)
- Tannins
- Alkaloid (jambosine)
- Triterpenoids
- Volatile oil

KEY ACTIONS

- Lowers blood sugar levels
- Astringent
- Carminative
- Diuretic

RESEARCH

- **Lowering blood sugar levels**
Research has shown that in common with a number of other medicinal plants, jambul appears to have a significant hypoglycemic action, helping to lower blood glucose levels. It is therefore of value in diabetes. Jambul is also known to reduce glucose levels in the urine.

TRADITIONAL & CURRENT USES

- **Diabetes treatment** A number of herbal medicines from all over the world, of which jambul is one and bilberry (*Vaccinium myrtillius*, p. 278) another, have been found to have the ability to lower blood sugar levels. Jambul is prescribed by herbal practitioners to counter the effects of diabetes, where the islet cells of the pancreas cease to produce sufficient insulin (a chemical that enables glucose to enter the cells of the body). Type II diabetes, which commonly develops in middle-to old-age, is becoming increasingly prevalent throughout the world, and in its early, mild stages can respond well to herbal treatment, provided the patient follows a strict diet.

- **Indian diabetes remedy**
In India, powdered jambul seeds, or occasionally the tincture, are given for diabetes and the frequent urination that accompanies it.

- **Diarrhea & dysentery** Jambul is a strongly astringent herb and may be taken to treat diarrhea and dysentery. In Ayurvedic medicine, jambul and mango seeds are combined and ground into a powder as a treatment for these conditions.

- **Indigestion** Jambul has useful carminative properties and is an effective remedy for the symptoms of indigestion. It is taken to help to soothe stomachache and cramps and to disperse gas.

- **Epilepsy** In parts of Southeast Asia, jambul roots are sometimes given as a treatment for epilepsy.

☒ PARTS USED

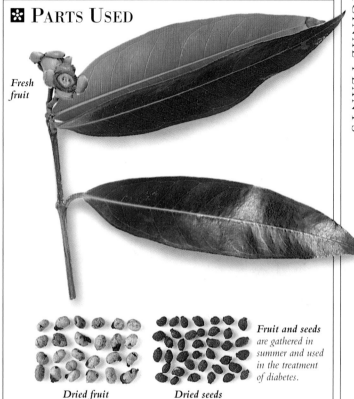

Fresh fruit

Dried fruit   *Dried seeds*

***Fruit and seeds** are gathered in summer and used in the treatment of diabetes.*

☕ KEY PREPARATIONS & THEIR USES

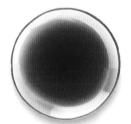

***Decoction** of seeds. For diarrhea, simmer ½ tsp and 1 cup water for 5 minutes (p. 290). Take 3 times a day.*

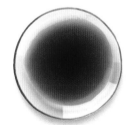

***Tincture** of seeds (to make, p. 291). For colic, take 40 drops with water 3 times a day.*

POWDER For flatulence, mix 1 g with water and take 3 times a day.

Tabebuia spp. *(Bignoniaceae)*

LAPACHO (SPANISH), PAU D'ARCO (PORTUGUESE)

LAPACHO
An evergreen tree (deciduous in cold climates) reaching 100 ft (30 m), with pink flowers.

BARK FROM THE LAPACHO tree has been valued for centuries within traditional South American herbal medicine for its remarkable health benefits. Today, it is given as a remedy for inflammatory and infectious problems, including viral conditions such as chronic fatigue syndrome (ME). It is also used for other conditions and has a significant reputation in the treatment of cancer, including leukemia.

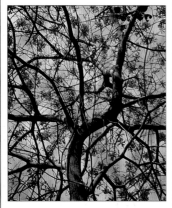

Lapacho is valued for its durable wood and for its bark that has important therapeutic properties.

HABITAT & CULTIVATION

An indigenous South American tree, lapacho grows well in mountainous terrains. In Peru and Argentina it is found growing high up in the Andes. Lapacho is also found in low-lying areas (in Paraguay and Brazil), where it is thought to have originated. A number of *Tabebuia* species are used in herbal medicine. *T. avellanedae* is considered to be the most therapeutically effective, but *T. impetignosa* is the species that is most commonly available. Lapacho is not normally cultivated – the inner bark is collected from wild trees throughout the year.

KEY CONSTITUENTS

- Quinones (lapachol)
- Bioflavonoids
- Lapachenole
- Carnosol
- Indoles
- Coenzyme Q
- Alkaloids (tecomine)
- Steroidal saponins

KEY ACTIONS

- Antibiotic
- Antifungal
- Immune stimulant
- Anti-inflammatory
- Cleansing
- Tonic
- Antitumor

RESEARCH

Antitumor properties

Lapacho's anticancer action is controversial, but research in Brazil, which started during the 1960s, indicates that the bark may be therapeutically useful in treating cancer and leukemia. Many of the herb's constituents play a part in counteracting the growth of tumors, notably lapachol, which inhibits the growth of tumor cells by preventing them from metabolizing oxygen.

Other research
Lapacho is known to be strongly anti-inflammatory. It also counters the effects of diabetes (an action that is due in part to the constituent tecomine) and it lowers blood pressure.

TRADITIONAL & CURRENT USES

Early cure-all
The Incas, the Callawaya in Brazil, and other Native South American peoples prized lapacho as a cure-all. They used it to treat a variety of conditions including wounds, fever, dysentery, intestinal inflammation, certain types of cancer, and snakebites.

Infections
Given the large number of active constituents in lapacho, it is not surprising that this beneficial herb is used in South America and by herbal practitioners throughout the world. It is an important, natural antibiotic for bacterial and viral infections, especially of the nose, mouth, and throat and is considered helpful for chronic conditions such as ME. Lapacho is also used to treat fungal conditions, including ringworm and yeast infections and is considered especially useful for treating chronic fungal conditions, including candidiasis.

Anti-inflammatory action
Lapacho reduces and relieves inflammatory problems, especially in the stomach and intestines. It is used to treat a wide range of inflammatory conditions, including cystitis, inflammation of the cervix, and prostatitis.

Cancer remedy
Lapacho is beneficial in the treatment of cancer, including leukemia. Clinical experience in Brazil, combined with its traditional use for cancer, suggests that lapacho should be more intensively researched for its therapeutic value in the treatment of this disease.

✤ PARTS USED

Dried inner bark

Bark has important antibiotic properties

Inner bark is prized for its immune-stimulant properties. It is used to treat many inflammatory conditions.

✍ KEY PREPARATIONS & THEIR USES

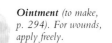

Ointment (to make, p. 294). For wounds, apply freely.

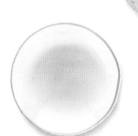

Decoction (to make, p. 290) is a traditional preparation in South America. For candidiasis, take 1 cup 3 times a day.

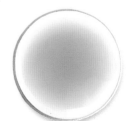

Tincture (to make, p. 291) is suitable for long term use. For ME, take 2 ml with water 3 times a day.

Tanacetum parthenium (Compositae)
FEVERFEW

FEVERFEW'S MAIN TRADITIONAL use was as a woman's herb. Nicholas Culpeper in *The English Physitian* (1653) sang its praises as "a general strengthener of [the] womb.... it cleanseth the womb, expelleth the after-birth and doth the woman all the good she can desire of a herb." Feverfew is now used principally as a treatment for migraine, but has also long been thought of as an herb for arthritis and rheumatism.

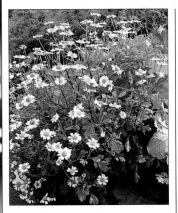

Feverfew has daisylike flowers that bloom all summer.

HABITAT & CULTIVATION
Originally from southeastern Europe, feverfew is now common throughout Europe, Australia, and North America. It can be propagated from seed or cuttings, and prefers well-drained soil and sun. The leaves are picked as required, and the aerial parts as a whole are harvested in summer when the plant is in flower.

RELATED SPECIES
Feverfew is a close relative of tansy (*Tanacetum vulgare*, p. 272), and the chrysanthemum and chamomile species.

KEY CONSTITUENTS
- Volatile oil (alpha-pinene)
- Sesquiterpene lactones (parthenolide)
- Sesquiterpenes (camphor)

KEY ACTIONS
- Analgesic
- Reduces fever
- Antirheumatic
- Promotes menstrual flow
- Bitter

RESEARCH
■ **Migraine** When the wife of a Welsh doctor ended her 50-year-old history of migraine with a course of feverfew, a detailed scientific investigation of feverfew got underway, and in clinical trials in Britain during the 1980s the herb was demonstrated to be an effective remedy for migraine. Despite extensive research, the exact nature of its action is not yet understood, but the constituent parthenolide appears to inhibit the release of the hormone serotonin, which is thought to trigger migraine.

■ **Rheumatoid arthritis** Feverfew's effectiveness in the treatment of rheumatoid arthritis is being investigated.

TRADITIONAL & CURRENT USES
■ **Fevers** As its name indicates, feverfew may be used to lower temperature and cool the body.

■ **Gynecological uses** The herb has been used since Roman times to induce menstruation. It is given in difficult births to aid expulsion of the placenta.

■ **Migraine & headaches** In small quantities, feverfew is now used as a preventive for migraine. It has to be taken regularly and at the first signs of an attack. It is useful for migraines associated with menstruation and for headaches.

■ **Arthritis remedy** The herb can help arthritic and rheumatic pain, especially in combination with other herbs.

SELF-HELP USE
■ **Migraine prevention**, p. 309.

✿ PARTS USED

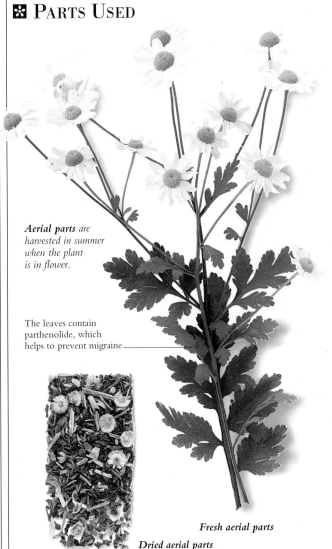

Aerial parts are harvested in summer when the plant is in flower.

The leaves contain parthenolide, which helps to prevent migraine

Fresh aerial parts

Dried aerial parts

☙ KEY PREPARATIONS & THEIR USES

Cautions Eating fresh leaves may cause canker sores. Do not take feverfew if taking warfarin or other blood-thinning drugs. Do not take during pregnancy.

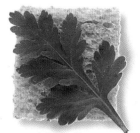

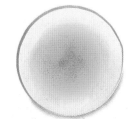

Fresh leaves To prevent migraine, eat 2–3 leaves daily on a piece of bread.

Tincture (to make, p. 291). For long-term prevention of migraine, take 5 drops with water up to 3 times a day.

🖉 CAPSULES (to make, p. 291). For symptomatic relief of headaches take a 100 mg capsule per day.

◎ TABLETS often contain other herbs. Take for headaches.

KEY MEDICINAL PLANTS

Taraxacum officinale (Compositae)
DANDELION

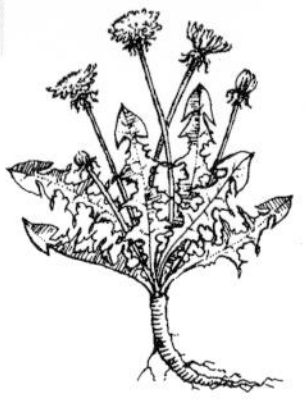

DANDELION
A perennial growing to 20 in (50 cm), with ragged basal leaves, hollow stalks, and golden flowers.

KNOWN PRINCIPALLY AS A WEED, dandelion has an astonishing range of health benefits. In Western folk medicine, the leaves, which can be eaten in salads, have long been used as a diuretic. They were recommended in the works of Arab physicians in the 11th century and in an herbal written by the physicians of Myddfai in Wales in the 13th century. The root, which has a shorter history of medicinal use, is good for the liver.

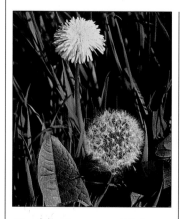

Dandelion's name, which is a corruption of the Latin dens leonis, *meaning "lion's teeth," derives from the appearance of its flowers.*

HABITAT & CULTIVATION
Dandelion grows wild in most parts of the world and is cultivated in Germany and France. It is propagated from seed in spring. The young leaves are picked in spring for tonic salads and later as a medicine. The root of 2-year-old plants is unearthed in autumn.

RELATED SPECIES
Pu gong ying (T. mongolicum) is used in Chinese herbal medicine to "clear heat" and relieve toxicity, especially of the liver.

KEY CONSTITUENTS
- Sesquiterpene lactones
- Triterpenes
- Vitamins A, B, C, and D

Leaf only:
- Coumarins
- Carotenoids
- Minerals (especially potassium)

Root only:
- Taraxacoside
- Phenolic acids
- Minerals (potassium, calcium)

KEY ACTIONS
- Diuretic
- Detoxifying
- Bitter

RESEARCH
- **Leaves** Research published in the journal *Planta Medica*, in 1974, confirmed that dandelion leaves are a powerful diuretic, though their exact mode of action is not understood. Unlike many conventional diuretics, which cause loss of potassium, dandelion leaves contain high levels of potassium, giving a net gain of the mineral.
- **Root** German research published in 1959 showed that the root has a significant cleansing action on the liver and stimulates bile production. It is also mildly bitter and a gentle laxative.

TRADITIONAL & CURRENT USES
- **Diuretic** Dandelion leaf is used as a diuretic and to treat high blood pressure by reducing the volume of fluid in the body.
- **Detoxifying remedy** Dandelion root is one of the most effective detoxifying herbs. Working principally on the liver and gallbladder to help remove waste products, it also stimulates the kidneys to remove toxins in the urine. A remarkably well-balanced remedy, the root encourages steady elimination of toxins due to infection or pollution. It has major therapeutic benefits for many conditions, including constipation, skin problems such as acne, eczema, and psoriasis, and arthritic conditions, including osteoarthritis, and gout.

�֍ PARTS USED
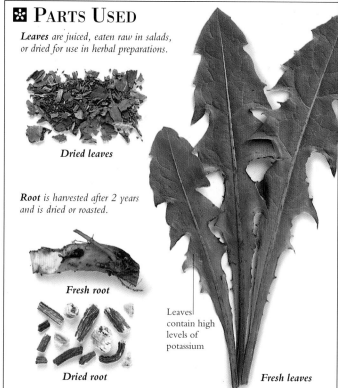

Leaves are juiced, eaten raw in salads, or dried for use in herbal preparations.

Dried leaves

Root is harvested after 2 years and is dried or roasted.

Fresh root

Leaves contain high levels of potassium

Dried root

Fresh leaves

🥣 KEY PREPARATIONS & THEIR USES

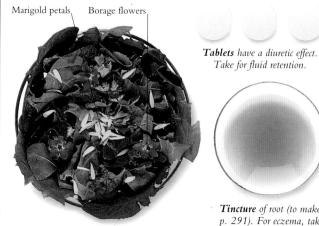

Marigold petals Borage flowers

Tonic salad made with dandelion leaves. Eat regularly for its cleansing benefits.

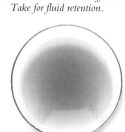

Tablets have a diuretic effect. Take for fluid retention.

Tincture of root (to make, p. 291). For eczema, take ½ tsp diluted with 100 ml water 3 times a day.

- **DECOCTION** of root (p. 290). For acne, take ½ cup 3 times a day.
- **INFUSION** of leaves (p. 290). For swollen ankles, take 500 ml daily.
- **JUICE** made from leaves. For fluid retention, take 20 ml 3 times a day.

- **Gallbladder problems** Both dandelion root and leaf have a marked action on the gallbladder and are used to prevent gallstones. The leaf may also help to dissolve already formed gallstones.

SELF-HELP USES
- **Acne & boils**, p. 305.
- **Constipation**, p. 307.
- **Detoxification for hangover**, p. 309.
- **Fluid retention**, p. 315.
- **Nettle rash**, p. 303.

Terminalia arjuna (Combretaceae)
ARJUNA

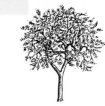

ARJUNA
An evergreen tree reaching 100 ft (30 m), with pale yellow flowers and cone-shaped leaves.

THE BARK OF THE ARJUNA TREE has been used in Indian herbal medicine for at least 3,000 years and has always been valued as a remedy for the heart. The first person credited with prescribing arjuna for heart disease was Vagbhata, an Indian physician of the 7th century AD. Arjuna is an example of an herb for which the traditional use has been confirmed by modern pharmacological research.

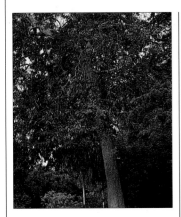

Arjuna is a handsome evergreen tree. Its bark is prescribed to help heart and circulation problems.

HABITAT & CULTIVATION
Arjuna is found throughout most of the Indian subcontinent, from Sri Lanka to the foothills of the Himalayas. It thrives in wet, marshy areas and on riverbanks. The tree is grown from seed and the bark is cut in late winter.

RELATED SPECIES
A number of other *Terminalia* species are also used medicinally, notably beleric myrobalan and chebulic myrobalan (*T. belerica* and *T. chebula*, p. 273). Both are close relatives of arjuna and are among the most used herbal medicines in India.

KEY CONSTITUENTS
- Tannins
- Triterpenoid saponins
- Flavonoids
- Sterols

KEY ACTIONS
- Cardiac tonic
- Lowers blood pressure
- Reduces cholesterol levels

RESEARCH
■ **Cardiac tonic** Research has been going on into arjuna in India since the 1930s. The results have been highly conflicting, with some studies indicating that it increases heart rate and blood pressure, and others suggesting the reverse. It seems that the herb is best used to treat conditions where the blood supply to the heart is poor – for example, in ischemic heart disease and angina. Arjuna is also of value in helping to maintain a regular heartbeat.
■ **Cholesterol** Indian research has demonstrated that arjuna reduces blood cholesterol levels.

TRADITIONAL & CURRENT USES
■ **Traditional heart remedy** In Indian herbal medicine, arjuna has always been taken as a heart tonic. It has a long history of treating heart failure and edema (a condition in which fluid accumulates in the ankles and legs because the heart is not pumping adequately).
■ **Other traditional uses** In Indian folk medicine, juice was extracted from arjuna leaves as a traditional remedy for earache. The herb is also traditionally believed to be an aphrodisiac.
■ **Ayurvedic medicine** Ayurvedic physicians use arjuna to restore balance when any of the 3 humors, *kapha*, *pitta*, or *vata* (see pp. 35), is present in excess. As a decoction, the bark is given to treat diarrhea and dysentery. Powdered bark is part of a traditional Ayurvedic treatment for asthma. Arjuna is also given in Ayurveda for bile duct problems, as well as for poisoning and scorpion stings.
■ **Modern heart remedy** Arjuna is beneficial for angina and poor coronary circulation. It is also of benefit if the heart's rate and rhythm are abnormal. By lowering blood cholesterol levels, reducing blood pressure, and supporting normal heart function, arjuna improves the health of the circulation and reduces the risk of developing a serious heart problem.

✦ PARTS USED

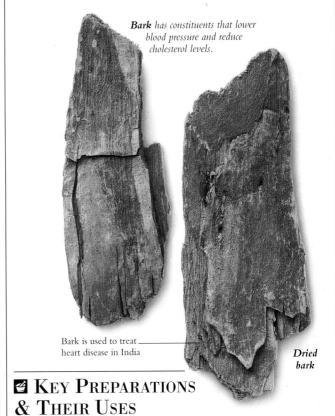

Bark has constituents that lower blood pressure and reduce cholesterol levels.

Bark is used to treat heart disease in India

Dried bark

✍ KEY PREPARATIONS & THEIR USES

Caution Take only under professional supervision.

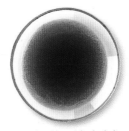

Decoction is used by herbalists to treat poor circulation to the heart.

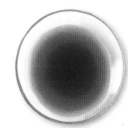

Tincture is a valuable cardiac tonic. Herbalists prescribe it to treat angina.

Powder is a traditional Ayurvedic remedy, prescribed for asthma.

Thymus vulgaris (Labiatae)

THYME, GARDEN THYME

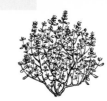

THYME
An aromatic shrub growing to 16 in (40 cm) with woody stems, small leaves, and pink flowers.

THYME WAS PRAISED by the English herbalist Nicholas Culpeper (1616–1654) as "a notable strengthener of the lungs, as notable a one as grows; neither is there a better remedy growing for that disease in children which they commonly call chin-cough [whooping cough]." Thyme is an excellent antiseptic and tonic, and today is still used as a respiratory remedy, as well as being important for a variety of other ailments.

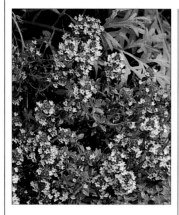

Thyme's *pink flowers attract bees in profusion and give a distinctive flavor to the honey.*

HABITAT & CULTIVATION

Thyme is related to mother of thyme, also known as wild thyme (*T. serpyllum*, p. 274), which is native to southern Europe. Now cultivated worldwide, it is grown from seed or by root division in spring. It prefers light, chalky soils. The aerial parts are harvested in mid-to-late summer.

RELATED SPECIES

There are many *Thymus* species, each with a different volatile oil content. Wild thyme (*T. serpyllum*, p. 274) is often used in the same way as thyme.

KEY CONSTITUENTS

- Volatile oil with variable content (thymol, methylchavicol, cineole, borneol)
- Flavonoids (apigenin, luteolin)
- Tannins

KEY ACTIONS

- Antiseptic
- Tonic

- Relieves muscle spasms
- Expectorant
- Expels worms

RESEARCH

- **Volatile oil** Thyme volatile oil is strongly antiseptic – the constituent thymol, in particular, is a most effective antifungal. The oil is also an expectorant, and it expels worms.
- **Muscle spasms** Thymol, methylchavicol, and the flavonoids relieve muscle spasms.
- **Anti-aging** Research in the 1990s in Scotland suggests that thyme and its volatile oil have a markedly tonic effect, supporting the body's normal function and countering the effects of aging.

TRADITIONAL & CURRENT USES

- **Infections** The antiseptic and tonic properties of thyme make it a useful tonic for the immune system in chronic, especially fungal, infections, as well as an effective remedy for chest infections, such as bronchitis, whooping cough, and pleurisy. The pleasant-tasting infusion can be taken for minor throat and chest infections, and the fresh leaves may be chewed to relieve sore throats.
- **Asthma & hay fever** Thyme is prescribed with other herbs for asthma, especially in children. Its invigorating qualities balance the sedative effect of many herbs used for asthma. The herb is also helpful in hay fever.
- **Worms** Thyme is often used to treat worms in children.
- **External uses** Applied to the skin, thyme relieves bites and stings, and helps sciatica and rheumatic aches and pains. It helps ringworm, athlete's foot, thrush, and other fungal infections, as well as scabies and lice. The infusion may be added to bathwater as a stimulant.

PARTS USED

Aerial parts are harvested in summer. They contain antiseptic volatile oil.

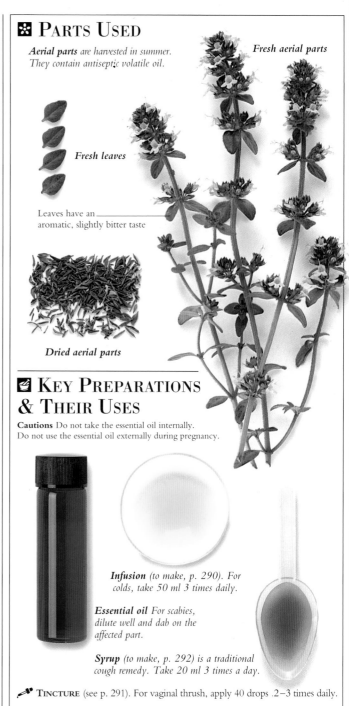

Fresh aerial parts

Fresh leaves

Leaves have an aromatic, slightly bitter taste

Dried aerial parts

KEY PREPARATIONS & THEIR USES

Cautions Do not take the essential oil internally. Do not use the essential oil externally during pregnancy.

Infusion (to make, p. 290). For colds, take 50 ml 3 times daily.

Essential oil For scabies, dilute well and dab on the affected part.

Syrup (to make, p. 292) is a traditional cough remedy. Take 20 ml 3 times a day.

TINCTURE (see p. 291). For vaginal thrush, apply 40 drops .2–3 times daily.

SELF-HELP USES

- **Back pain**, p. 313.
- **Bites & stings**, p. 303.
- **Colds & flu**, p. 311.
- **Congestion**, p. 300.
- **Coughs & bronchitis**, p. 310.
- **Earache**, p. 312.
- **Fungal infections**, pp. 304, 314
- **Maintaining vitality**, p. 319.
- **Mild asthma**, p. 301.
- **Tired & aching muscles**, p. 312.

Turnera diffusa syn. *T. diffusa* var. *aphrodisiaca* (Turneraceae)

DAMIANA

DAMIANA
An aromatic shrub growing to 6 ft (2 m), with smooth, pale green leaves and small yellow flowers.

DAMIANA IS A TRADITIONAL aphrodisiac of the Mayan people in Central America. It continues to be considered valuable as an aphrodisiac and general tonic, and its stimulant, tonic action also makes it a valuable remedy for people with mild depression. Damiana has a strongly aromatic, slightly bitter taste, and the leaves are used in Mexico as a substitute for tea and as a flavoring for liqueurs.

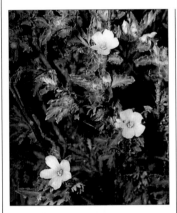

Damiana's tonic action makes it an excellent remedy for physical weakness and nervous exhaustion.

HABITAT & CULTIVATION

Damiana is native to the Gulf of Mexico, southern California and the northern Caribbean Islands, and Namibia. It grows wild and is also cultivated in these areas, preferring a hot, humid climate. The leaves are harvested when the herb is in flower in summer.

RELATED SPECIES

T. opifera and *T. ulmifolia* are used as tonics in Brazil and Central America respectively.

KEY CONSTITUENTS

- Arbutin (up to 7%)
- Volatile oil (about 0.5%), containing delta-cadinene (10%) and thymol (4%)
- Cyanogenic glycoside (tetraphyllin)
- Resin
- Gums

KEY ACTIONS

- Tonic
- Stimulant
- Mild laxative & diuretic
- Antidepressant
- Testosterogenic
- Reputed aphrodisiac

RESEARCH

- **Inconclusive research**
Virtually no detailed research has yet been undertaken. What little research there has been is inconclusive in its findings, but in the words of *Potter's New Cyclopaedia of Botanical Drugs and Preparations* (1988), "The aphrodisiac activity has not yet been demonstrated experimentally, however this is very difficult to do."

TRADITIONAL & CURRENT USES

- **Tonic** Damiana is a tonic and restorative for the nervous system, and has always been considered an aphrodisiac. Its tonic action is partly due to the constituent, thymol, which has an antiseptic and tonic action.
- **Antidepressant** Technically, damiana is a thymoleptic (having a life-enhancing and stimulating action on the body and mind). It is given people suffering from mild to moderate depression and nervous exhaustion. Its stimulating and restorative properties make it valuable when anxiety and depression occur together, as often happens after long-term stress.
- **Sexual restorative** Due to its testosterogenic quality, damiana has always been seen principally as an herb for men, helpful in treating premature ejaculation and impotence. It is, however, beneficial for both men and women, being considered restorative to the reproductive organs of both sexes.

✦ PARTS USED

Leaves are harvested in summer. They make a pleasant tasting tea and are used for a wide range of medicinal preparations.

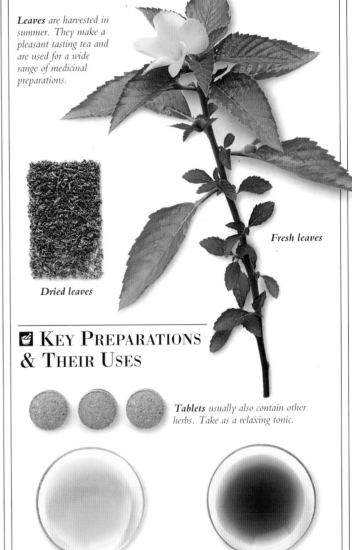

Fresh leaves

Dried leaves

✎ KEY PREPARATIONS & THEIR USES

Tablets usually also contain other herbs. Take as a relaxing tonic.

Tincture (to make, p. 291) is a nerve tonic and antidepressant. For mild depression, take 30 drops with water 4 times a day.

Infusion (to make, p. 290) is a tonic and is useful for urinary infections. Drink 1 cup daily as a general tonic.

- **Gynecological problems** Damiana is often given for painful and delayed periods, and is used specifically for headaches connected to menstruation.
- **Urinary antiseptic** Being a diuretic and urinary antiseptic, damiana is useful in the treatment of urinary infections such as cystitis and urethritis. This action is partly due to the constituent arbutin, which is converted into hydroquinone, a strong urinary antiseptic, in the urinary tubules. This constituent is also found in number of other plants, notably uva-ursi (*Arctostaphylos uva-ursi*, p. 168).
- **Laxative** Damiana is a mild laxative, useful in the treatment of constipation due to poor bowel muscle tone.

SELF-HELP USE

- **Anxiety, depression & tension**, p. 308.

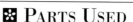

KEY MEDICINAL PLANTS

SLIPPERY ELM
A large tree growing
to 60 ft (18 m) with
a brown trunk and
rough, gray-white
bark on the branches.

Ulmus rubra (Ulmaceae)
SLIPPERY ELM

THIS MARVELOUS HERB is a gentle and effective remedy for irritated states of the mucous membranes of the chest, urinary tubules, stomach, and intestines. It was used in many different ways by Native Americans – as a poultice for wounds, boils, ulcers, and inflamed eyes, and internally for fevers, colds, and bowel complaints. Slippery elm has a strongly mucilaginous "slippery" taste and texture.

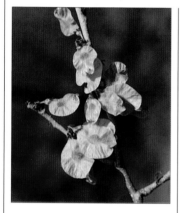

Slippery elm produces red-brown fruit, each consisting of a single seed, in summer.

HABITAT & CULTIVATION
Slippery elm is a native of the US and Canada, and is found most commonly in the Appalachian Mountains. The tree thrives on high ground and dry soil. The inner bark of the trunk and branches is collected in spring.

RELATED SPECIES
White elm (*U. americana*) is used in a similar way to slippery elm and was taken for coughs by the Mohicans. In Europe, the dried bark of elm (*Ulmus* spp.) was used as a demulcent and was first mentioned by Dioscorides in the 1st century AD.

KEY CONSTITUENTS
- Mucilage
- Starch
- Tannins

KEY ACTIONS
- Demulcent
- Emollient
- Nutritive
- Laxative

RESEARCH
■ **Mucilage** There is limited research into slippery elm, but its action as an herb with large quantities of mucilage is well understood. When the herb comes into direct contact with inflamed surfaces such as the skin or the intestinal membranes, it soothes and coats the irritated tissue, protects it from injury, and draws out toxins or irritants.
■ **Reflex action** When slippery elm is taken internally, it is thought likely that it causes a reflex stimulation of nerve endings in the stomach and intestines that leads to secretion of mucus by the membranes of the urinary tract.

TRADITIONAL & CURRENT USES
■ **Nourishing** Taken regularly, slippery elm is nutritious and soothing. It is an excellent food in convalescence and debilitated states, especially if the digestion is weak or overly sensitive. It is also a good baby food.
■ **Digestive disorders** Slippery elm is a particularly soothing herb and can bring instant relief from acidity, diarrhea, and gastroenteritis. It will also help alleviate conditions such as colic, inflammation of the gut, constipation, hemmorhoids, diverticulitis, and irritable bowel syndrome.
■ **Urinary problems** This herb is a useful remedy for urinary problems such as chronic cystitis.
■ **Respiratory conditions** Slippery elm has been used to treat all manner of chest conditions and has a soothing effect on everything from coughs and bronchitis to pleurisy and tuberculosis.
■ **External uses** Applied externally, the herb softens and protects the skin. It also works very well as a "drawing" poultice for boils and splinters.

✦ PARTS USED

Inner bark of 10-year-old slippery elm trees is collected in spring and powdered.

Fresh bark

Bark contains mucilage that soothes irritated tissues

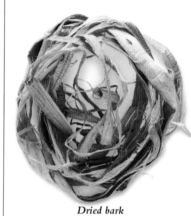

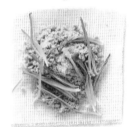

Dried bark

✎ KEY PREPARATIONS & THEIR USES

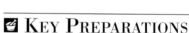

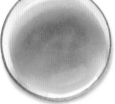

Infusion Mix 1 heaped tsp with 750 ml of warm water. Infuse for 5 minutes. For diarrhea, drink a whole dose 1–2 times a day.

Poultice For wounds, add several drops of calendula tincture to 1 tsp of powder. Mix into a paste and apply (see p. 294).

Capsules (to make, p. 291). For bronchitis, take a 200 g capsule 2–3 times a day.

🌰 **POWDER** For acid indigestion, take 1 tsp with water 2–3 times daily.
◯ **TABLETS** Take for diarrhea.

SELF-HELP USES
- **Acidity & indigestion**, p. 307.
- **Acne & boils**, p. 305.
- **Constipation in children**, p. 318.
- **Hemorrhoids**, p. 302.

144

Urtica dioica (Urticaceae)

NETTLE

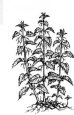

WELL KNOWN FOR ITS STING, nettle has long been appreciated for its medicinal uses. In the 1st century AD, the Greek physician, Dioscorides, listed a range of uses – the fresh, chopped leaves as a plaster for septic wounds, the juice for nosebleeds, and the cooked leaves mixed with myrrh to stimulate menstruation. Today, nettle is used for hay fever, arthritis, anemia, and, surprisingly, even for some skin conditions.

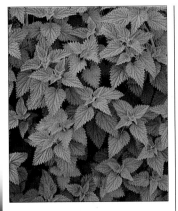

Nettle can be cooked as a vegetable and tastes like spinach.

HABITAT & CULTIVATION

Nettle grows in temperate regions throughout the northern hemisphere, southern Africa, the Andes, and Australia. Young shoots are picked in spring for use as a tonic and a vegetable. Aerial parts and leaves are picked in summer when the plant is in flower. The root is harvested in autumn.

RELATED SPECIES

The annual nettle (*U. urens*) is used in similar ways to *U. dioica*, and is also used in homeopathy. Roman nettle (*U. pilulifera*) was the species most used by the Romans for "urtication" (beating with nettles to encourage blood to the surface), which they did to keep themselves warm.

KEY CONSTITUENTS

Aerial parts:
- Flavonoids (quercitin)
- Amines (histamine, choline, acetylcholine, serotonin)
- Glucoquinone
- Minerals (calcium, potassium, silicic acid, iron)

Root:
- Plant sterols (stigmast-4-en-zone and stigmasterol)
- Phenols

KEY ACTIONS

- Diuretic
- Tonic
- Astringent
- Prevents hemorrhaging
- Antiallergenic
- Increases breast-milk production (leaf)
- Reduces prostate enlargement (root)

RESEARCH

- **Root** Research into nettle root in the US, Germany, and Japan has established its value as a medicine for benign prostate hypertrophy (enlargement).

TRADITIONAL & CURRENT USES

- **Cleansing** Nettle's key use is as a cleansing, detoxifying herb. It has a diuretic action, possibly due to its flavonoids and high potassium content, and increases urine production and the elimination of waste products. It helps many skin conditions – for example, childhood eczema – and arthritic problems, especially when poor kidney function and fluid retention are features.
- **Astringent** Nettle slows or stops bleeding from wounds and nosebleeds, and is good for heavy menstrual bleeding.
- **Allergies** Nettle is antiallergenic. It treats hay fever, asthma, itchy skin conditions, and insect bites. The juice can be used to treat nettle stings.
- **Additional uses** The leaves help anemia and improve breast-milk production. The root is now used to treat enlarged prostate.

SELF-HELP USES

- **Allergic rhinitis including hay fever**, p. 300.

PARTS USED

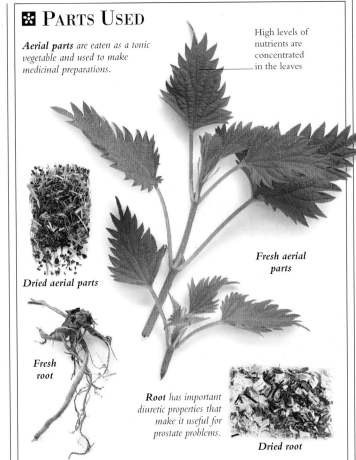

Aerial parts are eaten as a tonic vegetable and used to make medicinal preparations.

High levels of nutrients are concentrated in the leaves

Fresh aerial parts

Dried aerial parts

Fresh root

Root has important diuretic properties that make it useful for prostate problems.

Dried root

KEY PREPARATIONS & THEIR USES

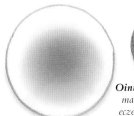

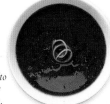

Decoction of root (to make, p. 290). For enlarged prostate, take 1 cup daily.

Ointment of leaves (to make, p. 294). For eczema, rub liberally.

Soup with nettle leaves, carrots, and onions is rich in iron. Drink regularly.

- **CAPSULES** of root (to make, p. 291). For heavy menstruation, take a 100 mg capsule 3 times a day.
- **INFUSION** of leaves (to make, p. 290). Drink 200 ml daily as a tonic.
- **TINCTURE** of root (to make, p. 291) helps allergies and skin conditions. For hay fever, take 1 tsp diluted with 100 ml water twice a day.

Valeriana officinalis (*Valerianaceae*)
VALERIAN

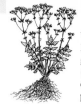

VALERIAN
Erect perennial growing to 4 ft (1.2 m) with pinnate, divided leaves and pink flowers.

VALERIAN HAS BEEN USED as a sedative and relaxant at least since Roman times. It was known to Dioscorides in the 1st century AD, who named it *phu*, the sound of the word reflecting its unpleasant smell. Valerian helps to relieve stress and has become an increasingly popular remedy in recent decades. It is a safe, non-addictive relaxant that reduces nervous tension and anxiety and promotes restful sleep.

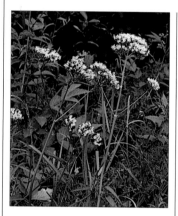

Valerian helps to reduce stress. Its name is thought to be derived from the Latin valere, *"to be well."*

HABITAT & CULTIVATION
Native to Europe and northern Asia, valerian grows wild in damp conditions. It is cultivated in central and eastern Europe. The plant is grown from seed in spring, and the root and rhizome of 2-year-old plants are unearthed in autumn.

RELATED SPECIES
V. capensis is given in South Africa for hysteria and epilepsy; *V. hardwickii*, found in China and Indonesia, is taken as an antispasmodic; *V. ulginosa* was used for cramps and menopausal symptoms by the Menominee people in North America; and *V. wallichi* is used in the Himalayas in almost exactly the same way as valerian.

KEY CONSTITUENTS
- Volatile oil (up to 1.4%), including bornyl acetate, beta-caryphyllene
- Iridoids (valepotriates) – valtrate, isovaltrate
- Alkaloids

KEY ACTIONS
- Sedative
- Relaxant
- Relieves muscle spasms
- Relieves anxiety
- Lowers blood pressure

RESEARCH
- **Therapeutic properties** Extensive research in Germany and Switzerland has confirmed that valerian encourages sleep, improves sleep quality, and lowers blood pressure.
- **Active constituents** The valepotriates are sedative and depressant, inducing sleep. Other constituents are also responsible for valerian's action, but they have not yet been identified.
- **Nervous system** Valerian reduces nervous activity by prolonging the action of an inhibitory neurotransmitter.

TRADITIONAL & CURRENT USES
- **Historical uses** Known as "all-heal" in the Middle Ages, valerian was credited with many virtues – in particular with healing epilepsy. In 1592, Fabius Calumna published a detailed work on herbal medicine in which he claimed to have cured his epilepsy with the herb.
- **Stress-related disorders** Valerian reduces mental over-activity and nervous excitability, helping people who find it hard to "switch off." It is beneficial for almost any stress-related condition, and, in general, has a calming, rather than directly sedative, effect on the mind.
- **Anxiety & insomnia** Many symptoms of anxiety, including tremors, panic, palpitations, and sweating, can be relieved with valerian. It is a useful remedy for insomnia, whether caused by anxiety or overexcitement.
- **Effective relaxant** Valerian relaxes overcontracted muscles, and is helpful for shoulder and neck tension, asthma, colic, irritable bowel syndrome, muscle spasms, and menstrual pain.
- **High blood pressure** Valerian is used with other herbs in remedies for high blood pressure caused by stress and anxiety.

✢ PARTS USED

Root and rhizome *are harvested in autumn when they contain the highest level of active ingredients.*

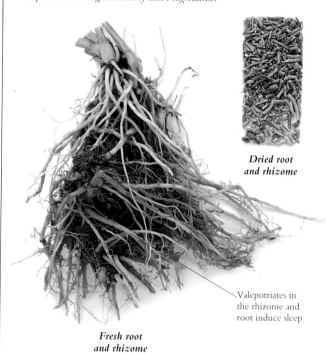

Dried root and rhizome

Valepotriates in the rhizome and root induce sleep

Fresh root and rhizome

☕ KEY PREPARATIONS & THEIR USES

Cautions Can cause drowsiness. Do not take valerian if already taking sleep-inducing drugs.

Tablets often also contain other herbs. Take for stress or anxiety.

Powder can be taken as capsules (to make, p. 291). For insomnia, take 1–2 × 500 mg at night.

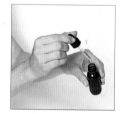

Tincture (to make, p. 291). For anxiety, take 20 drops in hot water up to 5 times a day.

🥣 DECOCTION (to make, p. 290). Take 25–100 ml as a sedative at night.

SELF-HELP USES
- **Chronic anxiety**, p. 308.
- **Insomnia**, p. 309.
- **Nervous exhaustion**, p. 309.
- **Premenstrual tension**, p. 315.
- **Sleeplessness due to backache**, p. 313.

Verbena officinalis (*Verbenaceae*)
VERVAIN, MA BIAN CAO (CHINESE)

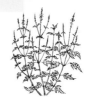

VERVAIN
A slender perennial
growing to 3 ft (1 m),
with stiff, thin stems
and spikes of small
lilac flowers.

VERVAIN HAS LONG BEEN credited with magical properties and was used in ceremonies by the Druids of ancient Britain and Gaul. It is a traditional herbal medicine in both China and Europe. Dioscorides in the 1st century AD called vervain the "sacred herb," and for many centuries it was taken as a cure-all. It has tonic, restorative properties, and is used to relieve stress and anxiety and to improve digestive function.

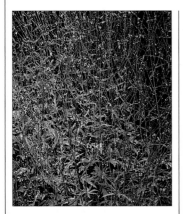

Vervain was carried in the Middle Ages to bring good luck.

HABITAT & CULTIVATION

Vervain grows wild throughout much of Europe and North Africa as well as in China and Japan. It is propagated from seed in spring or autumn and thrives in well-drained soil in a sunny position. The aerial parts are harvested in summer when the plant is in flower.

RELATED SPECIES

In the Caribbean, the related *V. domingensis* is taken as a bitter tonic for the digestion, and is used for wounds and headaches.

KEY CONSTITUENTS

- Bitter iridoids (verbenin, verbenalin)
- Volatile oil
- Alkaloids
- Mucilage
- Tannins

KEY ACTIONS

- Nervine
- Tonic
- Mild sedative
- Stimulates bile secretion
- Mild bitter

TRADITIONAL & CURRENT USES

■ **Established properties** Though poorly researched, some of vervain's properties are well known. It affects the parasympathetic nervous system and has a stimulant action on the uterus. Vervain is bitter and stimulates the digestion, causing vomiting at high doses. The constituent verbenalin, a mild purgative, may be responsible.

■ **Digestive tonic** A tonic for the digestion, vervain improves the absorption of food.

■ **Nervous system** Vervain is prized as a restorative for the nervous system and is especially helpful for nervous tension. It is thought to have a mild antidepressant action, and is used specifically to treat anxiety and the nervous exhaustion that follow long-term stress.

■ **Convalescence** By aiding the digestion and restoring the nervous system, vervain is an ideal tonic for people recovering from chronic illness.

■ **Headaches & migraine** Vervain alleviates headaches and in Chinese herbal medicine it is used for migraine connected with the menstrual cycle.

■ **Other uses** Vervain has an array of other medicinal uses. It is given for jaundice, gallstones, asthma, insomnia, premenstrual tension, and fevers (especially for the onset of flu). Vervain also helps labor contractions and increases breast-milk production.

SELF-HELP USES

■ **Nervous exhaustion**, p. 309.
■ **Premenstrual tension**, p. 315.

❖ PARTS USED

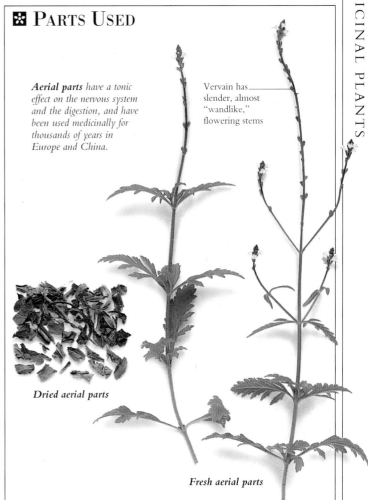

Aerial parts have a tonic effect on the nervous system and the digestion, and have been used medicinally for thousands of years in Europe and China.

Vervain has slender, almost "wandlike," flowering stems

Dried aerial parts

Fresh aerial parts

❖ KEY PREPARATIONS & THEIR USES

Cautions Do not exceed the stated dose. Vervain can cause vomiting if taken in excess. Do not take during pregnancy.

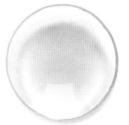

Tincture (to make, p. 291) is a relaxing, calming tonic. For stress and anxiety, take ½ tsp diluted in a glass of water 3 times a day.

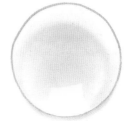

Infusion (to make, p. 290) helps to stimulate the digestion and improves effective absorption of food. Drink a cup regularly, particularly after heavy meals.

Powder can be used as a toothpaste. Rub on the teeth regularly to clean and protect them.

Viburnum opulus (Caprifoliaceae)
CRAMPBARK, GUELDER ROSE

CRAMPBARK
A deciduous shrub or tree growing to 13 ft (4 m), with lobed leaves, white flowers, and red oval fruits.

NATIVE TO BOTH NORTH AMERICA and Europe, crampbark was recognized in the *US National Formulary* as recently as 1960 as a sedative for nervous conditions and an antispasmodic in the treatment of asthma. As its name implies, the herb's primary medicinal use is to relieve cramps and other conditions, such as colic or painful menstruation caused by overcontraction of muscles.

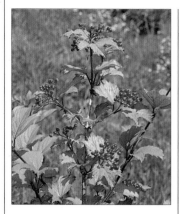

***Crampbark** has distinctive bright red berries in autumn.*

HABITAT & CULTIVATION
Crampbark grows in woodlands, hedges, and thickets in Europe and eastern North America. It is propagated by seed sown in autumn. Bark from the branches is collected in spring and summer when the plant is in flower.

RELATED SPECIES
Black haw (*V. prunifolium*, p. 279) is often used interchangeably with crampbark, but it is thought to have a more specific action on the uterus.

KEY CONSTITUENTS
- Hydroquinones (arbutin)
- Coumarins (scopoletin)
- Tannins (3%)
- Resin

KEY ACTIONS
- Antispasmodic
- Sedative
- Astringent
- Nervine

RESEARCH
- **Active constituents** To date, crampbark has been poorly researched, and there is also some confusion over which active constituents it contains, and which occur in the closely related black haw (*V. prunifolium*).

TRADITIONAL & CURRENT USES
- **Native American remedy** The Meskwaki people of North America took crampbark for cramps and pains throughout the body, while the Penobscot used it to treat swollen glands and mumps.
- **Muscle relaxant** Crampbark is effective at relieving any over-tense muscle, whether smooth muscle in the intestines, airways, or uterus, or striated muscle (attached to the skeleton) in the limbs or back. It may be taken internally or applied topically to relieve muscle tension. The herb also treats symptoms arising from excess muscle tension, including breathing difficulties in asthma, and menstrual pain caused by excessive contraction of the uterus. For night cramps and back pain, lobelia (*Lobelia inflata*, p. 108) is often mixed with crampbark. The herb also relieves constipation, colic, and irritable bowel syndrome, as well as the physical symptoms of nervous tension.
- **Arthritis** In some cases of arthritis, where joint weakness and pain have caused muscles to contract until they are almost rigid, crampbark can bring remarkable relief. As the muscles relax, blood flow to the area improves, waste products such as lactic acid are removed, and normal function can return.
- **Other uses** Crampbark is commonly used in treatments for high blood pressure and other circulatory conditions.

SELF-HELP USES
- **Back pain**, p. 313.
- **Breathing difficulties**, p. 301.

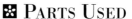

✦ PARTS USED

Bark is peeled off the tree in strips during spring and summer. Care must be taken to leave enough bark for the tree to stay alive.

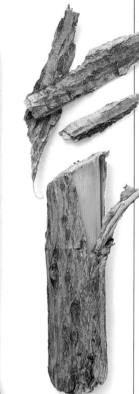

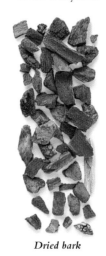

Dried bark

Fresh bark

⚗ KEY PREPARATIONS & THEIR USES

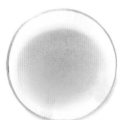

Decoction (to make, p. 290). For menstrual pain, take ½ cup every 3 hours.

Tincture (to make, p. 291) is used for long-term treatment of muscular tension. For irritable bowel syndrome, take ½ tsp diluted with hot water twice a day.

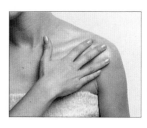

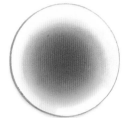

Lotion (to make, p. 295) relieves aching muscles. Rub into tense neck and shoulders.

- **Cramps & muscle spasms**, p. 312.
- **Menstrual pain**, p. 313
- **Poor circulation to the hands & feet**, p. 302.
- **Spastic constipation**, p. 307.
- **Stomach spasm**, p. 305.

Vitex agnus-castus (Verbenaceae)
AGNUS CASTUS, CHASTE TREE

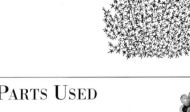

AGNUS CASTUS
A deciduous, aromatic tree growing to 22 ft (7 m), with palm-shaped leaves and small lilac flowers.

AGNUS CASTUS WAS WELL KNOWN in ancient times and featured in Homer's 6th-century BC epic, the *Iliad*, as a symbol of chastity capable of warding off evil. As the name "chaste tree" implies, it was thought to reduce sexual desire, and traditionally it was chewed by monks to reduce unwanted libido. Research has confirmed that agnus castus has a hormonal action, and today it is used for menstrual problems and infertility.

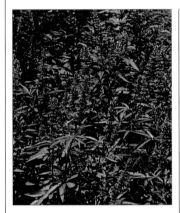

Agnus castus has small, fragrant, lilac flowers in summer, which grow in whorls on long spikes.

HABITAT & CULTIVATION
Agnus castus is native to the Mediterranean region and western Asia. It is cultivated in subtropical areas around the world, and has become naturalized in many regions. It is grown from seed in spring or autumn. The ripe berries are collected in autumn.

RELATED SPECIES
As a member of the *Verbenaceae* genus, agnus castus is a distant relative of vervain (*Verbena officinalis*, p. 147) and lemon verbena (*Lippia citriodora*, p. 227).

KEY CONSTITUENTS
- Volatile oil (cineol)
- Alkaloids (viticine)
- Flavonoids (casticin)
- Iridoids (aucubin, agnoside, eurostoside)

KEY ACTIONS
- Regulates hormones
- Progesterogenic
- Increases breast-milk production

RESEARCH
■ **Hormonal properties**
Researchers have been investigating agnus castus for over 30 years in the UK and Germany, and it is clear that the berries have a distinct hormonal effect on the body. However, the constituents responsible have not been isolated.
■ **Male sex hormones** Agnus castus berries are thought to be antiandrogenic, inhibiting the action of male androgens (sex hormones).
■ **Female sex hormones** A research study in Germany in 1988 indicated that the berries have a progesterogenic effect, acting on the pituitary gland, which regulates the menstrual cycle. Some trials have shown agnus castus to be valuable in treating premenstrual syndrome (PMS) and in increasing fertility.

TRADITIONAL & CURRENT USES
■ **Hormone regulator** Agnus castus is one of the most important herbs for regulating female hormones. By increasing progesterogenic activity, agnus castus can help to balance progesterone and estrogen production by the ovaries throughout the menstrual cycle.
■ **Menstrual problems** Agnus castus is prescribed by Western herbalists to treat menstrual problems, ranging from premenstrual syndrome and many of the symptoms that accompany it, to irregular or absent periods. For premenstrual syndrome, the herb should be taken for some months to see the full benefit,

which can often be significant – with bloating, breast swelling and tenderness, irritability, and depression all reduced.
■ **Irregular periods** The herb helps to regulate irregular periods, tending to shorten a long cycle and lengthen a short one.
■ **Other menstrual symptoms** Agnus castus is valuable in treating other problems that can be linked to the menstrual cycle, such as migraine and acne.

■ **Infertility** Agnus castus can help some women trying to conceive if infertility is due to low progesterone levels.
■ **Difficulty in breast-feeding** The berries are taken to increase breast-milk production.

SELF-HELP USES
- **Aiding conception**, p. 316.
- **Decreased estrogen & progesterone levels**, p. 316.
- **Irregular cycle**, p. 315.

✜ PARTS USED

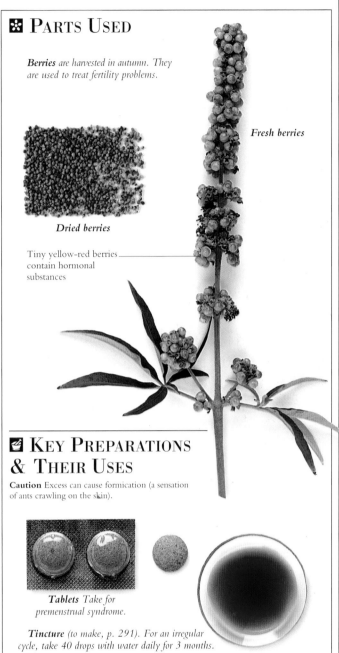

Berries are harvested in autumn. They are used to treat fertility problems.

Dried berries

Tiny yellow-red berries contain hormonal substances

Fresh berries

✍ KEY PREPARATIONS & THEIR USES

Caution Excess can cause formication (a sensation of ants crawling on the skin).

Tablets *Take for premenstrual syndrome.*

Tincture *(to make, p. 291). For an irregular cycle, take 40 drops with water daily for 3 months.*

Withania somnifera (Solanaceae)
WITHANIA, ASHWAGANDHA (HINDI)

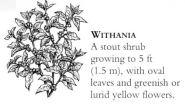

WITHANIA
A stout shrub growing to 5 ft (1.5 m), with oval leaves and greenish or lurid yellow flowers.

WITHANIA HAS BEEN CALLED "Indian ginseng" because it is used in Ayurveda in much the same way that ginseng is used in Chinese medicine: to improve vitality and to aid recovery after chronic illness. Its Hindi name means "horse smell," and refers not just to its smell but to a horse's strength, indicating its use as a tonic, strengthening, and aphrodisiac herb. Its traditional uses have been confirmed by research.

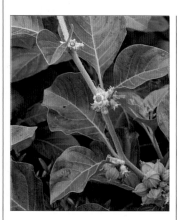

Withania has powerful medicinal properties proven by research.

HABITAT & CULTIVATION
Withania is found in India, the Mediterranean, and the Middle East. It is propagated from seed or cuttings in spring. The leaves are harvested in spring and the fruit and root in autumn.

KEY CONSTITUENTS
- Alkaloids
- Steroidal lactones (withanolides)
- Iron

KEY ACTIONS
- Adaptogenic
- Tonic
- Sedative

RESEARCH
- **Indian research** Withania has been widely researched in India.
- **Alkaloids** Studies in 1965 indicated that the alkaloids are sedative, reduce blood pressure, and lower the heartbeat rate.
- **Withanolides** Research in 1970 showed that withanolides, which are similar to the body's own steroid hormones, are anti-inflammatory. They also inhibit the growth of cancer cells. The herb may be of use in chronic inflammatory diseases such as lupus and rheumatoid arthritis, and as a cancer preventive.
- **Further research** Trials in 1980 indicated that withania increases hemoglobin levels, reduces graying of hair, and improves sexual performance. It also helps recovery from chronic illness.

TRADITIONAL & CURRENT USES
- **Ayurvedic tonic** Withania is valued in Ayurveda for its tonic, strengthening properties, and particularly for its ability to restore vitality in those suffering from overwork or nervous exhaustion. It is considered to reduce *vata* and *kapha* (*see p. 35*). Robert Svoboda in *Ayurveda, Life, Health and Longevity* (Arkana, 1992) states that it "clarifies the mind, calms and strengthens the nerves, and promotes sound restful sleep."
- **Restorative** Dioscorides in the 1st century AD recommended withania as a tonic. Today, it is mainly used in the West as a restorative for the elderly and the chronically ill.
- **Long-term stress** By reducing overactivity and encouraging rest and relaxation, withania is useful in countering the debility that accompanies long-term stress.
- **Anemia** Withania's high iron content makes it useful for anemia.

SELF-HELP USES
- **Long-term stress & convalescence**, pp. 308 & 319.
- **Male fertility**, p. 316.

✣ PARTS USED

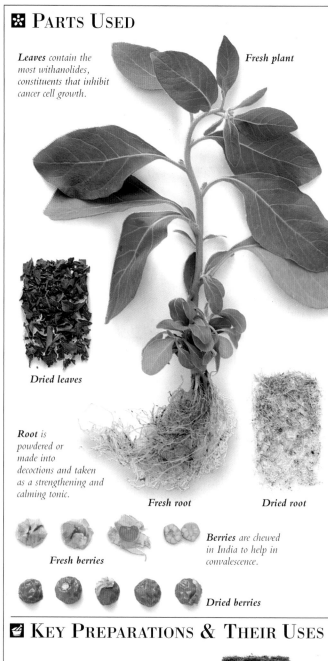

Leaves contain the most withanolides, constituents that inhibit cancer cell growth.

Fresh plant

Dried leaves

Root is powdered or made into decoctions and taken as a strengthening and calming tonic.

Fresh root

Dried root

Berries are chewed in India to help in convalescence.

Fresh berries

Dried berries

🥄 KEY PREPARATIONS & THEIR USES

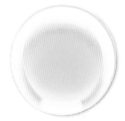

Decoction of the root (to make, p. 290). For stress, decoct 5 g with 100 ml water and take over 2 days.

Powder made from the leaves. For anemia, take ½ tsp in some water once a day.

🔎 **CAPSULES** of powdered root (to make, p. 291). For nervous exhaustion, take 1–2 g a day with water.

Zanthoxylum americanum (Rutaceae)
PRICKLY ASH, TOOTHACHE TREE

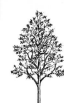

PRICKLY ASH
A deciduous shrub growing to 10 ft (3 m), with thorny gray branches and compound leaves.

KEY MEDICINAL PLANTS

INDIGENOUS TO NORTH AMERICA, prickly ash is a warming, stimulating herb for the circulation. It was esteemed by Native North Americans for its medicinal properties and both the bark and berries were chewed to alleviate rheumatism and toothache. Today, prickly ash is mainly given for arthritic and rheumatic conditions, but it is also helpful for certain digestive problems and for leg ulcers.

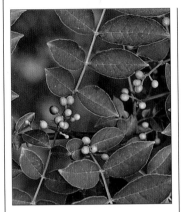

Prickly ash is antirheumatic and improves the circulation.

HABITAT & CULTIVATION
Prickly ash is native to southern Canada and northern, central, and western parts of the US, preferring moist, shady sites, such as woodlands. It is propagated from seed in autumn. The bark is harvested in spring, and the berries are collected in summer.

RELATED SPECIES
Southern prickly ash (*Z. clava-herculis*) grows in central and southern US, where it is used interchangeably with prickly ash. *Chuan jiao* (*Z. bungeanum*) is given in Chinese herbal medicine for "cold" patterns of illness causing abdominal pain. *Z. capense* is taken for colic in South Africa. *Z. zanthoxyloides* is a traditional West African herb for rheumatic conditions.

KEY CONSTITUENTS
- Alkaloids (chelerythrine)
- Herclavin
- Lignans (asarinin)
- Neoherculin
- Tannins
- Resins
- Volatile oil

KEY ACTIONS
- Circulatory stimulant
- Increases sweating
- Antirheumatic
- Carminative

TRADITIONAL & CURRENT USES
- **North American herb** Prickly ash was a Native North American remedy for toothache and rheumatism. It was used in the US during the 19th century as a circulatory stimulant and to treat arthritis. The bark was listed in the *Pharmacopoeia of the United States* from 1820 to 1926.
- **Arthritic conditions** Western herbalists regard prickly ash as a prime remedy for rheumatic and arthritic problems. It stimulates blood flow to painful and stiff joints, promoting the supply of oxygen and nutrients to the area and removing waste products.
- **Circulation** Prickly ash improves the circulation in both intermittent claudication and Raynaud's disease, conditions where the arteries of the limbs have narrowed, preventing sufficient blood reaching the hand or leg muscles.
- **Other uses** Prickly ash relieves gas and diarrhea and tones the digestion. It is applied topically to treat leg ulcers and chronic pelvic inflammatory disease.

SELF-HELP USES
- **Back pain**, p. 313.
- **Poor circulation**, p. 302.

✤ PARTS USED

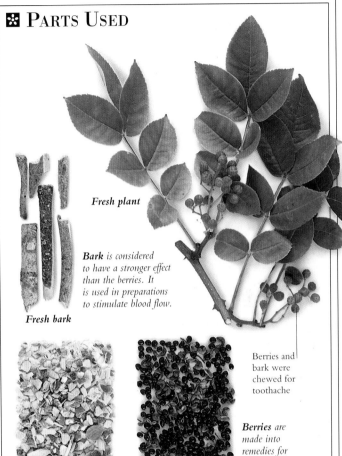

Fresh plant

Bark *is considered to have a stronger effect than the berries. It is used in preparations to stimulate blood flow.*

Fresh bark

Berries and bark were chewed for toothache

Berries *are made into remedies for poor circulation.*

Dried chopped bark   *Dried berries*

⊡ KEY PREPARATIONS & THEIR USES

Cautions Do not use during pregnancy. Do not take internally if suffering from inflammatory stomach conditions.

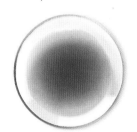

Tincture of bark (to make, p. 291). For arthritis, take 20 drops with water 3 times a day.

Decoction For poor circulation, decoct 3 tsp ginger and 3 tsp prickly ash berries with 750 ml water (see p. 290). Drink 1 cup twice a day.

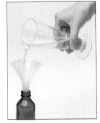

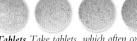

Tablets Take tablets, which often contain other herbs, for arthritis and rheumatism.

Lotion For poor circulation in the legs, make a decoction of bark (p. 291) and apply.

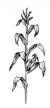

CORN
An annual grass reaching 10 ft (3 m), with plumelike male flowers. Female flowers produce cobs.

Zea mays (Gramineae)
CORN, MAIZE, CORNSILK, YU MI SHU (CHINESE)

THE STAPLE FOOD OF CENTRAL and South America for at least 4,000 years, corn is also used medicinally in countless different ways. The Aztecs gave a corn meal decoction for dysentery, "heat in the heart," and to increase breast-milk production. Cornsilk (the silky fronds wrapped around the cob) has always been the part most used medicinally, and is of particular value in treating urinary conditions.

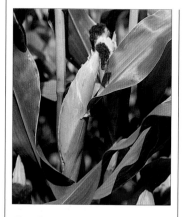

Corn's Latin name reflects its value – zea *means "cause of life" and* mays *means "our mother."*

HABITAT & CULTIVATION

Cultivated almost universally as a food crop, corn is native to the Andes and Central America, possibly originating in Peru. It is propagated from seed in spring. The cornsilk is harvested with the ripe cob in summer, then separated and dried.

OTHER SPECIES

Cornsmut (*Ustilago zeae*), a fungus that grows on corn, is used by the Zuni of New Mexico to speed childbirth and stop uterine hemorrhage.

KEY CONSTITUENTS

- Flavonoids (maysin)
- Alkaloids
- Allantoin
- Saponins
- Volatile oil (about 0.2%)
- Mucilage
- Vitamins C and K
- Potassium

KEY ACTIONS

- Urinary demulcent
- Diuretic

- Mildly stimulates bile secretion
- Gently lowers blood pressure

RESEARCH

- **Bile production** Cornsilk is thought to stimulate production of bile, improving its flow from the liver through the bile ducts.
- **Circulatory remedy** Research in China indicates that cornsilk lowers blood pressure and reduces blood-clotting time.

TRADITIONAL & CURRENT USES

- **Traditional herb** Corn meal has been used by Native Americans for a wide range of ailments. It makes an effective poultice and has been used in Mayan, Incan, and American folk medicine to treat bruises, swellings, sores, boils, and similar conditions. Vogel in *American Indian Medicine* (1970) stated that "the Chickasaw Indians treated itching skin, followed by sores when scratched, by burning old corncobs and holding the affected part over the smoke."
- **Urinary remedy** Partly due to its significant potassium content, cornsilk is a useful diuretic for almost all problems of the urinary system. It soothes and relaxes the lining of the urinary tubules and bladder, relieving irritation and improving urine flow and elimination. It is also helpful for frequent urination caused by irritation of the bladder and urethral walls, and for difficulty in passing urine such as in prostate disorders.
- **Kidney stones** Cornsilk is thought to have a beneficial effect on the kidneys, reducing kidney stone formation and

PARTS USED

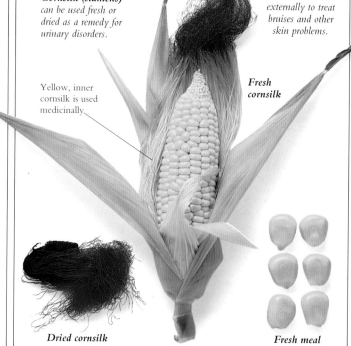

Cornsilk (stamens) can be used fresh or dried as a remedy for urinary disorders.

Meal is used externally to treat bruises and other skin problems.

Yellow, inner cornsilk is used medicinally

Fresh cornsilk

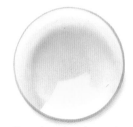

Dried cornsilk

Fresh meal

KEY PREPARATIONS & THEIR USES

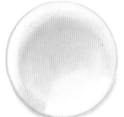

Infusion of cornsilk (to make, p. 290) is soothing. For cystitis, drink 500 ml daily.

Decoction of meal (to make, p. 290). Apply as a poultice (see p. 294) to sores and boils.

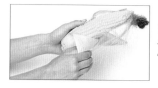

The outer leaves of corn are stripped to reveal the cornsilk and meal.

CAPSULES of cornsilk (to make, p. 291). For edema, take 2 g daily.

TINCTURE of cornsilk (to make, p. 291). For cystitis, combine 80 ml with 20 ml of buchu tincture and take 1 tsp with water 3 times a day.

relieving some of the symptoms of existing stones.
- **Cystitis** Chronic cystitis can be relieved with cornsilk and and it is a useful adjunct to other treatments for acute cystitis.
- **Chinese remedy** In China,

cornsilk is used to treat fluid retention and jaundice.

SELF-HELP USES

- **Fluid retention in pregnancy**, p. 317.
- **Urinary infections**, p. 314.

Zingiber officinale (Zingiberaceae)

GINGER, SHENG JIAN (CHINESE), SINGABERA (SANSKRIT)

GINGER
A perennial growing to 2 ft (60 cm), with lance-shaped leaves and stalks of white or yellow flowers.

FAMILIAR AS A SPICE AND FLAVORING, ginger is also one of the world's best medicines. It has been revered in Asia since the earliest times, and in medieval Europe it was thought to have derived from the Garden of Eden. Ginger brings relief to digestions troubled by motion sickness, morning sickness, and other causes, and the herb is also an important circulatory remedy. Fresh ginger has a pungent, slightly lemony taste.

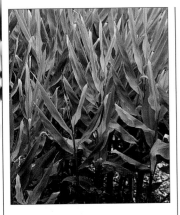

Ginger, widely used as a spice, is also an important digestive remedy.

HABITAT & CULTIVATION

Native to Asia, ginger is grown throughout the tropics. It is propagated by dividing the rootstock. Ginger flourishes in fertile soil and needs plenty of rain. The rhizome is unearthed when the plant is 10 months old. It is washed, soaked, and sometimes boiled and peeled.

RELATED SPECIES

Various *Zingiber* species are used medicinally, but no other has benefits equal to ginger. Turmeric (*Curcuma longa*, p. 88) is a close relative.

KEY CONSTITUENTS

- Volatile oil, (1–3%)
  – zingiberene (20–30%)
- Oleoresin (4–7.5%)
  – gingerol, shogaols

KEY ACTIONS

- Antiemetic
- Carminative
- Circulatory stimulant
- Inhibits coughing
- Anti-inflammatory
- Antiseptic

RESEARCH

■ Therapeutic properties

Ginger is well researched, and its therapeutic benefits are largely due to its volatile oil and oleoresin content. Gingerol is an acrid constituent, responsible for much of the herb's hot taste and stimulating properties. The shogaols, formed as the plant dries, are more strongly irritant and acrid than the constituents present in the fresh rhizome.

■ Antiemetic
Ginger is highly effective for motion sickness. Trials at St. Bartholomew's Hospital in London in 1990 found the herb more effective than conventional medicines in relieving postoperative nausea.

■ Antiseptic
In a trial in China 70% of patients with bacillary dysentery who were given ginger made a full recovery.

TRADITIONAL & CURRENT USES

■ Digestive problems
Ginger is an excellent remedy for many digestive complaints, such as indigestion, nausea, gas, and colic. It relieves motion sickness and morning sickness. Ginger's antiseptic qualities also make it highly beneficial for gastro-intestinal infections, including some types of food poisoning.

■ Circulatory stimulant
Ginger stimulates the circulation, and helps blood to flow to the surface, making it an important remedy for chilblains and poor circulation to the hands and feet. By improving the circulation, ginger helps high blood pressure. It also increases sweating and helps reduce body temperature in fevers.

■ Respiratory conditions
Ginger is warming and soothing for coughs, colds, flu, and other respiratory problems.

■ Chinese herb
Fresh and dried ginger are different remedies in China. Fresh ginger is given for fever, headaches, and aching muscles. Dried ginger is used for "internal cold," with symptoms such as cold hands, a weak pulse, and a pale complexion.

❁ PARTS USED

Rhizome contains high levels of a volatile oil that is warming and stimulating.

Yellowish fresh rhizome is strongly aromatic

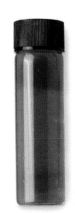

Fresh rhizome

Sliced, dried rhizome

🍃 KEY PREPARATIONS & THEIR USES

Cautions Do not take ginger medicinal doses if suffering from peptic ulcers. Do not take the essential oil internally except under professional supervision.

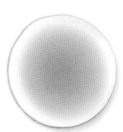

Infusion (to make, p. 290). For nausea, drink 1 cup 3 times a day.

Essential oil For arthritic aches and pains dilute 5 drops in 20 drops carrier oil and apply (see p. 296).

✆ **CAPSULES** (to make, p. 291). For morning sickness, take a 75 mg capsule every hour.

✒ **TINCTURE** (to make, p. 291). To improve digestion, take 30 drops twice a day.

SELF-HELP USES

- **Chilblains**, p. 302.
- **Colds, flu & fever**, p. 311.
- **Cold sores**, p. 304.
- **Constipation**, p. 307.
- **Digestive upsets, gas & colic**, p.318.
- **High blood pressure & arteriosclerosis**, p. 301.
- **Morning sickness**, p. 317.
- **Nausea & motion sickness**, p. 306.

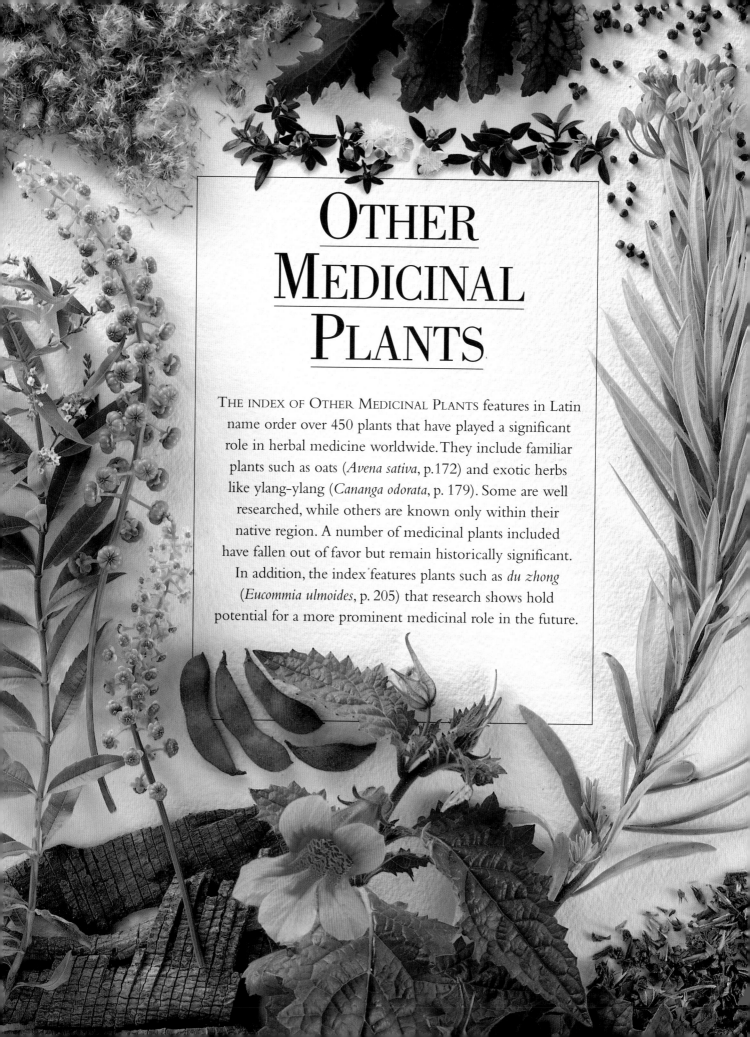

OTHER MEDICINAL PLANTS

THE INDEX OF OTHER MEDICINAL PLANTS features in Latin
name order over 450 plants that have played a significant
role in herbal medicine worldwide. They include familiar
plants such as oats (*Avena sativa*, p.172) and exotic herbs
like ylang-ylang (*Cananga odorata*, p. 179). Some are well
researched, while others are known only within their
native region. A number of medicinal plants included
have fallen out of favor but remain historically significant.
In addition, the index features plants such as *du zhong*
(*Eucommia ulmoides*, p. 205) that research shows hold
potential for a more prominent medicinal role in the future.

ABOUT THE ENTRIES

PLANT NAMES
The Latin name given is the one by which the plant is most generally known in medical herbalism. Latin synonyms are also provided. The first part of the Latin name designates the plant's genus (sub-family). The second part specifies the species name. In brackets after the Latin name(s) comes the plant's family name, the broader class to which the genus belongs. The plant's common name(s) are beneath the family name. If more than one common name is in popular use, they are listed in order of importance. Where appropriate, the origins of common names are given in brackets.

DESCRIPTION
Lists significant botanical information including whether the plant is evergreen or deciduous and whether it is annual, biennial, or perennial. Gives identifying characteristics of the plant.

HABITAT & CULTIVATION
Includes the plant's origins, its distribution, preferred growing conditions, and the seasons when it is propagated and harvested.

PARTS USED
Lists those parts of the plant that are used medicinally in order of importance.

CONSTITUENTS
Gives the key active constituents of the plant in order of significance. Sometimes includes details of a constituent's specific medicinal action on the body. *Note* To find out more about constituents and their actions, see *How Medicinal Plants Work*, pp. 10–15.

HISTORY & FOLKLORE
Provides information such as the derivation of the herb's name, traditional lore, and quotations from old herbals showing how the plant was regarded in the past, and how it was used medicinally. Also includes details of the plant's other uses.

MEDICINAL ACTIONS & USES
Encompasses both the confirmed and presumed actions of the whole plant (as opposed to isolated active constituents). Discusses the symptoms and illnesses that the plant is used to treat and the varying ways that the herb is used medicinally in different herbal traditions.

RESEARCH
Gives details of scientific research into the plant, its constituents, and its extracts, including the results of any clinical trials.

RELATED SPECIES
Provides information on related species that have a medicinal use. Gives a cross-reference to those species that have an entry in the *Encyclopedia*.

CAUTIONS
Gives cautions about using the herb medicinally and about the plant in general. States if the plant, its constituents, or its extracts are legally restricted.

SELF-HELP USES
Cross-refers to the self-help treatments in *Remedies for Common Ailments*. *Note* Always read the cautions about the herb and the information on pp. 289 & 298–299 before attempting a self-help use.

OTHER MEDICINAL PLANTS

Abies balsamea
(Pinaceae)
BALSAM FIR

DESCRIPTION Conical evergreen tree growing to 180 ft (55 m). Has aromatic needlelike leaves and purple fir cones.

HABITAT & CULTIVATION Native to North America, balsam fir is commercially grown for its lumber. The resin is tapped from 60- to 80-year-old trees in spring.

PARTS USED Oleo-resin, leaves.

CONSTITUENTS Balsam fir leaves contain a liquid oleo-resin.

HISTORY & FOLKLORE Balsam fir resin, often known as Canada balsam, was used for many illnesses by both Native Americans and settlers. The Penobscot smeared the resin on burns, cuts, and sores, whereas others applied it to the chest and back for colds and chest problems. The Pillagers used the aromatic needles in their sweat lodges, inhaling smoke from the burning leaves. Dr. Wooster Beech (1794–1868), founder of the Eclectic healing movement, regarded balsam fir as a stimulant and a laxative when taken internally, an emollient and coolant when used externally. The leaves, cones, and resin are commonly added to potpourri.

MEDICINAL ACTIONS & USES Balsam fir is an antiseptic and stimulant, and has been used in North America and Europe for congestion, chest infections such as bronchitis, and urinary tract conditions such as cystitis and frequent urination. Externally, balsam fir was rubbed on the chest or applied as a plaster for respiratory infections. It is not used much in herbal medicine today.

Abrus precatorius
(Leguminosae)
JEQUIRITY

DESCRIPTION Deciduous climber growing to 12 ft (4 m). Has compound leaves, clusters of pink flowers, and seed pods containing scarlet or (rarely) white seeds.

HABITAT & CULTIVATION Jequirity is native to India, and now grows in hedges and among bushes in all tropical regions.

PARTS USED Root, leaves, seeds.

CONSTITUENTS Jequirity seeds contain abrin, indole alkaloids, and anthocyanins. The root and leaves contain glycyrrhizin and traces of abrin. Abrin is extremely toxic. Glycyrrhizin is expectorant, anti-inflammatory, and anti-allergenic.

HISTORY & FOLKLORE Jequirity seeds have been used since ancient times in India to help weigh precious materials, including the famous Koh-i-noor diamond. The seeds are notorious as a poison.

MEDICINAL ACTIONS & USES Jequirity seeds have been used medicinally in the past as a contraceptive, abortifacient (induce a miscarriage), and as a treatment for chronic conjunctivitis. However, they are so poisonous that even external application is no longer justifiable. Even small amounts brought into contact with an open wound can prove fatal. The leaves and roots can be substituted for licorice (*Glycyrrhiza glabra*, p. 99), and have been used in the Ayurvedic tradition in the treatment of asthma, bronchitis, and other chest conditions. They have been used in Chinese medicine to treat fever.

CAUTIONS Never use the seeds. Use the leaves and roots only under professional supervision. Jequirity is subject to legal restrictions in some countries.

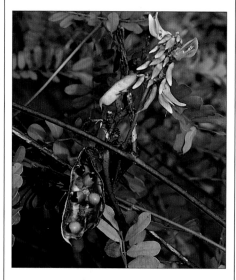

JEQUIRITY seeds were used medicinally in former times but are extremely poisonous.

Abutilon indicum
(Malvaceae)
KANGHI, INDIAN MALLOW

DESCRIPTION Upright, woody plant growing to 5 ft (1.5 m). Has a downy, slightly oily surface, single yellow flowers, and kidney-shaped seeds.

HABITAT & CULTIVATION Kanghi grows throughout much of India and also in Southeast Asia.

PARTS USED Root, bark, leaves, seeds.

CONSTITUENTS Kanghi contains mucilage, tannins, and asparagine. Asparagine is diuretic.

MEDICINAL ACTIONS & USES Also known as Indian mallow, kanghi is used in much the same way as marsh mallow (*Althaea officinalis*, p. 163), one of the main European demulcent herbs. The root and bark of kanghi are mucilaginous and are used to soothe and protect the mucous membranes of the respiratory and urinary systems. A decoction

of the root is given for chest conditions such as bronchitis. The mucilaginous effect benefits the skin; an infusion, poultice, or paste made from the powdered root or bark is applied to wounds and used for conditions such as boils and ulcers. The seeds are laxative and "useful in killing threadworms, if the rectum of the affected child be exposed to the smoke of the powdered seeds" (*Herbs that Heal*, H. K. Bakhru, 1992). The plant has an antiseptic effect within the urinary tract and can be used to treat urinary infections.

RELATED SPECIES *A. trisulcatum*, native to Central America, is used to treat asthma in children and is applied as a poultice for treating cancerous sores and ulcers, especially of the mouth and cervix.

Acacia arabica
(Leguminosae)
BABUL

DESCRIPTION Tree growing to 70 ft (20 m), with hard, woody, rust-brown bark and feathery leaves. Small, bright yellow flower heads produce pods up to 6 in (15 cm) long.

HABITAT & CULTIVATION Babul is native to North Africa. Today it is commonly found in Egypt and is cultivated in India.

PART USED Bark.

CONSTITUENTS Babul contains tannins, mucilage, and flavonoids.

HISTORY & FOLKLORE In ancient Egypt, the wood of the babul tree was used to make dwellings, wheels, and tool handles. The leaves, flowers, and pods were used as medicines to expel worms and to staunch and heal wounds, alleviate diarrhea, and suppress the coughing up of blood.

MEDICINAL ACTIONS & USES Strongly astringent, babul is used to contract and toughen mucous membranes throughout the body in much the same way as witch hazel (*Hamamelis virginiana*, p. 100) or oak bark (*Quercus robur*, p. 258) does. Babul may be made into a variety of preparations: for instance, a lotion for bleeding gums, a gargle for sore throats, a wash for eczema, an eyewash for conjunctivitis and other eye problems, and a douche for excessive vaginal discharge. The herb is taken internally to treat diarrhea, mainly in the form of a decoction. In Ayurvedic medicine, babul is considered a remedy that is helpful for treating premature ejaculation.

RELATED SPECIES Black wattle (*A. decurrens*), native to Australia, is used in much the same way as babul. Black wattle's bark contains 30–50% tannins. *See also* black catechu (*A. catechu, following entry*).

CAUTIONS Do not take babul for more than a few days at a time. *Acacia* species are subject to legal restrictions in some countries.

Acacia catechu
(Leguminosae)
BLACK CATECHU, CUTCH

DESCRIPTION Tree growing to 40 ft (12 m), with thorny branches and divided, feathery leaves.

HABITAT & CULTIVATION Native to India, Myanmar (Burma), Sri Lanka, and East Africa, this tree is cultivated for its lumber. It grows to altitudes of 5,000 ft (1,500 m).

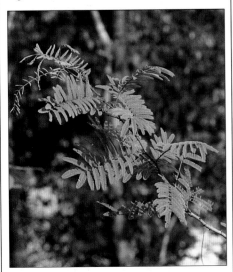

BLACK CATECHU is an astringent and antiseptic.

PARTS USED Bark, heartwood, leaves, shoots.

CONSTITUENTS The shiny, black-brown extract of leaves and young shoots, called "cutch," becomes a brittle solid when dried, and is the form in which black catechu is generally sold. Cutch contains 25–60% tannins, 20–30% mucilage, flavonoids, and resins.

MEDICINAL ACTIONS & USES Black catechu is a strong astringent and clotting agent. It helps reduce excess mucus in the nose, the large bowel, or vagina. It also treats eczema, hemorrhages, diarrhea, and dysentery. It may be used as an infusion, tincture, powder, or ointment. A small piece of cutch dissolved in the mouth is an excellent remedy for bleeding gums and canker sores. The powder and tincture are also applied to infected gums and have been used to clean the teeth. In Ayurvedic medicine, decoctions of the bark and heartwood are used for sore throat.

RESEARCH Cutch has been shown to lower blood pressure.

RELATED SPECIES *See also* babul (*A. arabica*, *preceding entry*).

CAUTIONS Do not take for more than 2–3 weeks at a time or if suffering from kidney inflammation. Cutch is subject to legal restrictions in some countries.

SELF-HELP USE Diarrhea, p. 307.

Acanthus mollis
(Acanthaceae)
ACANTHUS, BEAR'S BREECHES

DESCRIPTION Perennial growing to 3 ft (1 m). Has a black, branched taproot, white, purple, or blue flowers, and dark green basal leaves up to 3 ft (1 m) in length.

HABITAT & CULTIVATION Native to Europe, acanthus is most commonly found as a garden plant. It prefers damp sites and low-lying ground. The leaves are gathered in early summer and the roots in autumn.

PARTS USED Leaves, roots.

CONSTITUENTS Acanthus contains large quantities of mucilage and a tannin.

HISTORY & FOLKLORE Acanthus was well known in the ancient world. Callimacus, a Greek architect of the 5th century BC, reputedly created the decorative pattern of foliage at the top of Corinthian columns after being inspired by the perfect symmetry of acanthus leaves. In the 1st century AD, the Greek physician Dioscorides recommended the roots in the form of a plaster to treat burns and to wrap around dislocated joints. As an infusion, acanthus was thought to be diuretic. It was also used to relieve gas, spasms, and

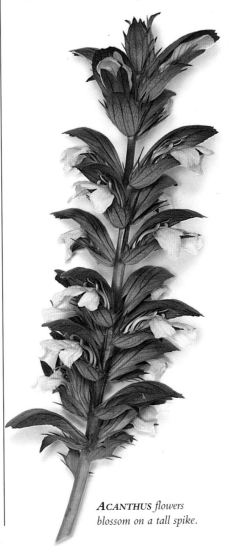

ACANTHUS flowers blossom on a tall spike.

digestive upsets, and to soothe damaged nerves and alleviate tension.

MEDICINAL USES & ACTIONS The herb's appreciable quantities of mucilage and tannin substantiate its traditional use as a treatment for dislocated joints and burns. These constituents are found in many wound-healing plants – for example, comfrey (*Symphytum officinale*, p. 136) and plantain (*Plantago major*, p. 249). Acanthus paste applied to a dislocated joint tends to normalize the affected muscles and ligaments, alternately relaxing and tightening them to encourage the joint back into its proper place and to precipitate the healing process. The plant's soothing, emollient properties are also useful in the treatment of irritated mucous membranes within the digestive and urinary tracts. Acanthus is similar to marsh mallow (*Althaea officinalis*, p. 163) in that it can be used externally to ease irritation, and internally to heal and protect.

Achyranthes bidentata
(Amaranthaceae)
NIU XI

DESCRIPTION Erect perennial herb growing to 3 ft (1 m). Has slender rambling branches, elliptical leaves, and greenish white flowers on terminal spikes.

HABITAT & CULTIVATION *Niu xi* is found in China at the edge of forests, along streams, and amid bushes. Grown commercially in the eastern provinces, the root is unearthed in winter once the foliage has died back.

PART USED Root.

CONSTITUENTS *Achyranthes* species contain triterpenoid saponins.

HISTORY & FOLKLORE *Niu xi's* potent ability to bring on menstruation led the 13th-century Chinese gynecologist Chen Ziming to prohibit its use during pregnancy to avoid causing miscarriage.

MEDICINAL ACTIONS & USES In traditional Chinese medicine, *niu xi* is believed to invigorate blood flow. It is used to stimulate menstruation when a period is delayed or scanty. The herb is also prescribed to ease menstrual pain. *Niu xi* is used to relieve pain in the lower back, especially where the discomfort is attributable to kidney stones. The herb is also taken as a treatment for canker sores, toothache, bleeding gums, and nosebleeds.

RESEARCH Research suggests that *niu xi* may lower blood pressure by reducing heart rate and dilating the peripheral arteries.

RELATED SPECIES *A. aspera* is used in Ayurvedic medicine to treat chest conditions such as asthma and coughs.

CAUTION Do not take *niu xi* during pregnancy.

Aconitum napellus
(Ranunculaceae)

ACONITE, MONKSHOOD

DESCRIPTION Perennial herb growing to 5 ft (1.5 m). Has dark green lobed leaves and violet or blue delphinium-like flowers on long spikes.

HABITAT & CULTIVATION Aconite grows mainly in southern or central Europe and is also found in Kashmir. It prefers damp and shady sites, and is cultivated as a garden plant. The root is unearthed in autumn.

PARTS USED Root.

CONSTITUENTS Aconite contains 0.3–2% terpenoid alkaloids, principally aconitine.

HISTORY & FOLKLORE *Aconitum* species have traditionally been used as arrow poisons.

MEDICINAL ACTIONS & USES Aconite is poisonous in all but the smallest doses and is rarely prescribed for internal use. More commonly, it is applied to unbroken skin to relieve pain from bruises or neurological conditions. In Ayurvedic medicine, aconite is used to treat neuralgia, asthma, and heart weakness. Aconite is also used extensively in homeopathy as an analgesic and sedative.

RELATED SPECIES Chinese aconite (*A. carmichaelii*) is used in China to treat shock and to support the circulatory system in emergencies. Trials in China indicate that it is helpful in congestive heart failure.

CAUTIONS Aconite is a deadly poison at the wrong dosage. Use only under professional supervision. The herb is subject to legal restrictions in some countries.

Adhatoda vasica
syn. *Justicia adhatoda*
(Acanthaceae)

MALABAR NUT

DESCRIPTION Evergreen tree growing to 3 m (10 ft), with lance-shaped leaves, white or purple flowers, and 4-seeded fruit.

HABITAT & CULTIVATION Native to tropical India, malabar nut grows in low-lying regions up to the Himalayan foothills.

PARTS USED Leaves, root, flowers, fruit (nut).

CONSTITUENTS Malabar nut contains alkaloids and an unidentified volatile oil.

HISTORY & FOLKLORE The bitter-tasting malabar nut is a traditional Ayurvedic remedy for chest problems.

MEDICINAL ACTIONS & USES Because of its expectorant qualities, malabar nut is useful for bronchitis and other chest conditions. An Ayurvedic preparation that includes malabar flowers is used for tuberculosis. A poultice of fresh leaves is applied to wounds and to inflamed joints in rheumatism.

CAUTION Do not take during pregnancy.

Adiantum capillus-veneris
(Polypodiaceae)

MAIDENHAIR FERN

DESCRIPTION Fern with delicate fronds growing to 1 ft (30 cm) long.

HABITAT & CULTIVATION Native to Europe and North America, maidenhair fern grows in moist, shady sites.

PARTS USED Aerial parts.

CONSTITUENTS Maidenhair fern contains flavonoids (including rutin and isoquercitin),

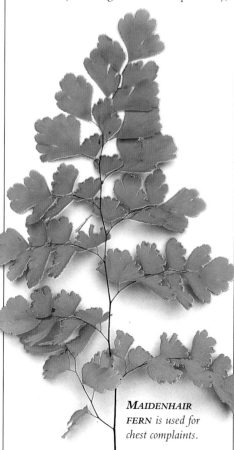

MAIDENHAIR FERN is used for chest complaints.

terpenoids (including adiantone), a tannin, and mucilage.

HISTORY & FOLKLORE Maidenhair fern has been used as a remedy since ancient times. The 18th-century herbalist K'Eogh stated: "It helps cure asthma, coughs, and shortness of breath. It is good against jaundice, diarrhea, spitting of blood and the biting of mad dogs. It also provokes urination and menstruation and breaks up stone in the bladder, spleen and kidneys."

MEDICINAL ACTIONS & USES Still used by Western herbalists to treat coughs, bronchitis, excess mucus, sore throat, and chronic nasal congestion, the plant also has a longstanding reputation as a remedy for conditions of the hair and scalp.

RELATED SPECIES *A. caudatum* has been shown to act as an antispasmodic and could be useful in the treatment of asthma.

Adonis vernalis
(Ranunculaceae)

FALSE HELLEBORE,
YELLOW PHEASANT'S EYE

DESCRIPTION Perennial herb growing to 8 in (20 cm). Has a scaly stem and feathery compound leaves. Stem bears large, bright yellow flowers up to 3 in (8 cm) across.

HABITAT & CULTIVATION Originating from the steppes of Russia and from the Black Sea region, this herb is native to much of Europe but not to Britain. It grows in mountain pasture undergrowth. It is rare and legally protected in Western Europe.

PARTS USED Aerial parts.

CONSTITUENTS False hellebore contains cardiac glycosides, including adonitoxin.

HISTORY & FOLKLORE False hellebore's botanical name refers to Adonis, a figure in Greek mythology associated with the seasonal renewal of plant life.

MEDICINAL ACTIONS & USES False hellebore contains cardiac glycosides similar to those found in foxglove (*Digitalis purpurea*, p. 199). These substances increase the heart's efficiency by increasing its output while slowing its rate. Unlike foxglove, however, false hellebore's effect on the heart is slightly sedative, and it is generally prescribed for patients with hearts that are beating too fast or irregularly. False hellebore is recommended as a treatment for certain cases of low blood pressure. False hellebore is strongly diuretic and can be used to counter water retention, particularly if this condition can be attributed to poor circulatory function. False hellebore is used in homeopathic medicine as a treatment for angina.

CAUTIONS False hellebore is poisonous at the wrong dosage. Take only under professional supervision. Gathering wild plants and their medicinal use are subject to legal restrictions in some countries.

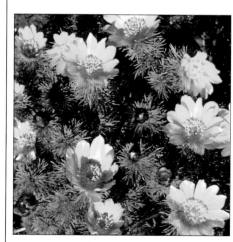

FALSE HELLEBORE'S cardiac glycosides help to slow down heart rate.

158

Aegle marmelos
(Rutaceae)
BAEL, BENGAL QUINCE

DESCRIPTION Thorny deciduous tree growing to 25 ft (8 m). Has aromatic oval- to lance-shaped leaves, greenish white flowers, and yellow plum-shaped fruit.

HABITAT & CULTIVATION Native to India, bael grows throughout much of Southeast Asia in dry forests. It is also cultivated throughout the region.

PARTS USED Fruit, leaves, root, twigs.

CONSTITUENTS Bael contains coumarins, flavonoids, alkaloids, tannins, and fixed oil.

HISTORY & FOLKLORE The bael tree is sacred to the Hindu deities Lakshmi (the goddess of wealth and good fortune) and Shiva (the god of health). It is commonly planted near temples. Its medicinal virtues are described in the *Charaka Samhita*, an herbal text written *c.* 700 BC.

MEDICINAL ACTIONS & USES The astringent half-ripe bael fruit reduces irritation in the digestive tract and is excellent for diarrhea and dysentery. The ripe fruit is a demulcent and laxative, with a significant vitamin C content. It eases stomach pain and supports the healthy function of this organ. Bael's astringent leaves are taken to treat peptic ulcers. The tree's most unusual application is for earache. A piece of dried root is dipped in the oil of the neem tree (*Azadirachta indica*, p. 173) and set on fire. Oil from the burning end is dripped into the ear. (This is not a recommended practice.)

SELF-HELP USE Diarrhea, p. 307.

Aesculus hippocastanum
(Hippocastanaceae)
HORSE CHESTNUT

DESCRIPTION Sturdy deciduous tree growing to 80 ft (25 m), with a large domed crown. Has leaves with 5–7 narrowly oval leaflets, clusters of white and pink flowers, and spiny green fruit with up to 3 rounded, shiny brown seeds about 1½ in (4 cm) across.

HABITAT & CULTIVATION Native to mountain woods in the Balkans and western Asia, this tree is cultivated in temperate regions worldwide. The bark and seeds are collected in autumn.

PARTS USED Seeds, leaves, bark.

CONSTITUENTS Horse chestnut contains triterpenoid saponins (notably aescin), coumarins, and flavonoids. Aescin, the main active constituent, has anti-inflammatory properties. In Germany and other European countries, specialized aescin preparations are used because aescin is not easily absorbed from the gut.

HISTORY & FOLKLORE Horse chestnut was first documented as a medicinal plant in 1565, in Pierandrea Matthioli's translation of Dioscorides' *Materia Medica*.

MEDICINAL ACTIONS & USES Horse chestnut is astringent, an anti-inflammatory, and an aid to toning the vein walls, which, when slack or distended, may become varicose, hemorrhoidal, or otherwise problematic. Horse chestnut also reduces fluid retention by increasing the permeability of the capillaries and allowing the reabsorption of excess fluid back into the circulatory system. The bark can be used to reduce fever. The herb has been taken internally in small to moderate doses for leg ulcers, varicose veins, hemorrhoids, and frostbite, and applied externally as a lotion, ointment, or gel. In France, an oil extracted from the seeds has been used externally for rheumatism. In the US, a decoction of the leaves has been given for whooping cough.

CAUTIONS Potentially toxic if ingested. Do not use for self-treatment except as a lotion, ointment, or gel applied to unbroken skin.

Aframomum melegueta
(Zingiberaceae)
GRAINS OF PARADISE

DESCRIPTION Perennial growing to 8 ft (2.5 m), with reedlike stems and narrow leaves. Single mauve flowers bear scarlet fruits growing to 4 in (10 cm) across. Seeds are small, reddish brown, and oyster-shaped, with a distinctly pungent, aromatic taste.

HABITAT & CULTIVATION This plant grows in tropical West Africa and is gathered when ripe.

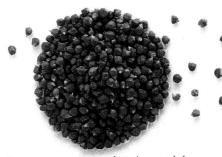

GRAINS OF PARADISE have been traded as a spice since the Middle Ages.

PARTS USED Seeds.

CONSTITUENTS The seeds contain a volatile oil (0.3 to 0.5%), a pungent principle called paradol (related to gingerol in ginger, *Zingiber officinale*, p. 153), and tannins.

MEDICINAL ACTIONS & USES Principally used as a condiment, the seeds also are a stimulant that strengthens and warms the stomach. Like other members of the ginger family, this plant is used to alleviate indigestion, gas, and bloating (the latter more commonly in livestock). Grains of paradise also ease abdominal discomfort due to colic or cramps. The seeds can help to reduce or prevent vomiting and to bring relief from nausea. The plant's stimulant properties make it an invigorating herb, especially helpful for those with weak digestions.

RELATED SPECIES *Sha ren*, the seeds of the closely related *A. villosum*, are used in Chinese medicine for similar complaints.

Agastache rugosa
(Labiatae)
HUO XIANG (CHINESE),
GIANT HYSSOP

DESCRIPTION Aromatic perennial or biennial herb growing to 4 ft (1.2 m). Has a square stem, triangular leaves, and purple flowers growing in dense spikes.

HABITAT & CULTIVATION Native to China and also found in Japan, Korea, Laos, and Russia, *huo xiang* grows wild on slopes and along roadsides. It is cultivated throughout China and gathered in summer.

PARTS USED Aerial parts.

CONSTITUENTS *Huo xiang* contains a volatile oil, including methyl chavicol, anethole, anisaldehyde, and limonene.

HISTORY & FOLKLORE *Huo xiang* was first mentioned in a Chinese medicinal text in Tao Hongjing's revision of the *Divine Husbandman's Classic (Shen'nong Bencoajing)*, which he wrote in about AD 500.

MEDICINAL ACTIONS & USES The acrid *huo xiang* is considered a slightly warming herb in Chinese herbal medicine (*see* pp. 38–41). It is employed in situations where there is excessive "dampness" within the digestive system, resulting in poor digestion and reduced vitality. The herb stimulates and warms the digestive tract, relieving symptoms such as abdominal bloating, nausea, indigestion, and vomiting. It is commonly used to relieve or prevent vomiting and morning sickness. *Huo xiang* is used to treat the early stages of viral infections that feature symptoms such as stomachache and nausea. *Huo xiang* is combined with Baical skullcap (*Scutellaria baicalensis*, p. 133) and other herbs for symptoms such as malaise, fever, aching muscles, and lethargy. A lotion containing *huo xiang* may be used externally to treat fungal conditions such as ringworm.

RESEARCH Laboratory experiments indicate that *huo xiang* is indeed effective against fungal infections.

OTHER SPECIES In southern China and Taiwan, *Pogostemon cablin* is used interchangeably with *huo xiang*. *P. cablin* is a close relative of the Indian plant *P. patchouli*, from which patchouli is produced.

Agave americana
(Agavaceae)
AGAVE, CENTURY PLANT

DESCRIPTION Succulent perennial with large rosette of 30–60 fleshy, sharply toothed leaves that reach a height of 6 ft (2 m). Clusters of yellow flowers, growing to 3 in (7 cm) across, bloom on a polelike stem after 10 years or more.

HABITAT & CULTIVATION Agave is native to deserts of Central America. It is now grown as an ornamental plant in tropical and subtropical areas around the world.

PART USED Sap.

CONSTITUENTS Agave sap contains estrogenlike isoflavonoids, alkaloids, coumarins, and vitamins pro-A, B_1, B_2, C, D, and K.

HISTORY & FOLKLORE Unlike Europeans at the time of the Spanish conquest of America, the Aztec and Maya people were skilled in wound healing. They used agave sap (often with egg white) to bind powders and gums in pastes or poultices to be applied to wounds. The *Badianus Manuscript* (1552), the first herbal to list the plants of the New World, described an Aztec treatment for diarrhea and dysentery, in which agave juice, combined with fresh-ground corn (*Zea mays*, p. 152) and extract of bladderwort (*Utricularia* species), is given as an enema, using a syringe made from the bladder of a small animal and a hollow bone or reed. Both tequila and mescal, Mexican alcoholic drinks, are distilled from the fermented sap or juice of agaves. These drinks were used by Mexican Indians to treat nervous conditions.

MEDICINAL ACTIONS & USES A demulcent, laxative, and antiseptic, agave sap is a soothing and restorative remedy for many digestive ailments. It is used to treat ulcers and inflammatory conditions affecting the stomach and intestines, protecting these parts from infection and irritation and encouraging healing. Agave has also been employed to treat a wide range of other conditions, including syphilis, tuberculosis, jaundice, and liver disease.

RELATED SPECIES Agave is a fairly close relative of aloe (*Aloe vera*, p. 57). The two plants have similar medicinal uses. The sisal agave (*A. sisalana*) is cultivated in subtropical America and in Kenya as a source of hecogenin, the substance that is the starting point in the production of corticosteroids (steroid hormones). Fiber from the sisal agave is used to make rope and hammocks.

CAUTIONS Do not use during pregnancy. Do not exceed the prescribed dose because it may cause digestive irritation and can lead to eventual liver damage. External use may cause skin irritation and should be avoided by people with sensitive skin.

Agrimonia eupatoria
(Rosaceae)
AGRIMONY

DESCRIPTION Erect, downy, and slightly aromatic perennial growing to 3 ft (1 m). Has paired leaves, green above and silvery green beneath, and small 5-petaled yellow flowers growing on terminal spikes.

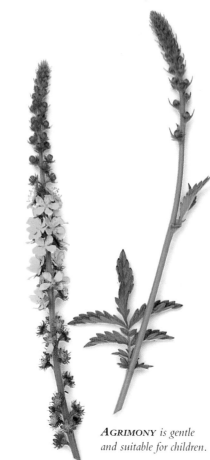

AGRIMONY is gentle and suitable for children.

HABITAT & CULTIVATION Agrimony is a native European herb commonly found in marshes, wet meadows, and in open areas. It is harvested when in flower in summer.

PARTS USED Aerial parts.

CONSTITUENTS Agrimony contains tannins, coumarins, flavonoids, including luteolin, volatile oil, and polysaccharides.

HISTORY & FOLKLORE The species name *Eupatoria* has regal associations. Mithridates Eupator (d. 63 BC), King of Pontus in northern Turkey, was said to have had a profound knowledge of plant lore.

MEDICINAL ACTIONS & USES Agrimony has long been used to heal wounds because it staunches bleeding and encourages clot formation. Astringent and mildly bitter, it is also a helpful remedy for diarrhea and a gentle tonic for the digestion as a whole. Combined with other herbs such as corn silk (*Zea mays*, p. 152), it is a valuable remedy for cystitis and urinary incontinence, and has also been used for kidney stones, sore throats, rheumatism, and arthritis.

RELATED SPECIES Xian he cao (*A. pilosa*) is a similar herb used in China to treat comparable conditions.

RESEARCH Agrimony's blood-staunching and anti-inflammatory properties have been established by experiments in China.

SELF-HELP USES Diarrhea, p. 307; **Infants & children – diarrhea**, p. 318.

Agropyron repens
syn. *Elymus repens*
(Gramineae)
COUCH GRASS

DESCRIPTION Vigorous perennial growing to 32 in (80 cm). Has a long, creeping rhizome, slender leaves, and erect spikes bearing green flowers aligned in two rows.

HABITAT & CULTIVATION Found in Europe, the Americas, northern Asia, and Australia, couch grass is an invasive weed. It is harvested throughout the year.

PARTS USED Rhizome, seeds, root.

CONSTITUENTS Couch grass contains polysaccharides (such as triticin), a volatile oil (mainly agropyrene), mucilage, and nutrients. Agropyrene has antibiotic properties.

HISTORY & FOLKLORE In classical times, both Dioscorides (AD 40–90) and Pliny (AD 23–79) recommended couch grass root for poor urine flow and kidney stones. In 1597, the herbalist John Gerard wrote that "Couch-grasse be an unwelcome guest to fields and gardens, yet his physicke virtues do recompense those hurts; for it openeth the stoppings of the liver and reins [ureters] without heat." In times of famine, the root has been roasted and ground as a substitute for coffee and flour.

MEDICINAL ACTIONS & USES A gentle, effective diuretic and demulcent, couch grass is most commonly used for urinary tract infections such as cystitis and urethritis. It both protects the urinary tubules against infection and irritants, and increases the volume of urine, thereby diluting it. It can be taken, usually with other herbs, to help treat kidney stones, reducing the irritation and laceration they cause. Couch grass is also thought to dissolve kidney stones (insofar as possible), and in any case will help to prevent their further enlargement. Both an enlarged prostate and prostatitis will benefit from a couch grass decoction taken over the course of several months. It has been used in the past for the treatment of gout and rheumatism. In German herbal medicine, heated couch grass seeds are used in a hot and moist pack that is applied to the abdomen to soothe peptic ulcers. Juice from the roots of couch grass has been used to treat jaundice and other liver complaints.

Ailanthus altissima syn. *A. glandulosa*
(Simaroubaceae)
TREE OF HEAVEN, CHUN PI

DESCRIPTION Deciduous tree growing to 70 ft (20 m). Has large leaves with up to 12 lance-shaped leaflets, and small greenish yellow flowers. Exudes an unpleasant odor.

HABITAT & CULTIVATION Native to China and India, it is now naturalized in some parts of Europe, Australia, and North America. It is cultivated as a garden tree. The bark and root bark are harvested in spring. When planted in marshy areas, it drains the soil and removes breeding sites for mosquitos.

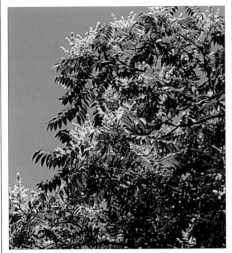

TREE OF HEAVEN has an unpleasant, bitter taste.

PARTS USED Bark, root bark.

CONSTITUENTS The bark contains quassinoids (such as ailanthone and quassin), alkaloids, flavonols, and tannins. Quassinoids are intensely bitter, antimalarial, and act against cancerous cells.

MEDICINAL ACTIONS & USES In Chinese herbal medicine, tree of heaven is used to treat diarrhea and dysentery, especially if there is blood in the stool. The bark of the tree has been employed in Asian and Australian medicine to counter worms, excessive vaginal discharge, gonorrhea, and malaria, and it has also been given for asthma. Tree of heaven has marked antispasmodic properties and acts on the body as a cardiac depressant.

RESEARCH Chinese researchers gave tree of heaven to 82 patients with acute dysentery and cured 81. Abdominal pain generally eased within 2 days. Quassinoids' anticancer properties are being extensively investigated.

RELATED SPECIES *A. malabrica* is used in Southeast Asia as a tonic and to reduce fever.

CAUTION Use tree of heaven only under professional supervision.

Ajuga reptans
(Labiatae)
BUGLE

DESCRIPTION Low-growing, creeping perennial up to 1 ft (30 cm) in height. Has rooting runners, erect hairy stems, oblong to oval leaves, and purplish blue flowers.

HABITAT & CULTIVATION Native to Europe, North Africa, and parts of Asia, bugle has become naturalized in North America. It prefers damp woods and grassy and mountainous areas, and is usually gathered when in flower in early summer.

PARTS USED Aerial parts.

CONSTITUENTS Bugle contains iridoid glycosides including harpagide, which is also found in devil's claw (*Harpagophytum procumbens*, p. 101).

HISTORY & FOLKLORE In the European tradition, bugle has long been valued as a wound-healing herb. Nicholas Culpeper praised it in 1652: "The decoction of the leaves and flowers made in wine and taken, dissolveth the congealed blood in those that are bruised inwardly by a fall or otherwise, and is very effectual for any inward wounds, thrusts or stabs into the body or bowels."

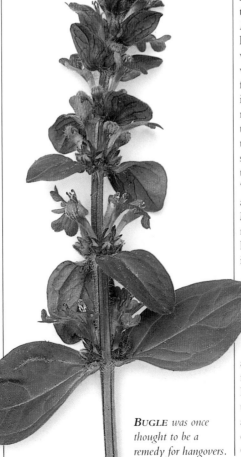

BUGLE was once thought to be a remedy for hangovers.

The herbalist Mrs. Grieve, writing in 1931, reported that it lowers the pulse rate and "equalizes the circulation."

MEDICINAL ACTIONS & USES Bugle is bitter, astringent, and aromatic, but opinion varies as to its value as a medicine. It has mild analgesic properties, and it is still used occasionally as a wound healer. It is also mildly laxative and traditionally has been thought to help cleanse the liver.

RELATED SPECIES Ground pine (*A. chamaepitys*) is used to treat gout and rheumatism. It is believed to have diuretic, menstruation-inducing, and stimulant properties. *A. decumbens* is used in Chinese medicine as an analgesic.

Alchemilla vulgaris
(Rosaceae)
LADY'S MANTLE

DESCRIPTION Herbaceous perennial growing to 1 ft (30 cm). Has a basal rosette of lobed leaves and insignificant green flowers ¼ in (3–5 mm) across in loose clusters.

HABITAT & CULTIVATION Lady's mantle is native to Britain and continental Europe. It is gathered in summer.

PARTS USED Aerial parts, root.

CONSTITUENTS Lady's mantle contains tannins, a glycoside, and salicylic acid.

HISTORY & FOLKLORE Andres de Laguna's translation (1570) of Dioscorides' *Materia Medica* recommended two preparations of lady's mantle – the root, powdered and mixed with red wine, for internal and external wounds, and an infusion of the aerial parts, for "greenstick" fractures and broken bones in babies and young children. When taken regularly for 15 days, lady's mantle was said to reverse sterility due to "slipperiness" of the womb. The plant's astringent effect is sufficiently marked that the infusion was used to contract the female genitalia, and it was "a thousand times sold" to those wishing to appear to be virgins!

MEDICINAL ACTIONS & USES Lady's mantle has always been prized as a wound healer. Its astringency ensures that blood flow is staunched and the first stage of healing soon gets under way. As the name implies, it is a valuable herb for women, taken principally to reduce heavy menstrual bleeding, to relieve menstrual cramps, and to improve regularity of the cycle. It is prescribed for conditions such as fibroids and endometriosis. It is also used as a douche for excess vaginal discharge. Lady's mantle has been used to facilitate childbirth, and is thought to act as a liver decongestant. Its astringency makes it a useful herb for treating diarrhea and gastroenteritis.

CAUTION Do not use during pregnancy.

Aletris farinosa
(Liliaceae)
STAR GRASS,
TRUE UNICORN ROOT, COLIC ROOT

DESCRIPTION Perennial growing to 3 ft (1 m). Has a flowering stem, smooth lance-shaped leaves, and white bell-shaped flowers that appear to be covered with frost.

HABITAT & CULTIVATION Native to eastern North America, star grass grows mainly in swamps and wet, sandy woodland, especially near the seashore. It is harvested commercially in Virginia, Tennessee, and North Carolina.

PARTS USED Rhizome, leaves.

CONSTITUENTS Star grass contains steroidal saponins based on diosgenin, as well as a bitter principle, volatile oil, and a resin.

HISTORY & FOLKLORE The Catawba used a cold-water infusion of star grass leaves for stomachache. Star grass was also advocated for snake bite.

MEDICINAL ACTIONS & USES It is difficult to gain a clear picture of star grass's medicinal value. Due to an apparent estrogenic action, it has been employed in this century chiefly for gynecological problems, particularly during menopause. It is also given for menstrual pain and irregular periods. Some authorities hold that it prevents threatened miscarriage. Star grass is also a good digestive herb, proving beneficial in treating loss of appetite, indigestion, flatulence, and bloating. The herb has also been employed in the treatment of rheumatism.

CAUTIONS Use only under professional supervision. The dried, and especially the fresh, rhizome can be toxic in overdose, causing colic, diarrhea, and vomiting.

Allium cepa
(Liliaceae)
ONION

DESCRIPTION Bulbous perennial growing to 3 ft (1 m). Has hollow stems and leaves, and white or purple flowers.

HABITAT & CULTIVATION Native to the northern hemisphere, onion has been cultivated in the Middle East for millennia. It is now grown worldwide as a vegetable.

PART USED Bulb.

CONSTITUENTS Onion contains a volatile oil with sulfurous constituents, sulfur-containing compounds such as allicin (an antibiotic) and alliin, flavonoids, phenolic acids, and sterols.

HISTORY & FOLKLORE Authorities throughout the ancient world recommended onion for a variety of health problems. Bunches were hung on doors to ward off the plague in medieval Europe. Wild onion (*A. sibiricum*) was used extensively by Native North American people to treat stings and help relieve colds.

MEDICINAL ACTIONS & USES Onion boasts a long list of medicinal actions – diuretic, antibiotic, anti-inflammatory, analgesic, expectorant, and antirheumatic. It is also beneficial to the circulation. Onions are taken the world over for colds, flu, and coughs. Like garlic (*A. sativum*, p. 56), onion offsets tendencies to angina, arteriosclerosis, and heart attack. It is also useful in preventing oral infection and tooth decay. The warmed juice can be dropped into the ear for earache, and baked onion is used as a poultice to drain pus from sores. Onion has a longstanding reputation as an aphrodisiac, and it is also used cosmetically to stimulate hair growth.

RELATED SPECIES In Chinese herbal medicine, the scallion (*A. fistulosum*) is given to encourage sweating, to unblock the nose, and to relieve bloating. It is also used to help drain boils and abscesses.

SELF-HELP USE Mild fever, p. 311.

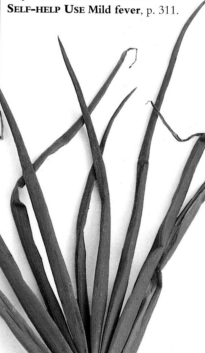

ONION juice is mixed with honey as a remedy for colds.

Allium ursinum
(Liliaceae)
RAMSONS

DESCRIPTION Bulbous perennial smelling strongly of garlic, growing to 11 in (28 cm). Has a triangular stem and broad, elliptical leaves. Clusters of white, starlike flowers grow from a common stem.

HABITAT & CULTIVATION Ramsons are native to Europe and Asia. They carpet shady sites in damp woods and by streams. The plants are gathered in early summer.

PARTS USED Bulb, aerial parts.

CONSTITUENTS Ramsons contain volatile oil, vinyl sulfide, aldehydes, and vitamin C.

HISTORY & FOLKLORE Ramsons (and many other onionlike plants) have been highly regarded as preventative medicines, as an old English rhyme attests: "Eat leeks in Lide and ramsons in May/And all the year after physicians may play!"

MEDICINAL ACTIONS & USES Used mainly as a folk remedy and as a food, ramsons are similar to garlic (*A. sativum*, p. 56) but weaker in action. They lower high blood pressure and help to prevent arteriosclerosis. Because ramsons ease stomach pain and are tonic to the digestion, they have been used for diarrhea, colic, gas, indigestion, and loss of appetite. The whole herb is used in an infusion against threadworms, either ingested or given as an enema. Ramsons are also thought to be beneficial for asthma, bronchitis, and emphysema. The juice is used as an aid to losing weight. Applied externally, the juice is a mild irritant. It stimulates local circulation and therefore may be of benefit in treating rheumatic and arthritic joints.

Alnus glutinosa
syn. *A. rotundifolia*
(Betulaceae)
ALDER

DESCRIPTION Small tree with fissured bark, growing to 70 ft (20 m). Has notched, oval leaves and male and female catkins.

HABITAT & CULTIVATION Alder is native to Europe, Asia, and North Africa. It thrives in damp places and along riverbanks. The bark and leaves are gathered in spring.

PARTS USED Bark, leaves.

CONSTITUENTS Alder contains lignans, tannin (10 to 20%), emodin (an anthraquinone), and glycosides.

HISTORY & FOLKLORE Water-resistant, alder was used in the construction of Venice. Wooster Beech (1794–1868), founder of the Eclectic healing movement, used a decoction of the bark to "purify the blood."

MEDICINAL ACTIONS & USES The astringent alder is employed most often as a mouthwash and gargle for tooth, gum, and throat problems. The drying action of a decoction of the bark helps to contract the mucous membranes and reduce inflammation. A decoction may also be used to staunch internal or external bleeding and to heal wounds. It is also used as a wash for scabies. In Spain, alder leaves are smoothed and placed on the soles of the feet to relieve aching. Leaves are used to help reduce breast engorgement in nursing mothers.

Alstonia spp.
(Apocynaceae)
FEVER BARK

DESCRIPTION Evergreen trees growing to 50 ft (15 m). Have glossy oblong leaves and creamy white, star-shaped flowers.
HABITAT & CULTIVATION *A. constricta* is native to Australia, and *A. scholaris* to Australia and Southeast Asia. Both are now found in tropical regions around the world.
PARTS USED Stem bark, root bark.
CONSTITUENTS The bark of both species contains indole alkaloids. *A. constricta* contains reserpine, a powerful hypotensive.
MEDICINAL ACTIONS & USES Fever bark has been taken to treat malarial fever (and has been called Australian quinine), but its efficacy against malaria remains unclear. The bark is antispasmodic and lowers blood pressure, and is now used mainly to reduce high blood pressure. Strongly bitter, the bark is also taken to treat diarrhea.
CAUTIONS Take only under professional supervision. Fever bark is toxic in large doses. The herb is subject to legal restrictions in some countries.

Althaea officinalis
(Malvaceae)
MARSH MALLOW

DESCRIPTION Downy perennial growing to 7 ft (2.2 m). Has thick white roots, heart-shaped leaves, and pink flowers.
HABITAT & CULTIVATION Native to Europe, marsh mallow is naturalized in the Americas. It prefers marshy fields and tidal zones, and is cultivated for medicinal use. The aerial parts are gathered in summer as the plant begins to flower, and the root is unearthed in autumn.
PARTS USED Root, leaves, flowers.
CONSTITUENTS Marsh mallow root contains about 37% starch, 11% mucilage, 11% pectin, flavonoids, phenolic acids, sucrose, and asparagine.

HISTORY & FOLKLORE Theophrastus (*c.* 372–286 BC) reported that marsh mallow root was taken in sweet wine for coughs. Marsh mallow was once a key ingredient in the sweets of the same name.
MEDICINAL ACTIONS & USES Useful whenever a soothing effect is needed, marsh mallow protects and soothes the mucous membranes. The root counters excess stomach acid, peptic ulceration, and gastritis. Marsh mallow is also mildly laxative and beneficial for many intestinal problems, including regional ileitis, colitis, diverticulitis, and irritable bowel syndrome. Taken as a warm infusion, the leaves treat cystitis and frequent urination. Marsh mallow's demulcent qualities bring relief to dry coughs, bronchial asthma, bronchial congestion, and pleurisy. The flowers, crushed fresh or in a warm infusion, are applied to help soothe inflamed skin. The root is used in an ointment for boils and abscesses, and in a mouthwash for inflammation. The peeled root may be given as a chewstick to teething babies.
OTHER SPECIES Hollyhock (*A. rosea*) and common mallow (*Malva sylvestris*, p. 230) are used in a similar fashion.
SELF-HELP USES Allergic rhinitis, p. 300; **Earache due to chronic congestion**, p. 312; **Urinary infections**, p. 314.

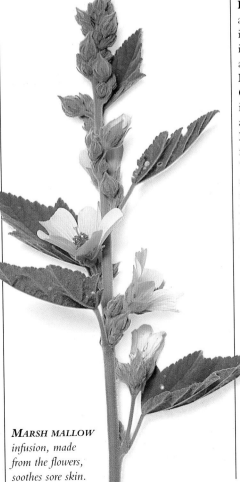

MARSH MALLOW infusion, made from the flowers, soothes sore skin.

Amaranthus hypochondriacus
(Amaranthaceae)
AMARANTH

DESCRIPTION Sturdy, upright annual growing to about 3 ft (1 m). Has deeply veined, lance-shaped, purple-green leaves that grow to 6 in (15 cm) and tufts of small, deep crimson flowers on long spikes.

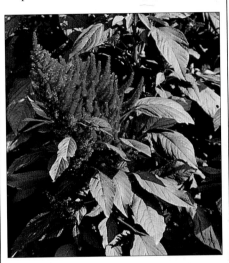

AMARANTH's long-lasting flowers gave rise to its name, meaning "unwithering" in Greek.

HABITAT & CULTIVATION Native to India, amaranth grows wild in many countries, including the US. A common garden plant, it is harvested when in flower in late summer and early autumn.
PARTS USED Aerial parts.
CONSTITUENTS Amaranth contains tannins, including a red pigment used to dye foods and medicines.
HISTORY & FOLKLORE Amaranth comes from the Greek word meaning "unwithering." The plants were used by the ancient Greeks to decorate tombs and signify immortality.
MEDICINAL ACTIONS & USES Amaranth is an astringent herb that is used primarily to reduce blood loss and to treat diarrhea. A decoction is taken to counter heavy menstrual bleeding, excessive vaginal discharge, diarrhea, and dysentery. It is also used as a gargle to soothe inflammation of the pharynx and to hasten the healing of canker sores.
RELATED SPECIES Quinoa (*A. caudatus*, also known as Inca wheat) is a nutritious Andean grain. It is used to make bread and is eaten in salads. The seeds of *A. grandiflorus* are used as a foodstuff by Australian Aborigines. In Ayurvedic medicine, *A. spinosus* is taken to reduce heavy menstrual bleeding and excessive vaginal discharge, and to arrest the coughing up of blood.

163

Ammi majus
(Umbelliferae)
BISHOP'S WEED

DESCRIPTION Erect annual herb growing to 32 in (80 cm), with tangled leaflets and umbels of small white flowers.

HABITAT & CULTIVATION Bishop's weed is native to the Mediterranean region and as far east as Iran. It is cultivated for its seeds, which are harvested in late summer.

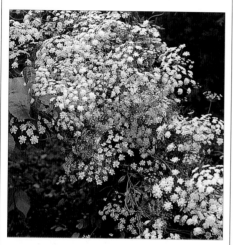

BISHOP'S WEED, like most members of the carrot family, has highly aromatic seeds.

PART USED Seeds.

CONSTITUENTS The seeds contain furanocoumarins (including bergapten), flavonoids, and tannins.

HISTORY & FOLKLORE Bishop's weed has been grown as a medicinal plant since the Middle Ages, but has been less often used than its cousin, visnaga (*A. visnaga*, p. 59).

MEDICINAL ACTIONS & USES Bishop's weed produces strongly aromatic seeds. In an infusion or as a tincture, they calm the digestive system. They are also diuretic, and, like visnaga, have been used to treat asthma and angina. Bishop's weed reputedly helps treat patchy skin pigmentation in vitiligo. It has also been used for psoriasis.

CAUTIONS Some people suffer nausea, vomiting, and headache after using bishop's weed. It can also cause allergic reactions to sunlight. Bishop's weed is subject to legal restrictions in some countries.

Anacardium occidentale
(Anacardiaceae)
CASHEW

DESCRIPTION Evergreen tree growing to 30 ft (10 m). Has large oval leaves and pink-streaked yellow flowers on long spikes. Its greenish gray "fruit" or "apple" is in fact a thickened stem. The true fruit hangs immediately below and contains the nut, which is encased in red or yellow flesh.

HABITAT & CULTIVATION This tree is native to tropical American forests and grasslands. It is now cultivated for its highly prized nuts throughout the tropics, especially in India and eastern Africa.

PARTS USED Nuts, leaves, bark, root, gum.

CONSTITUENTS The gum contains anacardic acid, which is bactericidal, fungicidal, and kills worms and protozoa.

HISTORY & FOLKLORE The "apple" is made into jams, and, in Brazil, into a liquor called *cajuado*. The gum exuded by the stem wards off ants and other insects.

MEDICINAL ACTIONS & USES Though many parts of the plant have a medicinal use, cashew nut is chiefly a food – after removal of its toxic lining. The nut is highly nutritious, containing 45% fat and 20% protein. The leaves are used in Indian and African herbal medicine for toothache and gum problems, and in West Africa for malaria. The bark is used in Ayurvedic medicine to detoxify snake bite. The roots are purgative. The gum is applied externally for leprosy, corns, and fungal conditions. The oil between the outer and inner shells of the nut is caustic and causes an inflammatory reaction even in small doses. In folk medicine in the tropics, the oil is used very sparingly to eliminate warts, corns, ringworm, and ulcers.

CAUTION The shell oil and its vapor are highly irritant – do not use in any form.

Anacyclus pyrethrum
(Compositae)
PELLITORY

DESCRIPTION Perennial herb growing to 1 ft (30 cm). Has smooth alternate leaves and large white flowers with yellow centers.

HABITAT & CULTIVATION Pellitory is native to the Mediterranean region as far east as the Middle East. The root is unearthed in autumn.

PARTS USED Root, essential oil.

CONSTITUENTS Pellitory contains anacycline, inulin, and volatile oil.

HISTORY & FOLKLORE The herbalist Nicholas Culpeper wrote in 1652 that pellitory "purgeth the brain of phlegmatic humours … easing pains in the head and teeth." It has been listed in the *British Pharmacopoeia* and was used to relieve a dry mouth. It was also taken to help ease neuralgia and paralysis of the tongue or lips.

MEDICINAL ACTIONS & USES The pungent pellitory root is taken as a decoction or chewed to relieve toothache and increase saliva production. The decoction may also be used as a gargle to soothe sore throats. In Ayurvedic medicine, the root is considered tonic, and is used to treat paralysis and epilepsy. The diluted essential oil is used in mouthwashes and to treat toothache.

CAUTION Do not take the oil internally except under professional supervision.

Anagallis arvensis
(Primulaceae)
SCARLET PIMPERNEL

DESCRIPTION Creeping annual growing to 2 in (5 cm), with oval- to lance-shaped leaves and scarlet 5-petaled flowers on long stems.

HABITAT & CULTIVATION Scarlet pimpernel is found in Europe and in temperate regions of Asia, North Africa, North America, and Australia. It prefers open areas and untended sandy ground, and is gathered in summer toward the end of its flowering period.

PARTS USED Aerial parts.

CONSTITUENTS The herb contains saponins (including anagalline), tannins, and cucurbitacins. The latter are cytotoxic (damaging to cells).

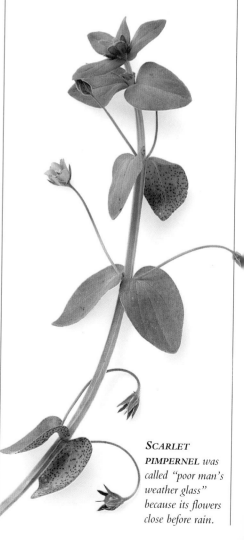

SCARLET PIMPERNEL was called "poor man's weather glass" because its flowers close before rain.

HISTORY & FOLKLORE Classical Greek writers believed scarlet pimpernel helped melancholy. In her *Modern Herbal* (1931), Mrs. Grieve quoted an old saying: "No heart can think, no tongue can tell/The virtues of the pimpernel." It has been employed in European folk medicine as a treatment for gallstones, liver cirrhosis, lung problems, kidney stones, urinary infections, gout, and rheumatism. This pattern of use suggests a detoxifying action for the plant.

MEDICINAL ACTIONS & USES Not used much by medical herbalists today, scarlet pimpernel has diuretic, sweat-inducing, and expectorant properties. As an expectorant, it was used to stimulate the coughing up of mucus and help recovery from colds and flu. It has been used to treat epilepsy and mental problems for 2,000 years, but there is little evidence to support its efficacy.

CAUTION Scarlet pimpernel is not recommended for medicinal use for more than 2-3 weeks at a time.

Anamirta cocculus
(Menispermaceae)
COCCULUS

DESCRIPTION Large woody climbing plant, with alternate oval leaves and long hanging clusters of greenish flowers. Male and female flowers on separate plants. Bears red-brown kidney-shaped fruit.

HABITAT & CULTIVATION Cocculus is found in forests in Southeast Asia from India and Sri Lanka across to Indonesia.

PARTS USED Leaves, fruit.

CONSTITUENTS Cocculus contains picrotoxin (up to 5%) and alkaloids. Picrotoxin is a powerful poison and nerve stimulant.

HISTORY & FOLKLORE The fruit is used as a fish poison. Scattered in the water, it stupefies fish in the surrounding area, causing them to float to the surface.

MEDICINAL ACTIONS & USES Cocculus fruit is sold commercially as a remedy for parasites. It is mainly applied externally to kill parasites such as lice, and it is also used to treat other skin afflictions. In Ayurvedic medicine, cocculus fruit is classified as an astringent, antifungal, and anthelmintic (de-worming), and is used for skin ulcers and fungal conditions such as ringworm. The plant is so toxic that it is rarely taken internally, but it has been used in this way in the past in Indian folk medicine to contract the uterus after childbirth. The herb is also used in homeopathy as a remedy for heart conditions.

CAUTIONS Cocculus is highly toxic. Do not take internally. Use externally only under professional supervision.

Ananas comosus
(Bromeliaceae)
PINEAPPLE

DESCRIPTION Herbaceous perennial growing to 3 ft (1 m). Has a short sturdy stem, spiny lance-shaped leaves, and succulent reddish yellow fruit.

HABITAT & CULTIVATION Pineapple is native to South America. It is cultivated throughout the tropics for its fruit and, to a lesser extent, its leaf fiber.

PARTS USED Fruit, juice, leaves.

CONSTITUENTS Pineapple fruit contains bromelain, a protein-splitting enzyme that aids digestion. It has significant levels of vitamins A and C.

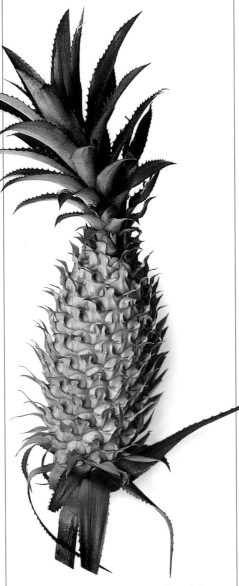

PINEAPPLE contains an enzyme, bromelain, which acts as an aid to digestion.

MEDICINAL ACTIONS & USES The sour, unripe fruit improves digestion, increases appetite, and relieves dyspepsia. In Indian herbal medicine, it is thought to act as a uterine tonic. The ripe fruit cools and soothes, and is used to settle gas and reduce excessive gastric acid. Its significant fiber content makes it useful in constipation. The juice of the ripe fruit is both a digestive tonic and a diuretic. The leaves are considered to be useful in encouraging the onset of menstrual periods and easing painful ones.

Anemarrhena asphodeloides
(Liliaceae)
ZHI MU

DESCRIPTION Perennial herb with thick rhizome, thin leaves up to 28 in (70 cm) long, and clusters of small white or light purple flowers.

HABITAT & CULTIVATION Native to northern China, *zhi mu* grows wild on exposed slopes and hills. It is cultivated in the northern and northeastern provinces.

PART USED Rhizome.

CONSTITUENTS *Zhi mu* contains triterpenoid saponins (timosaponin and sarsasapogenin).

HISTORY & FOLKLORE *Zhi mu* has been used in Chinese medicine for many centuries. It was first mentioned in the 1st-century AD herbal, the *Divine Husbandman's Classic (Shen'nong Bencaojing)*.

MEDICINAL ACTIONS & USES *Zhi mu* is used in Chinese herbal medicine for "excess heat" – fever, night sweats, and coughs. It has a bitter taste and a "cold temperament," and is used to treat canker sores, particularly in combination with rehmannia (*Rehmannia glutinosa*, p. 123) and *Scrophularia ningpoensis*.

Anemone pulsatilla
syn. *Pulsatilla vulgaris*
(Ranunculaceae)
PULSATILLA,
PASQUE FLOWER

DESCRIPTION Hairy perennial growing to 6 in (15 cm). Has feathery leaves and large, purple-blue bell-shaped flowers with bright yellow anthers.

HABITAT & CULTIVATION Native to Europe, this herb thrives in dry grassland in central and northern parts of the continent, preferring chalky soil. The aerial parts are harvested when it flowers in spring.

PARTS USED Dried aerial parts.

CONSTITUENTS Pulsatilla contains the lactone protoanemonin (which on drying forms anemonin), triterpenoid saponins, tannins, and volatile oil.

HISTORY & FOLKLORE In Greek mythology,

PULSATILLA *continued on following page*

the goddess Flora was jealous of her husband's attentions to the nymph Anemone and so transformed her into the "wind flower," at the mercy of the North Wind. The name "pasque flower," by which the plant is sometimes known, derives from the French name for Easter, when it is often in flower.

MEDICINAL ACTIONS & USES Pulsatilla is less commonly used now in herbal medicine than in the past, though it is still considered a worthwhile remedy for cramps, menstrual problems, and distress. It is considered a specific treatment for spasmodic pain of the reproductive system, both male and female, and is given quite frequently for premenstrual tension and period pain, especially when these are accompanied by nervous exhaustion. It also relieves headaches. In France, it has traditionally been used for treating coughs and as a sedative for sleep difficulties. Pulsatilla is also used to treat eye problems such as cataracts. The fresh plant is not used because it is strongly irritant. Pulsatilla is one of the most commonly used of all homeopathic remedies.

RELATED SPECIES The meadow anemone (*A. pratensis*) is used interchangeably with pulsatilla; wood anemone (*A. nemorosa*) is now rarely used in herbal medicine except occasionally as a counterirritant applied externally in arthritis and rheumatism.

CAUTIONS Take only under professional supervision. Do not take during pregnancy. Do not take the fresh plant, which is toxic.

Anethum graveolens
syn. Peucedanum graveolens
(Umbelliferae)

DILL

DESCRIPTION Aromatic annual growing to 30 in (75 cm). Has an erect hollow stem, feathery leaves, and numerous yellow flowers in umbels. Fruit is lightweight and pungent.

HABITAT & CULTIVATION Dill is a native of the Mediterranean region, southern Russia, and central and southern Asia, growing wild in open areas. It is also widely cultivated, notably in England, Germany, and North America. The leaves are picked as a culinary herb in spring and summer. The seeds are harvested in late summer.

PARTS USED Seeds, essential oil, leaves.

CONSTITUENTS Dill seeds contain up to 5% volatile oil (about half of which is carvone), flavonoids, coumarins, xanthones, and triterpenes.

HISTORY & FOLKLORE An ancient Egyptian remedy in the Ebers papyrus (*c.* 1500 BC) recommends dill as one of the ingredients in a pain-killing mixture. The ancient Greeks are believed to have covered

their eyes with fronds of the herb to induce sleep. Dill was commonly used as a charm against witchcraft in the Middle Ages, and was burned to clear thunderclouds. Its name comes from the Norse *dylla* – "to soothe."

MEDICINAL ACTIONS & USES Dill has always been valued as a remedy for the stomach, relieving gas and calming the digestion. Dill's essential oil relieves intestinal spasms and cramps and helps to settle colic. Chewing the seeds improves bad breath. Dill makes a useful addition to cough, cold, and flu remedies, and is a mild diuretic. Like caraway (*Carum carvi*, p. 182), it can be used with antispasmodics, such as crampbark (*Viburnum opulus*, p. 148), for period pain. Dill increases milk production, and when taken regularly by nursing mothers, helps to avoid colic in their babies.

RELATED SPECIES Indian dill (*A. sowa*), native to India and tropical Asia, is used to soothe indigestion.

CAUTION Do not take the essential oil internally except under professional supervision.

Seeds

Aerial parts

DILL *was used as a remedy by the ancient Greeks to encourage a good night's sleep.*

Angelica archangelica
(Umbelliferae)

ANGELICA

DESCRIPTION Aromatic biennial herb growing to 6 ft (2 m). Has ridged upright hollow stems, large bright green leaves, and greenish white flowers in umbels.

HABITAT & CULTIVATION Angelica grows in temperate regions as far apart as western Europe, the Himalayas, and Siberia. It prefers damp sites, especially near running water. Leaves and stems are harvested in early summer, seeds as they ripen in late summer, and roots in late autumn after one year's growth has taken place.

PARTS USED Root, leaves, stems, seeds.

CONSTITUENTS Angelica root contains a volatile oil (consisting mainly of beta-phellandrene), lactones, and coumarins. An extract of the root has been shown to be an anti-inflammatory.

HISTORY & FOLKLORE Angelica has a longstanding record as a prized medicinal herb. The *British Flora Medica* (1877) reported that "the Laplanders considered this plant as one of the most important productions of the soil … They are subject to a severe kind of colic, against which the root of angelica is one of their chief remedies." The stems are candied for culinary use.

MEDICINAL ACTIONS & USES Angelica is a warming and tonic remedy and is useful in a wide range of illnesses. All parts of the plant will help relieve indigestion, gas, and colic. Angelica can also be useful in cases of poor circulation since it improves blood flow to the peripheral parts of the body. It is considered a specific treatment for Buerger's disease, a condition that narrows the arteries of the hands and feet. By improving blood flow and stimulating the coughing up of phlegm, angelica's warm, tonic properties bring relief from bronchitis and debilitating chest conditions. For respiratory conditions, the roots are most commonly used, but the stems and seeds may be employed as well.

CAUTION Do not take angelica as a medicine during pregnancy.

SELF-HELP USE Stomach spasm, p. 305.

Angelica dahurica
(Umbelliferae)

BAI ZHI

DESCRIPTION Aromatic perennial growing to 8 ft (2.5 m). Has a hollow stem, large 3-branched leaves, and umbels bearing many white flower heads.

HABITAT & CULTIVATION Grows wild in thickets in China, Japan, Korea, and Russia.

Cultivated mainly in central and eastern regions of China.

PART USED Root.

CONSTITUENTS *Bai zhi* contains a volatile oil and the coumarins imperatorin, marmesin, and phellopterin.

HISTORY & FOLKLORE *Bai zhi* was first mentioned in Chinese herbal medicine in the *Divine Husbandman's Classic (Shen'nong Bencaojing)* of the 1st century AD. The famous military physician Zhang Congzheng (1150–1228) classified *bai zhi* as a sweat-inducing herb able to counter harmful external influences on the skin, such as cold, heat, dampness, and dryness.

MEDICINAL ACTIONS & USES The pungent, bitter *bai zhi* is used for headaches and aching eyes, nasal congestion, and toothache. Like its cousins angelica (*A. archangelica, see preceding entry*) and Chinese angelica (*A. sinensis*, p. 60), it is warming and tonic, and it is still given for problems attributed to "damp and cold" conditions, such as sores, boils, and ulcers affecting the skin. *Bai zhi* also appears to be valuable in treating the facial pain of trigeminal neuralgia.

RELATED SPECIES *A. pubescens* is used in a similar fashion in Chinese herbal medicine.

CAUTION Do not take during pregnancy.

Annona squamosa
(Annonaceae)
CUSTARD APPLE

DESCRIPTION Tree growing to 30 ft (10 m). Has oblong- to lance-shaped leaves, greenish flowers, and segmented green fruit.

HABITAT & CULTIVATION Native to tropical America and the Caribbean, this herb is cultivated throughout the tropics.

PARTS USED Leaves, bark, fruit, seeds.

CONSTITUENTS Custard apple contains fruit sugars and mucilage.

MEDICINAL ACTIONS & USES In the West Indies, the young shoots are used to treat colds and chills. In Cuban medicine, the leaves are taken to reduce uric acid levels. The leaves, bark, and unripe fruit are used to treat diarrhea and dysentery.

CAUTION Use only under professional supervision.

Anthemis cotula
(Compositae)
MAYWEED,
STINKING MAYWEED

DESCRIPTION Annual or perennial resembling German and Roman chamomile (*Chamomilla recutita*, p. 76 and *Chamaemelum nobile*, p. 184). Has slightly hairy stems and large, solitary, daisy-type flowers. As the name stinking mayweed suggests, this plant has an unpleasant smell and taste.

HABITAT & CULTIVATION This herb commonly grows wild in Europe, the Americas, Australia, New Zealand, and Siberia. The flowers and leaves are gathered in summer.

PARTS USED Flowers, leaves.

CONSTITUENTS Mayweed contains sesquiterpene lactones (including anthecotulide).

HISTORY & FOLKLORE In his *Irish Herbal* of 1735, the herbalist K'Eogh stated that mayweed is "good for women with the falling down of the womb, if they but wash their feet with a decoction of it. A hot wet application of it will ease the swelling of haemorrhoids."

MEDICINAL ACTIONS & USES Although it is similar in appearance to Roman and German chamomile, mayweed is far less effective as a medicine. It has been used as an antispasmodic and to induce menstruation, and was traditionally employed for supposedly hysterical conditions relating to the uterus. It is rarely used in contemporary herbal medicine.

CAUTIONS The whole plant can cause blistering if applied fresh to the skin. Do not take during pregnancy or breast-feeding.

Anthriscus cerefolium
(Umbelliferae)
CHERVIL

DESCRIPTION Annual herb growing to 2 ft (60 cm). Has finely grooved stems, opposite leaves, and many small white flowers arranged in compound umbels.

HABITAT & CULTIVATION Native to Europe, Asia Minor, Iran, and the Caucasus, chervil grows freely on roadsides and in open areas. It is cultivated in many countries worldwide, including New Zealand and Australia. The herb is gathered when in flower in summer.

PARTS USED Aerial parts.

CONSTITUENTS Chervil contains a volatile oil, coumarins, and flavonoids.

HISTORY & FOLKLORE A basket of chervil seeds was one of the items found in Tutankhamun's tomb. The herb is traditionally used as a "spring tonic" in central Europe. Chervil is used extensively in cooking.

MEDICINAL ACTIONS & USES Chervil is a good remedy for settling the digestion, and is also used to "purify the blood" and to help lower blood pressure. Chervil is considered a diuretic. Juice from the fresh plant is applied to a variety of skin conditions, including wounds, eczema, and abscesses.

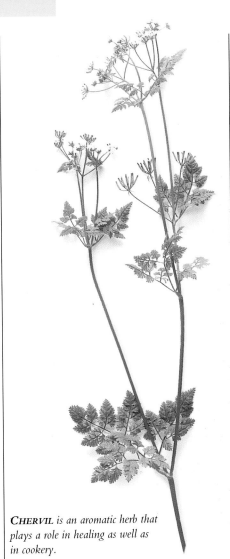

CHERVIL is an aromatic herb that plays a role in healing as well as in cookery.

Aphanes arvensis
(Rosaceae)
PARSLEY PIERT

DESCRIPTION Prostrate, hairy annual growing to 4 in (10 cm). Has small wedge-shaped leaves and tiny green flowers in tufts.

HABITAT & CULTIVATION Parsley piert is native to Europe, North Africa, and North America. It grows to an altitude of 1,600 ft (500 m), thriving in dry sites, including the top of walls. The herb is harvested when in flower in summer.

PARTS USED Aerial parts.

CONSTITUENTS Parsley piert contains tannins.

MEDICINAL ACTIONS & USES Astringent, diuretic, and demulcent, parsley piert is used to treat kidney and bladder problems, especially bladder stones (gravel), which cause irritation and obstruct urine flow. Best taken in an infusion, the herb is also a useful remedy for cystitis and recurrent urinary infections. It is often combined with marsh mallow (*Althaea officinalis*, p. 163) where a demulcent action is needed.

OTHER MEDICINAL PLANTS

Aralia racemosa
(Araliaceae)
AMERICAN SPIKENARD

DESCRIPTION Aromatic perennial bush growing to 6 ft (2 m). Has thick fleshy roots, large leathery leaves, small greenish white flowers, and red or purple berries.

HABITAT & CULTIVATION American spikenard is native to North America. The root is unearthed in summer or autumn.

PART USED Root.

CONSTITUENTS This herb contains a volatile oil, tannins, and diterpene acids.

HISTORY & FOLKLORE The Cherokee and New World settlers made a tea for backache from American spikenard. The Shawnee used it for flatulence, coughs, asthma, and breast pain; the Menominee, as a cure for blood poisoning. The plant was included in the *US National Formulary* from 1916 to 1965.

MEDICINAL ACTIONS & USES Many of American spikenard's current uses come directly from Native American precedents. The herb encourages sweating, and is stimulant and detoxifying. It is taken for rheumatism, asthma, and coughs. Applied externally as a poultice, American spikenard is used to treat a number of different skin conditions, including eczema.

RELATED SPECIES Wild sarsaparilla (*A. nudicaulis*) is a North American relative used medicinally in much the same way as American spikenard. The leaves and stalks of two East Asian *Aralias*, *A. chinensis* and *A. cordata*, are eaten as vegetables.

Arbutus unedo
(Ericaceae)
STRAWBERRY TREE

DESCRIPTION Evergreen shrub growing to 20 ft (6 m). Has an upright stem with reddish bark, leathery serrated leaves, white or pink bell-shaped flowers, and round warty red fruit resembling strawberries.

HABITAT & CULTIVATION Native to Mediterranean coasts, strawberry tree also grows in western Ireland, Australia, and Africa. The leaves are gathered in late summer, the fruit in autumn.

PARTS USED Leaves, fruit.

CONSTITUENTS Strawberry tree contains up to 2.7% arbutin, methylarbutin, and other hydroquinones, a bitter principle, and tannins. Arbutin is powerfully antiseptic in the urinary system.

HISTORY & FOLKLORE The fruit is made into liqueurs and preserves. It is unpalatable fresh – the Latin *unedo* derives from *un ede* meaning "[only] one I eat."

MEDICINAL ACTIONS & USES Strawberry

tree is valued as an astringent and antiseptic herb. Its antiseptic action within the urinary tract makes it a useful remedy for treating cystitis and urethritis. Its astringent effect has been put to use in the treatment of diarrhea and dysentery. Like many other astringent plants, it makes a gargle that is helpful for sore and irritated throats.

CAUTIONS Do not take during pregnancy or if suffering from kidney disease.

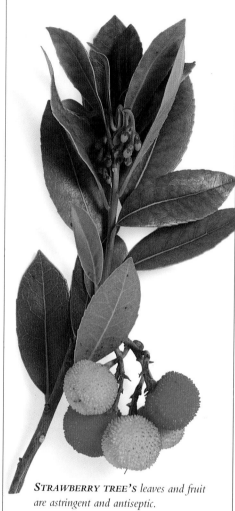

STRAWBERRY TREE'S leaves and fruit are astringent and antiseptic.

Arctostaphylos uva-ursi
(Ericaceae)
UVA-URSI, BEARBERRY

DESCRIPTION Low-lying evergreen shrub growing to 20 in (50 cm). Has long trailing stems, dark green leaves that are glossy on the upper side, bell-shaped pink flowers, and small glossy red berries.

HABITAT & CULTIVATION Uva-ursi is native to Europe and is naturalized throughout the northern hemisphere up to the Arctic. It grows in damp conditions in undergrowth, heathland, and grassland. The leaves are gathered in autumn. While not particularly palatable, the berries have been harvested in autumn as fruit.

PARTS USED Leaves, berries.

CONSTITUENTS The leaves contain hydroquinones (mainly arbutin, up to 17%), tannins (up to 15%), phenolic glycosides, and flavonoids. Arbutin and other hydroquinones have an antiseptic effect in the urinary tract.

HISTORY & FOLKLORE The name uva-ursi means "bear's grape" in Latin. Bears are fond of the fruit. The plant was first documented in *The Physicians of Myddfai*, a 13th-century Welsh herbal. Native American people enjoyed smoking a blend of uva-ursi leaves and tobacco (*Nicotiana tabacum*, p. 237).

MEDICINAL ACTIONS & USES Uva-ursi is one of the best natural urinary antiseptics. It has been used extensively in herbal medicine to disinfect and astringe the urinary tract in cases of acute and chronic cystitis and urethritis. However, it is not a suitable remedy if there is a simultaneous infection of the kidneys.

RESEARCH Experiments have shown that uva-ursi extracts have an antibacterial effect. This action is thought to be stronger in alkaline urine – thus the efficacy of uva-ursi is likely to increase if it is taken in combination with a vegetable-based diet.

CAUTIONS Do not take during pregnancy or if suffering from kidney disease. It is generally advisable to take uva-ursi for no more than 7–10 days at a time.

Arenaria rubra
(Carophyllaceae)
SANDWORT, SAND SPURREY

DESCRIPTION Herbaceous, low-growing, sticky, and hairy annual. Has small thin leaves and pale pink flowers growing to ¼ in (6 mm) across.

HABITAT & CULTIVATION Found in the wild throughout Europe, Asia, and Australia, sandwort thrives in sandy and gravelly places, especially close to the sea.

PARTS USED Aerial parts.

MEDICINAL ACTIONS & USES Sandwort is a diuretic herb that is thought to relax the muscle walls of the urinary tubules and bladder. Sandwort is most commonly taken in the form of an infusion to treat kidney stones, acute and chronic cystitis, and other conditions of the bladder.

RELATED SPECIES Seabeach sandwort (*A. peploides*), a closely related northern plant, is eaten by the Inuit of Alaska as a fresh, pickled, or oil-preserved vegetable. In Iceland, this plant is fermented and eaten like sauerkraut. Rupturewort (*Herniaria glabra*, p. 218), a European plant, has medicinal properties that are similar to those found in sandwort.

Argemone mexicana
(Papaveraceae)
MEXICAN POPPY

DESCRIPTION Prickly annual growing to 3 ft (1 m). Has spiny white-veined leaves and large yellow flowers with delicate petals.

HABITAT & CULTIVATION Mexican poppy grows in tropical regions from the southernmost US to South America. It favors dry soil and is often found in tobacco fields.

PARTS USED Aerial parts, latex, seeds.

CONSTITUENTS Mexican poppy contains isoquinoline alkaloids similar to those in the opium poppy (*Papaver somniferum*, p. 242).

HISTORY & FOLKLORE Like most poppies, this plant exudes a milky latex, which was traditionally used in Ecuador to treat cataracts.

MEDICINAL ACTIONS & USES The fresh latex of Mexican poppy contains protein-dissolving constituents, and is used to treat warts, cold sores, and blemishes on the lips. The whole plant acts as a mild painkiller. An infusion of the seeds – in small quantities – is used in Cuba as a sedative for children suffering from asthma. In greater quantities, the oil in the seeds is purgative. The flowers are expectorant, and are good for treating coughs and other chest conditions.

RELATED SPECIES In Hawaii, the latex of *A. glauca* is also used to treat warts.

CAUTION Use Mexican poppy only under professional supervision.

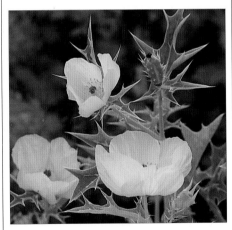

MEXICAN POPPY flowers have expectorant properties and are useful for treating coughs.

Arisaema consanguineum
(Araceae)
TIAN NAN XING

DESCRIPTION Perennial herb growing to 3 ft (1 m). Has star-shaped leaves and purple-white or green, pitcherlike bracts.

HABITAT & CULTIVATION *Tian nan xing* grows wild in eastern Asia, especially in China, where it is widely cultivated. The rhizome is unearthed in autumn or winter.

PART USED Dried rhizome.

CONSTITUENTS *Tian nan xing* contains triterpenoid saponins and benzoic acid.

HISTORY & FOLKLORE The herb was first mentioned in the 1st century AD *Divine Husbandman's Classic (Shen'nong Bencaojing)*.

MEDICINAL ACTIONS & USES In Chinese herbal medicine, *tian nan xing* is thought to encourage the coughing up of phlegm. The dried rhizome is used principally for chest problems. When prescribed internally it is always combined with fresh ginger root (*Zingiber officinale*, p. 153). The fresh rhizome is only ever used externally, for ulcers and other skin conditions.

RELATED SPECIES *A. amurense* and *A. heterophyllum* are used interchangeably with *tian nan xing*. *A. speciosum*, native to the Himalayas, is used as an antidote to toxic snake bite. Jack-in-the-pulpit or Indian turnip (*A. triphyllum*), a North American species, is a treatment for chest conditions.

CAUTIONS Take only under professional supervision. The fresh rhizome is very toxic; use only the dried rhizome internally.

Aristolochia clematitis
(Aristolochiaceae)
BIRTHWORT

DESCRIPTION Unpleasant-smelling perennial with heart-shaped leaves and tubular yellow flowers with flattened lips.

HABITAT & CULTIVATION Native to central and southern Europe, birthwort is also found in southwestern Asia. The root is unearthed in spring or autumn.

PARTS USED Root, aerial parts.

CONSTITUENTS Birthwort contains aristolochic acids, a volatile oil, and tannins. While stimulating white blood cell activity, aristolochic acid is also carcinogenic and damaging to the kidneys.

HISTORY & FOLKLORE *Aristolochia* means "excellent birth," and refers to the traditional use of the fresh juice to induce labor. Theophrastus (*c.* 372–286 BC) records that the plant was used to treat disorders of the uterus, reptile bites, and sores on the head. *Aristolochia* species were used by Native Americans to treat snake bite, stomachache, toothache, and fevers.

MEDICINAL ACTIONS & USES Not used much today, birthwort was formerly used to treat wounds, sores, and snake bite. It has been taken after childbirth to prevent infection and is also a potent menstruation-inducing herb and a (very dangerous) abortifacient. A decoction was taken to encourage healing of ulcers. Birthwort has also been used for asthma and bronchitis.

RESEARCH Chinese research into aristolochic acid has shown it to be an effective wound healer. *Aristolochia* species are used in China, but their medicinal use has been banned in Germany because of the toxicity of aristolochic acid.

RELATED SPECIES In the Amazon, a poultice and infusion of *A. klugii* are used for snake bite. In North America, Virginian snake root (*A. serpentaria*) was used in a similar way, and was also considered a strong fever remedy. *A. bracteata* is used in the Sudan for scorpion bites. *A. rotunda*, a European and Asian plant, is used in Iran as a tonic and to induce menstruation. The Chinese *A. kaempferi* and *A. fangchi* are used for lung disorders, pain, and fluid retention. Indian birthwort (*A. indica*) acts as a contraceptive.

CAUTION Until their safety has been clearly established, do not use birthwort or other *Aristolochia* species medicinally.

Armoracia rusticana
syn. *Cochlearia armoracia*
(Cruciferae)
HORSERADISH

DESCRIPTION Perennial growing to 20 in (50 cm). Has a deep root, large leaves, and clusters of 4-petaled white flowers.

HABITAT & CULTIVATION Native to Europe and western Asia, this herb is widely cultivated for its root, unearthed in autumn.

PARTS USED Root, leaves.

CONSTITUENTS Horseradish root contains glucosilinates (mainly sinigrin), asparagine, resin, and vitamin C. On being crushed, sinigrin produces allyl isothiocyanate, an antibiotic substance.

HISTORY & FOLKLORE Pliny (AD 23–79) probably had horseradish in mind when describing a plant that warded off scorpions, but, for most of its long history, horseradish has been used mainly as a diuretic herb. It is a popular condiment, particularly in Britain and central Europe.

MEDICINAL ACTIONS & USES Now undervalued as a medicinal herb, horseradish has many healing properties. It strongly stimulates the digestion, increasing gastric secretions and appetite. It is a good diuretic and promotes perspiration, making it useful in fevers, colds, and flu. It is also an expectorant and mildly antibiotic, and can be of use in both respiratory and urinary tract infections. A sandwich of freshly grated root is a home remedy for hay fever. Externally, a poultice of the root can soothe chilblains.

CAUTIONS Overconsumption of horseradish may irritate the gastrointestinal tract. The plant should be avoided by those with low thyroid function. A horseradish poultice may cause blistering.

Arnica montana
(Compositae)
ARNICA

DESCRIPTION Aromatic perennial growing to 1 ft (30 cm). Has downy egg-shaped leaves and bright yellow daisylike flowers.

HABITAT & CULTIVATION Arnica grows in mountain woods and pastures in central Europe, the Pyrenees, Siberia, Canada, and the northwestern US. Its flowers are harvested when in full bloom; the rhizomes, after the plant has died back in autumn.

PARTS USED Flowers, rhizome.

CONSTITUENTS Arnica contains sesquiterpene lactones, flavonoids, and a volatile oil that includes thymol, mucilage, and polysaccharides.

HISTORY & FOLKLORE Arnica has been used extensively in European folk medicine. Johann Wolfgang von Goethe (1749–1832), the German philosopher and poet, drank arnica tea to ease his angina in old age.

MEDICINAL ACTIONS & USES An effective ointment and compress for bruises, sprains, and muscle pain, arnica improves the local blood supply and speeds healing. It is anti-inflammatory and increases the rate of reabsorption of internal bleeding. Generally the plant is now taken internally only at a homeopathic dilution, principally for shock, injury, and pain. If taken as a decoction or tincture, it stimulates the circulation and is valuable in the treatment of angina and a weak or failing heart. It can be toxic even at low dosage and thus is rarely used in this way.

RELATED SPECIES In North America *A. fulgens* is used in place of arnica.

CAUTIONS Poisonous. Do not take internally. Arnica preparations should not be applied to broken skin. Dermatitis may result from external use. Arnica is subject to legal restrictions in some countries.

SELF-HELP USES Bruises, p. 304; **Sprains**, p. 312; **Tired & aching muscles**, p. 312.

Artemisia abrotanum
(Compositae)
SOUTHERNWOOD

DESCRIPTION Strongly aromatic, shrubby perennial growing to 3 ft (1 m). Has woody stems, feathery silver-green leaves, and yellow flowers.

HABITAT & CULTIVATION Native to southern Europe, this herb is rare in the wild but is cultivated for the perfume industry and, to a lesser extent, for herbal medicine. The aerial parts are harvested in late summer.

PARTS USED Aerial parts.

CONSTITUENTS Southernwood contains a volatile oil, abrotanin, and tannins.

HISTORY & FOLKLORE Much prized during the Middle Ages and the Renaissance, southernwood is now used infrequently in herbal medicine. The closely related wormwood (*A. absinthium*, p. 63) is considered superior. Like wormwood, southernwood contains a strong volatile oil that repels insects, and the leaves are placed among clothes to repel moths. Mrs. Grieve (*A Modern Herbal*, 1931) reported that in England "even in the early part of the last century a bunch of southernwood and rue [*Ruta graveolens*, p. 262] was placed next to the prisoner in the dock as a preventive from the contagion of jail fever."

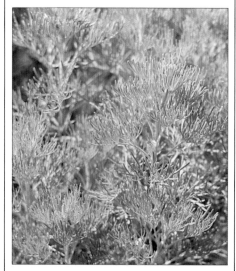

SOUTHERNWOOD leaves were traditionally placed among clothing to repel moths.

MEDICINAL ACTIONS & USES A bitter tonic, southernwood strengthens and supports digestive function by increasing secretions in the stomach and intestines. An infusion of southernwood has been given to children as a treatment for worms, but this is not recommended without professional supervision. Like other *Artemisias*, southernwood stimulates menstruation and is commonly taken to encourage the onset of irregular or absent periods.

CAUTIONS Do not take during pregnancy. Not suitable for children under 12 unless prescribed professionally.

Artemisia capillaris
(Compositae)
YIN CHEN HAO

DESCRIPTION Medium-sized perennial herb, with an erect stem, thin feathery leaves, and clusters of small composite flowers.

HABITAT & CULTIVATION Native to Southeast Asia, *yin chen hao* is cultivated in China and other Far Eastern countries. The young plants are gathered in spring.

PARTS USED Aerial parts.

CONSTITUENTS *Yin chen hao* contains a volatile oil and coumarins. The volatile oil is antifungal.

HISTORY & FOLKLORE *Yin chen hao* has been used in Chinese herbal medicine for more than 2,000 years. Its medicinal properties were first listed in the 1st-century AD *Divine Husbandman's Classic (Shen'nong Bencaojing)*.

MEDICINAL ACTIONS & USES *Yin chen hao* is an effective remedy for liver problems, being specifically helpful for treating hepatitis with jaundice. Traditional Chinese medicine (*see* pp. 38–41) holds that it is bitter and cooling, clearing "damp heat" from the liver and gall ducts and relieving fevers. *Yin chen hao* is also anti-inflammatory and diuretic. It was formerly used in a plaster for headaches.

RESEARCH Investigation in China indicates that, like many *Artemisia* species, *yin chen hao* has a tonic and strengthening effect on the liver, gallbladder, and digestive system.

CAUTIONS Do not take during pregnancy. Unsuitable for children under 12 unless prescribed professionally.

Artemisia cina
(Compositae)
LEVANT WORMWOOD

DESCRIPTION Shrubby perennial with long, thin leaves and tiny, round tufts of flowers.

HABITAT & CULTIVATION This herb is native to the region stretching from the eastern Mediterranean to Siberia. The unopened flower heads are gathered from wild and cultivated plants.

PARTS USED Flower heads.

CONSTITUENTS Levant wormwood contains santonin (a sesquiterpene lactone), artemisin, and a volatile oil (with up to 80% cineole). Santonin is directly toxic to roundworms and, to a lesser extent, threadworms.

HISTORY & FOLKLORE Levant wormwood was known to the classical Greek world as a remedy for intestinal worms, and it has been used for this purpose ever since. Its active constituent, santonin, was first isolated in 1830 and is now more commonly employed than the plant itself.

MEDICINAL ACTIONS & USES Almost exclusively used to expel worms, levant wormwood is strongly bitter and aromatic, and has a tonic and stimulant effect on the digestion. The dried flower heads are occasionally mixed with honey to disguise their bitterness.

CAUTIONS Do not take during pregnancy. Not suitable for children under 12 unless prescribed professionally.

Artemisia dracunculus
(Compositae)

TARRAGON

DESCRIPTION Aromatic perennial growing to 3 ft (1 m). Has narrow lance-shaped leaves and small greenish flower heads in long drooping clusters.

HABITAT & CULTIVATION Native to Russia, western Asia, and the Himalayas, tarragon is now cultivated as a culinary herb in gardens around the world. The aerial parts are picked in summer.

PARTS USED Aerial parts, root.

CONSTITUENTS Tarragon contains tannins, coumarins, and flavonoids, and up to 0.8% volatile oil, consisting of up to 70% methyl chervicol (estragole), which is toxic and potentially carcinogenic.

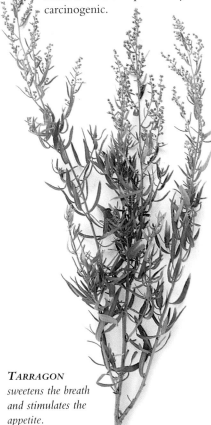

TARRAGON sweetens the breath and stimulates the appetite.

HISTORY & FOLKLORE Tarragon is widely used as an herb in cooking. In French, it is sometimes known as *herbe au dragon*, because of its reputed ability to cure the bites of serpents and mad dogs.

MEDICINAL ACTIONS & USES While tarragon stimulates the digestion, it is also reputed to be a mild sedative and has been taken to aid sleep. With its mild menstruation-inducing properties, it is also taken if periods are delayed. The root has traditionally been applied to aching teeth.

CAUTIONS Do not take during pregnancy. Do not exceed the dose, and do not take for longer than 4 weeks at a time.

Artemisia vulgaris
(Compositae)

MUGWORT

DESCRIPTION Shrubby perennial growing to about 3 ft (1 m). Has dark green deeply indented leaves and numerous clusters of small reddish or yellow flower heads.

HABITAT & CULTIVATION Mugwort is found in temperate regions of the northern hemisphere. It flourishes in open areas and along roads, and is gathered in late summer just before flowering.

PARTS USED Leaves, root.

CONSTITUENTS Mugwort contains a volatile oil, a sesquiterpene lactone, flavonoids, coumarin derivatives, and triterpenes.

HISTORY & FOLKLORE Mugwort was used from the earliest times in Europe and Asia. Roman centurions reputedly placed it in their sandals to keep the soles of their feet in good shape. The Greek physician Dioscorides (1st century AD) recounted that the goddess Artemis (who inspired the plant's genus name) was believed to give succor to women in childbirth. The 13th-century Welsh herbal *The Physicians of Myddfai* recommended: "If a woman be unable to give birth to her child let the mugwort be bound to her left thigh. Let it be instantly removed when she has been delivered, lest there should be haemorrhage."

An 18th-century Spanish herbalist, Diego de Torres, recommended the application of a mugwort plaster below the navel as an effective method of inducing labor. In China, mugwort has been valued for millennia. It is the principal ingredient of *moxa*, used in moxibustion – in which heat from a burning, cigar-shaped roll of chopped leaves is applied to acupuncture points.

MEDICINAL ACTIONS & USES A digestive and tonic herb, mugwort has a wide variety of traditional uses. Milder in action than most other *Artemisia* species, it can be taken over the long term at a low dose to improve appetite, digestive function, and absorption of nutrients. In addition to encouraging the elimination of worms, mugwort increases bile flow and mildly induces the onset of menstruation. The European conception of mugwort as a uterine stimulant is contradicted by Chinese usage, in which it is prescribed to prevent miscarriage and to reduce or stop menstrual bleeding. Mugwort is also an antiseptic and has been used in the treatment of malaria.

RELATED SPECIES *A. argyii* and *A. lavandulaefolia*, found growing in China, have been used in Chinese herbal medicine to treat many of the conditions treated by mugwort in Europe.

CAUTION Do not take during pregnancy.

Asclepias tuberosa
(Asclepiadaceae)

PLEURISY ROOT

DESCRIPTION Perennial, upright herb growing to 3 ft (1 m). Has narrow lance-shaped leaves and spikes of numerous 5-petaled orange or yellow flowers.

HABITAT & CULTIVATION This herb is native to the southern US. The root is unearthed in spring.

PART USED Root.

CONSTITUENTS Pleurisy root contains cardenolides and flavonoids. It is estrogenic.

HISTORY & FOLKLORE In North American herbal medicine, pleurisy root was considered a cure-all. It was used to treat conditions as diverse as pleurisy, typhoid, pneumonia, congestion, dysentery, colic, eczema, and hysteria. The Omaha ate the raw root for bronchitis and other chest conditions. Many tribes thought pleurisy root was a good remedy for hot, dry fevers.

MEDICINAL ACTIONS & USES Although its most specific usage is relieving the pain and inflammation of pleurisy, pleurisy root has other applications. It is useful for hot, dry, and tight conditions in the chest. It promotes the coughing up of phlegm, reduces inflammation, and helps reduce fevers by stimulating perspiration. The root is also taken for chronic diarrhea and dysentery.

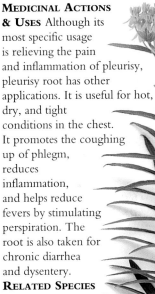

RELATED SPECIES *A. incarnata* and *A. syriaca* have been used in Native American herbal medicine to treat asthma.

CAUTIONS Do not take during pregnancy. Excessive doses may cause vomiting.

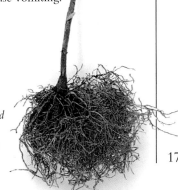
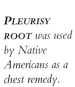

PLEURISY ROOT was used by Native Americans as a chest remedy.

Asparagus officinalis
(Liliaceae)
ASPARAGUS

DESCRIPTION Slender-stemmed perennial growing to 6 ft (2 m). Has long fronds of delicate needlelike leaves and bell-shaped yellow-green flowers that produce small bright red berries.

HABITAT & CULTIVATION Native to temperate regions in Europe, North Africa, and Asia, asparagus is cultivated worldwide as a vegetable. The shoots grow into tender (and, if sheltered from sunlight, white) stems in spring. The root is gathered after the shoots have been cut.

PARTS USED Root, shoots.

CONSTITUENTS Asparagus contains steroidal glycosides (asparagosides), bitter glycosides, asparagine, and flavonoids. Asparagine is a strong diuretic.

HISTORY & FOLKLORE To judge from ancient Egyptian tomb drawings, asparagus was cultivated as long ago as 4000 BC. It has long been known to be a diuretic. In the 1st century AD, the Greek physician Dioscorides recommended a decoction of asparagus root to improve urine flow and to treat kidney problems, jaundice, and sciatica. He also recommended holding the chewed root against aching teeth.

MEDICINAL ACTIONS & USES Asparagus is a strong diuretic that is useful for a variety of urinary problems, including cystitis. It is also useful for rheumatic conditions, helping to hasten the "flushing" of waste products accumulated in the joints out of the body in the urine. Asparagus is also bitter, mildly laxative, and sedative.

Asperula odorata
syn. Galium odoratum
(Rubiaceae)
SWEET WOODRUFF

DESCRIPTION Perennial growing to 18 in (45 cm). Has a square stem, whorls of narrow elliptical leaves, and small white flowers.

HABITAT & CULTIVATION Sweet woodruff is native to Europe, and is also found in Asia and North Africa. It grows in woodlands and shaded places. The herb is gathered when in flower in late spring.

PARTS USED Aerial parts.

CONSTITUENTS Sweet woodruff contains iridoids, coumarins (0.6%), tannins, anthraquinones, and flavonoids. The flavonoids act on the circulation and are diuretic.

HISTORY & FOLKLORE When it dries, sweet woodruff takes on the scent of newly cut grass, and it has often been placed between clothes to impart its aroma. In his *Irish Herbal* of 1735, K'Eogh recorded that "It is good in healing wounds if bruised and then applied, and also in curing boils and inflammations." In Germany *Maiwein*, made

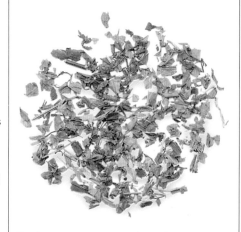

SWEET WOODRUFF is gathered from the wild when in flower in late spring.

of sweet woodruff steeped in white wine, is drunk to celebrate May Day.

MEDICINAL ACTIONS & USES Sweet woodruff is considered tonic, with significant diuretic and anti-inflammatory effects. Its coumarin and flavonoid constituents make it helpful for varicose veins and phlebitis. It has been used as an antispasmodic, and it is given to children and adults for insomnia.

CAUTIONS In excessive doses, sweet woodruff can cause internal bleeding. Do not use if taking conventional medication for circulatory problems or in pregnancy.

Aspidosperma
quebracho-blanco
(Apocynaceae)
QUEBRACHO

DESCRIPTION Tree growing to 100 ft (30 m). Has thick corky bark, leathery leaves, and tubular white flowers.

HABITAT & CULTIVATION Quebracho is found in the southern half of South America. The bark and lumber are used commercially.

PART USED Bark.

CONSTITUENTS Quebracho contains indole alkaloids (including yohimbine) and tannins.

HISTORY & FOLKLORE The name quebracho comes from the Spanish *quebrar* (to break) and *hacha* (axe), an allusion to the hardness of this tree's wood.

MEDICINAL ACTIONS & USES With its antispasmodic effect on the bronchial tubes, quebracho is used to treat asthma and emphysema. It is also a tonic and reduces fever. This herb is an astringent and has been used externally on wounds and burns.

RELATED SPECIES Many other species of *Aspidosperma* are grown for tanning and lumber in South America. Some are also considered fever remedies. One, *A. excelsum*, is used to relieve gas, stomach problems, flatulence, and indigestion.

CAUTIONS Take only under professional supervision. Quebracho is toxic in excessive doses. The herb is subject to legal restrictions in some countries.

Atractylodes macrocephala
(Compositae)
BAI ZHU

DESCRIPTION Erect perennial herb growing to 2 ft (60 cm). Has alternate oval- to lance-shaped leaves and purple flowers.

HABITAT & CULTIVATION *Bai zhu* is rare in the wild. It is cultivated in China, Japan, and Korea. The rhizome is unearthed in late autumn or winter.

PART USED Rhizome.

CONSTITUENTS *Bai zhu* contains a volatile oil (0.35–1.35%), which includes atractylol, and the lactones atractylenolide II and III. Atractylol has a liver protective activity.

HISTORY & FOLKLORE The first record of *bai zhu's* use is in the *Tang Materia Medica*, written in China in AD 659. Later, it was one of the 4 herbs that made up the "decoction of the 4 rulers," a mixture prescribed by Wang Ji (1463–1539) for syphilis.

MEDICINAL ACTIONS & USES *Bai zhu* has traditionally been used as a tonic, building *qi* (see p. 38–41) and strengthening the spleen. The rhizome has a sweet, pungent taste, and is used to relieve fluid retention (it is a powerful diuretic), excessive sweating, and digestive problems such as diarrhea and vomiting. Combined with Baical skullcap (*Scutellaria baicalensis*, p. 133), it is employed to prevent miscarriage.

Avena sativa
(Gramineae)
OATS

DESCRIPTION Annual grass growing to 3 ft (1 m). Has straight hollow stems, bladelike leaves, and small spikes holding seeds (grain).

HABITAT & CULTIVATION Native to northern Europe, oats are now grown worldwide in temperate regions as a cereal crop. They are harvested in late summer.

PARTS USED Seeds, straw (dried stems).

CONSTITUENTS Oats contain saponins, alkaloids, sterols, flavonoids, silicic acid, starch, proteins (including gluten), vitamins (especially B vitamins), and minerals (especially calcium).

HISTORY & FOLKLORE Formerly, oat straw was used to fill mattresses, proving beneficial to those suffering from rheumatism. In *The English Physitian* (1652) Nicholas Culpeper stated that "a poultice made of meal of oats and some oil of bay helpeth the itch and the leprosy." Earlier, in 1597, John Gerard was less enthusiastic: "Oatmeal is good to make a fair and well-coloured maid to look like a cake of tallow."

MEDICINAL ACTIONS & USES Oats are best known as a nutritious cereal, but they benefit the health in numerous other ways. Oat bran lowers cholesterol, and an oat-based diet may improve stamina (see *Research*, below). Oats, and oat straw in particular, are tonic when taken medicinally.

Oat straw is prescribed by medical herbalists to treat general debility and a wide variety of nervous conditions. The grains and straw are mildly antidepressant, gently raising energy levels and supporting an over-stressed nervous system. Oats are used to treat depression and nervous exhaustion, as well as the profound lethargy that results from multiple sclerosis, chronic neurological pain, and insomnia. With insomnia, oats are thought to stimulate sufficient nervous energy to make sleep possible.

Oats are one of the principal herbal aids to convalescence after a long illness. Externally, the grain is emollient and cleansing, and a decoction strained into a bath can help soothe itchiness and eczema.

RESEARCH In research in Australia, athletes who were placed on an oat-based diet for 3 weeks showed a 4% increase in stamina. Oats are thought to help maintain muscle function during training and exercise.

SELF-HELP USES Depression & decreased vitality, p. 316; Eczema, p. 300; Nervous exhaustion & stress, p. 319.

Azadirachta indica syn. *Melia azadirachta, M. indica*
(Meliaceae)
NEEM

DESCRIPTION Large evergreen tree growing to 52 ft (16 m). Has compound leaves and small white flowers.

HABITAT & CULTIVATION Native to forests and woody areas throughout India and Sri Lanka, neem is now naturalized in other tropical regions, including Indonesia, Australia, and West Africa.

PARTS USED Bark, leaves, twigs, seeds, sap.

CONSTITUENTS Neem contains meliacins, triterpenoid bitters, tannins, and flavonoids.

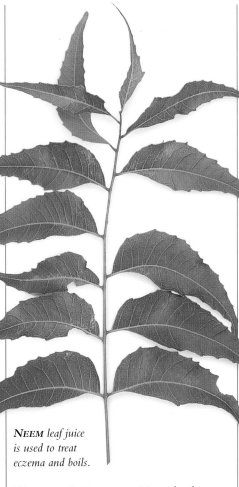

NEEM leaf juice is used to treat eczema and boils.

HISTORY & FOLKLORE Neem has been a part of Ayurvedic and folk medicine in India since the earliest times, and it still provides some of the most frequently used herbal remedies.

MEDICINAL ACTIONS & USES Considered a pharmacy in its own right in India, every part of the neem tree may be used medicinally. The bitter, astringent bark is applied as a decoction for hemorrhoids. The leaves are steeped for malaria, peptic ulcers, and intestinal worms. Neem juice (expressed from the leaves), infusion, or ointment is applied externally to ulcers, wounds, boils, and eczema. The twigs are used to clean the teeth, firming up the gums and preventing gum disease. Neem oil, expressed from the seeds, is commonly used as a hair dressing. Strongly antifungal and antiviral, it prevents lice and other infestations. This oil is also used to treat leprosy and may be used as a vehicle for other active ingredients. The sap is another traditional external remedy for leprosy. The seeds are spermicidal.

RESEARCH Recent research indicates that neem oil is anti-inflammatory and antibacterial, and to some degree reduces fever and lowers blood sugar levels. Currently, it is under investigation as a contraceptive for both men and women.

CAUTION Neem should not be given to infants, the elderly, or the debilitated.

Bacopa monnieri
(Scrophulariaceae)
WATER HYSSOP,
BRAHMI (HINDI)

DESCRIPTION Creeping succulent perennial growing to 20 in (50 cm). Has spatula-shaped fleshy leaves and pale blue or white flowers on long slender stalks.

HABITAT & CULTIVATION Water hyssop grows in warmer temperate and tropical climates, especially in southern Asia. It thrives in marshland, developing into dense mats on mudflats and at the edges of mangrove swamps.

PARTS USED Aerial parts.

CONSTITUENTS Water hyssop contains steroidal saponins (including bacosides).

MEDICINAL ACTIONS & USES In India, water hyssop is used principally for nervous system disorders such as neuralgia, epilepsy, and mental illness, but it is also employed for a wide range of other disorders, including indigestion, ulcers, gas and constipation, asthma and bronchitis, and infertility. In China, it is taken as a *yang* tonic for impotence, premature ejaculation, infertility, and rheumatic conditions. In Indonesia, the plant is a remedy for filariasis (a tropical disease caused by worms). In Cuba, water hyssop is used as a purgative, and a decoction of the whole plant is taken as a diuretic and laxative. The expressed juice is mixed with oil and applied as a rub for arthritic pain.

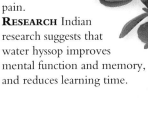

RESEARCH Indian research suggests that water hyssop improves mental function and memory, and reduces learning time.

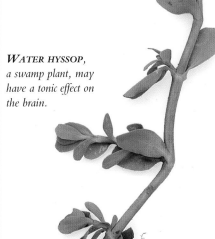

WATER HYSSOP, a swamp plant, may have a tonic effect on the brain.

Ballota nigra
(Labiatae)
BLACK HOREHOUND

DESCRIPTION Straggling, strong-smelling perennial growing to 3 ft (1 m). Has oval, toothed leaves and pink-purple flowers in whorls at the base of the upper leaves.

HABITAT & CULTIVATION This herb is found throughout much of Europe, in North America, and in Asia. It thrives in open areas, in pavement cracks, and by roadsides, mostly near human habitation. It is harvested when in flower in summer.

PARTS USED Aerial parts.

CONSTITUENTS Black horehound contains diterpenoids, including marrubiin, which is also a constituent of white horehound (*Marrubium vulgare*, p. 231).

HISTORY & FOLKLORE The Greek physician Dioscorides (1st century AD) recommended a plaster of black horehound leaves and salt for dog bites. He also advocated a balm, made from the dried leaves and honey, to purify infected wounds and ulcers.

MEDICINAL ACTIONS & USES Although it has long been considered a remedy for convulsions, low spirits, and menopausal

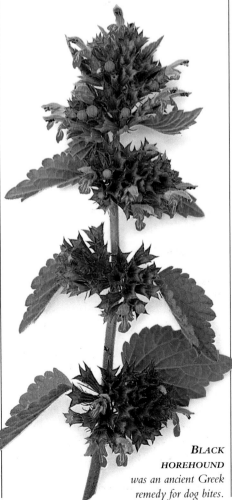

BLACK HOREHOUND was an ancient Greek remedy for dog bites.

problems, black horehound is not as commonly used today as it was in the past. Authorities differ over whether there is any substance to claims for its earlier uses. The herb is currently used by Anglo-American herbalists as an antiemetic – preventing or reducing nausea or vomiting. It is perhaps most useful when nausea stems from disorders of the inner ear (such as Ménière's disease) as opposed to those of the digestive system. Black horehound is thought to be mildly sedative and antispasmodic and is occasionally taken for arthritis and gout. It may be substituted for white horehound, but its medicinal effect is inferior.

Bambusa arundiaceae
(Gramineae)
SPINY BAMBOO

DESCRIPTION Perennial tree growing to 100 ft (30 m). Multiple stems grow from its base. Has narrow pointed leaves and very long loose clusters of yellow to yellowish green flowers.

HABITAT & CULTIVATION Found throughout tropical Asia, especially in India and China, spiny bamboo thrives up to 7,000 ft (2,100 m) above sea level.

PARTS USED Root, leaves, sprouts.

CONSTITUENTS Spiny bamboo juice contains high levels of silica.

HISTORY & FOLKLORE Spiny bamboo is arguably the most useful plant on earth, being used to make scaffolding, rafts, furniture, paper, and dozens of other items. It also has an important role to play in herbal medicine.

MEDICINAL ACTIONS & USES The various parts of spiny bamboo are used in many different ways in Indian and Ayurvedic medicine. The root is considered astringent and cooling, and is used to treat joint pain and general debility. The leaves are used to stimulate menstruation, and, being antispasmodic, to help relieve menstrual pain. The leaves also are used to tone and strengthen stomach function, are taken to expel worms, and have the reputation of being an aphrodisiac. The young sprouts are eaten to relieve nausea, indigestion, and gas, and a poultice of the sprouts is applied to help drain wounds that have become infected. The juice is rich in silica, and aids in the strengthening of cartilage in conditions such as osteoarthritis and osteoporosis.

RELATED SPECIES In Chinese herbal medicine, the juice and shavings of the black bamboo (*B. breviflora*) are prescribed to counter "excess heat," coughs, and a congested chest. Its roots are used as a diuretic and to treat fevers.

Banisteriopsis caapi
(Malpighiaceae)
AYAHUASCA

DESCRIPTION Woody vine growing to 100 ft (30 m). Has smooth bark, oval leaves, and bunches of small red or yellow flowers.

HABITAT & CULTIVATION Ayahuasca is native to jungles of the Amazon basin. It is cultivated by indigenous peoples, but the wild herb is preferred for medicinal use.

PART USED Bark.

CONSTITUENTS Ayahuasca contains beta-carboline alkaloids (including harmine, harmaline, and delta-tetrahycroharmine), which stimulate hallucinations.

HISTORY & FOLKLORE In the Quechua language, widely spoken in Peru and neighboring countries, *ayahuasca* means "spirit of the dead," indicating the awesome powers attributed to this plant. Another native Indian name is *nixi honi xuma*, meaning "vine from which the vision extract is made." Ayahuasca bark, often in combination with members of the *Datura* genus, is the primary hallucinogen of many Amazonian tribes, being prepared as part of complex ritual ceremonies.

MEDICINAL ACTIONS & USES Though known as a powerful hallucinogen, ayahuasca is also a medicine, being used as a remedy to cure a range of diagnosed conditions. However, ayahuasca is taken by the healer rather than by the patient. In the shamanistic societies of the Amazon, ayahuasca allows the healer to communicate with the spirit world where illness arises, interceding on behalf of the ill person and the community to restore health and harmony to all – quite unlike the individualized approach of Western medicine. Beyond its ability to affect the mood, the bark is emetic and purgative. At low doses it is used as a mild detoxifier.

CAUTIONS Ayahuasca is taken traditionally as part of a rich, complex ritual that affects the healing experience. Medicinal use of this plant is not advised.

Baptisia tinctoria
(Leguminosae)
WILD INDIGO

DESCRIPTION Herbaceous perennial growing to 3 ft (1 m). Has a smooth stem, cloverlike leaves, and purplish blue flowers in small terminal clusters.

HABITAT & CULTIVATION Native to eastern parts of North America, wild indigo grows from North Carolina to southern Canada in dry, hilly woods.

PARTS USED Root, leaves.

CONSTITUENTS Wild indigo contains isoflavones, flavonoids, alkaloids, coumarins, and polysaccharides. The isoflavones are estrogenic.

HISTORY & FOLKLORE Wild indigo was commonly used as a poultice by Native Americans and New World settlers to treat snake bite. The Mohicans used a decoction of the root to bathe cuts and wounds.

MEDICINAL ACTIONS & USES Wild indigo is an immunostimulant and a strong antiseptic. It is considered particularly effective for upper respiratory infections such as tonsillitis and pharyngitis, and is also valuable in treating infections of the chest, gastrointestinal tract, and skin. Its anti-microbial and immunostimulant properties combat lymphatic problems. When used with detoxifying herbs such as burdock (*Arctium lappa*, p. 62), it helps to reduce enlarged lymph nodes. Wild indigo is prescribed along with echinacea (*Echinacea angustifolia*, p. 90) for chronic viral conditions or chronic fatigue syndrome. A decoction of the root soothes sore or infected nipples and infected skin conditions. Used as a gargle or mouthwash, the decoction treats canker sores, gum infections, and sore throats.

CAUTION Take only under professional supervision.

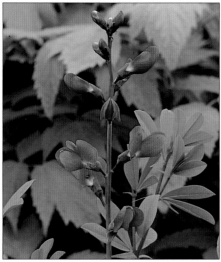

WILD INDIGO, *a North American plant, was used by the Penobscot people to treat wounds.*

Benincasa hispida
syn. *B. cerifa*
(Cucurbitaceae)
WAX GOURD, PETHA

DESCRIPTION Hairy annual climber. Has 3-lobed leaves, tendrils, and large yellow flowers. Produces rounded fruit (gourds) about 16 in (40 cm) long.

HABITAT & CULTIVATION This herb is native to tropical Asia and Africa, and

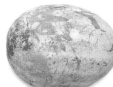

Wax gourd

cultivated in India and China as a vegetable. The fruit is harvested in late summer.

PARTS USED Fruit rind, fruit, seeds.

CONSTITUENTS Wax gourd contains saponins and guaridine.

HISTORY & FOLKLORE Wax gourd has been used as a food and medicine for thousands of years. It was first documented in the *Tang Materia Medica*, written in AD 659.

MEDICINAL ACTIONS & USES In Chinese herbal medicine, a decoction of wax gourd seeds is used to "drain dampness" and "clear heat." It is given for chest conditions and for vaginal discharge. In combination with Chinese rhubarb (*Rheum palmatum*, p. 124), it is prescribed for intestinal abscesses. In Ayurvedic medicine, the seeds are used to treat coughs, fever, and excessive thirst, and to expel tapeworms. The fruit is classified as cooling, diuretic, and laxative. It is thought to act as an aphrodisiac and is used for peptic ulceration and debility. In an ancient Indian recipe, the juice from the fruit is mixed with lime juice (*Citrus aurantiifolia*) to prevent or stop bleeding.

RESEARCH The fruit appears to have an anticancerous effect.

Berberis aquifolium
(Berberidaceae)
OREGON GRAPE

DESCRIPTION Evergreen shrub growing to 6 ft (2 m). Has shiny leaves, small yellowish green flowers, and purple berries in autumn.

HABITAT & CULTIVATION Native to North America, Oregon grape grows in the Rocky Mountains up to 7,000 ft (2,000 m), and in woods from Colorado to the Pacific coast. It is abundant in Oregon and northern California.

PART USED Root.

CONSTITUENTS Oregon grape contains isoquinoline alkaloids (including berberine, berbamine, and hydrastine). These alkaloids are strong antiseptics and are thought to reduce the severity of psoriasis.

HISTORY & FOLKLORE California Native peoples took a decoction or tincture of the bitter-tasting root for loss of appetite and debility. In the 19th and early 20th centuries, Oregon grape was an important herb in the Physiomedicalist movement, based on a combination of orthodox and Native American practices. In this context, it was

prescribed as a detoxifier and tonic.

MEDICINAL ACTIONS & USES Oregon grape is chiefly used for gastritis and general digestive weakness, to stimulate gallbladder function, and to reduce congestion problems (mainly of the gut). It also treats eczema, psoriasis, acne, boils, and herpes, and skin conditions linked to poor gallbladder function.

RELATED SPECIES Barberry (*B. vulgaris, see following entry*) is similar to Oregon grape in its overall action, but it is generally stronger in the effect it produces.

CAUTION Do not take during pregnancy.

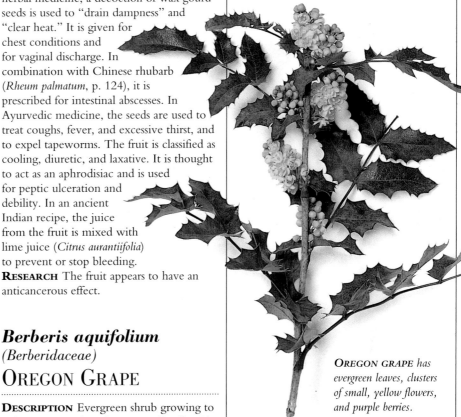

OREGON GRAPE *has evergreen leaves, clusters of small, yellow flowers, and purple berries.*

Berberis vulgaris
(Berberidaceae)
BARBERRY

DESCRIPTION Thorny, deciduous shrub growing to 10 ft (3 m), with leathery leaves, yellow flowers, and red berries in autumn.

HABITAT & CULTIVATION Native to Europe, barberry is naturalized in North America. It is cultivated as a garden plant and medicinal herb. The bark is gathered in spring or autumn, and the berries in autumn.

PARTS USED Stem bark, root bark, berries.

CONSTITUENTS Barberry contains isoquinoline alkaloids, including berberine and berbamine. Berberine is strongly antibacterial and amebicidal, and stimulates

BARBERRY *continued on following page*

bile secretion. Berbamine is strongly antibacterial. Many of the alkaloids are thought to be cancer-inhibiting.

HISTORY & FOLKLORE In ancient Egypt, *Berberis* berries were macerated with fennel seed (*Foeniculum vulgare*, p. 210) to make a drink for fevers. The berries are extremely sour but have been used in the past to make preserves – the French *confiture d'épine vinette* is one example. After the plant was introduced from Europe to the eastern US, it was used by the Catawba for peptic ulcers.

MEDICINAL ACTIONS & USES Barberry acts on the gallbladder to improve bile flow and ameliorate conditions such as gallbladder pain, gallstones, and jaundice. Barberry's strongly antiseptic property is of value in cases of amebic dysentery, cholera, and other similar gastrointestinal infections. Barberry is also thought to have a positive effect on the liver and is prescribed by herbalists for hepatitis.

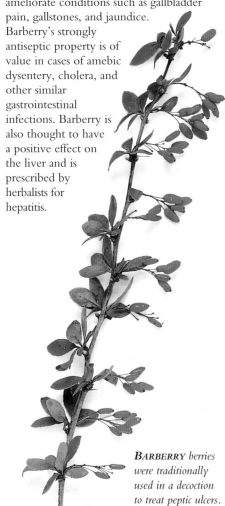

BARBERRY berries were traditionally used in a decoction to treat peptic ulcers.

The bark is astringent, antidiarrheal, and healing to the intestinal wall – in short, barberry has a strong, highly beneficial effect on the digestive system as a whole. Like Oregon grape (*B. aquifolium, see preceding entry*) and goldenseal (*Hydrastis canadensis*, p. 103), barberry helps in the treatment of chronic skin conditions such as eczema and psoriasis. The decoction makes a gentle and effective wash for the eyes, although it must be diluted sufficiently before use.

CAUTIONS Take only under professional supervision, for not more than 4–6 weeks at a time. Do not take during pregnancy.

Beta vulgaris
(Chenopodiaceae)
RED BEET, WHITE BEET

DESCRIPTION Perennial with swollen edible red or white root, upright shoots, large deep green leaves tinged with red, and spikes of green-petaled flowers.

HABITAT & CULTIVATION Sea beet (the wild subspecies) is native to coastal regions of Europe, North Africa, and Asia from Turkey to the East Indies. Varieties of red beet are cultivated worldwide as a vegetable; white beet, as a source of sugar.

PART USED Root.

CONSTITUENTS White beet contains betaine, which promotes the regeneration of liver cells and the metabolism of fat cells. Red beet contains betanin – an anthocyanin similar to those found in red wine – which is partly responsible for red beet's immune-enhancing effect.

HISTORY & FOLKLORE The 1st-century AD *Materia Medica* by Dioscorides gave the following prescription for clearing the head and relieving earache – mix beet juice with honey and sniff it up the nose. The herbal also noted that a decoction of the leaves and roots removes dandruff and nits. Nicholas Culpeper in *The English Physitian* (1652) recommended beets for erysipelas, a bacterial infection of the skin. Sugar was first extracted from white beet in 1760 by the Berlin apothecary Margraff.

MEDICINAL ACTIONS & USES White beet acts to support the liver, bile ducts, and gallbladder, influencing fat metabolism and helping to lower blood fat levels and cholesterol. It also alleviates headaches and can be used to counteract hair loss. Red beet juice is thought to stimulate the immune system, but only when taken in very large quantities – at least a liter a day, according to one authority. Red beet juice is also taken as part of a special diet in the treatment of cancer.

Betula pendula
syn. *B. verrucosa*
(Betulaceae)
SILVER BIRCH

DESCRIPTION Handsome slender deciduous tree growing to 100 ft (30 m). Has pale gray papery bark, toothed leaves, and catkins in spring.

HABITAT & CULTIVATION Silver birch is common in Europe, in temperate regions of Asia, and in North America. It flourishes in woods and thickets, and is also planted as a garden ornamental. The leaves are gathered in late spring.

PARTS USED Leaves, bark, sap.

CONSTITUENTS Silver birch contains saponins, flavonoids, tannin, and a volatile oil that includes methyl salicylate.

HISTORY & FOLKLORE Silver birch has been used as a medicinal herb in northern Europe and Asia since the earliest times. Its name is thought to derive from the Sanskrit word *bhurga*, meaning "tree whose bark is used for writing on." In the highlands of Scotland, silver birch sap – tapped in the spring – was drunk as a treatment for bladder and kidney complaints. Although the tree was known to classical writers, Hildegard of Bingen, a medieval abbess and mystic who wrote about herbal medicine, was the first European to document its medicinal properties.

MEDICINAL ACTIONS & USES An infusion made with silver birch leaves hastens the removal of waste products in the urine, and is beneficial for kidney stones and bladder stones (gravel), rheumatic conditions, and gout. The leaves are also used, in combination with diuretic herbs, to reduce fluid retention and swelling. Silver birch sap is a mild diuretic. The oil distilled from the leaves is antiseptic and is commonly used in preparations to help treat eczema and psoriasis. A decoction of silver birch bark can be used as a lotion for chronic skin problems. The bark can also be macerated in oil and applied to rheumatic joints.

RELATED SPECIES The Himalayan silver birch (*B. utilis*), a close relative, is used in Ayurvedic medicine as a treatment for convulsions, dysentery, hemorrhages, and skin diseases.

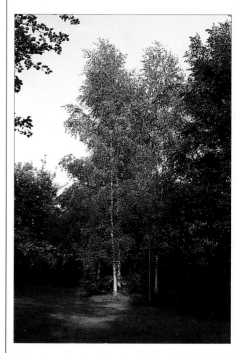

SILVER BIRCH is widespread in temperate regions throughout the northern hemisphere. Its leaf oil is used to improve eczema and psoriasis.

Bidens tripartita
(Compositae)
STICKTIGHTS, BUR MARIGOLD

DESCRIPTION Annual growing to 2 ft (60 cm). Has toothed lance-shaped leaves, yellow buttonlike flower heads, and burlike fruit.

HABITAT & CULTIVATION Sticktights grow throughout Europe, North America, and other temperate regions including Australia and New Zealand. They are found in damp places and near fresh water.

PARTS USED Aerial parts.

CONSTITUENTS Sticktights contain flavonoids, xanthophylls, volatile oil, acetylenes, sterols, and tannins.

HISTORY & FOLKLORE Nicholas Culpeper, writing in 1652, extolled this plant: "It helps the cachexia or evil disposition of the body, the dropsy and yellow jaundice, it opens obstructions of the liver, and mollifies the hardness of the spleen being applied outwardly."

MEDICINAL ACTIONS & USES Sticktights are not much used medicinally today, but they were once esteemed as a medicine. As an astringent and diuretic, they may be employed to treat bladder and kidney problems. They also quickly staunch blood flow, and can be used for uterine hemorrhage and conditions producing blood in the urine. Their astringency helps counteract peptic ulceration, diarrhea, and ulcerative colitis. When used to treat digestive tract ailments, sticktights are usually combined with an herb that reduces flatulence, such as ginger (*Zingiber officinale*, p. 153).

RELATED SPECIES *B. pilosa* is a South American herb that now grows throughout much of Africa and Australia. In Africa, it is used as a food crop, although it is considered very unappetizing. In Africa, the plant is used to treat diarrhea. In the Caribbean, the leaves are used to induce menstruation.

Bignonia catalpa syn. *Catalpa bignonioides*
(Bignoniaceae)
CATALPA, INDIAN BEAN TREE

DESCRIPTION Deciduous tree growing to 70 ft (20 m). Has large oval leaves in whorls of 3, white flowers in conical clusters, and long thin fruits (bean pods).

HABITAT & CULTIVATION Native to the southeastern US, this tree is often planted in gardens in southern and western Europe.

PARTS USED Bark, fruit.

CONSTITUENTS The bark contains catalpine, and oxylenzoic and protocatechetic acids.

HISTORY & FOLKLORE Catalpa bark was formerly used as a substitute for quinine in treating malaria.

MEDICINAL ACTIONS & USES The mildly sedative and narcotic bark is used to treat asthma, whooping cough, and other spasmodic coughs in children. The distilled water of the fruit, in combination with herbs commonly used to treat eye problems, such as eyebright (*Euphrasia officinalis*, p. 208) and rue (*Ruta graveolens*, p. 262), makes an effective eyewash for conjunctivitis and other eye infections.

CAUTION Never use the root, which is highly poisonous.

Bixa orellana
(Bixaceae)
ANNATTO

DESCRIPTION Evergreen tree growing to 25 ft (8 m). Has large leaves, pink or white flowers, and red fruit capsules containing red seeds.

HABITAT & CULTIVATION Native to tropical forests in the Americas and the West Indies, annatto is widely cultivated in similar climatic zones, notably in India. Seeds are collected as the fruit splits open.

PARTS USED Seeds, leaves, root.

CONSTITUENTS The seed pulp contains carotenoid coloring principles.

HISTORY & FOLKLORE In tropical South America, the brilliant red pigment in the seed pulp has traditionally been used in body painting. Annatto dye is also used as a colorant for margarine and cheese.

MEDICINAL ACTIONS & USES In the Caribbean, annatto leaves and roots are used to make an astringent infusion that is taken to treat fever, epilepsy, and dysentery. The infusion is also taken as an aphrodisiac. The leaves alone make an infusion that is used as a gargle. The seed pulp reduces blistering when applied immediately to burns. Taken internally, the seed pulp acts as an antidote for poisoning.

Borago officinalis
(Boraginaceae)
BORAGE

DESCRIPTION Hairy annual growing to 2 ft (60 cm). Has a pulpy stem, large basal leaves, and blue flowers in summer.

HABITAT & CULTIVATION Borage is a common Mediterranean weed thought to originate from southern Spain and Morocco. Often grown as a garden herb, it is also extensively cultivated for its seed oil.

PARTS USED Aerial parts, flowers, seed oil.

CONSTITUENTS Borage contains mucilage, tannins, and pyrrolizidine alkaloids, which are toxic to the liver.

HISTORY & FOLKLORE The herbalist John Gerard, writing in 1597, extoled borage's virtues: "A syrup made of the flowers of borage comforteth the heart, purgeth melancholy, and quieteth the phreneticke or lunaticke person." Gerard also quoted the old saying, "I, Borage, bring always courage."

MEDICINAL ACTIONS & USES With its high mucilage content, borage is a demulcent and soothes respiratory problems. Its emollient qualities make it helpful for sore and inflamed skin – prepared either as freshly squeezed juice, in a poultice, or as an infusion. The flowers encourage sweating, and the leaves are diuretic. The seed oil is particularly rich in polyunsaturated fats and is superior in this respect to evening primrose oil (*Oenothera biennis*, p. 239). Borage seed oil is used to treat premenstrual complaints, rheumatic problems, eczema, and other chronic skin conditions.

CAUTIONS Due to the presence of toxic pyrrolizide in alkaloids, there is uncertainty over borage's safety as a medicine. It is subject to legal restrictions in some countries and should not be taken internally. These restrictions and cautions do not apply to borage seed oil.

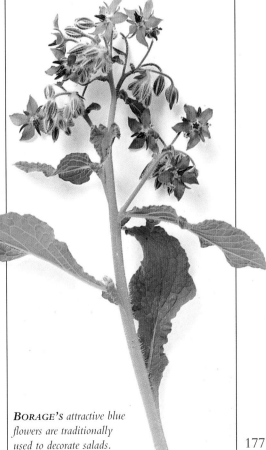

BORAGE'S attractive blue flowers are traditionally used to decorate salads.

Brassica oleracea
(*Cruciferae*)

CABBAGE

DESCRIPTION Biennial or perennial herb growing to 8 ft (2.5 m). Has a thick stem, gray leaves, and 4-petaled yellow flowers. Within the first year, it produces a greatly enlarged terminal bud that develops into the familiar cabbage head in late summer.

HABITAT & CULTIVATION Wild cabbage is native to coasts of the English Channel and the Mediterranean. Cultivated varieties are produced worldwide as a vegetable.

PARTS USED Leaves.

CONSTITUENTS Cabbage is rich in vitamins A, B_1, B_2, and C.

HISTORY & FOLKLORE The wholesome cabbage is one of the oldest vegetables. According to Greek myth, the plant sprang into existence from the perspiration of Zeus. In a Greek ritual, cabbage was given to expectant mothers shortly before birth in order to establish good breast-milk production. The Romans used cabbage as an antidote, especially to alcohol, believing it countered intoxication and prevented or reduced a hangover. They also used cabbage leaves to cleanse infected wounds. One traditional method of making a cabbage poultice, which is still used today, is to cut out the midrib of a leaf and iron it, placing it while still hot on the area to be treated.

Cabbage

MEDICINAL ACTIONS & USES Cabbage's best-known medicinal use is as a poultice – the leaves of the wild or cultivated plant are blanched, crushed, or chopped, and applied to swellings, tumors, and painful joints. Wild cabbage leaves eaten raw or cooked aid digestion and the breakdown of toxins in the liver – so the Romans' eating it to ease a hangover was in fact quite sensible. Cabbage is also detoxifying and helpful in the long-term treatment of arthritis. The high vitamin C content of cabbage has made it useful in the prevention of scurvy.

CAUTION A cabbage poultice may cause blisters if left on for several hours.

Bryonia dioica
syn. ***B. cretica*** subsp. ***dioica***
(*Cucurbitaceae*)

WHITE BRYONY

DESCRIPTION Perennial climbing vine with fleshy taproot. Has straggling stem with tendrils, greenish flowers, and red berries.

HABITAT & CULTIVATION White bryony is native to southern England and parts of Europe. The root is dug up in autumn.

PART USED Root.

CONSTITUENTS White bryony contains cucurbitacins, glycosides, volatile oil, and tannins. The cucurbitacins kill cells and act on tumors.

HISTORY & FOLKLORE From prehistory to the Middle Ages, the thick roots of white bryony were cut into a human shape as a substitute (or a counterfeit) for mandrake root (*Mandragora officinarum*, p. 230), which was believed to afford magical protection. The Greek physician Dioscorides (1st century AD) reported that the leaves, fruit, and root of white bryony were applied to gangrenous wounds. In medieval England, the plant was used to treat leprosy.

MEDICINAL ACTIONS & USES A powerful cathartic and purgative, white bryony is used with great caution in herbal medicine today. Principally prescribed for painful rheumatic conditions, it may be taken internally or applied externally as a counterirritant, causing swelling and increased blood flow to the area. It is also given for other inflammatory conditions such as duodenal ulcers, asthma, bronchitis, and pleurisy, and may be used to reduce high blood pressure. The whole herb has an antiviral effect.

RELATED SPECIES *B. alba* is used in homeopathy. Black bryony (*Tamus communis*) is an unrelated plant with approximately similar uses.

CAUTIONS Bryony is a toxic plant. Use only under professional supervision. Do not take during pregnancy.

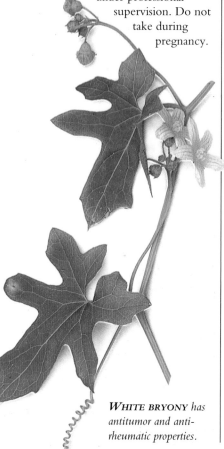

WHITE BRYONY has antitumor and anti-rheumatic properties.

Butea monosperma
(*Fabaceae*)

PALAS, FLAME OF THE FOREST, BENGAL KINO

DESCRIPTION Deciduous tree growing to 50 ft (15 m). Has 3-lobed leaves and large orange-red flowers in clusters.

HABITAT & CULTIVATION Palas is native to India and Malaysia. It grows in forests and open areas to altitudes of 4,000 ft (1,200 m).

PARTS USED Bark, flowers, leaves, gum, seeds.

CONSTITUENTS All parts of the tree except the seeds contain tannins.

MEDICINAL ACTIONS & USES The gum oozing from incisions in the bark is known as Bengal kino. Mildly astringent, it is used as a substitute for the kino derived from bastard teak (*Pterocarpus marsupium*). Bengal kino is taken as a decoction or a tincture for acid indigestion, diarrhea, and dysentery, and used as a gargle for sore throats and as a douche for vaginitis. The gum is mild in effect and is commonly given to children. A decoction of the astringent leaves and flowers is taken for diarrhea, heavy menstrual bleeding, and fever, and is applied to hemorrhoids and skin conditions. A decoction of leaves, bark, or flowers is also thought to be aphrodisiac, while the flowers are believed to have a contraceptive effect. The seeds are purgative, and are mainly used externally to treat herpes and ringworm.

CAUTION Do not take during pregnancy.

Caesalpina bonducella
(*Leguminosae*)

NIKKAR NUT

DESCRIPTION Thorny bush growing to 28 ft (9 m) with spiny compound leaves, yellow flowers in dense clusters, and prickly pods containing yellow seeds (nuts).

HABITAT & CULTIVATION Nikkar nut grows throughout India in grasslands and open areas, and in tropical areas throughout the world. The seeds are gathered when ripe.

PARTS USED Seeds.

CONSTITUENTS The seeds contain a fixed oil (25%), a bitter principle (bonducin), and tannins.

MEDICINAL ACTIONS & USES Nikkar seeds are used to treat fevers and are taken as a tonic and aphrodisiac. In India, they are often mixed with black pepper (*Piper nigrum*, p. 248) for medicinal use. The seeds are also taken for arthritis. Roasted nikkar seeds are used to treat diabetes. The oil from the seeds is used in cosmetics to soften the skin.

RELATED SPECIES A decoction of the bark of the Caribbean *C. bahamensis* is used for liver and kidney infections, and a decoction of the wood is used for diabetes. An infusion of the leaves of *C. pulcherrima* (native to Asia and Africa) is taken for liver problems and canker sores, and a decoction of the root is used in Angola to treat intermittent fever.

Calamintha ascendens syn. *C. sylvatica*, *C. officinalis* (Labiatae)
CALAMINT

DESCRIPTION Mint-scented perennial growing to 2 ft (60 cm). Has hairy oval leaves and purple flowers in late summer.
HABITAT & CULTIVATION Calamint grows wild in Europe and Asia from the British Isles eastward to Iran, especially in the Mediterranean region. It flourishes along roadsides and in dry places.
PARTS USED Aerial parts.
CONSTITUENTS Calamint contains a volatile oil (about 0.35%) consisting mainly of pulegone.
HISTORY & FOLKLORE In classical legend, calamint had the power to drive away the Basilisk, a serpent credited with the ability to kill with its gaze or breath.
MEDICINAL ACTIONS & USES Calamint stimulates sweating and hence helps lower fevers. It also settles gas and indigestion. It is an expectorant, and is a good cough and cold remedy. This range of applications makes it a good medicinal herb for mild respiratory infections, preferably mixed with other herbs such as yarrow (*Achillea millefolium*, p. 54) and thyme (*Thymus vulgaris*, p. 142).
CAUTION Do not take during pregnancy.

Calluna vulgaris (Ericaceae)
HEATHER

DESCRIPTION Small, branched shrub growing to 2 ft (60 cm). Has tiny leaves and white or pink to pale purple flowers growing on spikes.
HABITAT & CULTIVATION Heather grows in temperate regions of the northern hemisphere. It is found on heaths, moors, bogs, and in open woods. The herb is gathered when in flower in late summer.
PARTS USED Flowering tips.
CONSTITUENTS Heather contains flavonoids, arbutin, tannin, and an alkaloid, ericodin. This constituent has a strongly disinfectant effect within the bladder and urinary tubules.

HISTORY & FOLKLORE If the "erica" that Dioscorides discussed in his 1st-century AD *Materia Medica* is indeed heather, as has been surmised, then the flowering tips were used in classical times to treat snake bite. Galen (AD 131–200) wrote of the plant's ability to induce sweating. The rootstock of heather is made into musical pipes, the foliage provides mattress stuffing, and the flowers produce a delicate honey.
MEDICINAL ACTIONS & USES Heather is a good urinary antiseptic and diuretic, disinfecting the urinary tract and mildly increasing urine production. Besides its role in treating cystitis and inflammatory bladder conditions, heather has been used to treat kidney and bladder stones. It is a cleansing and detoxifying herb, helpful for rheumatism, arthritis, and gout. The macerated flowering tips produce a liniment to be rubbed on affected joints. A hot poultice of heather tips is a traditional remedy for chilblains.

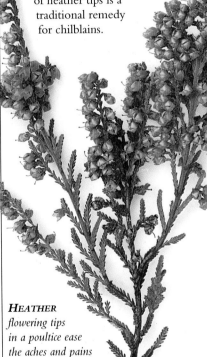

HEATHER flowering tips in a poultice ease the aches and pains of rheumatism.

Camellia sinensis syn. *Thea sinensis* (Theaceae)
TEA

DESCRIPTION Evergreen shrub clipped to 5 ft (1.5 m) in cultivation, with leathery, dark green leaves and fragrant white flowers.
HABITAT & CULTIVATION Cultivated principally in India, Sri Lanka, and China, tea has been grown since the earliest times.
PART USED Leaves and buds.
CONSTITUENTS Tea contains xanthines,

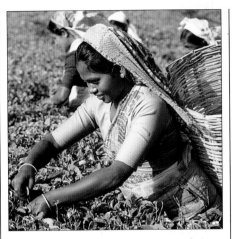

TEA leaves are picked throughout the year and used both as a beverage and a medicine.

caffeine (1–5%), theobromine, tannins, flavonoids, fats, and vitamin C.
HISTORY & FOLKLORE In China, many rituals have developed around tea.
MEDICINAL ACTIONS & USES Tea is useful in treating infections of the digestive tract. In Ayurveda, tea is considered astringent, sweat-inducing, and a nerve tonic, and is used for eye problems, hemorrhoids, tiredness, and fever. Tea leaves may be used externally to soothe insect bites and sunburn.
RESEARCH Research in China suggests that green tea can help hepatitis. Research in Japan in 1990 showed that tea contains constituents that inhibit tooth decay.

Cananga odorata syn. *Canangium odoratum* (Annonaceae)
YLANG-YLANG

DESCRIPTION Evergreen tree growing to 80 ft (25 m). Has lance-shaped leaves and strongly scented yellow-green flowers.
HABITAT & CULTIVATION Native to Indonesia and the Philippines, ylang-ylang is cultivated in tropical Asia and Africa.
PARTS USED Flowers, essential oil.
CONSTITUENTS The volatile oil contains linalool (11–30%), safrole, eugenol, geraniol, and sesquiterpenes (including 15–25% germacrene).
HISTORY & FOLKLORE The flowers are a traditional adornment in the Far East. Their scent is thought to have aphrodisiac qualities.
MEDICINAL ACTIONS & USES The flowers and essential oil are sedative and antiseptic. The oil has a soothing effect, and its main therapeutic uses are to slow an excessively fast heart rate and to lower blood pressure. Ylang-ylang has a reputation as an aphrodisiac and may be helpful in treating impotence.
CAUTION Do not take the essential oil internally without professional supervision.

Canella winterana
syn. *C. alba*
(Canellaceae)

CANELLA, WILD CINNAMON

DESCRIPTION White-barked tree growing to 50 ft (15 m). Has elliptical leaves, red flowers, and purple-black berries.

HABITAT & CULTIVATION Native to the Caribbean and Florida, canella is found in coastal swamps and scrubland. The bark is collected by gently beating the branches.

PART USED Bark.

CONSTITUENTS Canella contains about 1% volatile oil (including eugenol, alpha-pinene, and caryophyllene), alpha-aldehydes (including canellal), resin, and mannitol.

HISTORY & FOLKLORE Canella has long been used as a flavoring for tobacco (*Nicotiana tabacum*, p. 237).

MEDICINAL ACTIONS & USES Canella is cytotoxic (kills cells), antifungal, and repels insects. It is also strongly aromatic, stimulant, and antiseptic. Canella is often used in the West Indies and Latin America as a substitute for cinnamon (*Cinnamomum zeylanicum*, p. 80). The infusion is drunk both for its pleasant flavor and tonic effect (the bark is thought a sexual stimulant). Canella is also used for stomach problems, indigestion, and puerperal fever following childbirth.

Cannabis sativa
(Cannabinaceae)

MARIJUANA, HUO MA REN
(CHINESE)

DESCRIPTION Erect, branching annual growing to 12 ft (4 m). Has fine, serrated, segmented leaves. Both male and female plants flower; female plant produces seeds.

HABITAT & CULTIVATION Native to the Caucasus, China, Iran, and northern India, marijuana is cultivated the world over, both legally (for the fiber and seeds) and illegally (for use as a recreational drug).

PARTS USED Flowering tops of female plants, seeds.

CONSTITUENTS Marijuana contains over 60 different types of cannabinoids, including THC (delta 9-tetrahydrocannabinol). It also contains flavonoids, volatile oil, and alkaloids. It is the only plant to contain THC, one of the main psychoactive constituents.

Marijuana leaf

HISTORY & FOLKLORE In ancient Egypt, marijuana was used to treat inflammations of the eye and "to cool the uterus." First records of marijuana's use in India date back to about 800 BC, where it was recommended for congestion. Marijuana also appears in Chinese medicinal literature, in the *Divine Husbandman's Classic (Shen'nong Bencaojing)*, written in the 1st century AD. It was described as a treatment for "female weakness, gout, rheumatism, malaria, beri-beri, constipation and absent-mindedness." By the 3rd century AD, the leaves were taken in an infusion or eaten whole as an analgesic to relieve pain during surgery. Famously, Queen Victoria took marijuana as an analgesic – in the 19th century the plant was a standard painkiller for menstrual pain and cramps. From 1840 to 1900, over 100 papers were published recommending marijuana as a medicine.

MEDICINAL ACTIONS & USES In view of its long history as a medicinal treatment, it is hardly surprising that marijuana has, at one time or another, been recommended for almost every illness. As an analgesic, it appears to relieve pain with minimal side effects, being particularly helpful for cancer and AIDS patients undergoing chemotherapy. For those suffering from multiple sclerosis, cerebral palsy, and other muscular illnesses, marijuana can reduce neurological overactivity and muscle spasm.

The plant provides effective treatment for glaucoma, in which pressure within the eye is abnormally high, and is hypotensive, lowering blood pressure. Marijuana relieves asthma, menstrual pains, the pain of childbirth, and of arthritis and rheumatism, and may have value as an antidepressant. It encourages and induces sleep. The seeds are used in Chinese medicine as a strong but well-tolerated laxative, especially for constipation in the elderly.

RESEARCH Modern research shows marijuana to be an effective analgesic, sedative, and anti-inflammatory agent. Research has focused on the constituent THC, but it is clear that the complex of constituents within marijuana has a significantly wider range of applications.

CAUTION It is illegal to grow, possess, or use marijuana in many countries.

Capparis spinosa
(Capparaceae)

CAPER

DESCRIPTION Shrub growing to 3 ft (1 m) with spiny trailing stems, fleshy oval leaves, green buds, large white flowers, and red berries in autumn.

HABITAT & CULTIVATION Native to the Mediterranean region, caper thrives in open areas, often growing on stony terrain. The buds are harvested before the flowers open and are pickled for culinary use.

PARTS USED Root bark, bark, flower buds.

CONSTITUENTS Caper contains capric acid.

HISTORY & FOLKLORE Though much favored as a piquant food by the ancient Greeks, capers were said to disagree with the stomach. They remain a popular condiment to this day.

MEDICINAL ACTIONS & USES The unopened flower buds are laxative and, if prepared correctly with vinegar, are thought to ease stomach pain. The bark is bitter and diuretic, and can be taken immediately before meals to increase the appetite. The root bark is purifying and stops internal bleeding. It is used to treat skin conditions, capillary weakness, and easy bruising, and is also used in cosmetic preparations. A decoction of the plant is used to treat yeast and vaginal infections such as candidiasis.

RELATED SPECIES Various *Capparis* species are used as foods around the world. Some also have medicinal properties – for instance, the North American *C. cynophallophora*. A decoction of this plant is taken to encourage the onset of menstruation, used as a gargle for throat infections, and applied externally to treat herpes. *C. horrida* is thought to have sedative and sweat-reducing properties and to relieve stomach pain.

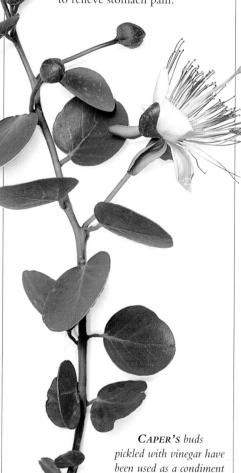

CAPER'S buds pickled with vinegar have been used as a condiment since ancient times.

Capsella bursa-pastoris syn. *Thlaspi bursa-pastoris*
(*Cruciferae*)
SHEPHERD'S PURSE

DESCRIPTION Annual or biennial with an erect stem, rosette of basal leaves, 4-petaled white flowers, and heart-shaped seed pods.

HABITAT & CULTIVATION Thought to be native to Europe and Asia, shepherd's purse is now found throughout most temperate regions, and grows profusely as a weed. It is harvested throughout the year.

PARTS USED Aerial parts.

CONSTITUENTS Contains flavonoids, polypeptides, choline, acetylcholine, histamine, and tyramine.

HISTORY & FOLKLORE This herb's name derives from the appearance of the seed pods, which resemble small, heart-shaped purses. During the First World War, when the standard herbal medicines for staunching blood – goldenseal (*Hydrastis canadensis*, p. 103) and ergot (*Claviceps purpurea*) – were unobtainable in Britain, shepherd's purse was used as an alternative.

MEDICINAL ACTIONS & USES One of the best remedies for preventing or arresting hemorrhage, shepherd's purse has long been a specific treatment for heavy uterine bleeding. While weaker-acting in this respect than ergot, shepherd's purse is less toxic and so better tolerated by the body. It may be used for bleeding of all kinds, from nosebleeds to blood in the urine. An astringent herb, it disinfects the urinary tract in cases of cystitis, and is taken for diarrhea. It is used in Chinese medicine for dysentery and eye problems.

RESEARCH Reports suggest that the plant is anti-inflammatory and reduces fever.

CAUTION Do not take during pregnancy.

SELF-HELP USE Heavy menstrual bleeding, p. 315.

Cardiospermum spp.
(*Sapindaceae*)
BALLOON VINE

DESCRIPTION Deciduous perennial climbers growing to 10 ft (3 m), with compound leaves, small white flowers, and black seeds.

HABITAT & CULTIVATION Balloon vine is found in tropical regions around the world.

PARTS USED Root, leaves, seeds.

CONSTITUENTS Most *Cardiospermum* species contain cyanogenic glycosides.

HISTORY & FOLKLORE Native Amazonians string balloon vine seeds into armbands that are worn to ward off snakes.

MEDICINAL ACTIONS & USES In Indian herbal medicine, balloon vine root is used to bring on delayed menstruation and to

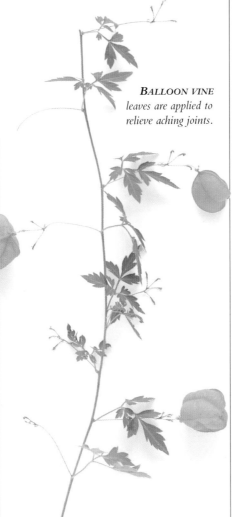

BALLOON VINE leaves are applied to relieve aching joints.

relieve backache and arthritis. The leaves stimulate local circulation and are applied to painful joints to help speed the clearing of toxins. The seeds are also thought to help in the treatment of arthritis. The plant as a whole has sedative properties.

CAUTION Do not take during pregnancy.

Carica papaya
(*Caricaceae*)
PAPAYA

DESCRIPTION Herbaceous tree growing very rapidly to 25 ft (8 m). Has segmented leaves, yellow flowers, and large black-seeded yellow to orange fruits weighing up to 11 lb (5 kg).

HABITAT & CULTIVATION Native to tropical America, papaya is now cultivated in tropical regions throughout the world.

PARTS USED Fruit, latex, leaves, flowers, seeds.

CONSTITUENTS Papaya fruit contains proteolytic enzymes (papain and chymopapain) and traces of an alkaloid, carpaine. Papain, found in the milky white latex that flows from incisions in the unripe fruit, is a protein-dissolving enzyme that aids digestion.

HISTORY & FOLKLORE Papaya juice, shoots, and latex were used in Mayan herbal medicine. In tropical Latin America, the leaves are used as a meat tenderizer.

MEDICINAL ACTIONS & USES Papaya's main medicinal use is as a digestive agent. The leaves and fruit can both be used to support sound digestion (the unripe fruit is especially effective). The latex from the trunk of the tree is also applied externally to speed the healing of wounds, ulcers, boils, warts, and cancerous tumors. The seeds gently expel worms. The latex has a similar but more violent effect. The flowers may be taken in an infusion to induce menstruation. A decoction of the ripe fruit is helpful for treating persistent diarrhea and dysentery in children. The ripe fruit is mildly laxative. The leaves are used to dress wounds.

Carthamus tinctorius
(*Compositae*)
SAFFLOWER, HONG HUA (CHINESE)

DESCRIPTION Annual herb growing to 3 ft (90 cm). Has long, spiny leaves with 6 oblong-oval leaflets, and groups of yellow flowers arising from the leaf axils.

HABITAT & CULTIVATION Thought to be native to Iran and northwestern India, and possibly Africa, this herb is also found in North America and the Far East. It grows in open areas and is gathered in summer.

PARTS USED Flowers, seeds, seed oil.

CONSTITUENTS Safflower contains carthamone, lignans, and a polysaccharide.

HISTORY & FOLKLORE In 19th-century North American herbal medicine, safflower was used to induce sweating, to promote the onset of a menstrual period, and as a treatment for measles.

MEDICINAL ACTIONS & USES In Chinese herbal medicine, the flowers are given to stimulate menstruation and to relieve abdominal pain. The flowers are also used to cleanse and heal wounds and sores and to treat measles. In the Anglo-American herbal tradition, the flowers are also given as a treatment for fever and skin rashes. The unpurified seed oil is purgative.

RESEARCH Chinese research indicates that safflower flowers can reduce the likelihood of coronary artery disease and lower cholesterol levels. Safflower contains a polysaccharide that has been shown to stimulate immune function in mice. Safflower oil also lowers cholesterol levels.

CAUTION Do not take the flowers or seeds during pregnancy (purified seed oil is safe).

Carum carvi
(Umbelliferae)
CARAWAY

DESCRIPTION Aromatic annual growing to 2 ft (60 cm). Has ridged stem, feathery leaves, and umbels of white flowers in midsummer. Exploding capsules contain 2 small narrow seeds.

HABITAT & CULTIVATION Caraway grows wild in Europe, North Africa, and Asia. It prefers sunny sites up to 6,600 ft (2,000 m) above sea level. It is cultivated in Europe, Russia, North Africa, and the US, and the seeds are harvested ripe in late summer.

PARTS USED Seeds, essential oil.

CONSTITUENTS Caraway contains a volatile oil high in carvone (40–60%), flavonoids, polysaccharides, and a fixed oil.

HISTORY & FOLKLORE Caraway seed is "conducive to all the cold griefs of the head and stomach … and has a moderate quality whereby it breaketh wind, and provoketh urine" (Nicholas Culpeper, *The English Physitian*, 1652). The seeds are commonly used in cooking.

MEDICINAL ACTIONS & USES Caraway is similar in action to anise (*Pimpinella anisum*, p. 246) and fennel (*Foeniculum vulgare*, p. 210).

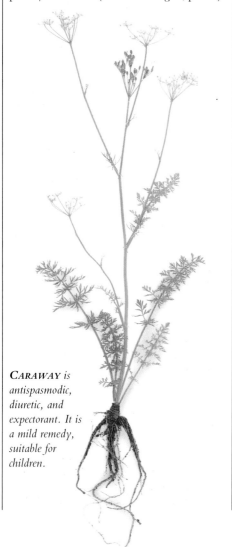

CARAWAY is antispasmodic, diuretic, and expectorant. It is a mild remedy, suitable for children.

Being antispasmodic and possessing carminative properties, the seeds soothe the digestive tract, acting directly on the intestinal muscles to relieve colic and cramps as well as all types of bloating and flatulence. They sweeten the breath, improve appetite, counter heart irregularity caused by excess digestive gas, and ease menstrual cramps. In addition, the seeds are diuretic, expectorant, and tonic, and are frequently used in bronchitis and cough remedies, especially those for children. Caraway has a reputation for increasing breast-milk production. The diluted essential oil is a useful remedy for scabies.

RESEARCH Caraway's beneficial effect on intestinal spasms and flatulence has been confirmed by research.

CAUTION Do not use the essential oil internally except under professional supervision.

Castanea sativa
(Fagaceae)
SWEET CHESTNUT

DESCRIPTION Deciduous tree growing to a height of 100 ft (30 m). Has smooth silver-gray bark, lance-shaped dark green leaves, male and female catkins, and spiny yellow-green seed cases containing 2 or 3 glossy brown nuts.

HABITAT & CULTIVATION Native to the Mediterranean, Asia Minor, and the Caucasus, sweet chestnut grows freely across Europe, including Britain. It is cultivated for its wood and for its nuts, which are collected in the autumn.

PARTS USED Leaves, bark.

CONSTITUENTS Sweet chestnut contains tannins, plastoquinones, and mucilage.

HISTORY & FOLKLORE Tradition has it that the sweet chestnut tree was carried from Turkey to Sardinia and from there it subsequently spread through Europe, arriving in Britain with the Romans. The nuts are a nutritious foodstuff that can be roasted, candied, or made into a flour. The flowers are sometimes added to blends of aromatic tobaccos.

MEDICINAL ACTIONS & USES An infusion of sweet chestnut leaves treats whooping cough, bronchitis, and bronchial congestion. The preparation tightens the mucous membranes and inhibits racking coughs. A decoction of leaves or bark is also valuable as a gargle for sore throats and may be taken for diarrhea. The leaves are also used to treat rheumatic conditions, lower back pain, and stiff joints or muscles.

RELATED SPECIES The Mohicans in North America used an infusion of American chestnut leaves (*C. dentata*) to treat whooping cough. In his *Natural History of North Carolina* (1737), John Brickell reported that the "leaves or bark of the tree boiled in wine are good against the bloody flux [excessive bleeding]."

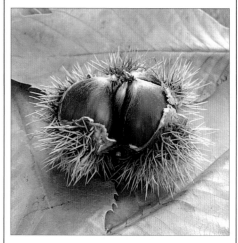

SWEET CHESTNUTS are a nutritious food, and the leaves are useful for treating coughs.

Catha edulis
(Celastraceae)
KHAT, CATHA

DESCRIPTION Tree growing to 50 ft (15 m). Has reddish twigs, oval leathery leaves, and small yellow or white flowers.

HABITAT & CULTIVATION Native to the Middle East and the Horn of Africa, khat prefers grassland and arid conditions. It is cultivated in Ethiopia, Somalia, East Africa, and the Arabian peninsula.

PARTS USED Leaves, twigs.

CONSTITUENTS Khat contains alkaloids similar to those in *Ephedra* species – norpseudoephedrine (up to 1%) and ephedrine, tannins, and a volatile oil. Ephedrine-type alkaloids strongly stimulate the central nervous system, are anti-allergenic, and suppress the appetite.

HISTORY & FOLKLORE Khat is taken in some African and Middle Eastern countries as a stimulant, tonic, and appetite suppressant. Infused, smoked, or chewed, khat produce an effect somewhat similar to that of coca leaves (*Erythroxylum coca*, p. 204). Whether khat is addictive is unclear, but withdrawal can produce lethargy.

MEDICINAL ACTIONS & USES Mainly used as a social drug, khat is also chewed fresh or taken in an infusion to treat ailments such as malaria. In Africa, it is taken in old age, stimulating and improving mental function. Khat is used in Germany to counter obesity.

CAUTIONS Khat may cause headaches, raised blood pressure, and general over-stimulation if used more than a few weeks at a time. Do not take during pregnancy.

Ceanothus americanus
(Rhamnaceae)
NEW JERSEY TEA

DESCRIPTION Deciduous shrub growing to about 5 ft (1.5 m). Has downy, oval, pale green leaves and clusters of white flowers.

HABITAT & CULTIVATION This herb is native to eastern North America. The root is harvested in spring, the leaves in summer.

PARTS USED Root, root bark, leaves.

CONSTITUENTS New Jersey tea contains tannins, alkaloids, resin, and a coagulant.

HISTORY & FOLKLORE New Jersey tea root and root bark were used extensively by Native Americans to treat fevers and problems of the mucous membranes such as congestion and sore throats. The Cherokee used a lotion made from the root to treat skin cancer. During the Revolutionary War, New Jersey tea leaves were brewed as a substitute for tea. The plant appears to encourage blood coagulation.

MEDICINAL ACTIONS & USES Being astringent, expectorant, and antispasmodic, New Jersey tea is used for sore throats, bronchitis, asthma, and coughs. Like other plants containing appreciable amounts of tannins, it has been employed to treat diarrhea and dysentery. It is also thought to be a sedative and to lower blood pressure.

RELATED SPECIES The Mexican *C. azurea* is a fever remedy.

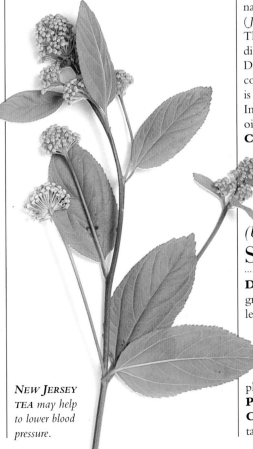

NEW JERSEY TEA may help to lower blood pressure.

Cedrus spp.
(Pinaceae)
CEDAR

DESCRIPTION Cedar of Lebanon (*C. libani*) is a majestic flat-topped tree growing to 130 ft (40 m). It has dark green needlelike leaves and oval cones. Himalayan cedar (*C. deodora*) grows to 280 ft (85 m).

HABITAT & CULTIVATION Cedar of Lebanon is native to mountain forests in Lebanon and southwest Turkey. Himalayan cedar is native to the Himalayan region, growing 3,500 to 12,000 ft (1,050–3,600 m) above sea level.

PARTS USED Leaves, wood, volatile oil.

CONSTITUENTS The volatile oil contains cedrene (50%), atlantol, and atlantone (*C. atlantica* only).

HISTORY & FOLKLORE The cedar of Lebanon was possibly used to build the Hanging Gardens of Babylon and Solomon's Temple. The oil has long been used in incense, perfumes, and embalming.

MEDICINAL ACTIONS & USES Cedar of Lebanon is an antiseptic and expectorant, acting to disinfect the respiratory tract. In Indian herbal medicine, Himalayan cedar leaves are used to treat tuberculosis. The heartwood is also given as a decoction for feverish chest ailments such as acute bronchitis, and for insomnia and diabetes. Cedarwood essential oil is generally distilled from the Atlas or African cedar (*C. atlantica*, native to Morocco) and the red cedar (*Juniperus virginia*, native to North America). The oil is strongly antiseptic, astringent, diuretic, an expectorant, and sedative. Diluted and massaged into the skin, it treats congestion, chest infections, and cystitis. It is also used to treat skin wounds and ulcers. In Ayurvedic medicine, cedarwood essential oil is prescribed for syphilis and leprosy.

CAUTION Do not take the essential oil internally except under professional supervision.

Celtis australis
(Ulmaceae)
SOUTHERN HACKBERRY

DESCRIPTION Dome-shaped deciduous tree growing to 80 ft (25 m). Has lance-shaped leaves, green flowers, and small round purple-black fruits.

HABITAT & CULTIVATION Southern hackberry is native to the Mediterranean region and southwestern Asia. It is also planted as a border tree in Italy and France.

PARTS USED Leaves, fruit.

CONSTITUENTS Southern hackberry contains tannins and mucilage.

HISTORY & FOLKLORE An ancient Egyptian recipe to make "scented ox fat" required 4 lb (2 kg) of hackberry seeds per 2 lb (1 kg) of ox fat. The fruit is edible (though rarely eaten today) and can be made into preserves.

MEDICINAL ACTIONS & USES Due to their astringent properties, both the leaves and fruit may be used as a remedy. Although the fruit is considered more effective, particularly before it has fully ripened, a decoction of both is taken to reduce heavy menstrual and intermenstrual uterine bleeding. The fruit and leaves may be used to astringe the mucous membranes in peptic ulcers, diarrhea, and dysentery.

Centaurea cyanus
(Compositae)
CORNFLOWER

DESCRIPTION Annual or biennial plant growing to 3 ft (90 cm). Has a multi-branched stem, a basal rosette of leaves, and sky-blue flowers in summer.

HABITAT & CULTIVATION Native to the Near East, cornflower grows wild in all temperate regions, often in cornfields. The flowers are gathered just after they open.

PARTS USED Flowers, seeds, leaves.

CONSTITUENTS Cornflower contains flavonoids, sesquiterpene lactones (including cnicin), acetylenes, and coumarins. Cnicin is slightly antibiotic.

HISTORY & FOLKLORE Cornflower's medicinal properties were first mentioned in the 12th-century writings of Hildegard of Bingen. Later, the herbalist Pierandrea Mattioli (1501–1577) recommended it on the basis of the Doctrine of Signatures, which held that a plant's appearance indicated the ailments it would cure. Cornflower's deep blue color symbolized healthy eyes – hence it became a treatment for eye ailments. (In France, the plant is called *casse-lunette*, or "break glasses.")

MEDICINAL ACTIONS & USES Cornflower is still used in French herbal medicine as a remedy for the eyes (the strained infusion is used as an eyewash, and the petals applied as a poultice), but opinion differs as to its efficacy. The petals are also taken as a bitter tonic and stimulant, improving digestion and possibly supporting the liver as well as improving resistance to infection. The seeds have been used as a mild laxative for children. A decoction of the leaves is used to treat rheumatic complaints.

RELATED SPECIES Greater knapweed (*C. scabiosa*) formed part of the medieval *salve*, an ointment applied to heal wounds and skin infections.

SELF-HELP USE Conjunctivitis, p. 310.

OTHER MEDICINAL PLANTS

Cephaelis ipecacuanha
(Rubiaceae)
IPECAC

DESCRIPTION Small shrub with a slender stem growing to 1 ft (30 cm). Has a few oblong leaves, small white flowers, and purple-black berries.

HABITAT & CULTIVATION This herb grows in South America, mainly Brazil. It prefers moist, shady woods. Cultivation has been attempted in Southeast Asia, but with limited success. The root of 3-year-old plants is unearthed when the plant is in flower, and is dried before use.

PARTS USED Root, rhizome.

CONSTITUENTS Ipecac contains isoquinoline alkaloids, tannins, and glycosides. The alkaloids are an expectorant and, at a larger dose, cause vomiting and diarrhea. They are also strongly amebicidal.

HISTORY & FOLKLORE Ipecac came to Europe in 1672 and achieved fame as a cure for dysentery. But the cure was not without controversy. It appeared to work well in some cases but to have no effect in others. Now it is possible to see why. There are two types of dysentery – amebic and bacillary. While the herb is strongly amebicidal, it has little effect against bacilli.

MEDICINAL ACTIONS & USES Ipecac is still used in both conventional and herbal medicine, and is listed in most national pharmacopoeias. One of the surest of emetics, even moderate doses will stimulate vomiting until the contents of the stomach are cleared – it is particularly useful for drug overdose. At a lower dose, ipecac is a strong expectorant. It is commonly found in many patent cough medicines, and is used in the treatment of bronchitis and whooping cough. Ipecac is also still used for amebic dysentery with good results.

CAUTIONS Do not use the root or rhizome. Take formulations containing ipecac carefully and only as instructed on the label. Several deaths have resulted from overdose.

Ceratonia siliqua
(Leguminosae)
CAROB

DESCRIPTION Evergreen tree growing to 30 ft (10 m). Has compound leaves, green flowers, and large violet-brown fruit (bean pods).

HABITAT & CULTIVATION Native to southeastern Europe, western Asia, and North Africa, carob flourishes in poor soil in warm temperate climates; it is said to "want sight of the sea." It is cultivated for its fruit, and harvested in late summer or autumn.

PARTS USED Fruit, bark.

CONSTITUENTS The fruit contains up to 70% sugars, fats, starch, proteins, vitamins, and tannins.

HISTORY & FOLKLORE In ancient Egypt, carob pods were combined with porridge, honey, and wax as a remedy for diarrhea. They also featured in recipes for expelling worms, and treating poor eyesight and eye infections. In the 1st century AD, the Greek physician Dioscorides wrote that carob acted to relieve stomach pain and settle the digestion. Carob was important in the rituals of the early Christian Church. Pulp from the pods has long been used as a sweet food and for making alcoholic drinks. As a flour, this pulp forms the basis of most cocoa-flavored drinks.

MEDICINAL ACTIONS & USES Carob pods are nutritious and, due to their high sugar content, sweet-tasting and mildly laxative. However, a decoction of the pulp is also

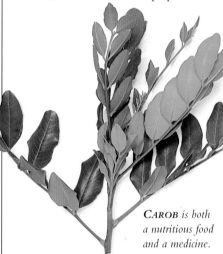

CAROB is both a nutritious food and a medicine.

antidiarrheal, gently helping to cleanse and relieve irritation within the gut. These appear to be contradictory effects, but carob is an example of how the body responds to herbal medicines in different ways, according to how the herb is prepared and according to the specific medical problem. The bark is strongly astringent, and a decoction of it is taken to treat diarrhea.

Cetraria islandica
(Parmeliaceae)
ICELAND MOSS

DESCRIPTION Yellow-green lichen growing in undulating, leathery tufts up to 3 in (8 cm) across.

HABITAT & CULTIVATION Iceland moss is native to northern and alpine areas of Europe. It flourishes in sub-Arctic and mountainous regions on rocks and on the bark of trees, especially conifers. It is harvested throughout the year.

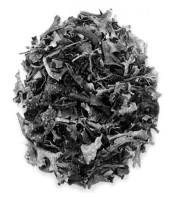

ICELAND MOSS is used to ease coughs and treat congestion. It also has a soothing and bitter tonic effect on the digestive tract.

PART USED Whole plant.

CONSTITUENTS Iceland moss contains lichen acids (including usnic acid), and about 50% polysaccharides. Usnic acid and the other lichen acids are powerful antibiotics.

HISTORY & FOLKLORE Iceland moss has been used since ancient times as a cough remedy, and has also been used in European folk medicine as a cancer treatment.

MEDICINAL ACTIONS & USES Strongly demulcent, Iceland moss soothes the mucous membranes of the chest, counters congestion, and calms dry and paroxysmal coughs, being particularly helpful as a treatment for elderly people. Iceland moss is also very bitter and, within the gut, has both a demulcent and bitter tonic effect – a combination almost unique in medicinal herbs. It is thus of value in all kinds of chronic digestive problems – for instance, irritable bowel syndrome. Iceland moss also gently expels worms, and, in view of recent European research, could prove useful for certain digestive infections.

SELF-HELP USE Acidity & indigestion, p. 307.

Chamaemelum nobile
syn. Anthemis nobilis
(Compositae)
ROMAN CHAMOMILE

DESCRIPTION Aromatic perennial growing to 20 in (50 cm). Has feathery leaves and daisylike flower heads.

HABITAT & CULTIVATION Native to western Europe, chamomile is now cultivated across Europe and also in other temperate regions. The flowers are harvested as they open in summer.

PARTS USED Flowers, essential oil.

CONSTITUENTS Roman chamomile contains up to 1.75% volatile oil (including tiglic and angelic acid esters and chamazulene), sesquiterpene lactones, flavonoids, coumarins, and phenolic acids.

HISTORY & FOLKLORE Roman chamomile has long been valued as a medicinal plant in Britain. Although called Roman chamomile, this herb was not cultivated in Rome until the 16th century, probably arriving there from Britain.

MEDICINAL ACTIONS & USES A remedy for the digestive system, Roman chamomile is often used interchangeably with German chamomile (*Chamomilla recutita*, p. 76). However, an infusion of Roman chamomile has a more pronounced bitter action than its German namesake. It is an excellent treatment for nausea, vomiting, indigestion, and loss of appetite. It is also sedative, antispasmodic and mildly analgesic, and will relieve colic, cramps, and other cramping pains. By stimulating digestive secretions and relaxing the muscles of the gut, it helps normalize digestive function. Roman chamomile may also be taken for headaches and migraine, even by children. Its anti-inflammatory and antiallergenic properties make it helpful for irritated skin.

Dried flower heads

CAUTIONS Do not use the essential oil internally except under professional supervision. The essential oil is subject to legal restrictions in some countries.

Chamaenerion angustifolia syn. *Epilobium angustifolium* (Onagraceae)
ROSEBAY WILLOWHERB

DESCRIPTION Perennial growing to 6 ft (2 m). Has an erect stem, narrow leaves, and long spikes of pink-purple flowers.
HABITAT & CULTIVATION This herb is found in Europe and western Asia, and grows in clearings, along roadsides, and in open areas. It is picked when in flower in late summer.
PARTS USED Aerial parts.
CONSTITUENTS Rosebay willowherb contains flavones and tannins.
HISTORY & FOLKLORE The leaves of rosebay willowherb were taken in Europe as an astringent tea. In Siberia, an alcoholic drink has been made from this herb and the fly agaric mushroom (*Amanita muscaria*).
MEDICINAL ACTIONS & USES Demulcent and astringent, rosebay willowherb treats diarrhea, mucous colitis, and irritable bowel syndrome. It has also been made into an ointment to soothe skin problems in children. Rosebay willowherb has been used in Germany and Austria to treat prostate problems.

Cheiranthus cheiri (Cruciferae)
WALLFLOWER

DESCRIPTION Evergreen perennial growing to 18 in (45 cm). Has lance-shaped leaves and yellow-orange flowers appearing in spring.
HABITAT & CULTIVATION Native to southern Europe, wallflower is now found throughout the continent. It grows on cliffs and old walls, and is a common garden plant.
PARTS USED Leaves, flowers.
CONSTITUENTS The herb contains cheiranthin and other cardioactive glycosides.
HISTORY & FOLKLORE In 1735, the Irish herbalist K'Eogh described wallflower thus: "It provokes urination and menstruation and expels a stillborn child, and the afterbirth if a decoction of the dried flowers or a little seed is drunk in wine."
MEDICINAL ACTIONS & USES Although wallflower was formerly used as a diuretic, there was no understanding of its powerful effect on the heart. In small doses it is cardiotonic, supporting a failing heart in a manner similar to foxglove (*Digitalis purpurea*, p. 199). In more than small doses it is toxic, and is therefore rarely used.
CAUTIONS Use only under professional supervision. Do not take during pregnancy.

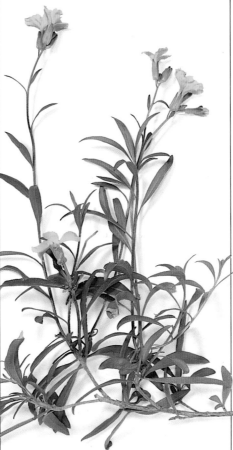

THE GREEK PHYSICIAN DIOSCORIDES (1st century AD) used wallflower roots to treat gout.

Chelidonium majus (Papaveraceae)
GREATER CELANDINE

DESCRIPTION Thin-stemmed perennial herb growing to a height of 3 ft (90 cm). Has indented yellow-green leaflets and 4-petaled flowers, which appear in clusters in late spring.
HABITAT & CULTIVATION Native to Europe, western Asia, and North Africa, greater celandine flourishes close to human habitation, preferring open areas, the banks of roadsides, and damp places. The aerial parts of the herb are collected in late spring or early summer.
PARTS USED Aerial parts, latex.
CONSTITUENTS Greater celandine contains isoquinoline alkaloids, including allocryptopine, berberine, chelidonine, and sparteine. Several of these alkaloids are analgesic. Chelidonine is antispasmodic and also lowers blood pressure. Sparteine, by contrast, raises it.
HISTORY & FOLKLORE In folk medicine, greater celandine has often been viewed as a cure-all. It has also been used for thousands of years to treat and clear the eyesight, especially for the removal of cataracts. According to Pliny and Dioscorides (both 1st century AD), swallows used the latex that flows from cuts in the stems or leaves as a means to sharpen their eyesight. In the 17th century, the herbalist Nicholas Culpeper tested this ancient belief by putting the latex into the eyes of young swallows to see if it would improve their eyesight.
MEDICINAL ACTIONS & USES Greater celandine acts as a mild sedative, relaxing the muscles of the bronchial tubes, intestines, and other organs. In both Western and Chinese herbal traditions, it has been used to treat bronchitis, whooping cough, and asthma. The herb's antispasmodic effect also extends to the gallbladder, where it helps to improve bile flow. This would partly account for its use in treating jaundice, gallstones, and gallbladder pain, as well as its longstanding reputation as a detoxifying herb. Greater celandine's sedative action does not, however, extend to the uterus – it causes the muscles of this organ to contract. The herb is applied externally to soothe and encourage the healing of conditions such as eczema. The latex of greater celandine is applied to warts, ringworm, and malignant skin tumors, which are slowly broken down by the effect of its protein-dissolving enzymes.
CAUTIONS Use only under professional supervision. Do not take greater celandine during pregnancy. The plant is subject to legal restrictions in some countries.

Chelone glabra
(Scrophulariaceae)

BALMONY

DESCRIPTION Perennial herb growing to 2 ft (60 cm). Has oblong leaves and short spikes of creamy white to purple double-lipped flowers.

HABITAT & CULTIVATION Native to eastern North America, balmony thrives in marshland, wet woodland, and on riverbanks. It is grown from seed in spring and is harvested when in flower in summer or fall.

PARTS USED Aerial parts.

CONSTITUENTS Balmony contains resins and bitters.

HISTORY & FOLKLORE Balmony's genus name, *Chelone*, means "tortoise" in Greek, referring to the flower head's supposed resemblance to the head of the tortoise.

MEDICINAL ACTIONS & USES A strongly bitter remedy, balmony is mainly used to treat gallstones and other gallbladder problems. It stimulates bile flow and has a mildly laxative action. It can relieve nausea and vomiting, intestinal colic, and expel worms, and may also be an antidepressant. Balmony is a suitable remedy for children.

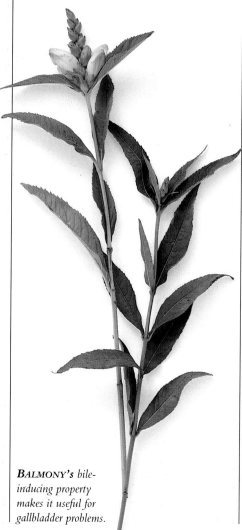

BALMONY's bile-inducing property makes it useful for gallbladder problems.

186

Chenopodium ambrosioides
(Chenopodiaceae)

WORMSEED

DESCRIPTION Annual herb growing to 3 ft (1 m) with toothed lance-shaped leaves. Yellow-green flowers in round clusters bloom in summer, producing small black seeds in autumn.

HABITAT & CULTIVATION Wormseed is native to Central and South America and the Caribbean. It has been extensively cultivated in the US – in Maryland. It is also grown in China.

PARTS USED Aerial parts, flowering tops.

CONSTITUENTS Wormseed contains a volatile oil (up to 90% ascaridol, plus geraniol and methyl salicylate) and triterpenoid saponins. Ascaridol is a powerful worm expellent.

HISTORY & FOLKLORE An herbal remedy that has been used for centuries, wormseed was used by the Maya tribe in Central America to expel worms. By the middle of the 18th century, medicinal use of the plant was firmly established in the eastern US – European settlers using it for the treatment of worms, especially in children. The Catawba made a poultice from the plant, which they used to detoxify snake bite and other poisonings.

MEDICINAL ACTIONS & USES Wormseed is principally known for its ability to expel worms, especially roundworms and hookworms. However, it also used in the Americas as a digestive remedy, being generally taken to settle colic and stomach pains. Wormseed leaves have antispasmodic properties. A decoction of the leaves or of the whole plant brings relief to a variety of gastrointestinal problems. Its muscle-relaxing action has led to its use in the treatment of spasmodic coughs and asthma. The plant also has external uses. Juice expressed from the whole herb is applied as a wash for hemorrhoids. In addition, the whole plant is thought to have wound-healing properties.

RELATED SPECIES Many species of *Chenopodium* are used as foods, and some medicinally. *C. quinoa* produces quinoa grain, eaten principally in Chile, Bolivia, and Peru, and now increasingly consumed elsewhere around the world. The seeds of *C. rhadinostachyum* are used as food by Aboriginal peoples in central Australia. Good King Henry (*C. bonus-henricus*), a species that is native to Europe, is both eaten as a vegetable and used medicinally to treat anemia.

CAUTIONS Use only under professional supervision. Wormseed is toxic in overdose. Do not take during pregnancy. The herb is subject to legal restrictions in some countries.

Chimaphila umbellata
(Ericaceae)

PIPSISSEWA

DESCRIPTION Evergreen plant with several stems, growing to 8 in (20 cm). Has shiny wedge-shaped leaves and small flat-topped clusters of white flowers tinged with red.

HABITAT & CULTIVATION Native to North America, Europe, and Asia, pipsissewa grows in woods and shady places, in sandy soils. The leaves are gathered in summer.

PARTS USED Leaves.

CONSTITUENTS Pipsissewa contains hydroquinones (including arbutin), flavonoids, triterpenes, methyl salicylate, and tannins. The hydroquinones have a pronounced disinfectant effect within the urinary tract.

HISTORY & FOLKLORE Pipsissewa was much used by Native North Americans to induce sweating and treat fevers, including typhus. European settlers used the herb for rheumatism and for urinary and kidney problems. It was listed in the *Pharmacopoeia of the United States* from 1820 to 1916.

MEDICINAL ACTIONS & USES Astringent, tonic, and diuretic, pipsissewa is mainly used in an infusion for urinary tract problems such as cystitis and urethritis. It has also been prescribed for more serious conditions such as gonorrhea and kidney stones. By increasing urine flow, it stimulates the removal of waste products from the body, and is therefore of benefit in treating rheumatism and gout. The fresh leaves may be applied externally to rheumatic joints or muscles, as well as to blisters, sores, and swellings.

RESEARCH In tests on animals, pipsissewa leaves appear to lower blood sugar levels.

Chionanthus virginicus
(Oleaceae)

FRINGE TREE

DESCRIPTION Deciduous shrub or tree growing to 30 ft (10 m). Has elliptical dark green leaves and long flowering stems with spikes of white flowers. Produces dark blue oval fruits.

HABITAT & CULTIVATION Native to the US, fringe tree grows from Pennsylvania south to Florida and Texas. It is also now found in eastern Asia, and thrives on riverbanks and in damp shrubby areas. The root is unearthed in spring or autumn, mostly in Virginia and North Carolina.

PARTS USED Root bark, bark.

CONSTITUENTS Fringe tree contains a saponin (chionanthin) and a glycoside (phyllirine).

HISTORY & FOLKLORE Fringe tree was commonly used by Native Americans and European settlers alike to treat inflammations of the eye, canker sores, and spongy gums. The Choctaw of Louisiana applied the mashed bark to cuts and bruises. Native Americans in Alabama used the bark as a treatment for toothache. In the 19th-century Anglo-American Physiomedicalist tradition, fringe tree was valued as a bitter tonic, and the bark was often used to aid recovery from long-term illness.

MEDICINAL ACTIONS & USES The root bark is a liver tonic, stimulates bile flow, and acts as a mild laxative. It is prescribed mainly for gallbladder pain, gallstones, jaundice, and chronic weakness. Although it appears to be beneficial to liver and gallbladder function, there is as yet no research to substantiate its effects. The root bark also appears to strengthen function in the pancreas and spleen. Anecdotal evidence indicates that it may substantially reduce sugar levels in the urine. Fringe tree also stimulates the appetite and digestion, and is an excellent remedy for chronic illness, especially where the liver has been affected. For external use, the crushed bark may be made into a poultice for treating sores and wounds.

Chondrodendron tomentosum
(*Menispermaceae*)
PAREIRA

DESCRIPTION Vine climbing to a great height in tropical rainforests. Reaches 100 ft (30 m). Has large leaves up to 1 ft (30 cm) long, and trailing clusters of flowers.

HABITAT & CULTIVATION Pareira grows wild in rainforests in the upper Amazon region and in Panama. It is collected from the wild as available.

PARTS USED Root, stem.

CONSTITUENTS Pareira contains alkaloids, including delta-tubocurarine and L-curarine. Tubocurarine is a potent muscle relaxant.

HISTORY & FOLKLORE Pareira and similar species are famous for being the source of curare, the paralyzing arrow poison used by Amazonian and other South American Indians to catch their prey. A dart or spear tipped with curare causes instantaneous paralysis on entering the bloodstream of the animal. Traditional recipes for toxins usually involve blending 10 or more different plants, but pareira or a plant with similar action is always present in the mix.

MEDICINAL ACTIONS & USES Pareira's notoriety as a poison hinges on the effect of its toxic derivative entering directly into the bloodstream. Provided there are no cuts or sores in the mouth, the plant is reasonably safe taken orally as a medicinal remedy. The bitter and slightly sweet-tasting roots and stems are mildly laxative, tonic, and diuretic, and also act to induce menstruation. The plant is chiefly used to relieve chronic inflammation of the urinary tubules.

In Brazil, it is also used for snake bite, for which an infusion of the root is taken internally while the bruised leaves are applied externally.

RESEARCH Pareira's powerful ability to paralyze has led to its being extensively researched, and it has been adopted by Western medicine. Tubocurarine – one of the many alkaloids within the plant – is now used (as tubocurarine chloride) to paralyze the body's muscles during operations.

RELATED SPECIES At least four other closely related species of *Chondrodendron* are used to produce the traditional poison curare. In Guyana, Venezuela, and Colombia, *Strychnos* species are used as a source of the toxin.

CAUTIONS Use only under professional supervision. Pareira and/or curare are subject to legal restrictions in some countries.

Chondrus crispus
(*Gigartinaceae*)
IRISH MOSS, CARRAGHEEN

DESCRIPTION Reddish brown seaweed growing to 10 in (25 cm). Plant body is flat and forked, with a fan-shaped outline.

HABITAT & CULTIVATION Irish moss is found on the Atlantic coasts of Europe and North America. It grows just below the waterline, attached to rocks and stones. In summer in North America and in the fall in Ireland, it is pulled up by hand or with a rake at low tide and dried in the sun.

PART USED Whole herb.

CONSTITUENTS Irish moss contains large amounts of polysaccharides, proteins (up to 10%), amino acids, iodine, and bromine. The polysaccharides become jellylike and demulcent when the plant is immersed in water.

HISTORY & FOLKLORE Irish moss is used extensively in the food and pharmaceutical industries as an emulsifying and binding agent – for example, in toothpastes.

MEDICINAL ACTIONS & USES A useful demulcent and emollient, Irish moss is mainly taken for coughs and bronchitis. Its expectorant effect encourages the coughing up of phlegm, and it soothes dry and irritated mucous membranes. It is of value for acid indigestion, gastritis, and urinary infections such as cystitis. For these conditions it is normally combined with other appropriate herbs. Mucilaginous in texture and slightly salty in taste, Irish moss makes a valuable nutrient in convalescence. Applied externally, this emollient herb soothes inflamed skin. Irish moss also acts to thin the blood.

CAUTION Due to its blood-thinning property, Irish moss should not be used by people taking anticoagulant medicines.

Cichorium intybus
(*Compositae*)
CHICORY

DESCRIPTION Deep-rooted perennial growing to 5 ft (1.5 m). Has a hairy stem, oblong leaves, and blue flowers.

HABITAT & CULTIVATION Native to Europe, chicory also grows in North Africa and western Asia. It flourishes along paths and roadsides, on banks, and in dry fields. The root is unearthed in spring or autumn.

PARTS USED Root, leaves, flowers.

CONSTITUENTS The root contains up to 58% inulin and sesquiterpene lactones, as well as vitamins and minerals.

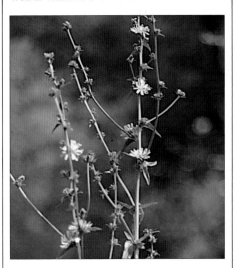

CHICORY leaves make a settling digestive tea.

HISTORY & FOLKLORE According to Pliny (AD 23–79), chicory juice was mixed with rose oil and vinegar as a remedy for headaches. The roasted root is commonly used as a coffee substitute. The young root can be boiled and eaten like parsnips.

MEDICINAL ACTIONS & USES Chicory is an excellent mild, bitter tonic for the liver and digestive tract. The root is therapeutically similar to dandelion root (*Taraxacum officinale*, p. 140), supporting the action of the stomach and liver and cleansing the urinary tract. Chicory is also taken for rheumatic conditions and gout, and as a mild laxative, one particularly appropriate for children. An infusion of the leaves and flowers also aids the digestion.

RELATED SPECIES The endive (*C. endiva*), has similar though milder effects.

Cnicus benedictus
syn. *Carbenia benedicta*
Carduus benedictus
(Compositae)
HOLY THISTLE

DESCRIPTION Erect, red-stemmed annual growing to 26 in (65 cm). Has spiny leathery leaves, a spiny stem, and yellow flowers in summer and autumn.

HABITAT & CULTIVATION This Mediterranean plant flourishes on dry stony ground and in open areas. The leaves and flowering tops are collected in summer.

PARTS USED Leaves, flowering tops.

CONSTITUENTS Holy thistle contains lignans, sesquiterpene lactones (including cnicin), volatile oil, polyacetylenes,

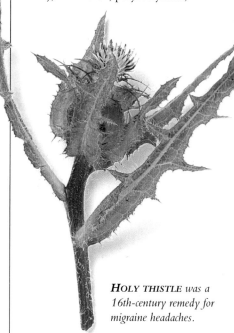

HOLY THISTLE was a 16th-century remedy for migraine headaches.

flavonoids, triterpenes, phytosterols, and tannins. Cnicin is bitter, anti-inflammatory, and antibiotic.

HISTORY & FOLKLORE Holy thistle was esteemed as a medicine in the Middle Ages, and was even thought capable of curing the plague. In his herbal of 1568, Nicholas Turner wrote: "There is nothing better for the canker [ulcerous sore] and old rotten and festering sores than the leaves, juice, broth, powder and water of holy thistle."

MEDICINAL ACTIONS & USES Holy thistle is a good bitter tonic, stimulating the secretions of the stomach, intestines, and gallbladder. It is taken for minor digestive complaints. It has also been a treatment for intermittent fevers. Holy thistle is mildly expectorant and is also antibiotic. It makes a healing balm for wounds and sores.

CAUTIONS In excessive doses, holy thistle may cause vomiting. It is subject to legal restrictions in some countries.

Cnidium monnieri
(Umbelliferae)
SHE CHUANG ZI

DESCRIPTION Upright plant typical of the carrot family. Has ridged stem, compound leaves, and clusters of flowers.

HABITAT & CULTIVATION *She chuang zi* is cultivated in China.

PARTS USED Seeds, essential oil.

CONSTITUENTS The volatile oil of *she chuang zi* contains pinene, camphene, bornyl isovalerate, and isoborneol.

HISTORY & FOLKLORE *She chuang zi* is first mentioned in the Chinese tradition in the *Divine Husbandman's Classic (Shen'nong Bencaojing)* in the 1st century AD. In the *Bencao Gangmu* by Li Shizhen (1564), the herb is classified in the same order of "sweet-smelling" plants as Chinese angelica (*Angelica sinensis*, p. 60) and *Ligusticum wallichii*, a lovage species.

MEDICINAL ACTIONS & USES The seeds of *she chuang zi* appear to have an antifungal action. *She chuang zi* is most often prescribed externally as a lotion, powder, or ointment for skin conditions such as eczema, ringworm, and scabies. The seeds are considered particularly helpful for problems affecting the genital area – for example vaginitis and vaginal discharge. *She chuang zi* is also taken internally for impotence, and infertility in both men and women, often combined with schisandra (*Schisandra chinensis*, p. 132).

RESEARCH Clinical research in China indicates that *she chuang zi* is indeed helpful in treating trichomonal vaginitis.

CAUTION Do not take the essential oil internally except under professional supervision.

Cochlearia officinalis
(Cruciferae)
SCURVY GRASS

DESCRIPTION Low-growing perennial with fleshy heart-shaped leaves, dense clusters of white 4-petaled flowers, and rounded swollen seedpods.

HABITAT & CULTIVATION Native to Europe and temperate regions of Asia and North America, but now rare, scurvy grass thrives in the salty soil of coastal areas and salt marshes. It is occasionally cultivated.

PARTS USED Leaves, aerial parts.

CONSTITUENTS Scurvy grass contains glucosilinates, a volatile oil, a bitter principle, tannin, vitamin C, and minerals.

HISTORY & FOLKLORE As the common name suggests, this plant has long been used for its high vitamin C content. It was used by sailors and others to prevent the onset of scurvy, a potentially fatal vitamin C deficiency marked by bleeding of the gums. The English physician Robert Turner, writing in the 17th century, recommended scurvy grass taken in ale as a remedy for a range of conditions, including "ague." Prior to the discovery of vitamins, the effectiveness of the plant in preventing scurvy was ascribed to its volatile oil.

MEDICINAL ACTIONS & USES Besides having a high vitamin C content, scurvy grass has antiseptic and mild laxative actions. The young plant, which has a general detoxicant effect and contains a wide range of minerals, is taken as a spring tonic. Like watercress (*Nasturtium officinale*, p. 237), it has diuretic properties and is useful for any condition in which poor nutrition is a factor. It can be used in the form of a juice as an antiseptic mouthwash for canker sores, and can also be applied externally to spots and pimples.

Coffea arabica
(Rubiaceae)
COFFEE

DESCRIPTION Evergreen shrub or small tree growing to 28 ft (9 m). Has dark green, shiny oval leaves and white star-shaped flowers. Produces small red fruit, each containing two seeds (beans).

HABITAT & CULTIVATION Native to tropical East Africa, coffee is now cultivated in tropical areas worldwide. The best-quality beans are produced by fermenting, sun-drying, and roasting the seeds.

PARTS USED Seeds.

CONSTITUENTS Coffee contains 0.06–0.32% caffeine, theobromine and theophylline, and tannins. Caffeine is strongly stimulant. Theophylline is stimulant and relaxes smooth muscle.

HISTORY & FOLKLORE Coffee has been drunk for approximately 1,000 years. The practice allegedly began after the Arab mullah Schadelih met a goatherd whose flock was jumping around in an excited fashion. When asked to explain their behavior, the goatherd told the mullah that the animals grew agitated every time they grazed on the leaves and fruit of the coffee bush. Schadelih then ate some of the fruit and immediately felt more alert. Later, he accidentally burned some beans. Their excellent flavor convinced him to continue to prepare them in this way in the future.

MEDICINAL ACTIONS & USES Although it is not often recognized as a medicinal herb, coffee is highly effective when taken as a general stimulant, having a particular effect on the central nervous system, temporarily improving perception and physical performance. Coffee increases heart output, stimulates digestive juices, and is a powerful diuretic. It can help in headaches and migraine. Coffee's active constituent, caffeine, is often combined with conventional

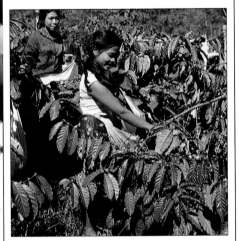

COFFEE, native to East Africa, is an important remedy for headaches.

analgesics in over-the-counter headache remedies. In Ayurvedic medicine, the unripe beans are used for headaches, and the ripe, roasted beans for diarrhea. Coffee enemas effectively cleanse the large bowel.

CAUTIONS Herbalists consider that coffee should be avoided by those prone to acid indigestion, diarrhea, high blood pressure, or palpitations. It is a short-term stimulant and in the long term is thought to weaken vitality. It should not be taken in excess as it can provoke insomnia.

Cola acuminata
(Sterculiaceae)
KOLA NUT, COLA NUT

DESCRIPTION Evergreen tree growing to 70 ft (20 m) with dark green leaves and yellowish white flowers. Large woody seed pods contain 5–10 white or red seeds (nuts).
HABITAT & CULTIVATION Native to West Africa, kola nut is cultivated widely in the tropics, especially in Nigeria, Brazil, and the West Indies. The seeds are harvested when ripe and dried in the sun.
PARTS USED Seeds.
CONSTITUENTS Kola nut contains up to 2.5% caffeine (generally higher than coffee), theobromine, tannins, phlobaphene, and an anthocyanin.
HISTORY & FOLKLORE Chewed for their digestive, tonic, and aphrodisiac properties, kola nuts have been an integral part of western and central African life for thousands of years. The plant is cultivated extensively in the West Indies and was probably first grown there by African slaves who had

managed to bring seeds with them across the Atlantic. Kola nuts are used in huge quantities today to flavor soft drinks.
MEDICINAL ACTIONS & USES Kola nut stimulates the central nervous system and the body as a whole. It increases alertness and muscular strength, counters lethargy, and has been used extensively both in western African and Anglo-American herbal medicine as an antidepressant, particularly during recovery from chronic illness. Like coffee (*Coffea arabica, see preceding entry*), kola is used to treat headaches and migraine. It is diuretic and astringent, and may be taken for diarrhea and dysentery.
RELATED SPECIES *C. nitida*, growing in Africa, Brazil, and the West Indies, is used in a similar fashion.
CAUTION Do not take if suffering from high blood pressure, peptic ulcers, or palpitations.

Colchicum autumnale
(Liliaceae)
MEADOW SAFFRON

DESCRIPTION Attractive perennial growing from bulblike corm to 4 in (10 cm). Has pointed lance-shaped leaves and tubular 6-petaled pink flowers in autumn.

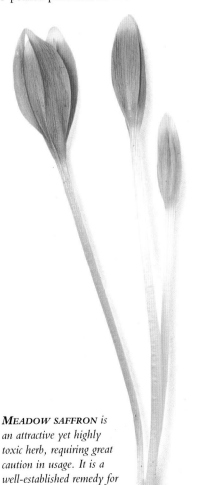

MEADOW SAFFRON is an attractive yet highly toxic herb, requiring great caution in usage. It is a well-established remedy for treating gout.

HABITAT & CULTIVATION Common in Europe and North Africa, meadow saffron grows wild in woods and damp meadows. It is also cultivated. The corm is gathered in early summer, the seeds in late summer.
PARTS USED Corm, seeds.
CONSTITUENTS Meadow saffron contains alkaloids (including colchicine) and flavonoids. Colchicine is anti-inflammatory and is used in conventional medicine for acute attacks of gout. As it affects cell division, it can cause fetal abnormality. Colchicine has been used in the laboratory to create new genetic strains.
HISTORY & FOLKLORE Meadow saffron was not used in classical times due to its poisonous nature. Arabian physicians used it in the Middle Ages to treat joint pain and gout, but otherwise herbalists disregarded the plant until the 19th century.
MEDICINAL ACTIONS & USES Despite its toxicity, meadow saffron is considered one of the best remedies for acute gout pain. Leukemia has been successfully treated with meadow saffron, and the plant has also been used with some success to treat Behçet's syndrome, a chronic disease marked by recurring ulcers and leukemia. Taken internally, the herb has significant side effects even at low dosage. Externally, it is applied to relieve neuralgia and itchiness.
CAUTIONS This herb is highly toxic. Use only under professional supervision. Do not use during pregnancy. Meadow saffron is subject to legal restrictions in some countries.

Collinsonia canadensis
(Labiatae)
STONE ROOT

DESCRIPTION Perennial herb growing to 3 ft (1 m). Has a square stem, oval leaves, and clusters of greenish yellow flowers.
HABITAT & CULTIVATION This herb is native to moist woodlands of eastern North America. The root is dug up in autumn.
PARTS USED Root, leaves.
CONSTITUENTS Stone root contains a volatile oil, tannins, and saponins.
MEDICINAL ACTIONS & USES Diuretic and tonic, stone root is chiefly employed in the treatment of kidney stones. It is also prescribed to counteract fluid retention. It has been used to reduce back pressure in the veins, which in turn helps prevent the formation or worsening of hemorrhoids and varicose veins. As an astringent, stone root contracts the inner lining of the intestines, and can be helpful in treating digestive system disorders such as irritable bowel syndrome and mucous colitis. The fresh leaves or roots of stone root are used as a poultice for bruises, cuts, and sores.

191

Conium maculatum
(Umbelliferae)
HEMLOCK

DESCRIPTION Graceful biennial growing to 8 ft (2.5 m). Has slender, red-speckled stems, finely divided leaves, small clusters of white flowers, and small seeds that have beaded ridges.

HABITAT & CULTIVATION Commonly found in Europe, hemlock also grows in temperate regions of Asia and North America. It flourishes in damp meadows, on riverbanks, and in open areas. The seeds are gathered when almost ripe in summer.

PARTS USED Leaves, seeds.

CONSTITUENTS Hemlock contains alkaloids, mainly coniine, and a volatile oil. Coniine is extremely toxic and causes congenital deformities.

HISTORY & FOLKLORE Hemlock is notorious as the poison used as a capital punishment in ancient Greece. The Greek philosopher Socrates died in 399 BC after drinking hemlock juice. According to an old English tradition, the stems took their color in sympathy with the mark placed on Cain's forehead after he murdered Abel. Dioscorides (AD 40–90) recommended applying the mashed plant or juice to tumors and ulcers, and to the genitals in cases of priapism (continual painful erection of the penis). In the 19th century, hemlock was used as a painkiller.

MEDICINAL ACTIONS & USES In extremely small quantities, hemlock is sedative and analgesic; in larger doses it causes paralysis and death. Rarely used today, it has been prescribed in the past as a treatment for epilepsy, Parkinson's disease, and Sydenham's chorea. Hemlock has also been used to treat acute cystitis.

CAUTIONS Deadly poison at the wrong dosage. Do not take internally. Use externally only under professional supervision. Hemlock is subject to legal restrictions in some countries.

Convallaria majalis
(Liliaceae)
LILY OF THE VALLEY

DESCRIPTION Attractive perennial growing to 9 in (23 cm). Has a pair of elliptical leaves, clusters of bell-shaped white flowers on one side of the stem, and red berries.

HABITAT & CULTIVATION Native to Europe, this herb is also distributed over North America and northern Asia. It is widely cultivated as a garden plant. The leaves and flowers are gathered in late spring as the plant comes into flower.

PARTS USED Leaves, flowers.

CONSTITUENTS Lily of the valley contains cardiac glycosides, including the cardenolides convallotoxin, convalloside, convallatoxol, and others, and flavonoid glycosides. The cardiac glycosides act to strengthen a weakened heart.

HISTORY & FOLKLORE The 2nd-century AD herbalist Apuleius recorded that Apollo gave lily of the valley as a gift to Aesculapius, the god of healing. In the 16th century, the herbalist John Gerard had this to say about its therapeutic value: "The flowers of the valley lillie distilled with wine, and drunke to the quantitie of a spoonful, restore speech unto those that have the dumb palsie and that are fallen into apoplexy, and are good against the gout, and comfort the heart."

MEDICINAL ACTIONS & USES Lily of the valley is used by European herbalists in place of common foxglove (*Digitalis purpurea*, p. 199). Both herbs have a profound effect in heart failure, whether due in the long term to a cardio-vascular problem or to a chronic lung problem such as emphysema. Lily of the valley encourages the heart to beat more slowly, regularly and efficiently. It is also strongly diuretic, reducing blood volume and lowering blood pressure. It is better tolerated than foxglove, since it does not accumulate within the body to the same degree. Relatively low doses are required to support heart rate and rhythm, and to increase urine production.

CAUTIONS Use only under professional supervision. Lily of the valley is subject to legal restrictions in some countries.

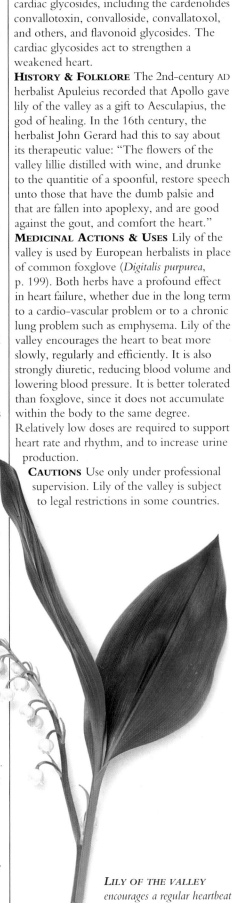

LILY OF THE VALLEY encourages a regular heartbeat and acts as a strong diuretic.

Copaifera spp.
(Leguminosae)
COPAIBA

DESCRIPTION Evergreen trees growing to 60 ft (18 m). Have compound leaves and small yellow flowers.

HABITAT & CULTIVATION Copaiba is native to tropical South America and also found in southern Africa. Holes drilled in the trunk yield oleo-resin, a blend of volatile oil and resin.

PART USED Oleo-resin.

CONSTITUENTS The oleo-resin contains a volatile oil (30–90%) containing alpha- and beta-caryophyllene, sesquiterpenes, resins, and terpenic acids.

HISTORY & FOLKLORE Copaiba was used by native Brazilians long before the arrival of Europeans. In 1625, the Portuguese monk Manoel Tristaon observed that it was employed to heal wounds and remove scars.

MEDICINAL ACTIONS & USES Antiseptic, diuretic, and stimulant, copaiba is still taken extensively in Brazil. Its primary use is to counter mucus in the chest and genitourinary system. It also irritates the mucous membranes and promotes the coughing up of mucus. A solution or tincture of copaiba is taken for bronchitis, chronic cystitis, diarrhea, and hemorrhoids. It has been frequently used in the past to treat gonorrhea. Eczema and other skin diseases reportedly benefit from its application.

RELATED SPECIES Several of the 40 *Copaifera* species yield the medicinal oleo-resin. *C. lansdorfii* is one of the main sources, but *C. coriacea, C. multijuga, C. officinalis,* and *C. reticulata* are tapped as well. In Zimbabwe, a decoction of *C. mopane* is inhaled for temporary insanity.

CAUTIONS Copaiba is toxic in overdose. Use only under professional supervision.

Coptis chinensis
(Ranunculaceae)
HUANG LIAN (CHINESE),
CHINESE GOLDTHREAD

DESCRIPTION Perennial herb growing to 20 in (50 cm). Has basal leaves and small whitish green flowers.

HABITAT & CULTIVATION This herb is native to the mountains of China and is most commonly cultivated in Szechwan province. The root is dug up in autumn.

PART USED Root.

CONSTITUENTS Contains isoquiniline alkaloids, including berberine, coptisine, and worenine. Berberine is antibacterial, amebicidal, and antidiarrheal.

MEDICINAL ACTIONS & USES A bitter-tasting herb, *huang lian* is given in the Chinese herbal tradition as a decoction to "clear heat" and "dry dampness," relieving fever, red and sore eyes, and sore throats. The herb is particularly helpful for diarrhea and dysentery, and has been used to quell vomiting. Skin problems such as acne, boils, abscesses, and burns are also treated with *huang lian*. Like the root of goldthread (*C. trifolia, see following entry*), *huang lian* is taken as a gargle for canker sores and tongue ulcers, and for swollen gums and toothache. Both herbs are also used as an eyewash to treat acute conjunctivitis.

RESEARCH In a Chinese trial, 30 patients with tuberculosis were given *huang lian*, and all of them showed marked improvement in their symptoms.

CAUTION Use only under professional supervision. Do not take during pregnancy.

Coptis trifolia
(Ranunculaceae)
GOLDTHREAD

DESCRIPTION Perennial growing to 6 in (15 cm). Has a slender golden root, 3-lobed leaves, and single small white flowers.

HABITAT & CULTIVATION Native to eastern North America from Labrador to Tennessee, this herb prefers damp sites. The rhizome is dug up in autumn.

PART USED Rhizome.

CONSTITUENTS Goldthread contains isoquiniline alkaloids (including berberine and coptisine).

HISTORY & FOLKLORE Though not used much in herbal medicine today, this herb was once highly valued. In a book recounting his travels in North America (1779), Jonathan Carver stated that the plant "was greatly esteemed both by the Indians and the colonists as a remedy for any soreness in the mouth, but the taste of it is exquisitely bitter." The Montagnais used a decoction of the root for problems of the mouth, lips, and eyes. The Menominee used the plant as a gargle for children's throat problems, and to treat canker sores and tumors in the mouth.

MEDICINAL ACTIONS & USES A strongly bitter tonic, goldthread has been prescribed in the North American tradition principally for indigestion and stomach weakness, though it has also come under consideration as a treatment for peptic ulcers and has been applied as a wash for vaginal yeast infections. Goldthread has been used as a mouthwash, gargle, or lotion for canker sores, sore lips, and throats. It can help to tighten mucous membranes. The herb's constituents (and to some degree its actions) are similar to those of goldenseal (*Hydrastis canadensis*, p. 103), and it has been used as a substitute for this herb.

RELATED SPECIES Huang lian (*C. chinesis, see preceding entry*) is a close relative with similar actions. The Indian *C. teeta* is used as a bitter tonic and for eye problems.

CAUTIONS Use only under professional supervision. Do not take during pregnancy.

Coriandrum sativum
(Umbelliferae)
CORIANDER, CILANTRO

DESCRIPTION Strongly aromatic annual growing to 20 in (50 cm). Has finely cut upper leaves (known as cilantro) and white or pink flowers producing little, round seeds (coriander) in beige seed coats.

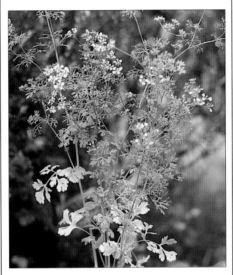

CORIANDER was used as a digestive aid and a treatment for measles in 6th-century China.

HABITAT & CULTIVATION Native to southern Europe and western Asia, this herb is cultivated throughout the world. The seeds are gathered ripe in late summer.

PARTS USED Seeds, essential oil, leaves.

CONSTITUENTS Coriander contains up to 1.5% volatile oil, consisting mainly of delta-linalool (at about 70%), alpha-pinene and terpinine. It also contains flavonoids, coumarins, phthalides, and phenolic acids.

HISTORY & FOLKLORE Coriander has been used throughout Asia, northern Africa, and Europe for well over 2,000 years. It is listed in the Ebers papyrus (dating to about 1500 BC), and apparently was much employed in ancient Egypt (partly as an aphrodisiac), and in ancient Greece by Hippocrates and other physicians. The herb reached China during the Han Dynasty (202 BC–AD 9). Pliny (AD 23–79) described its use "for spreading sores … diseased testes, burns, carbuncles, fluxes of the eyes, too, if woman's milk be added."

MEDICINAL ACTIONS & USES Coriander is more often used as a spice than as a medicine. Nevertheless, an infusion of the herb is a gentle remedy for flatulence, bloating, and cramps. It settles spasms in the gut and counters nervous tension. Coriander is also chewed to sweeten the breath, especially after consumption of garlic (*Allium sativum*, p.56). It is applied externally as a lotion for rheumatic pain. In Europe, it is considered an aphrodisiac.

CAUTION Do not take the essential oil internally.

Cornus officinalis
(Cornaceae)
SHAN ZHU YU

DESCRIPTION Deciduous tree reaching 12 ft (4 m) with glossy elliptical leaves and bright red oval berries.

HABITAT & CULTIVATION Native to China, Japan, and Korea, this tree is cultivated in central and eastern China. The fruit is harvested when ripe in autumn.

PART USED Fruit.

CONSTITUENTS *Shan zhu yu* contains an iridoid glycoside (verbenalin), saponins, and tannins. Verbenalin is known to have a mild effect on the involuntary nervous system, especially that governing the digestive system.

HISTORY & FOLKLORE Listed in the 1st-century AD *Divine Husbandman's Classic (Shen'nong Bencaojing)*, *shan zhu yu* is one of the constituents of the "Pill of Eight Ingredients," used to "warm up and invigorate the *yang* of the loins."

MEDICINAL ACTIONS & USES As an herb that "stabilizes and binds," *shan zhu yu* is used principally to reduce heavy menstrual bleeding and unusually active secretions, including copious sweating, excessive urine, spermatorrhea (involuntary discharge of semen), and premature ejaculation. *Shan zhu yu* is astringent, and like all herbs that suppress bodily fluids (even excessive ones), it will simply prolong or lead to a worsening of symptoms if used without tonic or detoxifying herbs. When used in combination with other herbs – for example, Chinese foxglove – *shan zhu yu* treats problems such as frequent urination, dizziness, and tinnitus.

RELATED SPECIES Several *Cornus* species are used medicinally around the world. In Europe, the fruit and bark of the cornelian cherry (*C. mas*), and the bark of common dogwood (*C. sanguinea*), are used as astringents and to relieve fever. The American boxwood (*C. florida*) was used by Native Americans as a fever remedy. The Central American *C. excelsa* was used as a traditional tonic and astringent.

OTHER MEDICINAL PLANTS

Crithmum maritimum
(Umbelliferae)
SAMPHIRE, SEA FENNEL

DESCRIPTION Maritime herb growing to 2 ft (60 cm). Has long succulent bright green leaves and clusters of small yellowish green flowers.

HABITAT & CULTIVATION Samphire grows on the Atlantic, Mediterranean, and Black Sea coasts of Europe and Asia Minor. It is found on rocks and cliffs close to the sea, and gathered in early summer.

PARTS USED Aerial parts.

CONSTITUENTS Samphire contains a volatile oil, pectin, vitamins (especially vitamin C), and minerals.

HISTORY & FOLKLORE A much valued herb in the past, samphire fell into disfavor but is slowly becoming popular again as a vegetable, either pickled or eaten fresh. The English herbalist John Gerard described it in 1597 as "the pleasantest sauce, most familiar, and best agreeing with man's body, both for the digestion of meates, breaking of stone, and voiding of gravel." Samphire was a well-known preventative against scurvy, and was pickled and taken on long sea journeys.

MEDICINAL ACTIONS & USES Though it is currently not used much in herbal medicine, samphire is a good diuretic, and it has potential as a treatment for obesity. Samphire has a high vitamin C and mineral content, and is thought to relieve flatulence and to act as a digestive remedy. In this, the plant resembles its inland namesake, fennel (*Foeniculum vulgare*, p. 210).

Crocus sativus
(Iridaceae)
SAFFRON

DESCRIPTION Perennial plant growing to 9 in (23 cm) from a bulblike corm. Has narrow leaves and mauve to purple flowers with 3 deep red threadlike stigmas.

HABITAT & CULTIVATION Native to India, the Balkans, and the eastern Mediterranean, saffron is cultivated in India, Spain, France, Italy, and the Middle East. It is harvested in early autumn and dried.

PARTS USED Stigmas and styles.

CONSTITUENTS Saffron contains a volatile oil composed of terpenes, terpene alcohols, and esters. The herb also contains bitter glycosides (including crocin), caretenoids, and vitamins B_1 and B_2.

HISTORY & FOLKLORE In the past, saffron was credited with an immense array of health benefits. In ancient Greece and Rome, it was used not only within medicine and cooking but as a cosmetic dye. Saffron peaked in popularity as a medicinal herb in Europe during the late Middle Ages. An example of the herb's acclaim was provided by the herbalist Christopher Catton: "Saffron has power to quicken the spirits, and the virtue thereof pierces by and by to the heart, provoking laughter and merriment."

MEDICINAL ACTIONS & USES Despite its long history as a medicinal herb, saffron has fallen out of favor as a treatment. Cheaper and superior herbs are easily found to replicate its ability to induce menstruation, treat period pain and chronic uterine bleeding, and calm indigestion and colic. In Chinese herbal medicine, saffron stigmas are occasionally used to treat painful obstructions of the chest, to stimulate menstruation, and to relieve abdominal pain.

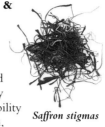
Saffron stigmas

CAUTION In very large doses, saffron may induce abortion. During pregnancy, take only in amounts normally used in cooking.

Cucurbita pepo
(Cucurbitaceae)
PUMPKIN

DESCRIPTION Annual plant with twining stems, lobed leaves, yellow flowers, and large orange fruit.

HABITAT & CULTIVATION Probably native to North America, pumpkin is now found worldwide. It is harvested in autumn.

PARTS USED Seeds, pulp.

CONSTITUENTS Pumpkin seeds contain 30% unsaturated fixed oil (which includes linoleic and oleic fatty acids). The seeds also contain cucurbitacins, vitamins, and minerals, notably zinc.

HISTORY & FOLKLORE The pumpkin has been much used as a medicine in Central

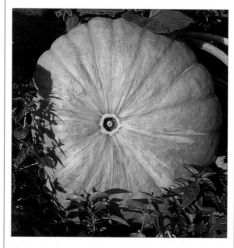
PUMPKIN *was a popular medicinal plant in the Americas; its seeds are still used to treat worms.*

and North America. The Maya applied the sap of the plant to burns, the Menominee used the seeds as a diuretic, and European settlers ground and mixed the seeds with water, milk, or honey to make a remedy for worms. This practice became so widespread in homes across North America that the medical profession eventually adopted it as a standard treatment.

MEDICINAL ACTIONS & USES Pumpkin seeds are taken principally as a safe deworming agent. They are particularly useful against tapeworms in pregnant women and in children, for whom stronger-acting and toxic preparations are unsuitable. The seeds are also mildly diuretic, and have been used in Central American herbal medicine as a treatment for nephritis and other urinary system problems. Varieties of pumpkin that are particularly diuretic, tonic to the bladder, and high in zinc have been recommended in the early stages of prostate problems. The pulp is used as a decoction to relieve intestinal inflammation, and is applied as a poultice or plaster for burns.

Cuminum cyminum
(Umbelliferae)
CUMIN

DESCRIPTION Small annual growing to 1 ft (30 cm). Has long narrow segmented leaves, clusters of pink or white flowers, and small oblong ridged fruits.

HABITAT & CULTIVATION Cumin is native to Egypt and is widely cultivated in southern Europe and Asia. The seeds are gathered when ripe in late summer.

PART USED Seeds.

CONSTITUENTS Cumin seeds contain 2–5% volatile oil, which consists of 25–35% aldehydes, pinene, and alpha-terpineol. The seeds also contain flavonoids (including apigenin).

HISTORY & FOLKLORE A popular spice and medicinal herb in ancient Egypt, cumin was used for illnesses of the digestive system, for chest conditions and coughs, as a painkiller, and to treat rotten teeth. The herb is mentioned in the Old Testament and was widely used in the Middle Ages. It has declined in popularity since that time, although it is still favored in contemporary Egyptian herbal medicine. In cooking, cumin is an ingredient of many Chinese, Indian, and Middle Eastern recipes, especially curries and pickles.

MEDICINAL ACTIONS & USES Cumin, like its close relatives caraway (*Carum carvi*, p. 182) and anise (*Pimpinella anisum*, p. 246), relieves flatulence and bloating, and stimulates the entire digestive process. Reducing abdominal gases and distension, it relaxes the gut as a whole. In Indian herbal medicine, cumin is used for insomnia, colds, and fevers, and, mixed into a paste with onion juice, has been applied to scorpion stings. The seeds are also taken to improve breast-milk production – a role it shares with fennel seeds (*Foeniculum vulgare*, p. 210).

Cupressus sempervirens
(Cupressaceae)
CYPRESS

DESCRIPTION Evergreen tree growing to 100 ft (30 m). Has tiny dark green leaves, and male and female cones.
HABITAT & CULTIVATION Native to Turkey and cultivated in the Mediterranean, this herb is gathered in spring.
PARTS USED Cones, branches, essential oil.
CONSTITUENTS Cypress contains a volatile oil (with pinene, camphene, and cedrol) and tannins.
HISTORY & FOLKLORE Ancient Greeks took the cones, mashed and steeped in wine, to treat dysentery, the coughing up of blood, asthma, and coughs.

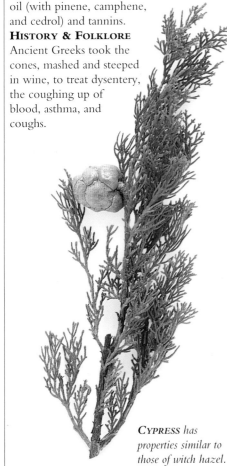

CYPRESS has properties similar to those of witch hazel.

MEDICINAL ACTIONS & USES Applied externally as a lotion or as a diluted essential oil, cypress astringes varicose veins and hemorrhoids, tightening up the blood vessels. A footbath of the cones is used to cleanse the feet and counter excessive sweating. Taken internally, cypress is an antispasmodic and general tonic, and is prescribed for whooping cough, the spitting up of blood, and spasmodic coughs.

Conditions such as colds, flu and sore throats, and rheumatic aches and pains also benefit from cypress.
CAUTION Do not take the essential oil internally without professional supervision.

Curcuma amada
(Zingiberaceae)
MANGO-GINGER

DESCRIPTION Aromatic perennial growing to 3 ft (90 cm). Has long tapering leaves and white or pale yellow flowers in spikes.
HABITAT & CULTIVATION Mango-ginger is found throughout most of the Indian sub-continent. It is cultivated for its rhizome, which is a food as well as a medicine
CONSTITUENTS Mango-ginger contains a volatile oil and pungent principles.
PART USED Rhizome.
HISTORY & FOLKLORE The rhizome, which has a scent similar to fresh mangoes, is pickled as a foodstuff, used in perfumery, and used medicinally.
MEDICINAL ACTIONS & USES A close relative of turmeric (*C. longa*, p. 88), mango-ginger is used in traditional Indian herbal medicine to treat flatulence, stomach pain, bad breath, loss of appetite, hiccups, indigestion, colic, and constipation. It is also given for coughs and other chest conditions such as bronchitis. The mashed or grated rhizome is applied externally to the skin to treat ulcers, bruises, wounds, and sprains.
RELATED SPECIES Zedoary (*C. zedoaria*, *see following entry*) and turmeric (*C. longa*, p. 88) are similar remedies.

Curcuma zedoaria
(Zingiberaceae)
ZEDOARY

DESCRIPTION Perennial herb with large tapering elliptical leaves, pink or yellow flowers, and an aromatic pale yellow root.
HABITAT & CULTIVATION Zedoary is a common Indian and East Asian plant. It is cultivated in India, Bangladesh, Indonesia, China, and Madagascar.
PART USED Rhizome.
CONSTITUENTS Zedoary contains a volatile oil, sesquiterpenes, curcumemone, curcumol, and curdione. Curcumol and curdione have anticancer properties.
HISTORY & FOLKLORE In India, the rhizome is used commmonly in perfumery and as a condiment.
MEDICINAL ACTIONS & USES An aromatic, bitter digestive stimulant, zedoary is used in much the same way as ginger (*Zingiber officinale*, p. 153) – to relieve indigestion,

nausea, flatulence, and bloating, and generally to improve the digestion. The rhizome is used in China to treat certain types of tumors.
RESEARCH In Chinese trials, zedoary has reduced cervical cancer, and increased the cancer-killing effects of radiotherapy and chemotherapy.
RELATED SPECIES In Chinese herbal medicine zedoary is often substituted for turmeric (*C. longa*, p. 88).

Cuscuta epithymum
(Convolvulaceae)
DODDER, HELLWEED, DEVIL'S GUTS

DESCRIPTION Leafless parasitic plant. Has threadlike stems, which are usually yellow-red in color, and small scented pale pink flowers.
HABITAT & CULTIVATION Dodder grows throughout Europe, Asia, and southern Africa. It prefers coastal and mountainous regions, and is gathered in summer.
PARTS USED Aerial parts.
CONSTITUENTS Dodder contains flavonoids (including kaempferol and quercitin) and hydroxycinnamic acid.
HISTORY & FOLKLORE Dodder has always been an unpopular country plant. It is also known as hellweed and devil's guts, due to its tendency to overrun and strangle the plant on which it feeds. This host can be thyme (*Thymus vulgaris*, p. 142), gorse (*Ulex europeaus*), or a crop such as beans. Dodder does, however, have medicinal benefits. In his *Materia Medica*, Dioscorides (1st century AD) noted its use in classical times in combination with honey to purge "black bile" and to lift a melancholy humor. In 1652, the herbalist Nicholas Culpeper similarly recommended it "to purge black or burnt choler." Culpeper further stated that dodder plucked off thyme is the most efficacious, making the interesting point that the parasite's medicinal benefits are determined in part by its host.
MEDICINAL ACTIONS & USES In line with its traditional use to purge black bile, dodder is still considered a valuable, though rarely used, herb for problems affecting the liver and gallbladder. It is thought to support liver function and is taken for jaundice. Dodder has a mildly laxative effect and is also taken for urinary problems.
RELATED SPECIES Greater dodder (*C. europaea*) and flax dodder (*C. epilinum*) may be used in the same way as *C. epithymum*. *C. reflexa* is employed in Ayurvedic medicine to treat difficulty in urinating, jaundice, muscle pain, and coughs.

195

Cyanopsis tetragonoloba
(Leguminosae)
GUAR GUM

DESCRIPTION Erect annual growing to 2 ft (60 cm), with hairy 3-lobed leaves, small purple flowers, and fleshy seed pods.

HABITAT & CULTIVATION Native to the Indian subcontinent, guar gum is cultivated extensively in India and Pakistan. The seed pods are harvested when ripe in summer.

PARTS USED Pods, seeds.

CONSTITUENTS Guar gum contains about 86% water-soluble mucilage, comprising mainly galactomannan.

HISTORY AND FOLKLORE Guar gum has been used as a filter in the mining industry, in paper manufacturing, and in cosmetics.

MEDICINAL ACTIONS & USES Guar gum is an effective bulk laxative similar in action to psyllium (*Plantago ovata*, p. 120). It delays the emptying of the stomach and thus slows down absorption of carbohydrates. Since this stabilizes blood sugar levels, it may be useful in prediabetic conditions and the early stages of late-onset diabetes. Guar gum also lowers cholesterol. In Indian medicine, the guar seed is used as a laxative and a digestive tonic.

CAUTION Guar gum use has caused esophageal obstruction. Do not exceed the dose. Guar gum can cause gas, abdominal distension, and intestinal obstruction. Use under medical supervision.

Cydonia oblonga
(Rosaceae)
QUINCE

DESCRIPTION Deciduous tree growing to 25 ft (8 m). Has green-gray oval leaves, pink or white flowers, and yellow pear-shaped sweet-smelling fruit.

HABITAT & CULTIVATION Native to southwest and central Asia, quince has become naturalized in Europe, especially in the Mediterranean region. It grows in damp, rich soils in hedges and copses. The fruit is harvested when ripe in autumn.

PARTS USED Fruit, seeds.

CONSTITUENTS The fruit contains tannin, pectin, and fruit acids; the seeds contain about 20% mucilage, cyanogenic glycosides (including amygdalin), fixed oil, and tannins.

HISTORY & FOLKLORE The quince has long been prized as a fruit and medicine in Greece and the eastern Mediterranean. It was used as an astringent in the time of Hippocrates (460–377 BC). The physician Dioscorides (AD 40–90) recorded a recipe for quince oil, which was applied to itchy and infected wounds and spreading sores.

In northerly climates, quince is often cooked to make a preserve. The English word "marmalade," which means citrus fruit jam, comes from the Portuguese word for quince, *marmelo*.

MEDICINAL ACTIONS & USES The great astringency of the unripe fruit makes it useful as a remedy for diarrhea, one that is particularly safe for children. The fruit and its juice can also be taken as a mouthwash or gargle to treat canker sores, gum problems, and sore throats. When cooked, much of the fruit's astringency is lost; quince syrup is recommended as a pleasant, mildly astringent, digestive drink. The seeds contain significant quantities of mucilage, and are helpful both in treating bronchitis and as a bulk laxative.

CAUTION Use the seeds only under professional supervision.

Cymbopogon citratus
(Graminaeae)
LEMON GRASS

DESCRIPTION Sweetly scented grass growing in large clumps up to 5 ft (1.5 m). Has narrow leaf blades and branched stalks of flowers.

HABITAT & CULTIVATION Native to southern India and Sri Lanka, lemon grass is now cultivated in tropical regions around the world.

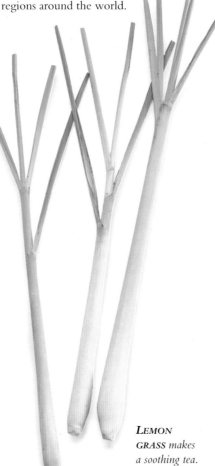

LEMON GRASS makes a soothing tea.

PARTS USED Leaves, essential oil.

CONSTITUENTS Lemon grass contains a volatile oil with citral (about 70%) and citronellal as its main constituents. Both are markedly sedative.

HISTORY & FOLKLORE Lemon grass is cultivated for its oil, which is a culinary flavoring, as a scent, and as a medicine.

MEDICINAL ACTIONS & USES Lemon grass is principally taken as a tea to remedy digestive problems. It relaxes the muscles of the stomach and gut, relieves cramping pains and flatulence, and is particularly suitable for children. In the Caribbean, lemon grass is primarily regarded as a fever-reducing herb (especially where there is significant congestion). Applied externally as a poultice or as diluted essential oil, it eases pain and arthritis. In India, a paste of the leaves is smeared on patches of ringworm.

RELATED SPECIES *C. martinii* and *C. nardus* yield essential oils that are widely used in soaps and detergents.

CAUTION Do not take the essential oil internally without professional supervision.

Cynara scolymus
syn. *C. cardunculus*
(Compositae)
ARTICHOKE

DESCRIPTION Perennial herb growing to 5 ft (1.5 m). Has large, thistlelike leaves, gray-green above and woolly white beneath, and very large purple-green flower heads.

HABITAT & CULTIVATION Native to the Mediterranean region, artichoke thrives in rich soil in warm temperate climates. Commercially grown plants are renewed after 4 years. The unopened flower heads and leaves are picked in early summer.

PARTS USED Flower heads, leaves, root.

CONSTITUENTS All parts of the plant contain the sesquiterpene lactone cynaropicrin (which is strongly bitter) and much inulin. The leaves also contain cynarin, which has liver-protective properties.

HISTORY & FOLKLORE Artichokes were greatly valued by the ancient Greeks and Romans. Dioscorides (1st century AD) recommended applying the mashed roots to the armpit or elsewhere on the body to sweeten offensive odors.

MEDICINAL ACTIONS & USES Artichoke is a valuable medicinal plant. Like milk thistle (*Carduus marianus*, p. 71), it benefits the liver, protecting against toxins and infection. Although the leaves are particularly effective, all parts of the plant are bitter and stimulate digestive secretions, especially bile. This makes artichoke useful for gallbladder problems, nausea, indigestion, and abdominal distension, with the added benefit that it lowers blood cholesterol levels.

A Mediterranean home recipe uses fresh artichoke leaf juice mixed with wine or water as a liver tonic. It is also taken during the early stages of late-onset diabetes. It is a good food for diabetics, since it significantly lowers blood sugar. It is also a useful diuretic, and in France it has been used to treat rheumatic conditions.

Cyperus esculentus
(Cyperaceae)
CHUFA, TIGER NUT

DESCRIPTION Erect, grasslike plant growing to 20 in (50 cm). Has cylindrical brown tubers, lance-shaped leaves, and rays of small spikes of green-brown flowers.

HABITAT & CULTIVATION Native to the Mediterranean region, chufa was first introduced to Spain and North Africa by the Arabs. It now grows worldwide, including in India. The tubers (called "nuts") are unearthed in winter and summer.

PARTS USED Tubers.

CONSTITUENTS Chufa contains 20–36% fixed oil, known as chufa or tiger nut oil.

HISTORY & FOLKLORE Chufa nuts have been found in the excavations of the earliest settlements in the Nile Valley, and since ancient times they have remained a popular food in the region. The 1st-century AD physician Dioscorides mentioned their ability to comfort the stomach.

MEDICINAL ACTIONS & USES Chufa is regarded as a digestive tonic. It has a heating and drying effect on the digestive system and alleviates flatulence. It also promotes urine production and menstruation. The juice is taken to heal canker sores of the mouth and gums. Ayurvedic medicine classifies the nuts as digestive, tonic, effective against flatulence, and aphrodisiac, and so they are given for flatulence, indigestion, colic, diarrhea, dysentery, debility, and excessive thirst.

RELATED SPECIES Many other species of *Cyperus* are used as foods or medicines. For example, in Chinese herbal medicine *C. rotundus* is used as a liver tonic, to counter indigestion, and to promote menstruation. *C. stolonifera,* native to tropical regions of Asia and Australia, is thought to ease stomach pain and act as a heart stimulant. Perhaps the most famous *Cyperus* species of all is papyrus (*C. papyrus*). This plant provided fiber for the first writing paper, invented by the ancient Egyptians. Papyrus was also chewed like sugar cane, and used medicinally in eye compresses, to bandage wounds, and to open and dry fistulae (abnormal openings from an internal organ to the surface of the body).

Cypripedium pubescens
(Orchidaceae)
LADY'S SLIPPER,
AMERICAN VALERIAN

DESCRIPTION Perennial orchid with several stems sheathed by broad lance-shaped leaves. Has beautiful, complex golden-yellow and purple flowers in late summer.

HABITAT & CULTIVATION This herb is native to eastern North America. Its natural habitat is woods and pastures, but due to overharvesting, it is rarely found in the wild. It is cultivated to a limited degree.

PART USED Rootstock.

CONSTITUENTS Lady's slipper is poorly researched, but it is known to contain a volatile oil, resins, glucosides, and tannins.

HISTORY & FOLKLORE Lady's slipper was held in high regard by Native Americans, who used it as a sedative and antispasmodic. It was commonly taken to ease menstrual and labor pains, and to counter insomnia and nervous conditions. The Cherokee used one variety to treat worms in children. In the Anglo-American Physiomedicalist tradition, lady's slipper had many uses. Swinburne Clymer (in *Nature's Healing Agents*, 1905) considered the plant "of special value in reflex functional disorders, or chorea, hysteria, nervous headache, insomnia, low fevers, nervous unrest, hypochondria and nervous depression accompanying stomach disorders."

MEDICINAL ACTIONS & USES Due to its scarcity and cost, lady's slipper is now used on a small scale. A sedative and relaxing herb, lady's slipper treats anxiety, stress-related disorders such as palpitations, headaches, muscular tension, panic attacks, and neurotic conditions generally. Like valerian (*Valeriana officinalis*, p. 146), lady's slipper is an effective tranquilizer. It reduces emotional tension and often calms the mind sufficiently to allow sleep. Indeed, its restorative effect appears to be more positive than that of valerian.

CAUTION In view of its rarity, lady's slipper should no longer be used medicinally.

Daphne mezereum
(Thymelaeaceae)
MEZEREON

DESCRIPTION Hardy deciduous shrub growing to 4 ft (1.2 m). Has oval to lance-shaped leaves, clusters of red or pink flowers, and small red berries.

HABITAT & CULTIVATION Mezereon is found in Europe, North Africa, and western Asia, flourishing in damp mountain woodlands. It is also cultivated as a garden plant. The root and bark of mezereon are gathered in autumn.

PARTS USED Root, root bark, bark.

CONSTITUENTS Mezereon contains diterpenes (including daphnetoxin and mezerein), mucilage, and tannins. Daphnetoxin and mezerein are highly toxic, but they have antileukemic properties, and have been used in a number of countries in the treatment of cancer.

HISTORY & FOLKLORE Mezereon was formerly well used in northern Europe, both internally as a purgative and externally as an ointment for cancerous sores and skin ulcers. The Swedish botanist Carolus Linnaeus (1707–1778) recorded that the bark was applied to the bites of poisonous reptiles and rabid dogs. People have reportedly died simply from eating birds that have eaten the highly poisonous berries.

MEDICINAL ACTIONS & USES Today mezereon is considered too poisonous to be ingested. It is used occasionally as an external counterirritant, increasing blood flow to the affected area. It has been considered effective for rheumatic joints.

CAUTIONS Under no circumstances should mezereon be taken internally. It should only be used externally under professional supervision and never on open wounds.

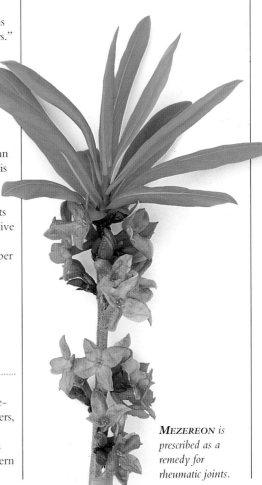

MEZEREON is prescribed as a remedy for rheumatic joints.

Datura stramonium
(Solanaceae)
THORNAPPLE

DESCRIPTION Robust annual growing to 3 ft (1 m). Has lobed oval leaves, long white or violet trumpet-shaped flowers, and spiny fruit capsules similar to those of the horse chestnut (*Aesculus hippocastanum*, p. 159).

HABITAT & CULTIVATION Thornapple grows in the Americas, Europe, Asia, and North Africa. It is cultivated for medicinal use in Hungary, France, and Germany. The leaves and flowering tops are harvested in summer, and the seeds in early autumn when the capsules burst.

PARTS USED Leaves, flowering tops, seeds.

CONSTITUENTS Thornapple contains 0.2–0.45% tropane alkaloids (especially hyoscyamine and hyoscine), flavonoids, withanolides, coumarins, and tannins. The tropane alkaloids are similar to those found in deadly nightshade (*Atropa belladonna*, p. 66), acting to reduce secretions and relax smooth muscle.

HISTORY & FOLKLORE Thornapple has a long history of medicinal use. If taken in sufficient doses, it causes hallucinations; the Delphic oracle in ancient Greece and the Inca in South America may have used it as an aid to making prophecies. Though it is hallucinogenic, thornapple has traditionally been used to treat insanity.

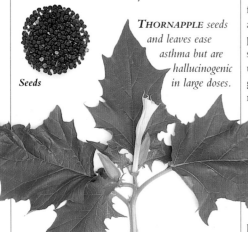

THORNAPPLE seeds and leaves ease asthma but are hallucinogenic in large doses.

Seeds

MEDICINAL ACTIONS & USES At low doses, thornapple is a common remedy for asthma, whooping cough, muscle spasm, and the symptoms of Parkinsonism. It relaxes the muscles of the gastrointestinal, bronchial, and urinary tracts, and reduces digestive and mucous secretions. Like deadly nightshade, it may be applied externally to relieve rheumatic pains and neuralgia.

RELATED SPECIES *D. metel* and *D. innoxia*, plants native to India, are similarly employed in the treatment of asthma, coughs, fevers, and skin conditions.

CAUTIONS Take only under professional supervision. Since it is toxic at more than small doses, thornapple is subject to legal restrictions in most countries.

Daucus carota
(Umbelliferae)
CARROT

DESCRIPTION Annual (cultivated varieties) or biennial (wild). Has erect stem growing to 3 ft (1 m), feathery leaves, small white flowers, and flat green seeds. Cultivated subspecies have fleshy orange taproots.

HABITAT & CULTIVATION Wild carrot is native to Europe. Cultivated subspecies are grown around the world. The root is harvested in late summer, and the seeds are gathered in late summer or early autumn.

PARTS USED Seeds, root, leaves.

CONSTITUENTS Wild carrot seeds contain flavonoids, and a volatile oil including asarone, carotol, pinene, and limonene. Cultivated carrot root contains sugars, pectin, carotene, vitamins, minerals, and asparagine. Carrot leaves contain significant amounts of porphyrins, which stimulate the pituitary gland and lead to the release of increased levels of sex hormones.

HISTORY & FOLKLORE The origins of the familiar garden carrot are a mystery – it has been cultivated as a nutritious and cleansing food at least as long ago as ancient Greece and Rome. In the 1st century AD, the physician Dioscorides recommended the seeds to stimulate menstruation, to relieve urinary retention, and to "wake up the genital virtue." The cultivated variety did not reach the shores of Britain until the 16th century. Women of the time used its beautiful, finely divided leaves to adorn their hair.

MEDICINAL ACTIONS & USES This common vegetable is also a wonderfully cleansing medicine. It supports the liver, and stimulates urine flow and the removal of waste by the kidneys. The juice of organically grown carrots is a delicious drink and a valuable detoxifier. Carrots are rich in carotene, which is converted to vitamin A by the liver. This nutrient acts to improve night blindness as well as vision in general. The raw root, grated or mashed, is a safe treatment for threadworms, especially in children. Wild carrot leaves are a good diuretic. They have been used to counter cystitis and kidney stone formation, and to diminish stones that have already formed. The seeds are also diuretic and carminative. They stimulate menstruation and have been used in folk medicine as a treatment for hangovers. Both leaves and seeds relieve

flatulence and gassy colic, and are a useful remedy for settling the digestion and upsets of the stomach.

CAUTION Do not take carrot seeds, which may be abortifacient, during pregnancy.

Desmodium gangeticum
(Leguminosae)
SALPAN

DESCRIPTION Bushy perennial growing to 4 ft (1.2 m). Has woody stems, oval leaves, white or lilac flowers, and beaded seed pods.

HABITAT & CULTIVATION Native to India, southern Asia, and Africa, salpan is found as undergrowth in tropical forests.

PART USED Root.

CONSTITUENTS Salpan contains a volatile oil and an alkaloid.

MEDICINAL ACTIONS & USES Salpan root is bitter and tonic, and is used in Ayurveda to improve poor appetite and digestion, and to treat dysentery and hemorrhoids. The plant is also given for feverish and congestive conditions such as bronchitis and asthma.

RELATED SPECIES *D. adscendens*, which grows in Africa, South America, and other tropical areas, is used in West Africa and Europe to treat asthma and liver problems such as hepatitis. Preliminary research in Ghana indicates that it has a significant protective effect on the liver.

Dianthus superbus
(Caryophyllacaea)
QU MAI, FRINGED PINK

DESCRIPTION Upright perennial herb growing to 20 in (50 cm) or more. Has narrow lance-shaped leaves and large, delicate, fragrant pink or lilac flowers.

HABITAT & CULTIVATION *Qu mai* grows in China, Japan, and Europe. It is found in clumps on hillsides and in crevices. Cultivated in eastern China, it is gathered in summer and autumn when in flower.

PARTS USED Aerial parts.

CONSTITUENTS *Qu mai* contains a volatile oil including eugenol, benzyl benzoate, and methyl salicylate.

HISTORY & FOLKLORE *Qu mai* was first mentioned in the 1st-century AD Chinese herbal known as the *Divine Husbandman's Classic (Shen'nong Bencaojing).*

MEDICINAL ACTIONS & USES In traditional Chinese medicine (see pp. 38–41), the bitter-tasting *qu mai* clears "damp-heat," and has been used principally to treat hot, painful conditions of the kidneys and urinary tubules, such as kidney stones, urinary tract infections, and blood in the urine. Not used much on its own, *qu mai* is commonly combined with *dan shen* (*Salvia militorhiza*, p. 129) to induce menstruation. The herb is also used for constipation and some types of eczema.

RESEARCH Research undertaken in China suggests that the flowering tops of *qu mai* are the most markedly diuretic part of the plant.

RELATED SPECIES The gillyflower (*D. caryophyllus*), of Mediterranean origin, has similar constituents and is traditionally prescribed in European herbal medicine for coronary and nervous disorders.

Dictamnus albus
(Rutaceae)
DITTANY, GAS PLANT

DESCRIPTION Strongly aromatic, bushy, and hairy perennial growing to 32 in (80 cm). Has compound leaves and spikes of 5-petaled white or pink flowers that are streaked with purple.

HABITAT & CULTIVATION This herb grows in southern and central Europe and northern Asia, preferring warm, wooded areas. The flowering tops are gathered in late summer; the root, generally in autumn.

PARTS USED Root, flowering tops.

CONSTITUENTS Dittany's potent volatile oil contains estragol and anethole, and a toxic alkaloid, dictamnin.

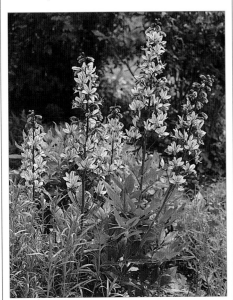

DITTANY flowers were formerly used to make a preparation that was sniffed up the nose as a treatment for head colds.

HISTORY & FOLKLORE Dittany exudes such large amounts of volatile oil that in hot, dry conditions, a match held close will cause the whole plant to burst into flames. The plant has been used to flavor liqueurs and has been brewed as a tea in parts of Siberia. In European folk medicine, this plant was considered an antidote to poison, pestilence, and the bites of all types of venomous animals.

MEDICINAL ACTIONS & USES Very rarely used today, dittany has an action similar to that of rue (*Ruta graveolens*, p. 262), in that it strongly stimulates the muscles of the uterus, inducing menstruation and sometimes causing abortion. By contrast, its effect on the gastrointestinal tract is antispasmodic. It relaxes the gut and acts as a mild tonic for the stomach. The plant has also been used as a treatment for nervous conditions.

CAUTIONS This herb is toxic. Take only under professional supervision. Do not take during pregnancy.

Digitalis lutea
(Scrophulariaceae)
YELLOW FOXGLOVE

DESCRIPTION Erect perennial growing to a height of 3 ft (1 m). Has narrow lance-shaped leaves and long spikes of yellow bell-shaped flowers.

HABITAT & CULTIVATION Native to western and central Europe, yellow foxglove grows in woodland areas, on roadsides, and in mountainous regions. It is cultivated for medicinal purposes in Russia. The leaves of the plant are harvested in the second summer of growth.

PART USED Leaves.

CONSTITUENTS Yellow foxglove contains cardiac glycosides (including the cardenolides alpha-acetyldigitoxin, acetyldigitoxin, and lanatoside). All act to strengthen the beating of a weakened heart.

HISTORY & FOLKLORE Unlike the closely related common foxglove (*D. purpurea, see following entry*), yellow foxglove does not appear to have played a significant role in European herbal medicine.

MEDICINAL ACTIONS & USES Yellow foxglove is not used much in herbal medicine, but it is a less toxic alternative to purple foxglove and wooly foxglove (*D. lanata*). It has similar medicinal actions, but its alkaloids are more readily metabolized and flushed out by the body. Like other foxgloves, this plant supports a weakened or failing heart, increasing the strength of contraction, slowing and steadying the heart rate, and lowering blood pressure by strongly stimulating the production of urine, which reduces overall blood volume.

RELATED SPECIES Common foxglove (*see following entry*).

CAUTIONS Excessive doses of yellow foxglove can prove fatal. This plant is subject to legal restrictions in some countries.

Digitalis purpurea
(Scrophulariaceae)
COMMON FOXGLOVE,
PURPLE FOXGLOVE

DESCRIPTION Perennial growing to 5 ft (1.5 m). Has a single erect stem, broad lance-shaped leaves, and bell-shaped purple-pink or white flowers in long spikes.

HABITAT & CULTIVATION This herb is native to western Europe. Though it is also cultivated, the wild plant is considered superior. The leaves are picked in summer.

PARTS USED Leaves.

CONSTITUENTS Foxglove contains cardiac glycosides (including digoxin, digitoxin, and lanatosides), anthraquinones, flavonoids, and saponins. Digitoxin rapidly strengthens the heartbeat but is excreted very slowly. Digoxin is preferred as a long-term medication.

HISTORY & FOLKLORE In medical history, foxglove is best known as the discovery of William Withering, an 18th-century English country doctor. Curious about the formula of a local herbalist, he explored the plant's potential medical uses. His work led to the production of a life-saving medicine.

MEDICINAL ACTIONS & USES Foxglove has a profound tonic effect on a diseased heart. Heart disease worsens when the heart's ability to maintain normal circulation decreases. Foxglove's cardiac glycosides enable the heart to beat more strongly, slowly, and regularly, without requiring more oxygen. At the same time, it stimulates urine production, which lowers the volume of blood, and thus lessens the load on the heart.

RELATED SPECIES Wooly foxglove (*D. lanata*) is today the main source of cardiac glycosides.

CAUTIONS Potentially fatal in overdose. Use only under professional supervision. This plant is subject to legal restrictions.

COMMON FOXGLOVE enables the heart to beat more evenly and is an invaluable remedy for heart disease.

Dioscorea opposita syn. *D. batatas*
(Dioscoreaceae)

SHAN YAO (CHINESE), CHINESE YAM

DESCRIPTION Climbing perennial herb growing to 15 ft (5 m). Has a thick fleshy root, ridged slender stem, triangular leaves, and single flower heads.

HABITAT & CULTIVATION *Shan yao* grows throughout China, Japan, and Southeast Asia, preferring sunny slopes both in the wild and in cultivation. *Shan yao* root is unearthed in winter.

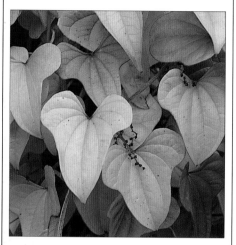

SHAN YAO is a twining plant found on sunny slopes in China, Japan, and Southeast Asia.

PART USED Root.

CONSTITUENTS Contains steroidal saponins.

HISTORY & FOLKLORE *Shan yao* has been used medicinally for at least 2,000 years. It forms part of "The Pill of Eight Ingredients," traditionally prescribed in Chinese medicine to treat hypothyroidism, nephritis, and diabetes. The root is also eaten as a vegetable.

MEDICINAL ACTIONS & USES A gentle tonic, *shan yao* is prescribed for tiredness, weight loss, and lack of appetite. The root strengthens a weak digestion, improves appetite, and may help bind watery stools. It counters excessive sweating, frequent urination, and chronic thirst, and it is also given for chronic coughs and wheezing. The traditional use of *shan yao*, like that of other yam species, indicates a hormonal effect. It is also taken to treat vaginal discharge and spermatorrhea (involuntary emission of semen).

RELATED SPECIES Many other species of yam are grown as foods, herbal medicines, and as sources of natural hormones. The wild yam (*D. villosa*, p. 89) of Mexico is the best known. It yields diosgenin, a precursor of the female hormones used in contraceptive pills.

Dipsacus fullonum
(Dipsacaceae)

TEASEL

DESCRIPTION Perennial with a spiny ridged stem growing to 6 ft (2 m). Has lance-shaped leaves and lilac-colored flowers blooming from hooked heads.

HABITAT & CULTIVATION Common throughout Europe and western Asia, teasel thrives in open areas, roadsides, and banks. It is cultivated only on a small scale. The root is unearthed in late summer.

PART USED Root.

CONSTITUENTS Teasel contains inulin, bitter substances, and a scabioside.

HISTORY & FOLKLORE Teasel heads are perhaps best known as implements to card wool, and they are still used to comb certain cloths, notably the green baize used on billiard tables. Medicinally, the root was used to treat conditions such as warts, fistulae (abnormal passages opening through the skin), and cancerous sores. The water that collects in the leaf was called "Venus's bath" by early herbalists, and was thought to be very beneficial for the eyes.

MEDICINAL ACTIONS & USES Teasel root is not much used medicinally today, and its therapeutic applications are disputed. It is thought to have diuretic, sweat-inducing, and stomach-soothing properties, cleansing the system and improving digestion. Due to its apparent astringency, teasel is considered helpful in diarrhea. It is also thought to increase appetite, to tone the stomach, and to act on the liver, helping with jaundice and gallbladder problems. There is no clear picture of teasel's actions, but its closeness to the thistle family means it might well reward careful investigation.

Dorema ammoniacum
(Umbelliferae)

AMMONIACUM

DESCRIPTION Very large perennial herb growing to a height of 10 ft (3 m), with a stout stem, compound leaves, and umbels of white flowers.

HABITAT & CULTIVATION Ammoniacum is native to central Asia, Iran, and northern Russia. When pierced, the stem exudes a milky gum, which is pressed into blocks and then ground into a powder.

PART USED Oleo-gum-resin.

CONSTITUENTS Ammoniacum contains a resin (60–70%), gum, volatile oil (including ferulene and linalyl acetate), free salicylic acid, and coumarins.

HISTORY & FOLKLORE Ammoniacum's medicinal value has been appreciated since ancient times, and was mentioned by Hippocrates (460–377 BC). The herb's common name reputedly derives from the Temple of Jupiter Ammon in Libya, in an area where it was commonly collected.

MEDICINAL ACTIONS & USES Used in both Western and Indian medicine, ammoniacum is still listed in the *British Pharmacopoeia* as an antispasmodic and as an expectorant that stimulates the coughing up of thick mucus. It is a specific treatment for chronic bronchitis, asthma, and persistent coughs. Ammoniacum is also occasionally used to induce sweating or menstruation.

OTHER SPECIES Ammoniacum is medicinally similar to asafoetida (*Ferula assa-foetida*, p. 208) and galbanum (*Ferula gummosa*, p. 209).

Dorstenia contrayerva
(Urticaceae)

CONTRAYERVA

DESCRIPTION Stemless, perennial herb growing to 1 ft (30 cm). Has palm-shaped leaves and long-stalked, greenish flowers.

HABITAT & CULTIVATION Native to Central and South America and the Caribbean islands, contrayerva is generally gathered from the wild.

PART USED Rhizome.

HISTORY & FOLKLORE Contrayerva means "antidote" in Spanish, indicating its traditional use in the treatment of poisoning and venomous bites. The herb was employed in Mayan and Aztec medicine for a variety of purposes, including as a poultice to draw pus.

MEDICINAL ACTIONS & USES Contrayerva rhizome is considered aromatic, stimulant, and sweat-inducing. Occasionally used in the early stages of serious fevers such as typhoid, it is also given for gastrointestinal problems such as diarrhea and dysentery. There is no scientific proof of its reputation as an antidote.

RELATED SPECIES *D. convexa*, native to Zaire, is used as a wound healer; *D. klainei* is used in tropical Africa as a gargle.

Drosera rotundifolia
(Droseraceae)

SUNDEW

DESCRIPTION Evergreen, insectivorous perennial growing to 6 in (15 cm). Has small white flowers. The hinged, spoon-shaped leaves edged with spines secrete a sticky fluid ("sundew"), which traps insects. They are digested when the leaf closes.

HABITAT & CULTIVATION Sundew grows in Europe, Asia, and North America, and is found in marshy ground at altitudes up to 6,000 ft (1,800 m). Formerly, it was picked while in flower in summer. Since it is now rare, it should not be gathered from the wild.

PARTS USED Aerial parts.

CONSTITUENTS Sundew contains naphthaquinones, enzymes, flavonoids, and volatile oil. The naphthaquinones are antimicrobial, antispasmodic, and also cough-suppressing.

HISTORY & FOLKLORE In the 16th and 17th centuries, sundew was thought to be a remedy for melancholy. In his _Irish Herbal_ (1735), K'Eogh advised using sundew to "eat away rotten sores."

MEDICINAL ACTIONS & USES Sundew is of greatest value in the treatment of

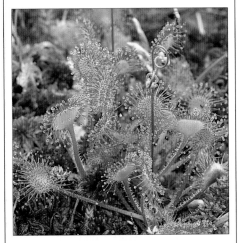

SUNDEW was once considered a refreshing herb because it maintained its "dew" even in full sun.

spasmodic chest conditions such as whooping cough, bronchial asthma, and asthma. In relaxing the muscles of the respiratory tract, the plant eases breathing, relieves wheezing, and lessens the spasms of whooping cough. Commonly mixed with thyme in a syrup, sundew is a helpful remedy for coughs in children. The herb is also prescribed for gastric problems.

RELATED SPECIES _D. peltata_, which grows in Asia and Australia, is used externally to stimulate blistering of the skin (which helps speed the clearance of toxins in arthritis and rheumatism) and internally to treat syphilis.

Dryopteris filix-mas syn. _Aspidium filix-mas_ (_Polypodiaceae_)
MALE FERN

DESCRIPTION Perennial fern growing to 3 ft (1 m). Has brown, tangled rootstock and wide, spreading fronds.

HABITAT & CULTIVATION Male fern is found throughout temperate regions of Europe, Asia, and the Americas. It prefers

damp and shady terrains. The rhizome is unearthed in autumn, and must be used within one year of harvesting or it loses its pharmacological efficacy.

PART USED Rhizome.

CONSTITUENTS Male fern contains an oleo-resin (6%) with phloroglucinol derivatives or "filicin," which is responsible for its deworming action. In addition, the fern contains triterpenes, alkanes, a volatile oil, and resins.

HISTORY & FOLKLORE In his 16th-century translation of the writings of Dioscorides, Andreas de Laguna recommended taking male fern root with honey-sweetened water to destroy tapeworms. Apart from male fern's medicinal use, European folk tradition considered the plant to be one of the surest remedies against witchcraft, a belief recorded in rural Germany well into the 19th century.

MEDICINAL ACTIONS & USES One of the most effective of all "worm herbs," male fern root, or the oleo-resin it yields, is a specific treatment for tapeworms. It acts by paralyzing the muscles of the worm, forcing it to relax its hold on the gut wall. Provided that the root is taken along with a nonoily purgative – Dioscorides recommended scammony (_Convolvulus scammonia_) or black hellebore (_Helleborus niger_, p. 217) – it will flush out the parasites.

CAUTIONS Male fern is highly toxic and should be administered only by a professional medicinal herbalist. Excessive doses can lead to liver damage and blindness. It is subject to legal restrictions in some countries.

Echium vulgare (_Boraginaceae_)
VIPER'S BUGLOSS

DESCRIPTION Abundantly hairy perennial growing up to 3 ft (1 m). Has narrow prickly leaves and pink to violet clusters of flowers in dense spikes.

HABITAT & CULTIVATION Native to Europe, viper's bugloss is commonly found on uncultivated land, by roadsides, and in low-lying and coastal regions. The flowering tops are gathered in late summer.

PARTS USED Flowering tops.

CONSTITUENTS Viper's bugloss contains pyrrolizidine alkaloids, allantoin, alkannins, and mucilage. In isolation, pyrrolizidine alkaloids are toxic to the liver. The alkannins are antimicrobial and allantoin helps wounds to heal.

HISTORY & FOLKLORE As its name suggests, viper's bugloss was once considered a preventative and remedy for viper bite. In his 1656 _The Art of Simpling_, herbalist William Coles described the plant: "its stalks all to be speckled like a snake or viper, and

is a most singular remedy against poison and the sting of scorpions." Four years earlier, the English herbalist Nicholas Culpeper had praised its action against "the biting of vipers" but also listed other uses: "the seeds being drunk in wine procureth abundance of milk in women's breasts. The same also being taken easeth the pains in the loins, back and kidneys."

MEDICINAL ACTIONS & USES In many respects, viper's bugloss is similar to borage (_Borago officinalis_, p. 177) in that both herbs have a sweat-inducing and diuretic effect if taken internally. Viper's bugloss has also been taken to treat chest conditions since its mucilage soothes dry coughs and encourages expectoration. The significant mucilage content in viper's bugloss has also proved helpful in treating skin conditions. Prepared in a poultice or plaster, it is an effective balm for boils and carbuncles. In recent times, this herb has fallen out of use, due partly to lack of interest in its medicinal potential, and partly to its pyrrolizidine alkaloids, which in isolation are toxic. Viper's bugloss may be safely used externally.

CAUTION Do not take viper's bugloss internally.

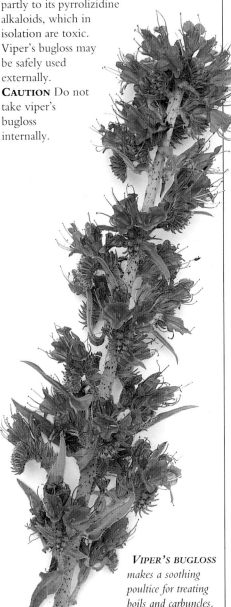

VIPER'S BUGLOSS makes a soothing poultice for treating boils and carbuncles.

Eclipta prostrata
syn. *E. alba*
(Compositae)
TRAILING ECLIPTA

DESCRIPTION Multibranched annual growing to 2 ft (60 cm). Has lance-shaped leaves and white flowers.

HABITAT & CULTIVATION Trailing eclipta is native to Africa, Asia, and Australia. It is now found throughout the tropics, being particularly common in India, China, and Queensland and New South Wales in Australia. It is harvested in early autumn.

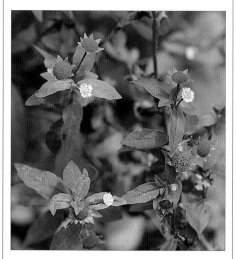

TRAILING ECLIPTA is taken in India and China to stop premature graying of the hair.

PARTS USED Aerial parts.

CONSTITUENTS Trailing eclipta contains saponins, including ecliptine and alpha-terthienylmethanol.

HISTORY & FOLKLORE Trailing eclipta was first mentioned in herbal literature in the Chinese *Tang Materia Medica* of AD 659. The herb contains a black pigment that has been used to color the hair in India, and mothers wash babies' heads in a decoction of the leaves to encourage hair growth. It has been used as ink for tattooing. The leaves are also eaten as a vegetable.

MEDICINAL ACTIONS & USES Trailing eclipta has remarkably similar uses in Ayurveda and in Chinese herbal medicine. In both of these traditions, a decoction is used to invigorate the liver, to prevent premature graying of the hair, and to staunch bleeding, especially from the uterus. In the Chinese tradition, the herb is considered a *yin* tonic; in Ayurvedic medicine it is thought to prevent aging. In the Caribbean, the juice is sometimes taken for asthma and bronchitis. Trailing eclipta is also used there as a treatment for enlarged glands, as well as for dizziness, vertigo, and blurred vision. The plant is employed externally for various skin problems and as a wound healer.

Embelia ribes
(Myrsinaceae)
EMBELIA

DESCRIPTION Climber with short elliptical leaves, white or white-green flowers, and round red or black fruits.

HABITAT & CULTIVATION Native to India and Southeast Asia, embelia grows in hilly regions. The fruit is harvested when ripe.

PART USED Fruit.

CONSTITUENTS Embelia contains naphthaquinones, including embelin. Embelin stimulates the production of estrogen and progesterone, and it may have a contraceptive effect.

MEDICINAL ACTIONS & USES Embelia has been used in Asia as a home remedy for expelling worms. The herb is also diuretic and relieves flatulence, and is used for indigestion, colic, constipation, and debility.

RESEARCH Embelia has been studied since the 1980s as a potential contraceptive.

CAUTIONS Use only under professional supervision. Do not take during pregnancy.

Emblica officinalis
(Euphorbiaceae)
INDIAN GOOSEBERRY

DESCRIPTION Deciduous tree with feathery leaves, pale green flowers, and round pale green or yellow fruit.

HABITAT & CULTIVATION Native to India and the Middle East, Indian gooseberry is cultivated for its fruit.

PART USED Fruit.

CONSTITUENTS Indian gooseberry contains a fixed oil, a volatile oil, and tannins.

HISTORY & FOLKLORE The Indian gooseberry was featured in a 7th-century Ayurvedic medical text. The sage Muni Chyawan reputedly restored his vitality with this fruit.

MEDICINAL ACTIONS & USES The astringent Indian gooseberry is given to allay the effects of aging and to restore the organs. In Ayurvedic medicine, the fruit juice is given to strengthen the pancreas of diabetics. The juice is also given to treat eye problems, joint pain, and diarrhea and dysentery.

Entada phaseoloides
(Leguminosae)
MATCHBOX BEAN

DESCRIPTION Woody vine with compound leaves and clusters of pea-type flowers. Huge, flat brown seed pods, containing black glossy seeds, grow to 5 ft (1.5 m) in length,

making them the largest-growing legumes in the world.

HABITAT & CULTIVATION Matchbox bean is native to Australia and tropical regions of Asia and Africa. The seeds are collected when the pods are ripe.

PARTS USED Seeds.

CONSTITUENTS Matchbox bean contains significant amounts of saponins.

HISTORY & FOLKLORE The young leaves and roasted seed pods are eaten as vegetables. Fiber from the stems is made into fishing nets, ropes, and sails. Due to the plant's high level of saponin (a substance that foams when agitated with water), it has been used to wash the hair.

MEDICINAL ACTIONS & USES Australian Aborigines use the seeds to treat female sterility and indigestion, and as a painkiller.

CAUTION Take only under professional advice. The seeds are toxic in large doses.

Equisetum arvense
(Equisetaceae)
HORSETAIL, BOTTLEBRUSH

DESCRIPTION Perennial plant with a yellowish fruiting stem growing to 14 in (35 cm), followed by a sterile segmented and toothed stem growing to 2 ft (60 cm). The latter has whorls of needle-shaped leaves.

HABITAT & CULTIVATION Native to Europe, North Africa, northern Asia, and the Americas, horsetail is a common plant, preferring damp soil. The sterile stems are harvested in summer and carefully dried, all discolored parts being discarded.

PARTS USED Aerial parts.

CONSTITUENTS Horsetail contains large amounts of silicic acid and silicates (about 15%), flavonoids, phenolic acids, alkaloids (including nicotine), and sterols. Much of the therapeutic effectiveness of this herb is due to its high silica content, a large proportion of which is soluble and can be absorbed. Silica supports the regeneration of connective tissue.

HISTORY & FOLKLORE Horsetail is a primitive plant, a descendant of huge trees that lived in the Paleozoic era (600–375 million years ago). The herb's high silica content makes it abrasive, and in the past it was used to polish metal and wood. Its common name, bottlebrush, indicates another of its uses. Horsetail was also tied to the tails of livestock to help them ward off flies. It was long considered a wound-healing herb. The English herbalist John Gerard, writing in 1597, recounted: "Dioscorides saith, that the horse-taile being stamped and laid to, doth perfectly cure wounds, yea although the sinues be cut in sunder, as Galen addeth."

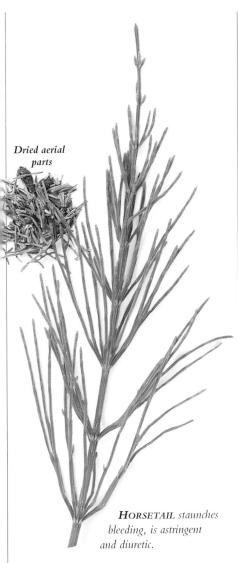

Dried aerial parts

HORSETAIL *staunches bleeding, is astringent and diuretic.*

MEDICINAL ACTIONS & USES As its traditional usage indicates, horsetail is an excellent clotting agent. It staunches wounds, stops nosebleeds, and reduces the coughing up of blood. In addition, horsetail has an astringent effect on the genitourinary system, proving especially valuable where there is bleeding within the urinary tract, and in cases of cystitis, urethritis, and prostate disease. Horsetail speeds the repair of damaged connective tissue, improving its strength and elasticity. The herb is also prescribed to treat rheumatic and arthritic problems, for chest ailments such as emphysema, for chronic swelling of the legs, and for various other conditions. A decoction of the herb added to a bath benefits slow-healing sprains and fractures, as well as certain skin conditions such as eczema.

CAUTIONS Do not use horsetail for more than 6 weeks except under professional supervision since the herb may cause irritation of the digestive tract. Do not confuse horsetail with the marsh horsetail (*E. palustre*), a similar but much larger plant containing toxic alkaloids.

Erigeron canadensis syn. *Conyza canadensis*
(Compositae)
CANADIAN FLEABANE

DESCRIPTION Erect, annual herb growing to 3 ft (1 m). Has narrow, dark green, lance-shaped leaves and clusters of small white flower heads that quickly fade into silky white tufts.

HABITAT & CULTIVATION Native to North America, Canadian fleabane is now common in South America and Europe. It thrives on uncultivated and recently cleared land, often invading in large swathes. It is gathered from the wild when in flower.

PARTS USED Aerial parts.

CONSTITUENTS Canadian fleabane contains a volatile oil (including limonene, terpineol, and linalool), flavonoids, terpenes, plant acids, and tannins.

HISTORY & FOLKLORE In traditional North American herbal medicine, Canadian fleabane was boiled to make steam for sweat lodges, taken as a snuff to stimulate sneezing during the course of a cold, and burned to create a smoke that warded off insects – hence its common name.

MEDICINAL ACTIONS & USES An astringent herb, Canadian fleabane is taken for gastrointestinal problems such as diarrhea and dysentery. A decoction of Canadian fleabane is reportedly a very effective treatment for bleeding hemorrhoids. The herb is occasionally used as a diuretic for bladder problems, to clear toxins in rheumatic conditions, and to treat gonorrhea and other urinogenital diseases.

RELATED SPECIES The Philadelphia fleabane (*E. philadelphicus*) was used by the Houma as a treatment for menstrual problems. *E. affinis*, a Mexican relative, is used to make a tooth powder and to treat toothache.

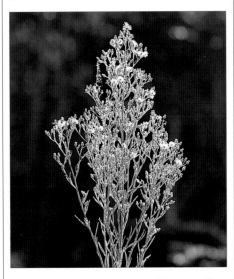

CANADIAN FLEABANE *was used both ritually and medicinally by Native North Americans.*

Eriodictyon californicum
(Hydrophyllaceae)
YERBA SANTA

DESCRIPTION Sticky evergreen shrub growing to 8 ft (2.5 m). Its narrow lance-shaped leaves are shiny green on the upper side and hairy white underneath. Trumpet-shaped white or blue flowers grow in clusters.

HABITAT & CULTIVATION Native to California and Oregon in the US, and northern Mexico, yerba santa flourishes on dry mountain slopes. It grows at altitudes of up to 4,000 ft (1,200 m).

PARTS USED Leaves.

CONSTITUENTS Yerba santa contains a volatile oil, flavonoids (including eriodictyol), and resin.

HISTORY & FOLKLORE The name *yerba santa* (holy weed) was given to this plant by Spanish colonists, who learned of its medicinal virtues from Native Americans. Traditionally, the leaves were infused and taken for coughs, colds, sore throats, mucus, and asthma. The infusion was also used as a wash to ease fever, and the mashed leaves were applied as a poultice to treat sores. The *Eclectic Medical Journal* featured an article on yerba santa in 1875, and it was listed in the *Pharmacopoeia of the United States* in 1894.

MEDICINAL ACTIONS & USES This aromatic herb, with its pleasant sweet taste, is a valuable expectorant that can be used to treat tracheitis, bronchitis, and asthma, and similar respiratory tract ailments.

Ervatamia coronaria
(Apocynaceae)
GRAPE JASMINE,
EAST INDIAN ROSEBAY

DESCRIPTION Perennial shrub growing to 6 ft (2 m). Has dark green elliptical leaves and strongly perfumed white flowers.

HABITAT & CULTIVATION Grape jasmine is grown in India, Malaysia, and Indonesia.

PARTS USED Root, leaves, latex, wood.

CONSTITUENTS Grape jasmine contains alkaloids and resins.

MEDICINAL ACTIONS & USES In Ayurvedic medicine, the root and the latex are used to expel worms. The root is also chewed to relieve toothache. The latex is used to treat cataracts (especially in the early stages), eye inflammations, and poor eyesight. The leaf juice makes a soothing treatment for skin irritations and wounds. The wood reduces fevers. In Indonesia, a decoction of the root is taken for diarrhea.

CAUTION Use grape jasmine only under professional supervision.

Eryngium maritimum
(Umbelliferae)
SEA HOLLY, ERYNGO

DESCRIPTION Evergreen perennial growing to 2 ft (60 cm). Has spiny silver leaves and tiny flowers in summer.

HABITAT Sea holly is found in coastal areas of Europe, preferring sandy soils. The root is unearthed in autumn.

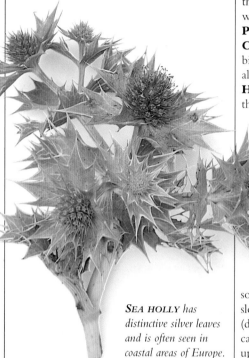

SEA HOLLY has distinctive silver leaves and is often seen in coastal areas of Europe.

PART USED Root.

CONSTITUENTS Sea holly contains saponins, coumarins, flavonoids, and plant acids.

HISTORY & FOLKLORE In 17th-century England, sea holly root was candied and eaten as a sweetmeat. It was also consumed as a means of preventing scurvy. In his *Irish Herbal* (1735), K'Eogh stated that the herb "provokes urination and menstruation, encourages flatulence, and removes obstructions of the liver, kidneys and bladder." In K'Eogh's time, sea holly was a popular medicinal herb, and was considered helpful in the treatment of a wide array of neurological conditions, including paralysis and convulsions. The plant was also used as an aphrodisiac.

MEDICINAL ACTIONS & USES In contemporary European herbal medicine, sea holly is used as a diuretic. It is prescribed as a treatment for cystitis and urethritis, and taken as a means to alleviate kidney stones. It is unlikely that the herb actually dissolves established stones, but it probably helps retard their formation. Sea holly is also used to treat enlargement or inflammation of the prostate gland, and may be of benefit in treating chest problems.

Erythraea centaurium
(Gentianaceae)
CENTAURY

DESCRIPTION Biennial herb growing to 10 in (25 cm) with a basal rosette of leaves and 5-petaled pink flowers in clusters.

HABITAT & CULTIVATION Native to Europe and southwestern Asia, centaury is now found in temperate regions throughout the world. The plant is harvested in summer when just about to flower.

PARTS USED Aerial parts.

CONSTITUENTS Centaury contains many bitter constituents, including secoiridoids, also found in gentian (*Gentiana lutea*, p. 97).

HISTORY & FOLKLORE In classical myth, the centaur Chiron used this herb to treat a poisoned arrow wound.

MEDICINAL ACTIONS & USES One of the most useful bitter herbs, centaury strengthens digestive function, especially within the stomach. By increasing stomach secretions, it hastens the breakdown of food. It also stimulates the appetite and increases bile production. Centaury needs to be taken over some weeks. The preparation should be slowly sipped so that the components (detectable at a dilution of up to 1:3,500) can stimulate reflex activity throughout the upper digestive tract.

SELF-HELP USES Weak digestion, p. 306; **Gas & bloating**, p. 306.

Erythrina variegata
(Leguminosae)
INDIAN CORAL TREE,
DADAP (HINDI)

DESCRIPTION Deciduous shrub growing to 20 ft (6 m). Has prickly stems, leaves with triangular leaflets, and pealike red flowers.

HABITAT & CULTIVATION Indian coral tree grows in deciduous forests throughout much of the Indian subcontinent. It is cultivated to support pepper plants.

PARTS USED Bark, leaves.

CONSTITUENTS This plant's constituents are unknown.

MEDICINAL ACTIONS & USES In Ayurveda, Indian coral tree is used to treat inflammatory conditions, menstrual pain, and problems related to eating and digestion, including anorexia, flatulence, colic, and worms. The bark is used for skin problems, fever, and leprosy. A paste made from the leaves is traditionally applied to heal wounds.

Erythronium americanum
(Liliaceae)
ADDER'S TONGUE

DESCRIPTION Perennial growing to 10 in (25 cm) from a small, bulblike corm. Has two oblong leaves mottled with purple and a large, bright yellow lily flower.

HABITAT & CULTIVATION Native to North America, adder's tongue is found mainly in the east, from New Brunswick to Florida. It prefers damp woodland and open ground. The leaves are gathered in summer.

PARTS USED Leaves.

CONSTITUENTS Very little is known about the constituents of this plant. It contains alpha-methylenebutyrolactone.

HISTORY & FOLKLORE Adder's tongue was not used much by Native Americans. European settlers considered its medicinal properties to be similar to those of meadow saffron (*Colchicum autumnale*, p. 191). Adder's tongue was listed in the *Pharmacopoeia of the United States* from 1820 to 1863 as a treatment for gout.

MEDICINAL ACTIONS & USES An infusion of the leaves is taken for the relief of skin problems such as ulcers and tumors, and for enlarged glands. Adder's tongue is often used to treat scrofulous skin arising from tubercular infection. The leaves (or whole plant) are applied as a poultice to treat skin conditions. Although the fresh leaves are strongly emetic, they are rarely used to stimulate vomiting.

CAUTION Take adder's tongue only under professional supervision.

Erythroxylum coca
(Erythroxylaceae)
COCA

DESCRIPTION Evergreen shrub growing to 10 ft (3 m). Has alternate oval leaves, small white flowers, and small red berries that each contain a single seed.

HABITAT & CULTIVATION Native to Peru and Bolivia, coca grows in high-rainfall areas of the eastern Andes to altitudes of 5,000 ft (1,500 m). It is mostly cultivated for the illegal market. The leaves are picked when they begin to curl.

PARTS USED Leaves.

CONSTITUENTS Coca contains cocaine and various other alkaloids, a volatile oil, flavonoids, vitamins A and B_2, and minerals. The plant's stimulant and anesthetic action is due largely to the cocaine it possesses.

HISTORY & FOLKLORE The indigenous peoples of the Andes carry pouches containing coca leaves and lime, which they chew throughout the day. Early European

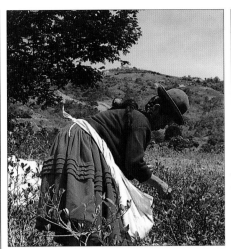

COCA is cultivated in the Andes and chewed as a tonic to help counter the effects of cold.

travelers noted that individuals chewing coca never suffered from tooth or gum problems, and local folk medicine considered the plant a treatment for toothache. Coca leaf extract is still used as a flavoring for cola drinks – but cocaine has long been banned from the formulas.

MEDICINAL ACTIONS & USES In Bolivia and Peru, coca leaves play an important part in the culture and herbal medicine of the indigenous Aymara and Quechua peoples. High altitudes, cold, and an impoverished diet place great physical demands on the population. Coca leaves, chewed with lime or ashes, release small amounts of the active constituents, which act as a tonic and help block the effects of cold, exhaustion, and poor nutrition. Coca leaves are also used in South American herbal medicine to treat nausea, vomiting, and asthma, and have been used to speed convalescence. In Colombia the leaf is used as a heart tonic. Cocaine extracted from coca leaves is used legally in conventional medicine as a local anesthetic. It is also taken illegally as a narcotic, stimulant drug. As an isolated chemical, cocaine is extremely addictive.

CAUTIONS Take only under professional supervision. Coca is subject to legal restrictions in most countries.

Eschscholzia californica
(*Papaveraceae*)
CALIFORNIA POPPY

DESCRIPTION Annual or perennial growing to 2 ft (60 cm). Has finely cut leaves and bright orange, yellow, pink, or red flowers.
HABITAT & CULTIVATION California poppy is native to western North America. Widely cultivated as a garden plant, it prefers sandy soils.
PARTS USED Aerial parts.

CONSTITUENTS California poppy contains alkaloids (including protopine, cryptopine, and chelidonine) and flavone glycosides.
HISTORY & FOLKLORE Native American peoples were known to use the sap of California poppy for its pain-killing properties, particularly for toothache.
MEDICINAL ACTIONS & USES Although California poppy is closely related to the opium poppy (*Papaver somniferum*, p. 242), it has a markedly different effect on the central nervous system. California poppy is not a narcotic. In fact, rather than disorientating the user, it tends to normalize psychological function. California poppy's gently antispasmodic, sedative, and analgesic effects make it a valuable herbal medicine for treating physical and psychological problems in children. California poppy may also prove beneficial in attempts to overcome bedwetting, difficulty in sleeping, and nervous tension and anxiety.

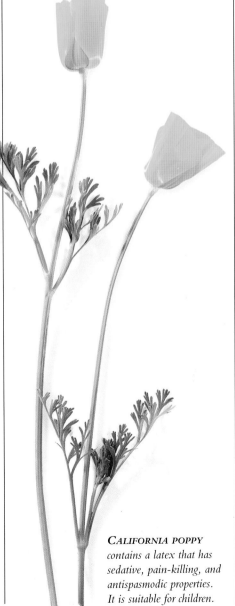

CALIFORNIA POPPY contains a latex that has sedative, pain-killing, and antispasmodic properties. It is suitable for children.

Eucalyptus smithii
(*Myrtaceae*)
EUCALYPTUS

DESCRIPTION Aromatic evergreen tree growing to 160 ft (50 m).
HABITAT & CULTIVATION Native to Australia, eucalyptus now grows in temperate and subtropical zones around the world.
PART USED Essential oil.
CONSTITUENTS The volatile oil contains about 70% eucalyptol (1, 8-cineole), as well as pinene, limonene, alpha-terpineol, and linalool. While it is similar to the oils of related species, this oil appears to be better tolerated by the skin.
MEDICINAL ACTIONS & USES Eucalyptus essential oil is used in aromatherapy, and also as a disinfectant and antiseptic for the treatment of viral conditions, skin and other infections, and as a decongestant.
CAUTION While the essential oil of *E. smithii* is less toxic than those of other eucalyptus species, it should nevertheless be used only according to label instructions or under the guidance of a professional practitioner.

Eucommia ulmoides
(*Eucommiaceae*)
DU ZHONG (CHINESE),
GUTTA PERCHA

DESCRIPTION Deciduous tree growing to 70 ft (20 m). Has elliptical leaves, with male flowers in loose clusters, and solitary female flowers in the leaf axils.
HABITAT & CULTIVATION *Du zhong* grows in temperate zones in China. It is cultivated, but only in small amounts.
PART USED Bark.
CONSTITUENTS *Du zhong* contains gutta percha, alkaloids, iridoids and other glycosides, and potassium.
HISTORY & FOLKLORE The herb was mentioned in the Chinese herbal, the *Divine Husbandman's Classic (Shen'nong Bencaojing)*, which was written in the 1st century AD.
MEDICINAL ACTIONS & USES *Du zhong* is considered an excellent tonic for the liver and kidneys. In particular it helps lower back pain, knee weakness, and frequent urination. *Du zhong* is said to "tonify the *yang*" and to invigorate the circulation. It is also thought to prevent miscarriage.
RESEARCH Much interest has been aroused by *du zhong's* ability to reduce high blood pressure. In a clinical trial in China involving 119 subjects treated with the herb, 46% of those tested showed a significant reduction in blood pressure level. However, *du zhong* has little effect in cases of severe hypertension.

Euonymus atropurpureus
(Celastraceae)
WAHOO BARK

DESCRIPTION Deciduous tree growing to 25 ft (8 m). Has smooth branches, serrated elliptical leaves, clusters of purple flowers, and 4-lobed scarlet fruit.

HABITAT & CULTIVATION Native to eastern North America, wahoo bark thrives in damp woods and close to water. The bark is gathered in autumn.

PARTS USED Stem bark, root bark.

CONSTITUENTS Wahoo bark contains cardenolides (cardiac glycosides) similar to digitoxin, alkaloids, including asparagine, sterols, and tannins.

HISTORY & FOLKLORE The Sioux, Cree, and other Native American peoples used wahoo bark in various ways, for example as an eye lotion, as a poultice for facial sores, and for gynecological conditions. Native Americans introduced the plant to early European settlers, and it became very popular in Britain as well as in North America in the 19th century.

MEDICINAL ACTIONS & USES Wahoo bark is considered a gallbladder remedy with laxative and diuretic properties. It is prescribed for biliousness and liver problems, as well as for skin conditions such as eczema (which may result from poor liver and gallbladder function), and for constipation. In the past, it was often used in combination with herbs such as gentian (*Gentiana lutea*, p. 97) as a fever remedy, especially if the liver was under stress. Following the discovery that it contains cardiac glycosides, wahoo bark has been given for heart conditions.

CAUTIONS Wahoo bark is toxic. Use only under professional supervision. Do not take during pregnancy or while breast-feeding.

Eupatorium cannabinum
(Compositae)
HEMP AGRIMONY

DESCRIPTION Perennial growing to 5 ft (1.5 m). Has a red stem, downy leaves, and dense bunches of pink to mauve florets.

HABITAT & CULTIVATION Native to Europe, hemp agrimony is now also found in western Asia and North Africa. It grows in damp woods, ditches, and marshes, as well as in open areas, and is gathered when in flower in summer.

PARTS USED Aerial parts, root.

CONSTITUENTS Hemp agrimony contains a volatile oil (with alpha-terpinene, p-cymene, thymol, and an azulene), sesquiterpene lactones (especially eupatoriopicrin), flavonoids, pyrrolizidine alkaloids, and polysaccharides. P-cymene is antiviral, while eupatoriopicrin has anti-cancer properties and inhibits cellular growth. The polysaccharides stimulate the immune system. In isolation, the pyrrolizidine alkaloids are toxic to the liver.

HISTORY & FOLKLORE Hemp agrimony was known to Avicenna (AD 980–1037) and other practitioners of Arabian medicine in the early Middle Ages. In her book *A Modern Herbal* (1931), Mrs. Grieve described how "people used to lay the leaves on bread, considering that they thus prevented it from becoming mouldy."

MEDICINAL ACTIONS & USES Hemp agrimony has been employed chiefly as a detoxifying herb for fever, colds, flu, and other acute viral conditions. It also stimulates the removal of waste products via the kidneys. The root is laxative, and the whole plant is considered to be tonic. Recently, hemp agrimony has found use as an immunostimulant, helping to maintain resistance to acute viral and other infections.

RELATED SPECIES *See also* boneset (*E. perfoliatum, following entry*) and gravel root (*E. purpureum, subsequent entry*).

CAUTION In view of hemp agrimony's pyrrolizidine alkaloid content, take only under professional supervision.

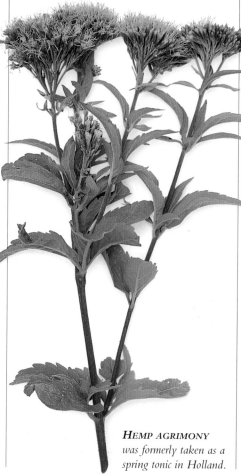

HEMP AGRIMONY
was formerly taken as a spring tonic in Holland.

Eupatorium perfoliatum
(Compositae)
BONESET

DESCRIPTION Erect perennial growing to 5 ft (1.5 m). Has tapering lance-shaped leaves and many white or purple florets.

HABITAT & CULTIVATION Native to eastern North America, boneset is found in meadows and marshland. It is gathered when in flower in summer.

PARTS USED Aerial parts.

CONSTITUENTS Boneset contains sesquiterpene lactones (including eupafolin), polysaccharides, flavonoids, diterpenes, sterols, and volatile oil. The sesquiterpene lactones and polysaccharides are significantly immunostimulant.

HISTORY & FOLKLORE Native American people used boneset to make an infusion for treating colds, fever, and arthritic and rheumatic pain. European settlers learned of the plant's benefits, and by the 18th and 19th centuries it was regarded as a virtual cure-all. Boneset's common name derives from its ability to treat "break-bone fever."

MEDICINAL ACTIONS & USES A hot infusion of boneset will bring relief to symptoms of the common cold. The plant stimulates resistance to viral and bacterial infections, and reduces fever by encouraging sweating. Boneset also loosens phlegm and promotes its removal through coughing, and it has a tonic and laxative effect. It has been taken for rheumatic illness, skin conditions, and worms.

RELATED SPECIES Wild horehound (*E. teucrifolium*) was used as a substitute for boneset. *E. occidentale* was used by the Zuni of the southwestern US to treat rheumatism. *See also* hemp agrimony (*E. cannabinum, preceding entry*) and gravel root (*E. purpureum, following entry*).

CAUTION Boneset can be toxic if taken in excessive doses.

SELF-HELP USES Allergic rhinitis with mucus, p. 300; Colds, influenza, & fevers, p. 311; High fever, p. 311.

Eupatorium purpureum
(Compositae)
GRAVEL ROOT, JOE PYE WEED

DESCRIPTION Erect perennial growing to 5 ft (1.5 m). Has whorls of pointed oblong leaves and clusters of purple-pink florets.

HABITAT & CULTIVATION Gravel root is native to eastern North America. The root is unearthed in autumn.

PART USED Root.

CONSTITUENTS Gravel root contains a volatile oil, flavonoids, and resin.

HISTORY & FOLKLORE The plant's alternative name, Joe Pye weed, is in honor of the Native American said to have used it to cure New Englanders of typhus. Native Americans used the herb as a diuretic and for conditions affecting the genitourinary system. It was listed in the *Pharmacopoeia of the United States* from 1820 to 1842.

MEDICINAL ACTIONS & USES As its common name indicates, gravel root is a valuable herb for urinary tract problems. It helps to prevent the formation of kidney and bladder stones and may diminish existing stones. Gravel root is also useful for cystitis, urethritis, prostate enlargement (and other forms of obstruction), and for rheumatism and gout. The root is thought to help the latter two conditions by increasing the removal of waste by the kidneys.

RELATED SPECIES *E. maculatum*, native to eastern North America, is used to treat kidney and urinary problems. See also *E. cannabinum* and *E. perfoliatum*, p. 206.

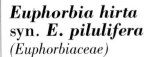

GRAVEL ROOT is especially helpful for urinary tract problems.

Euphorbia hirta
syn. *E. pilulifera*
(Euphorbiaceae)
PILL-BEARING SPURGE,
ASTHMA PLANT

DESCRIPTION Erect annual or perennial plant growing to 20 in (50 cm), with pointed oval leaves and clusters of small flowers.

HABITAT & CULTIVATION Native to India and Australia, pill-bearing spurge is now widespread throughout the tropics. The aerial parts of the plant are gathered when it is in flower.

PARTS USED Aerial parts.

CONSTITUENTS Pill-bearing spurge contains flavonoids, terpenoids, alkanes, phenolic acids, shikimic acid, and choline. The latter two constituents may be partly responsible for the antispasmodic action of this plant.

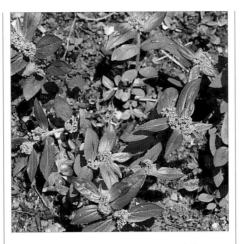

PILL-BEARING SPURGE is recommended as a treatment for asthma.

HISTORY & FOLKLORE As its name suggests, this plant was traditionally used in Asia to treat asthma.

MEDICINAL ACTIONS & USES A specific treatment for bronchial asthma, pill-bearing spurge relaxes the bronchial tubes and eases breathing. Mildly sedative and expectorant, it is also taken for bronchitis and other respiratory tract conditions. It is most often used along with other antiasthmatic herbs, notably gumplant (*Grindelia camporum*, p. 216) and lobelia (*Lobelia inflata*, p. 108). In the Anglo-American tradition, pill-bearing spurge is taken to treat intestinal amebiasis.

RELATED SPECIES The Cherokee used *E. maculata* to treat sore nipples and skin disorders. Many other North American *Euphorbia* species were used for constipation. A decoction of *E. lancifolia*, native to the West Indies, is used to stimulate breast-milk production. *E. atoto* is used in Malaysia and Indochina to induce delayed menstruation and as an abortifacient. Many species of *Euphorbia* are used as arrow poisons.

Euphorbia lathyrus
(Euphorbiaceae)
CAPER SPURGE

DESCRIPTION Vigorous biennial growing to 3 ft (1 m). Has a hollow stem, heart-shaped leaves, clusters of small green flowers, and green fruit.

HABITAT & CULTIVATION Common throughout much of Europe, Asia, and North America, caper spurge grows in low-lying areas. The fruit is picked in summer.

PARTS USED Seeds, latex.

CONSTITUENTS The seeds contain a fixed oil and resin; the latex contains euphorbone and resin.

HISTORY & FOLKLORE For thousands of years, caper spurge was taken as a violent purge. In the 1st century AD, the Greek physician Dioscorides recommended "6 or 7 grains of the seeds, in pill form or taken with figs or dates, which purges from below water, phlegm and choler." It was still used as a purgative in rural France in the 19th century. The leaves of caper spurge were formerly used by beggars to raise unsightly sores on their skin, thereby increasing their chances of eliciting pity and alms.

MEDICINAL ACTIONS & USES Caper spurge is so violent a purgative that it is rarely if ever used in contemporary herbal medicine. This indicates the extent to which medicine as a whole has changed in modern times. Purging was the first resort of many traditional medical systems, and never more enthusiastically so than in Western medicine in the 18th century. Caper spurge seeds were commonly employed, but an oil extracted from them was also used in very small doses (the oil is highly toxic). In the past, the milky latex of caper spurge was used as a depilatory and to remove corns, but is too irritant to be used safely.

CAUTION Caper spurge is a toxic plant. Do not use under any circumstances.

Euphorbia pekinensis
(Euphorbiaceae)
DA JI

DESCRIPTION Erect annual or perennial plant with oblong leaves and dense clusters of small flowers.

HABITAT & CULTIVATION Native to China, *da ji* is cultivated mainly in the eastern and central provinces. The root is unearthed in early spring.

PART USED Root.

CONSTITUENTS *Da ji* contains euphorbon.

MEDICINAL ACTIONS & USES *Da ji* is classified as a toxic herb in Chinese herbal medicine, and therefore it is prescribed only for relatively serious illnesses. It is taken as a cathartic to purge excess fluid in conditions such as pleurisy and ascites (excess fluid in the abdomen), and for the treatment of kidney problems, especially nephritis. *Da ji* is applied externally to inflamed sores to reduce swelling. The herb is incompatible with licorice species (*Glycyrrhiza glabra*, p. 99 and *G. uralensis*, p. 215) because it neutralizes their effects.

RESEARCH Research in China indicates that *da ji* is therapeutically useful in the treatment of ascites and nephritis; however, it produces significant side effects.

RELATED SPECIES *E. kansui* is similar to *da ji* but has a stronger cathartic action. In Chinese herbal medicine it is only given to people with strong constitutions.

CAUTION *Da ji* is a toxic plant. Take only under professional supervision.

Euphrasia spp.
(Scrophulariaceae)
EYEBRIGHT

DESCRIPTION Creeping, semiparasitic annual growing to 20 in (50 cm). Has tiny oval leaves and small scallop-edged white flowers with yellow spots and a black center, somewhat resembling an eye.

HABITAT & CULTIVATION Common in Europe, eyebright thrives in meadows and open grassland. It is gathered in summer when in flower.

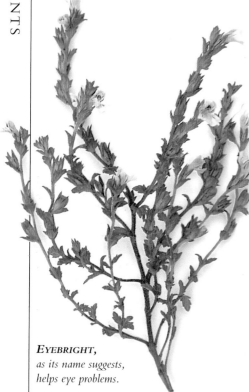

EYEBRIGHT,
as its name suggests,
helps eye problems.

PARTS USED Aerial parts.

CONSTITUENTS Eyebright contains iridoid glycosides (especially aucubin), tannins, phenolic acids, and volatile oil.

HISTORY & FOLKLORE Eyebright's use for eye problems was due in part to the Doctrine of Signatures, a 16th-century theory that held that a plant's appearance pointed to the ailments it treated.

MEDICINAL ACTIONS & USES Eyebright tightens the mucous membranes of the eye and appears to relieve the inflammation of conjunctivitis and blepharitis. Its ability to counter mucus means that it is often used for infectious and allergic conditions affecting the eyes, middle ear, sinuses, and nasal passages. Although eyebright counters liquid mucus, it should be used guardedly for dry and stuffy congestion, which tends to be made worse by the plant's astringency.

SELF-HELP USES Allergic rhinitis with mucus, p. 300; **Conjunctivitis**, p. 310; **Prevention of nosebleeds**, p. 310.

208

Evodia rutaecarpa
(Rutaceae)
EVODIA, WU ZHU YU (CHINESE)

DESCRIPTION Deciduous tree growing to 30 ft (10 m). Has compound leaves, clusters of white flowers, and greenish red fruit.

HABITAT & CULTIVATION Native to China, Tibet, and the eastern Himalayas, evodia is cultivated in China. The partially ripe fruit is gathered in late summer.

PART USED Fruit.

CONSTITUENTS Evodia contains evodine, evodiamine, and rutaecarpine.

HISTORY & FOLKLORE Evodia was listed in the *Divine Husbandman's Classic (Shen'nong Bencaojing)* of the 1st century AD.

MEDICINAL ACTIONS & USES Evodia has a marked warming effect on the body, helping to relieve headaches and a wide range of digestive problems. In Chinese herbal medicine, evodia is used mainly for abdominal pains, vomiting, diarrhea, headaches, and a weak pulse.

RESEARCH Chinese studies indicate that evodia is analgesic and reduces blood pressure.

CAUTION Use evodia only under professional supervision.

Fagopyrum esculentum
(Polygonaceae)
BUCKWHEAT

DESCRIPTION Annual growing to about 20 in (50 cm). Has arrow-shaped leaves and clusters of white or pink 5-petaled flowers.

HABITAT & CULTIVATION Buckwheat is native to central and northern Asia, and is cultivated extensively in temperate regions, especially the US. It is harvested in summer.

PARTS USED Leaves, flowers.

CONSTITUENTS Buckwheat contains bioflavonoids, especially rutin, which is strongly anti-oxidant. Rutin strengthens the inner lining of blood vessels.

HISTORY & FOLKLORE Buckwheat's French name, *blé Sarrasin*, alludes to its ancient Middle Eastern origins. The grain was either introduced to Europe during the crusades (11th and 12th centuries), or it was brought to Spain by the Arabs several centuries earlier.

MEDICINAL ACTIONS & USES Buckwheat is used to treat a wide range of circulatory problems. It is best taken as a tea or tablet, accompanied by vitamin C or lemon juice (*Citrus limon*, p. 81) to aid absorption. Buckwheat is used particularly to treat fragile capillaries (seen as small bruises with no apparent cause), but also helps strengthen varicose veins and heal chilblains. Often combined with linden flowers (*Tilia* spp., p. 275), buckwheat is a specific treatment

for hemorrhage into the retina. Buckwheat is also commonly taken in combination with other herbs for high blood pressure.

RELATED SPECIES Recent research has shown that the Chinese *F. dibotrys* and *F. cymosum* are immune-stimulant. They are prescribed for chronic bronchitis, inflamed gallbladder, and pulmonary abscesses.

SELF-HELP USES High blood pressure & arteriosclerosis, p. 301; **Poor circulation & high blood pressure**, p. 319.

Feronia limonia
(Rutaceae)
WOOD APPLE

DESCRIPTION Small, spiny tree growing to 70 ft (20 m). Has feathery leaves, red flowers, and round whitish fruit the size of oranges.

HABITAT & CULTIVATION Native to southern India, wood apple is cultivated in tropical Asia.

PARTS USED Fruit, leaves.

CONSTITUENTS The fruit contains fruit acids, vitamins, and minerals. The leaves contain tannins and a volatile oil.

MEDICINAL ACTIONS & USES Wood apple fruit is used mainly to stimulate the digestive system. In India, the fruit forms part of a paste applied to tone the breasts. The astringent leaves are used to treat indigestion, flatulence, diarrhea, dysentery (particularly in children), and hemorrhoids.

Ferula assa-foetida
(Umbelliferae)
ASAFOETIDA, DEVIL'S DUNG

DESCRIPTION Perennial plant growing to about 6 ft (2 m). Has a fleshy taproot, hollow stem, compound leaves, and many white flowers in umbels.

HABITAT & CULTIVATION Native to Iran, Afghanistan, and Pakistan, asafoetida produces a gum obtained in summer from 4-year-old plants. The stems are cut off, and successive slices are made through the roots. The gum wells up and is collected after it has hardened.

PART USED Oleo-gum-resin.

CONSTITUENTS Asafoetida exudate contains 6–17% volatile oil, as well as resin and gum. The volatile oil contains disulphides, which have an expectorant action. The oil also settles the digestion. Asafoetida resin contains sesquiterpenoid coumarins, including foetidin.

HISTORY & FOLKLORE In the 7th century BC, *Charaka Samhita*, a Hindu medical treatise, proclaimed asafoetida the best remedy for clearing gas and bloating. The name devil's dung notwithstanding, the plant is thought to have been the most popular spice in ancient Rome. Asafoetida is as persistent in aroma as garlic (*Allium sativum*, p. 56), and is still used as a flavoring, notably in Worcestershire sauce.

MEDICINAL ACTIONS & USES In Middle Eastern and Indian herbal medicine, asafoetida is used for simple digestive problems such as gas, bloating, indigestion, and constipation. Asafoetida's volatile oil, like that of garlic, has components that leave the body via the respiratory system and aid the coughing up of congested mucus. Asafoetida is taken (usually in tablet form) for bronchitis, bronchial asthma, whooping cough, and other chest problems. Asafoetida also lowers blood pressure and thins the blood. The herb has a reputation for helping in neurotic states. Improvement may be a psychosomatic response, since the herb's unpleasant smell suggests potency.

RELATED SPECIES *F. silphion* was used in ancient Rome as a contraceptive. It was overharvested and died out in about AD 300. *F. persica* is used in the Middle East for rheumatic problems and backache. The central Asian *F. sumbul* is used as a nerve tonic. *F. jaeschkeana* has recently been investigated as a potential contraceptive. See also *F. gummosa* (*following entry*).

CAUTION While safe in adults, asafoetida may be harmful to young babies.

Ferula gummosa
syn. *F. galbaniflua*
(*Umbelliferae*)
GALBANUM

DESCRIPTION Perennial with a smooth hollow stem, finely toothed compound leaves, and umbels of small white flowers.

HABITAT & CULTIVATION Native to central Asia, galbanum produces a gum that is obtained when stems are cut off and successive slices are made through the roots. Gum wells to the surface and is collected after it has hardened.

PART USED Oleo-gum-resin.

CONSTITUENTS Galbanum exudate contains a volatile oil, resins, gums, and a coumarin (umbelliferone).

HISTORY & FOLKLORE Galbanum has been used medicinally for centuries.

MEDICINAL ACTIONS & USES Galbanum is a digestive stimulant and antispasmodic, reducing flatulence, cramps, and colic. It is also an expectorant. Applied as an ointment, the gum may help heal wounds.

RELATED SPECIES See asafoetida (*F. assa-foetida*, *preceding entry*).

SELF-HELP USE Acidity & indigestion, p. 307.

Ficus benghalensis
(*Moraceae*)
BANYAN TREE

DESCRIPTION Tree growing to 70 ft (20 m) with oval leaves, fig-type fruit, and roots that grow into the ground from branches.

HABITAT & CULTIVATION Growing wild in India and Pakistan, the banyan tree is also cultivated across the Indian subcontinent.

PARTS USED Fruit, bark, leaves, latex, aerial roots.

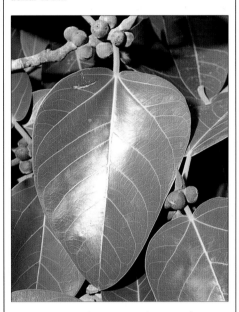

BANYAN TREE leaves are astringent and are used to tighten mucous membranes.

CONSTITUENTS Banyan tree contains ficusin and bergaptin.

HISTORY & FOLKLORE The banyan tree is sacred to Hindus.

MEDICINAL ACTIONS & USES The astringent leaves and bark of the tree are employed to relieve diarrhea and dysentery and to reduce bleeding. As with other *Ficus* species, the latex is applied to hemorrhoids, warts, and aching joints. The fruit is laxative and the roots are chewed to prevent gum disease. The bark is used in Ayurvedic medicine for diabetes.

RELATED SPECIES See *F. carica* (*following entry*).

CAUTION The latex is toxic and should not be taken internally.

Ficus carica
(*Moraceae*)
FIG

DESCRIPTION Deciduous tree growing to 12 ft (4 m). Has large leaves and fleshy receptacles that ripen into purple-brown pear-shaped fruit.

HABITAT & CULTIVATION Native to western Asia, fig now grows wild and often is cultivated in temperate and subtropical regions. Fruit is gathered in summer.

PARTS USED Fruit, latex.

CONSTITUENTS Figs contain about 50% fruit sugars (mainly glucose), flavonoids, vitamins, and enzymes.

HISTORY & FOLKLORE The fig leaf was used by Adam and Eve to hide their nakedness in the Garden of Eden. There are many other references to the plant in the Old Testament, mainly to the sweetness of the fruit and to its use as a medicine. Spartan athletes in ancient Greece were said to eat figs in order to improve their performance.

MEDICINAL ACTIONS & USES The fruit sugars within the fig (especially the dried fruit) have a pronounced but gentle laxative effect; syrup of figs is still a remedy for mild constipation. The fruit's emollient pulp helps relieve pain and inflammation, and it has been used to treat tumors, swellings, and gum abscesses – the fruit often being roasted before application. Figs are also mildly expectorant and, when used with herbs such as elecampane (*Inula helenium*, p. 105), are helpful in treating dry and irritable coughs and bronchitis. The milky latex from leaves and stems is reputed to be analgesic, and has long been used to treat warts, insect bites, and stings.

RELATED SPECIES The juice and powdered bark of the Central American *F. cotinifolia* are applied to wounds and bruises. *F. indica* is used in Ayurvedic medicine as a tonic, diuretic, and treatment for gonorrhea. *F. lacor* is used in Chinese herbal medicine to induce sweating, while *F. retusa*, which is native to China, Indonesia, and Australia, is used in the Chinese tradition to treat toothache and tooth decay. *See also* banyan tree (*F. benghalensis*, *preceding entry*) and peepal (*F. religiosa*, *following entry*).

CAUTIONS The latex is toxic and should not be used internally. Applied to the skin, it may cause an allergic reaction to sunlight.

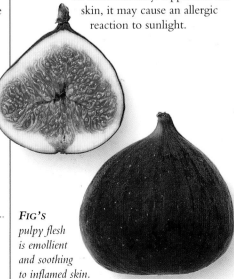

FIG'S pulpy flesh is emollient and soothing to inflamed skin.

Ficus religiosa
(Moraceae)
PEEPAL

DESCRIPTION Tree growing to about 25 ft (8 m) with large, leathery, heart-shaped leaves and purple fruit growing in pairs.

HABITAT & CULTIVATION Peepal grows in northern and central India, in forests and by water. It is also cultivated throughout the subcontinent and southern Asia. The fruit is gathered when ripe.

PARTS USED Fruit, leaves, bark, latex.

CONSTITUENTS The fruit contains fruit sugars, flavonoids, and enzymes.

HISTORY & FOLKLORE Sacred to Hindus and Buddhists, the peepal is the tree under which the Buddha attained enlightenment. It is a long-living tree; a peepal in Sri Lanka is thought to be over 2,000 years old.

MEDICINAL ACTIONS & USES Peepal's uses are similar to those of the banyan (*F. benghalensis*, p. 209). Its astringent bark and leaves are taken for diarrhea and dysentery, whereas the leaves alone are used for constipation. The leaves are applied with *ghee* (clarified butter) as a poultice to boils and to swollen salivary glands in mumps. The powdered fruit may be taken for asthma, and the latex is used to treat warts.

RELATED SPECIES See fig (*F. carica*, p. 209).

Foeniculum vulgare
(Umbelliferae)
FENNEL

DESCRIPTION Aromatic perennial growing to about 5 ft (1.5 m). Has dark green, feathery leaves, umbels of yellow flowers, and small, ridged oval-shaped seeds.

HABITAT & CULTIVATION Native to the Mediterranean region, fennel is now cultivated in temperate regions around the world. The seeds are gathered in autumn.

PARTS USED Seeds, essential oil.

CONSTITUENTS Fennel seeds contain about 8% volatile oil (about 80% anethole, plus fenchone and methyl chavicol), flavonoids, coumarins (including bergapten), and sterols. The volatile oil relieves gas and is antispasmodic.

HISTORY & FOLKLORE Some ancient authors considered fennel a remedy for snake bite. In the early Middle Ages the plant was considered to be an antidote to witchcraft.

MEDICINAL ACTIONS & USES The primary use of fennel seeds is to relieve bloating, but they also settle stomach pain, stimulate the appetite, and are diuretic and anti-inflammatory. Like anise (*Pimpinella anisum*, p. 246) and caraway (*Carum carvi*, p. 182), the seeds make an excellent infusion for

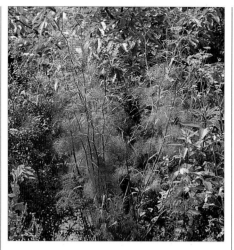

FENNEL has a long history of use as a remedy for ailments of the digestive tract.

settling the digestion and reducing abdominal distension. The seeds help in the treatment of kidney stones and, combined with urinary antiseptics such as uva-ursi (*Arctostaphylos uva-ursi*, p. 168), make an effective treatment for cystitis. An infusion of the seeds may be taken as a gargle for sore throats and as a mild expectorant. Fennel is safe for children and, as an infusion or syrup, can be given for colic and painful teething in babies. Fennel increases breast-milk production, and is still used as an eyewash for sore eyes and conjunctivitis. The seeds have a longstanding reputation as an aid to weight loss and to longevity. Essential oil from the sweet variety is used for its digestive and relaxing properties.

CAUTIONS Fennel seeds are potentially toxic; do not exceed recommended dose. Do not take the essential oil internally.

SELF-HELP USES Acidity & indigestion, p. 307; Gas & bloating, p. 306; Morning sickness & nausea, p. 317; Stomach spasm, p. 305.

Forsythia suspensa
(Oleaceae)
LIAN QIAO (CHINESE),
WEEPING FORSYTHIA

DESCRIPTION Deciduous shrub growing to 10 ft (3 m). Has toothed leaves, bright yellow flowers, and woody fruit.

HABITAT & CULTIVATION Native to China and Japan, *lian qiao* is cultivated in the northern and central areas of China and in other temperate regions. The fruit is harvested in autumn just before it is completely ripe.

PART USED Fruit.

CONSTITUENTS The fruit contains forsythin.

HISTORY & FOLKLORE *Lian qiao* was first listed in the *Divine Husbandman's Classic* (*Shen'nong Bencaojing*), written in the 1st century AD. *Lian qiao* was featured in a remedy for infections from the 18th century.

MEDICINAL ACTIONS & USES A bitter-tasting, pungent herb with an antiseptic effect, *lian qiao* is chiefly used to treat boils, carbuncles, mumps, and infected neck glands. It is also a remedy for colds, flu, sore throats, and tonsillitis, and for the early stages of fevers. It is given in combination with other herbs for dysentery and skin infections, and is used for "cold" swellings of the neck (as in tuberculosis of the lymph glands). In Chinese folk medicine, it is a treatment for breast cancer. The herb is sometimes taken to induce menstruation.

RESEARCH Research in China indicates that forsythin is significantly antimicrobial and reduces nausea and vomiting.

Fragaria vesca
(Rosaceae)
WILD STRAWBERRY

DESCRIPTION Low-growing perennial herb spread by runners. Has 3-lobed leaves, white flowers, and small red berries.

HABITAT & CULTIVATION Wild strawberry is native to Europe and temperate regions of Asia. The leaves and fruit are gathered in early summer.

PARTS USED Leaves, fruit.

WILD STRAWBERRY was said to "comfort fainting spirits."

CONSTITUENTS The leaves contain flavonoids, tannins, and a volatile oil. The fruit contains fruit acids, and a volatile oil with methyl salicylate and borneol.

HISTORY & FOLKLORE Wild strawberry appears to have not been much used medicinally until the Middle Ages. Writing in 1652, Nicholas Culpeper listed its benefits: "the berries are excellent good to cool the liver, the blood and the spleen or a hot cholerick stomach … the leaves and roots thereof [are] also good to fasten loose teeth and to heal spongy foul gums."

MEDICINAL ACTIONS & USES Wild strawberry leaves are mildly astringent and diuretic. The plant is rarely used medicinally today, but it can be taken to treat diarrhea and dysentery. The leaves were also used as a gargle for sore throats, and in a lotion for minor burns and scrapes. In Europe, the fruit is considered to have cooling and diuretic properties, and has been prescribed as part of a diet in cases of tuberculosis, gout, arthritis, and rheumatism.

Fraxinus excelsior
(Oleaceae)
ASH

DESCRIPTION Deciduous tree growing to 130 ft (40 m). Has pale gray bark, black conical leaf buds, and bright green leaves with 7–13 oval leaflets.

HABITAT & CULTIVATION Common in Europe, ash thrives in lowland and moorland. The leaves are gathered in summer, but the bark is gathered in spring.

PARTS USED Leaves, bark.

CONSTITUENTS Ash leaves and bark contain coumarins, flavonoids, tannins, sugars, and a volatile oil.

HISTORY & FOLKLORE The ash was the "world-tree" of Norse mythology, its roots spreading to the domain of the gods and its branches extending to the most remote corners of the universe. In Norse myth, the first man was carved from a piece of ash wood. Until the last century in the Highlands of Scotland, it was customary to give a spoonful of ash sap to every newborn child.

MEDICINAL ACTIONS & USES Ash bark is tonic and astringent. Rarely used in herbal medicine today, it is occasionally taken for fever. The leaves are also astringent, and they have a laxative and diuretic effect. They have been used as a mild substitute for senna (*Cassia senna*, p. 72).

RELATED SPECIES The bark of the American white ash (*F. americana*) has been used as a bitter tonic and astringent. The wax deposited by an insect on the Chinese *F. chinensis* is used to coat pills. Several ash species exude a nutritious sap, called "manna," which is used as a laxative for children. In particular, the manna ash (*F. ornus*) has been cultivated in southern Europe for its high yield of manna sap.

Fritillaria thunbergii
(Liliaceae)
ZHE BEI MU

DESCRIPTION Bulbous perennial with erect stems, long narrow leaves, and hanging bell-shaped flowers.

HABITAT & CULTIVATION Native to China and Siberia, *zhe bei mu* is cultivated in eastern China. The bulb is unearthed in early summer.

PART USED Bulb.

CONSTITUENTS The bulb contains alkaloids, including peimine, which affects the parasympathetic nervous system.

HISTORY & FOLKLORE *Zhe bei mu* was used in much the same way as *chuan bei mu* (*F. cirrhosa*, see *Related Species*) until 1765, when it was classified as having distinct actions. *Zhe bei mu* is considered more effective in acute conditions.

MEDICINAL ACTIONS & USES *Zhe bei mu* increases the coughing up of mucus and relieves irritability in the respiratory tract. It is given for the treatment of bronchitis and tonsillitis, and for fever and respiratory symptoms accompanying other acute infections such as flu. *Zhe bei mu* is thought to act specifically on tumors and swellings of the throat, neck, and chest, and is taken for thyroid gland nodules, scrofula (tuberculosis of the lymph glands of the neck), abscesses and boils, and breast cancer. It has also been used to treat dysentery, and to increase breast-milk production.

RELATED SPECIES *F. cirrhosa* grows in Sichuan and Tibet and is used medicinally to treat coughs of all kinds. *F. roylei*, also a Chinese herb, is occasionally used in the treatment of asthma. *F. imperialis*, native to Iran and Afghanistan, has been used as an expectorant and also to encourage increased breast-milk production.

CAUTION *Fritillaria* species are very toxic. Take only under professional supervision.

Fucus vesiculosus
(Fucaceae)
BLADDERWRACK, KELP

DESCRIPTION Brownish-green alga growing to 3 ft (1 m) in length. Has flat, usually forked, fronds containing air bladders.

HABITAT & CULTIVATION Bladderwrack is native to the shores of the North Atlantic and western Mediterranean, and is harvested throughout the year.

PART USED Whole plant.

CONSTITUENTS Bladderwrack contains phenols, polysaccharides, and minerals, especially iodine (up to 0.1%). The polysaccharides are immune-stimulant.

The iodine may stimulate the thyroid gland.

HISTORY & FOLKLORE Bladderwrack has been employed as a fuel, as a winter feed for cattle, and as a source of iodine and potash.

MEDICINAL ACTIONS & USES Due to its iodine content, bladderwrack is taken as an antigoiter remedy. The plant appears to raise the metabolic rate by increasing hormone production by the thyroid gland, but this increase may be limited to poorly functioning thyroids. Bladderwrack is reputedly helpful in rheumatic conditions.

RESEARCH In one clinical trial (Italy 1976), patients taking bladderwrack lost much more weight than the control group.

CAUTIONS Do not take if pregnant or breast-feeding. If suffering from a thyroid illness, take only under professional advice.

Fumaria officinalis
(Fumariaceae)
FUMITORY

DESCRIPTION Climbing annual growing to 1 ft (30 cm). Has compound leaves and maroon-tipped pink tubular flowers.

HABITAT & CULTIVATION Native to Europe and North Africa, fumitory also grows in Asia, North America, and Australia.

PARTS USED Flowering aerial parts.

CONSTITUENTS Fumitory contains isoquinoline alkaloids.

HISTORY & FOLKLORE Fumitory has a long history of use in Europe.

MEDICINAL ACTIONS & USES The herb has a stimulant action on the liver and gallbladder and is chiefly used to treat skin conditions such as eczema. It is also diuretic and mildly laxative.

RELATED SPECIES Fumitory is related to corydalis (*Corydalis yanhusuo*, p. 85) and *F. parviflora* from central Asia. The latter, like fumitory, is used as a detoxifying, laxative, and diuretic herb.

CAUTION Fumitory is toxic in excessive doses. Use only under professional advice.

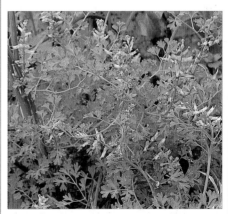

FUMITORY may be applied externally as a treatment for eczema.

OTHER MEDICINAL PLANTS

Galega officinalis
(Leguminosae)
GOAT'S RUE

DESCRIPTION Bushy perennial growing to about 3 ft (1 m). Has compound leaves with lance-shaped leaflets, delicate pink pea-type flowers on terminal spikes, and red-brown seed pods in autumn.

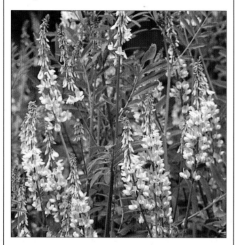

GOAT'S RUE *was once taken to treat the plague.*

HABITAT & CULTIVATION Native to Asia and continental Europe, and naturalized in Britain, goat's rue grows in damp and low-lying areas. It is harvested in summer.

PARTS USED Aerial parts.

CONSTITUENTS Goat's rue contains alkaloids (including galegine), saponins, flavonoids, and tannins. Galegine strongly reduces blood sugar levels.

HISTORY & FOLKLORE Formerly used as a treatment for the plague, goat's rue has been widely cultivated as a cattle feed.

MEDICINAL ACTIONS & USES Today, goat's rue is chiefly used as an antidiabetic herb, having the ability to reduce blood sugar levels. It is not a substitute for conventional treatments but can be valuable in the early stages of late-onset diabetes, and is best used as an infusion. The herb has the effect of increasing breast-milk production. It is also a useful diuretic.

CAUTION Use as part of the treatment of diabetes only under professional supervision.

Galipea officinalis
syn. *G. cusparia*
(Rutaceae)
ANGOSTURA

DESCRIPTION Evergreen tree growing to 50 ft (15 m) with gray bark, shiny bright green leaflets, and foul-smelling flowers.

HABITAT & CULTIVATION Angostura is native to some Caribbean islands and to tropical South America. The bark is gathered throughout the year.

PART USED Bark.

CONSTITUENTS Angostura bark contains bitter principles, alkaloids, including cusparine, and 1–2% volatile oil.

HISTORY & FOLKLORE Angostura is a traditional tonic and fever remedy in South America. Native Amazonians also use the plant as a fish poison. Angostura has been used as a source of "bitters," but it is no longer an ingredient of the cocktail flavoring bearing the same name.

MEDICINAL ACTIONS & USES A strong bitter with tonic properties, angostura stimulates the stomach and digestive tract as a whole. It is antispasmodic and is reported to act on the spinal nerves, helping in paralytic conditions. Angostura is typically given for weak digestion, and is considered valuable as a remedy for diarrhea and dysentery. In South America, it is sometimes used as a substitute for cinchona (*Cinchona* spp., p. 79) to control fevers.

Galium aparine
(Rubiaceae)
CLEAVERS, GOOSE GRASS

DESCRIPTION Straggling, square-stemmed annual growing to a height of 4 ft (1.2 m) with whorls of lance-shaped leaves, clusters of small white flowers, and small, round, green fruit with hooked prickles.

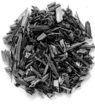

Dried aerial parts

HABITAT & CULTIVATION Common throughout Europe and North America, cleavers is found in many other temperate regions, including in Australia. It grows prolifically in gardens and along roadsides, and is gathered when it is just about to flower in late spring.

PARTS USED Aerial parts.

CONSTITUENTS Cleavers contains iridoids (including asperuloside), polyphenolic acids, anthraquinones (only in the root), alkanes, flavonoids, and tannins. Asperuloside is a mild laxative.

HISTORY & FOLKLORE The name cleavers refers to the plant's ability to cling (or cleave) to fur or clothing. Dioscorides, a Greek physician of the 1st century AD, considered it useful for countering weariness, and described how shepherds used the stems to make sieves for straining milk.

MEDICINAL ACTIONS & USES A valuable diuretic, cleavers is often taken for skin diseases such as seborrhea, eczema, and psoriasis; for swollen lymph glands; and as a general detoxifying agent in serious illnesses such as cancer. The plant is commonly prepared in the form of an infusion, but for conditions such as cancer, it is best taken as a juice, which is strongly diuretic. The juice and the infusion are also taken for kidney stones and other urinary problems.

RESEARCH According to French research (1947), an extract of the plant appears to lower blood pressure.

RELATED SPECIES The Mexican *G. orizabense* is used by the Mazatecs to treat intestinal parasites and to relieve fever. *G. umbrosum* from New Zealand has been used to treat gonorrhea. *See also* lady's bedstraw (*G. verum, following entry*).

Galium verum
(Rubiaceae)
LADY'S BEDSTRAW

DESCRIPTION Short, sprawling perennial growing to 32 in (80 cm). Has whorls of narrow dark green leaves and tufts of very small bright yellow flowers.

HABITAT & CULTIVATION Found throughout Europe and western Asia, and naturalized in North America, lady's bedstraw thrives in dry meadows, along roadsides, and in wayside places. It is gathered when in flower in summer.

PARTS USED Aerial parts.

CONSTITUENTS Lady's bedstraw contains iridoids (including asperuloside), flavonoids, anthraquinones, and alkanes.

HISTORY & FOLKLORE The name of this pleasant-scented herb derives from its traditional use as a stuffing for mattresses. In medieval times, it was used as a "strewing" herb on floors. Lady's bedstraw curdles milk and gives a yellow color to cheese produced from the curd. In his *Irish Herbal* (1735), K'Eogh stated, "when applied to burns, the crushed flowers alleviate inflammation, and when applied to wounds, they can heal them."

MEDICINAL ACTIONS & USES A slightly bitter-tasting remedy, lady's bedstraw is used mainly as a diuretic and for skin problems. Like its close relative, cleavers (*G. aparine, see preceding entry*), the herb is given for kidney stones, bladder stones, and other urinary conditions, including cystitis. It is occasionally used as a means to relieve chronic skin problems such as psoriasis, but, in general, cleavers is preferred as a treatment for this condition. Lady's bedstraw has had a longstanding reputation, especially in France, of being a valuable remedy for epilepsy, though it is rarely used for this purpose today.

RELATED SPECIES *G. elatum* has also been considered a remedy for epilepsy in France. (*See also G. aparine, above.*)

Gardenia jasminoides
syn. *G. augusta, G. florida*
(Rubiaceae)
ZHI ZI (CHINESE), GARDENIA

DESCRIPTION Evergreen shrub growing to 10 ft (3 m). Has green leaves, scented double flowers, and orange-red fruit.

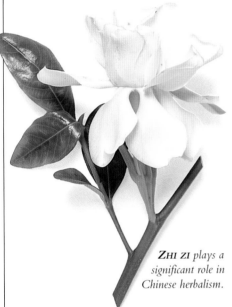

ZHI ZI plays a significant role in Chinese herbalism.

HABITAT & CULTIVATION Native to southeastern provinces of China, *zhi zi* prefers humid, tropical climates. The fruit is gathered when it turns reddish yellow.

PART USED Fruit.

CONSTITUENTS *Zhi zi* fruit contains a volatile oil, gardenin crocin, and geniposide.

HISTORY & FOLKLORE *Zhi zi* has been used in Chinese medicine for at least 2,000 years. It provides an important essential oil used to flavor teas. The oil is also used to make perfumes. Gardenia perfumes often blend *zhi zi*, jasmine, and tuberose.

MEDICINAL ACTIONS & USES In the Chinese herbal tradition (pp. 38–41), *zhi zi* is a "bitter, cold" herb used mostly to relieve symptoms associated with heat. These include fever, irritability and restlessness, insomnia, painful urination, and jaundice. The herb also treats cystitis, headaches, and difficulty in breathing. It staunches bleeding, and is taken for nosebleeds and for urinary and rectal bleeding. *Zhi zi* is mixed with egg white and applied as a powder to bruises.

RELATED SPECIES The fruit of the northern Indian *G. campanulata* is cathartic and used to expel worms. *G. gummifera*, from eastern India, is antiseptic and digestive. The Pacific region *G. taitensis* relieves headaches. The African *G. thunbergia* is used to relieve constipation.

CAUTION Do not take *zhi zi* if suffering from diarrhea.

Gaultheria procumbens
(Ericaceae)
WINTERGREEN

DESCRIPTION Aromatic, low-lying shrub growing to 6 in (15 cm). Has leathery oval leaves, small white or pale pink bell-shaped flowers, and brilliant red fruit.

HABITAT & CULTIVATION Native to North America, wintergreen is found in woodland and exposed mountainous areas. The leaves and fruit are gathered in summer.

PARTS USED Leaves, fruit, essential oil.

CONSTITUENTS Wintergreen contains phenols (including gaultherin and salicylic acid), 0.8% volatile oil (up to 98% methyl salicylate), mucilage, resin, and tannins.

HISTORY & FOLKLORE Wintergreen was popular with Native Americans, who used it for treating back pain, rheumatism, fever, headaches, sore throats, and many other conditions. Samuel Thomson, founder of the 19th-century Physiomedicalist movement, combined it with hemlock (*Conium maculatum*, p. 192) to treat severe fluid retention. Wintergreen leaves have been used as a substitute for tea (*Camellia sinensis*, p. 179) – for example during the Revolutionary War (1776–1783).

MEDICINAL ACTIONS & USES Wintergreen is strongly anti-inflammatory, antiseptic, and soothing to the digestive system. It is an effective remedy for rheumatic and arthritic problems, and, taken as a tea, it relieves flatulence and colic. The essential oil, in the form of a liniment or ointment, brings relief to inflamed, swollen, or sore muscles, ligaments, and joints, and can also prove valuable in treating neurological conditions such as sciatica (pain resulting from pressure

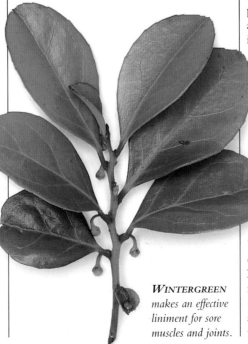

WINTERGREEN makes an effective liniment for sore muscles and joints.

on a nerve in the lower spine) and trigeminal neuralgia (pain affecting a facial nerve). The oil is sometimes used to treat cellulitis, a bacterial infection causing skin to become inflamed. The Inuit of Labrador and other native peoples eat the berries raw, and use the leaves to treat headaches, aching muscles, and sore throat.

CAUTIONS People who are sensitive to aspirin should not take wintergreen internally. Oil of wintergreen should never be taken internally, nor applied (even well diluted) to the skin of children under 12 unless under professional supervision.

Gelidium amansii
(Rhodophyceae)
AGAR

DESCRIPTION Seaweed with red-brown, translucent, multibranched ribbons and fronds growing to about 3 ft (1 m) in length. It has spherical fruit that appears in late autumn and winter.

HABITAT & CULTIVATION Agar is native to the Pacific coasts of China and Japan, and the coast of South Africa. It grows to a depth of 100 ft (30 m) below sea level. Commercial harvesters rake the plants from banks and rocks. The cleaned seaweed, after being boiled with sulphuric acid, yields agar, which sets to form a jelly. About 6,500 tons of processed agar are produced each year.

PART USED Seaweed extract (agar).

CONSTITUENTS Agar contains polysaccharides, mainly agarose and agaropectin (up to 90%), which are very mucilaginous.

HISTORY & FOLKLORE Agar is commonly used as a thickening agent in food preparation, but its most widespread application is in scientific research, where it is used as a culture medium for growing micro-organisms in petri dishes. Its Japanese name, *kanten*, means "cold weather." This is due to the fact that the seaweed used to be harvested during the winter months, because freezing and thawing were necessary for the manufacturing process.

MEDICINAL ACTIONS & USES Like most seaweeds and their derivatives, agar is nutritious and contains large amounts of mucilage. Its chief medicinal use is as a bulk laxative. In the intestines, agar absorbs water and swells, stimulating bowel activity and the subsequent elimination of feces.

RELATED SPECIES While *G. amansii* is the main agar-producing species, *G. cartilagineum* (found on the Pacific coast of North America) and other closely related species around the world are being used as alternative sources.

Gelsemium sempervirens
(Loganiaceae)
YELLOW JASMINE, GELSEMIUM

DESCRIPTION Evergreen, woody climber growing to 20 ft (6 m). Has shiny dark green leaves and clusters of fragrant trumpet-shaped yellow flowers.

HABITAT & CULTIVATION Native to southern US and Central America, yellow jasmine prefers damp sites. The rootstock is unearthed in autumn.

PART USED Rootstock.

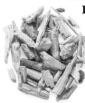

CONSTITUENTS Yellow jasmine contains indole alkaloids (including gelsemine and gelsedine), iridoids, coumarins, and tannins. The alkaloids found in the herb are toxic and act as a depressant to the central nervous system.

Dried rootstock

HISTORY & FOLKLORE It is unclear whether yellow jasmine was used by Native Americans. The plant came into regular use only in the middle of the 19th century. It was first employed by followers of the Eclectic herbal movement, and later became an official medicine. Yellow jasmine was listed in the *Pharmacopoeia of the United States* from 1863 to 1926.

MEDICINAL ACTIONS & USES A potent medicinal herb, yellow jasmine is prescribed in small doses as a sedative and antispasmodic, most commonly to treat neuralgia (pain caused by nerve irritation or damage). Yellow jasmine is often given for nerve pain affecting the face. The herb is also applied externally to treat intercostal neuralgia (nerve pain between the ribs) and sciatica (pain resulting from pressure on a nerve in the lower spine). Yellow jasmine's antispasmodic property is employed in treating whooping cough and asthma. The herb is occasionally taken to treat migraine, insomnia, and bowel problems, and also to reduce blood pressure. Yellow jasmine is also used in homeopathic medicine.

CAUTIONS Yellow jasmine is an extremely toxic plant that should be used only under professional supervision. The plant is subject to legal restrictions in some countries.

Gentiana macrophylla
(Gentianiaceae)
QIN JIAO

DESCRIPTION Perennial herb growing to 28 in (70 cm). Has opposite lance-shaped leaves, and bell-shaped violet flowers emerging from the leaf axils.

HABITAT & CULTIVATION *Qin jiao* is native to Mongolia and northeastern provinces of China, where the root is unearthed in spring or autumn.

PART USED Root.

CONSTITUENTS *Qin jiao* contains alkaloids such as gentianine and gentianindine, and bitter principles.

HISTORY & FOLKLORE *Qin jiao* is one of the 252 herbs listed in the *Divine Husbandman's Classic (Shen'nong Bencaojing)*, a Chinese herbal written in the 1st century AD.

MEDICINAL ACTIONS & USES Like its European cousin, gentian (*Gentiana lutea*, p. 97), *qin jiao* is a strongly bitter herb. It is commonly taken in the form of a tincture in order to stimulate the digestion and "cool" the body in general. Unlike gentian, however, *qin jiao* is also mildly pungent, and is therefore appropriate for a somewhat different range of illnesses. In Chinese herbal medicine, it is prescribed for the treatment of "wind-damp" conditions such as fever, jaundice, and "dry" constipation, and is used generally to help support the function of the liver and digestive system. Since it has anti-inflammatory and mildly sedative properties, *qin jiao* is also prescribed as a treatment for various rheumatic and arthritic conditions.

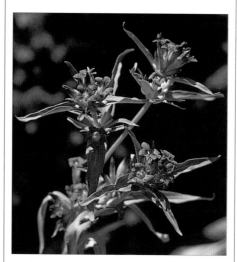

QIN JIAO shares anti-inflammatory and bitter properties with its European cousin, gentian.

RESEARCH Studies in China indicate that this herb has both an antibiotic and anti-inflammatory effect.

RELATED SPECIES Another Chinese species of gentian, *long dan cao* (*G. scabra*) is also used as a pure bitter. It promotes digestive secretions and treats a range of illnesses associated with the liver. *G. adsurgens*, native to Mexico, was used by the Maya to stimulate the stomach and to treat stomach pain. *G. andrewsii*, from eastern North America, was used as a remedy for snake bite and as a pure bitter. *See also* centaury (*Erythraea centaurium*, p. 204).

Geranium maculatum
(Geraniaceae)
AMERICAN CRANESBILL

DESCRIPTION Perennial growing to 2 ft (60 cm). Has deeply cleft leaves, pink-purple flowers, and beak-shaped fruit.

HABITAT & CULTIVATION Native to woodlands of eastern and central North America, the root is dug up in early spring, and the aerial parts are gathered in summer.

PARTS USED Root, aerial parts.

CONSTITUENTS American cranesbill contains up to 30% tannins.

HISTORY & FOLKLORE Native American people used American cranesbill for sore throats, canker sores, infected gums, and oral thrush. The herb was later used by European settlers for diarrhea, internal bleeding, cholera, and venereal diseases.

MEDICINAL ACTIONS & USES An astringent and clotting agent, American cranesbill is used today much as in earlier times. The herb is often prescribed for irritable bowel syndrome and hemorrhoids, and it is used to staunch wounds. It may also be used to treat heavy menstrual bleeding and excessive vaginal discharge.

RELATED SPECIES *See* Herb Robert (*G. robertianum, following entry*).

CAUTION American cranesbill should only be taken for a few weeks at a time.

Geranium robertianum
(Geraniaceae)
HERB ROBERT

DESCRIPTION Strong-smelling annual or biennial herb growing to 20 in (50 cm). Has deeply cleft red-green leaves, bright pink flowers, and pointed seed capsules.

HABITAT & CULTIVATION Native to Europe and Asia, Herb Robert is naturalized in North America. It is gathered in summer.

PARTS USED Aerial parts, root.

CONSTITUENTS Herb Robert contains tannins, a bitter principle (geraniin), traces of volatile oil, and citric acid.

HISTORY & FOLKLORE Herb Robert's unpleasant odor has earned it the name "stinking Bob" in parts of England.

MEDICINAL ACTIONS & USES Herb Robert is rarely used in contemporary European herbal medicine. It is occasionally employed in much the same way as American cranesbill (*G. maculatum, preceding entry*), as an astringent and wound healer. The herb bears closer investigation as a remedy. According to one authority, it is also effective against stomach ulcers and inflammation of the uterus, and it has potential as a treatment for cancer.

Geum urbanum
(Rosaceae)
AVENS

DESCRIPTION Downy perennial growing to 2 ft (60 cm). Has wiry stems, compound leaves, small yellow 5-petaled flowers, and fruit covered with hooks.

HABITAT & CULTIVATION Native to Europe and central Asia, avens is a common roadside plant. The root is dug up in spring; the aerial parts are picked in summer.

PARTS USED Aerial parts, root.

CONSTITUENTS Avens contains phenolic glycosides (including eugenol), tannins, a volatile oil, and possibly a sesquiterpene lactone (cnicin).

HISTORY & FOLKLORE Once known as *herba benedicta* (blessed herb), avens was credited with significant magical powers in the Middle Ages. According to tradition, the root should be unearthed on March 25th. The herbalist Nicholas Culpeper, writing in 1652, described avens as "good for the diseases of the chest or breast, for pains and stitches of the sides, and to expel crude and raw humours from the belly and stomach." The root has been used in the past as a mild sedative and to reduce fever.

MEDICINAL ACTIONS & USES Avens is an astringent herb, used principally for problems affecting the mouth, throat, and gastrointestinal tract. It tightens up soft gums, heals canker sores, makes a good gargle for infections of the pharynx and larynx, and reduces irritation of the stomach and gut. It may be taken for peptic ulcers, irritable bowel syndrome, diarrhea, and dysentery. Avens has been used in a lotion or ointment as a soothing remedy for hemorrhoids. The herb may also be used as a douche for treating excessive vaginal discharge. Avens reputedly has a mild quinine-type action in lowering fever.

Glechoma hederacea
syn. *Nepeta glechoma*
(Labiatae)
GROUND IVY

DESCRIPTION Creeping perennial herb growing to 6 in (15 cm). Has long rooting runners, notched kidney-shaped leaves, and purple-blue flowers in whorls.

HABITAT & CULTIVATION Native to Europe and western Asia, ground ivy is now naturalized in other temperate regions, including North America. It thrives on the outskirts of woods and along paths and hedges. It is gathered in summer.

PARTS USED Aerial parts.

CONSTITUENTS Ground ivy contains sesquiterpenes, flavonoids, a volatile oil, a bitter principle (glechomine), saponin, resin, and tannins.

HISTORY & FOLKLORE Known in parts of England as "alehoof," ground ivy was used to flavor and clarify ale, the traditional drink of the Anglo-Saxons. In medieval times, it was recommended for fever and was a popular treatment for chronic coughs. The 16th-century herbalist John Gerard considered it a valuable remedy for tinnitus.

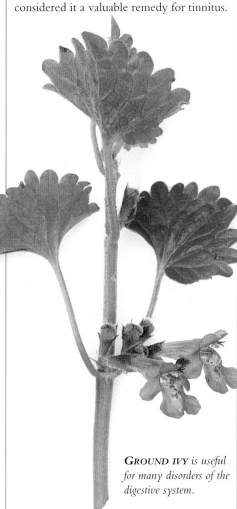

GROUND IVY is useful for many disorders of the digestive system.

MEDICINAL ACTIONS & USES Ground ivy is tonic, diuretic, and a decongestant, and is used to treat many problems involving the mucous membranes of the ear, nose, throat, and digestive system. A well-tolerated herb, it can be given to children to clear lingering congestion and to treat chronic conditions such as "glue ear" and sinusitis. Throat and chest problems, especially those due to excess mucus, also benefit from this remedy. Ground ivy is also a valuable treatment for gastritis and acid indigestion. Further along the gastrointestinal tract, its binding nature helps to counter diarrhea and to dry up watery and mucoid secretions. Ground ivy has been employed to prevent scurvy and as a spring tonic, and is considered beneficial in kidney disorders.

Glycine max
(Leguminosae)
SOY

DESCRIPTION Annual growing to 6 ft (2 m). Has leaves with 3 leaflets, white or purple flowers, and pods with 2–4 beans.

HABITAT & CULTIVATION Soy is native to southwestern Asia, and is cultivated in warm temperate regions. The pods are gathered when ripe.

PARTS USED Beans, sprouts.

CONSTITUENTS Soy beans contain protein, fixed oil, coumestrol, isoflavones, lecithin, vitamins, and minerals. Coumestrol and the isoflavones closely mimic estrogen within the body.

HISTORY & FOLKLORE A staple food in much of Asia, soy has become one of the world's most important food crops.

MEDICINAL ACTIONS & USES Although the soy bean has only a mild medicinal action, it is helpful in stimulating the circulation and acting as a general detoxicant. In Chinese medicine, the sprouts are thought to help relieve "summer heat" and fever.

Glycyrrhiza uralensis
syn. *G. viscida* *(Leguminosae)*
GAN CAO

DESCRIPTION Perennial herb growing to 3 ft (1 m). Has fibrous roots, a hairy stem, clusters of purplish flowers, and flat pods.

HABITAT & CULTIVATION *Gan cao* grows in China, Mongolia, and eastern Russia. The root is unearthed in spring or autumn.

PARTS USED Root, rhizome.

CONSTITUENTS *Gan cao* contains triterpene saponins (especially glycyrrhizin and glycyrrhetinic acid), flavonoids and isoflavonoids (including liquiritigenin and liquiritin), and chalcones.

HISTORY & FOLKLORE *Gan cao* has been used in China for more than 2,000 years.

MEDICINAL ACTIONS & USES *Gan cao* is one of the most important medicinal herbs in China. It is used to "harmonize" different herbs prescribed together, but it is also valuable in its own right. A sweet-tasting tonic with therapeutic properties similar to those of licorice (*G. glabra*, p. 99), *gan cao* is prescribed for sore throats, wheezing, coughs, canker sores, peptic ulcers, and gastritis. When prescribed for "deficient *qi*" states, it improves resistance and vitality. *Gan cao* also detoxifies inflamed skin.

CAUTIONS Take only under professional supervision. Long-term use may lead to increased blood pressure and fluid retention. Do not take if anemic or pregnant.

OTHER MEDICINAL PLANTS

Gnaphalium uliginosum
(Compositae)
MARSH CUDWEED

DESCRIPTION Annual plant growing to
8 in (20 cm). Has narrow silver-gray leaves
and tiny yellow flower heads.

HABITAT & CULTIVATION Marsh
cudweed is native to Europe, the Caucasus,
and western Asia, and is naturalized in
North America. It prefers damp areas and
is gathered in summer when in flower.

PARTS USED Aerial parts.

CONSTITUENTS Marsh cudweed contains
a volatile oil and tannins.

MEDICINAL ACTIONS & USES While not
used much medicinally today, marsh cudweed
has astringent, antiseptic, and decongestant
properties. In British herbal medicine, it is
occasionally taken for tonsillitis, sore throat,
and hoarseness, and for mucus in the throat,
nasal passages, and sinuses. Marsh cudweed
is used in Russia to treat high blood pressure.
It is thought to be an antidepressant and
aphrodisiac.

RELATED SPECIES Another European
species, *G. dioicum*, is used as an astringent
and to treat lung problems. A North
American relative, *G. polycephalum*, was used
to treat respiratory and intestinal congestion,
and was applied as a poultice for bruises.
G. keriense, native to New Zealand, is also
considered a remedy for bruises.

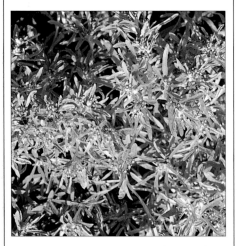

*MARSH CUDWEED is commonly found in damp
areas in Europe, North America, and Asia.*

Gossypium herbaceum
(Malvaceae)
COTTON

DESCRIPTION Biennial or perennial growing
to about 8 ft (2.5 m). Has lobed leaves, large
white or pink flowers, and seed capsules
surrounded by fluffy white tufts.

HABITAT & CULTIVATION Native to the
Indian subcontinent and the Arabian
peninsula, cotton thrives in warm temperate
and tropical climates. It is widely cultivated
for its fiber. The root and seeds are harvested
in autumn.

PARTS USED Root bark, seed oil.

CONSTITUENTS Cotton root bark contains
gossypol (a sesquiterpene) and flavonoids.
Cotton seed contains a fixed oil, which is
about 2% gossypol, and flavonoids. Gossypol
causes infertility in men.

HISTORY & FOLKLORE In India and the
Middle East, cotton has been cultivated since
the earliest times for its fiber and medicinal
properties. The plant was particularly valued
for its ability to induce menstruation. Cotton
seed oil's contraceptive effect in men was
first discovered in China when men became
infertile after eating food cooked in the oil.

MEDICINAL ACTIONS & USES Cotton root
bark is rarely used medicinally today. It was
once employed as a substitute for ergot
(*Claviceps purpurea*), the widely used labor-
inducing herb. Cotton root bark is both
milder-acting and safer in effect, stimulating
uterine contractions and hastening a difficult
labor. It also promotes abortion or the onset
of menstruation, and reduces menstrual
flow. The root bark encourages the blood to
clot and the secretion of breast milk. Cotton
seed oil is also used to treat heavy menstrual
bleeding and endometriosis.

RESEARCH Cotton seeds and seed oil cause
infertility in men, and have been tested as a
male contraceptive in China. In addition to
lowering sperm count, cotton seed oil causes
the degeneration of sperm-producing cells.

RELATED SPECIES The American species
G. hirsutum was used extensively as a
medicinal herb by the Maya and Aztecs, and
was also cultivated for its fiber. Columbus
carried samples of this species back to Europe
from his first voyage. Native American people
used the bark to ease the pain of childbirth,
and by the 19th century it was held to be an
inducer of menstruation and abortion.

CAUTIONS Cotton root bark and seed oil are
potentially toxic and should only be used
under professional supervision. Do not use
during pregnancy.

Grindelia camporum
syn. *G. robusta* var. *rigida*
(Compositae)
GUMPLANT

DESCRIPTION Perennial herb growing to
3 ft (1 m). Has triangular leaves and yellow-
orange daisy-type flowers.

HABITAT & CULTIVATION Native to the
southwestern US and Mexico, gumplant
grows in arid and saline soil. It is harvested
in late summer when in flower.

PARTS USED Leaves, flowering tops.

CONSTITUENTS Gumplant contains
diterpenes (including grindelic acid), resins,
and flavonoids.

HISTORY & FOLKLORE Gumplant was used
by Native Americans to treat bronchial
problems and skin afflictions such as
reactions to poison ivy. The plant's
medicinal value was not recognized by
orthodox practitioners in the US until the
mid-19th century. Gumplant was officially
recognized in the *Pharmacopoeia of the United
States* from 1882 to 1926.

MEDICINAL ACTIONS & USES Gumplant
is a valuable remedy for bronchial asthma,
and for states where phlegm in the airways
impedes respiration. Both antispasmodic and
expectorant, gumplant helps to relax the
muscles of the smaller bronchial passages
and to clear congested mucus. In addition,
it is thought to desensitize the nerve endings
in the bronchial tree and to slow the heart
rate, both leading to easier breathing.
Gumplant is also taken for bronchitis and
emphysema, and is of use in clearing mucus
build-up in the throat and nose. It has also
been used to treat whooping cough, hay
fever, and cystitis, and externally to help
speed the healing of skin irritation and burns.

RELATED SPECIES *G. squarrosa*, a North
American species used interchangeably with
G. camporum, was taken by Native Americans
to treat respiratory problems such as colds,
coughs, and tuberculosis.

CAUTIONS Gumplant is toxic in excessive
doses. Do not take if suffering from kidney
or heart problems.

Guaiacum officinale
(Zygophyllaceae)
LIGNUM VITAE

DESCRIPTION Evergreen tree growing to
30 ft (10 m). Has compound oval leaves,
small, deep blue, star-shaped flowers, and
heart-shaped seed capsules.

HABITAT & CULTIVATION Lignum vitae is
native to South America and the Caribbean
islands. It grows in tropical rainforests. The
tree is felled for its timber, and resin is
extracted from the heartwood.

PARTS USED Wood, resin.

CONSTITUENTS Lignum vitae contains
lignans (such as furoguaiacidin and guaiacin),
18–25% resin, vanillin, and terpenes.

HISTORY & FOLKLORE In 1519, Ulrich von
Hutten, a German satirist, was said to have
cured himself of syphilis after a 40-day regime
involving fasting, profuse sweating, and
drinking decoctions of lignum vitae.
Furthermore, in 1526, Oviedo, one of the
earliest chroniclers of American natural
history, wrote that "Caribbean Indians cure

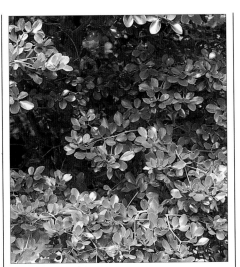

LIGNUM VITAE was once in high demand in Europe as a purported cure for syphilis.

themselves very easily" of venereal disease with this plant. For some years, lignum vitae was in great demand in Europe but it slowly fell into disrepute, its use as a cure for syphilis being seen as a long-lasting hoax. However, it is possible that the herb might have some effect if combined with an intensive naturopathic regime.

MEDICINAL ACTIONS & USES Used in Europe, especially in Britain, as a remedy for arthritic and rheumatic conditions, lignum vitae has anti-inflammatory properties that help to reduce joint pain and swelling. It is also diuretic, laxative, and sweat-inducing, and speeds the elimination of toxins, which makes it valuable for treating gout. Tincture of lignum vitae is used as a friction rub on rheumatic areas. Cotton balls moistened with the resin may be applied to aching teeth. A decoction of the wood chips acts as a local anesthetic, and is used to treat rheumatic joints and herpes blisters.

RELATED SPECIES G. sanctum, which grows in Central America and parts of Florida, and G. coulteri, native to Mexico, are used in the same manner as lignum vitae.

CAUTION Lignum vitae is subject to legal restrictions in some countries.

Guarea rusbyi
(Meliaceae)
COCILLANA

DESCRIPTION Evergreen tree with pale gray bark, compound, lance-shaped leaves, and green-white flowers.

HABITAT & CULTIVATION Cocillana is native to the eastern Andes. The bark is gathered throughout the year.

PART USED Bark.

CONSTITUENTS Cocillana contains beta-sitosterol, and probably also resins, a fixed oil, tannin, an alkaloid, and a glycoside.

HISTORY & FOLKLORE Cocillana has been used as an emetic in traditional South American and Caribbean medicine, probably for many centuries. The plant was first introduced to Western medicine by H. H. Rusby, who collected samples in Bolivia in 1886.

MEDICINAL ACTIONS & USES Cocillana is used in cough mixtures, being an even more powerful expectorant than ipecacuanha (*Cephaelis ipecacuanha*, p. 184). Cocillana is taken as a treatment for coughs, excessive mucus production in the throat and chest, and bronchitis. At a high dosage, the plant induces vomiting.

RELATED SPECIES A gum resin derived from the Caribbean *G. guara* is used as a clotting agent, and a decoction of the leaves is taken as a treatment for internal bleeding. The Brazilian *G. martiana* is used to purify and cleanse the system in general.

CAUTION Use cocillana only under professional supervision.

Haronga madagascariensis
(Guttiferae)
HARONGA

DESCRIPTION Small evergreen tree growing to 25 ft (8 m). Has black-dotted leaves with a dark green upper surface and red-brown hairs underneath, and clusters of rust-colored flowers.

HABITAT & CULTIVATION Haronga is native to Madagascar and East Africa, and grows in tropical areas. The leaves and bark are collected throughout the year.

PARTS USED Leaves, bark.

CONSTITUENTS Haronga bark contains phenolic pigments, triterpenes, anthraquinones, and tannins. The leaves contain phenolic pigments, hypericin, flavonoids, and tannins. Hypericin, which is also found in St. John's wort (*Hypericum perforatum*, p. 104), has antiviral and antidepressant properties.

HISTORY & FOLKLORE Haronga resin has traditionally been used in Africa to secure arrowheads onto shafts.

MEDICINAL ACTIONS & USES Thought to stimulate bile secretion, haronga is used in European herbal medicine to treat indigestion and poor pancreatic function. In African herbal medicine, haronga is chiefly employed as an astringent and mild laxative, and is also given for digestive system ailments such as diarrhea and dysentery.

RELATED SPECIES H. paniculata, which is also native to Madagascar and East Africa, and is found in central Africa as well, is used as the source of an oil that is commonly applied to all manner of skin disorders.

Helleborus niger
(Ranunculaceae)
BLACK HELLEBORE,
CHRISTMAS ROSE

DESCRIPTION Evergreen perennial growing to a height of 1 ft (30 cm). Has leathery basal leaves and large pink, purple, or white flowers.

HABITAT & CULTIVATION Native to Europe, black hellebore grows wild in south and central Europe and in Turkey. It is also widely cultivated as a garden plant. The leaves are picked in summer; the root and rhizome are unearthed in autumn.

PARTS USED Rhizome, root, leaves.

CONSTITUENTS Black hellebore contains cardiac glycosides (helleborin, helleborein, and hellebrin). These substances have an action similar to that of the glycosides found in common foxglove (*Digitalis purpurea*, p. 199).

HISTORY & FOLKLORE The natural historian Pliny (AD 23–79) claimed that black hellebore was used to treat mental conditions as early as 1400 BC. The plant was believed to expel black bile, which, according to the Theory of the Four Humors, causes insanity.

MEDICINAL ACTIONS & USES Toxic when taken in all but the smallest doses, the acrid black hellebore is purgative and cardiotonic, expels worms, and promotes menstrual flow. In the 20th century, the cardiac glycosides in the leaves came into use as a heart stimulant for the elderly. The herb has also been taken to stimulate delayed menstruation. However, black hellebore is now considered too strong to be safely used.

CAUTION Black hellebore is extremely toxic. Do not use under any circumstances.

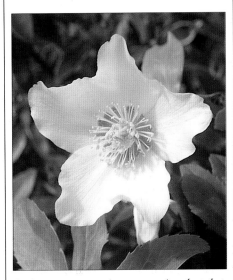

BLACK HELLEBORE is a strong-acting plant that was once taken for its cardiotonic properties.

Herniaria glabra
(Caryophyllaceae)
RUPTUREWORT

DESCRIPTION Prostrate annual or perennial with bright green oval leaves and clusters of green flowers.

HABITAT & CULTIVATION Rupturewort is found throughout Europe and western Asia. It thrives in barren areas, in lime, and sandy soils. It is gathered when in flower.

PARTS USED Aerial parts.

CONSTITUENTS Rupturewort contains coumarins (including 3% herniarin and scopoletin), flavonoids, phenolic acids, and saponins.

HISTORY & FOLKLORE Rupturewort was first documented in European herbals of the 16th century. Its genus name, *Herniaria*, refers to its reputed ability to heal hernias.

MEDICINAL ACTIONS & USES Rupturewort is of value chiefly as a diuretic herb. The fresh plant treats urinary problems such as cystitis, irritable bladder, and kidney stones. It is also astringent and has been applied as a poultice to speed the healing of ulcers. The whole plant appears to have an antispasmodic effect on the bladder.

Hieracium pilosella
syn. *Pilosella officinarum*
(Compositae)
MOUSE-EAR HAWKWEED

DESCRIPTION Perennial herb growing to a height of 8 in (20 cm) with a rosette of basal leaves and a solitary, bright yellow flower head.

HABITAT & CULTIVATION Mouse-ear hawkweed is common throughout much of Europe and temperate regions of Asia. It is naturalized in North America. Found growing in dry pastures and on sandy soil, it is collected when in flower in summer.

PARTS USED Aerial parts.

CONSTITUENTS Mouse-ear hawkweed contains a coumarin (umbelliferone), flavonoids, and caffeic acid. It is thought to be mildly antifungal.

HISTORY & FOLKLORE Mouse-ear hawkweed has been much used since the Middle Ages. In his *Irish Herbal* (1735), K'Eogh summarized its medicinal benefits: "good against the spitting of blood, all kinds of flow, coughs, ulcers of the lungs, mouth and eyes, and shingles."

MEDICINAL ACTIONS & USES Mouse-ear hawkweed relaxes the muscles of the bronchial tubes, stimulates the cough reflex, and reduces the production of mucus. This combination of actions makes the herb effective against all manner of respiratory problems, including asthma and wheezing, whooping cough, bronchitis, and other chronic and congested coughs. Mouse-ear hawkweed's astringency and its diuretic action also help to counter the production of mucus, sometimes throughout the respiratory system. The herb is used to control heavy menstrual bleeding and to ease the coughing up of blood. It may be applied as a poultice to hasten the healing of wounds.

Hippophae rhamnoides
(Elaeagnaceae)
SEA BUCKTHORN

DESCRIPTION Thorny deciduous shrub growing to 15 ft (5 m). Has narrow silvery leaves, male or female flowers, and clusters of brownish orange berries.

HABITAT & CULTIVATION Native to Europe and Asia, sea buckthorn grows mainly in sandy coastal areas and in dry riverbeds in mountainous regions. The berries are picked in autumn.

PARTS USED Berries.

CONSTITUENTS The fruit contains flavonoids, fruit acids, and vitamin C.

HISTORY & FOLKLORE The berries have traditionally been eaten with milk and cheese by Siberians and Tartars, who also used them to make a pleasant-tasting jelly.

MEDICINAL ACTIONS & USES Sea buckthorn berries are very high in vitamin C. They have principally been used to help improve resistance to infection. The berries are mildly astringent, and a decoction of them has been used as a wash to treat skin irritation and eruptions.

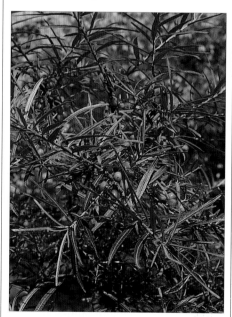

SEA BUCKTHORN is distinguished by its thorny stems and narrow silvery leaves. The berries help improve the body's resistance to infection.

Hordeum distichon
(Gramineae)
BARLEY

DESCRIPTION Annual grass growing to about 3 ft (1 m). Has an erect hollow stem, lance-shaped leaves, and ears bearing twin rows of seeds and long bristles.

HABITAT & CULTIVATION Barley is cultivated in temperate regions worldwide. It is harvested when the seeds are mature.

PARTS USED Seeds.

CONSTITUENTS Barley contains proteins, sugars, starch, fats, and B vitamins. The young seedlings also contain the alkaloids hordenine and gramine.

BARLEY has been eaten since Neolithic times.

HISTORY & FOLKLORE Barley has been consumed for many thousands of years. Dioscorides (1st century AD) recommended it "to weaken and restrain all sharp and subtle humours, and sore and ulcerated throats."

MEDICINAL ACTIONS & USES An excellent food for convalescence in the form of porridge or barley water, barley is soothing to the throat and provides easily assimilated nutrients. It can also be taken to clear mucus. Its demulcent quality also soothes inflammation of the gut and urinary tract. Barley aids in the digestion of milk and is given to babies to prevent the development of curds within the stomach. It is commonly given to children suffering from minor infections or diarrhea, and it is particularly recommended as a treatment for fever. Made into a poultice, barley is an useful remedy for soothing and reducing inflammation in sores and swellings.

RESEARCH Chinese research suggests that barley may be of aid in the treatment of hepatitis. Trials undertaken elsewhere in the early 1990's indicate that barley may help control diabetes, and that barley bran may have the effect of lowering cholesterol and preventing bowel cancer.

RELATED SPECIES Six-rowed barley (*H. vulgare*) is used in Chinese herbal medicine to strengthen digestion. It is also thought to reduce breast-milk production.

Hydrangea arborescens
(Hydrangeaceae)
WILD HYDRANGEA

DESCRIPTION Woody-stemmed deciduous shrub growing to a height of about 10 ft (3 m). Has oval leaves and clusters of small creamy-white flowers.

HABITAT & CULTIVATION Native to the eastern US from New York to Florida, wild hydrangea grows in woodland and on riverbanks. The root is dug up in autumn.

PART USED Root.

CONSTITUENTS Hydrangea is thought to contain flavonoids, a cyanogenic glycoside (hydrangein), saponins, and a volatile oil.

HISTORY & FOLKLORE The Cherokee used hydrangea as a remedy for kidney and bladder stones. The 19th-century Physiomedicalist herbal movement used a formula comprising hydrangea, couch grass (*Agropyron repens*, p. 160), and hollyhock (*Althaea rosea*) to treat serious kidney disorders, including nephritis.

MEDICINAL ACTIONS & USES Western herbal medicine considers the diuretic hydrangea as being particularly helpful in the treatment of kidney and bladder stones. It is thought both to encourage the expulsion of stones and to help dissolve those that remain. The herb is given for many other conditions that affect the genitourinary system, including cystitis, urethritis, enlarged prostate, and prostatitis.

Hygrophila spinosa
(Acanthaceae)
GOKULAKANTA

DESCRIPTION Thorny, red-stemmed annual growing to 2 ft (60 cm). Has bright blue flowers and small, flat, dark red seeds.

HABITAT & CULTIVATION Native to India, gokulakanta is now widely distributed throughout tropical regions. It is gathered when in flower.

PARTS USED Aerial parts, root.

CONSTITUENTS Gokulakanta contains mucilage, fixed and volatile oils, and an alkaloid.

MEDICINAL ACTIONS & USES Commonly used as a remedy in India, gokulakanta is taken chiefly for its reputed aphrodisiac properties. Both the aerial parts and ash of the burned plant are strongly diuretic, and are used to flush water from the body in cases of excess fluid retention. Gokulakanta root is demulcent and is used to alleviate the inflammation produced by urinary tract infections. The herb is also thought to support the liver in conditions such as jaundice and hepatitis.

Hyoscyamus niger
(Solanaceae)
HENBANE

DESCRIPTION Annual or biennial herb growing to 3 ft (1 m). Has delicate, slightly lobed leaves and bell-shaped flowers, pale yellow in color with fine purple veining.

HABITAT & CULTIVATION Native to western Asia and southern Europe, henbane is now found across much of western and central Europe, and North and South America. It is cultivated for therapeutic use in parts of Europe, including England, and in North America. The leaves and flowers are picked just after the plant has flowered, in the first year for the annual variety and in the second year for the biennial.

PARTS USED Leaves, flowering tops.

CONSTITUENTS Henbane contains 0.045–0.14% tropane alkaloids, especially hyoscyamine and hyoscine. Hyoscyamine and hyoscine are common to other members of the *Solanaceae* family, but henbane's relatively high hyoscine content gives it a more specifically sedative action than its relatives thornapple (*Datura stramonium*, p. 198) and deadly nightshade (*Atropa belladonna*, p. 66).

HISTORY & FOLKLORE Henbane has been used as a medicinal herb for thousands of years. Babylonian accounts and the Egyptian Ebers papyrus (*c.* 1500 BC) record that henbane was smoked to relieve toothache. In Greek myth, the dead were adorned with henbane when they arrived in Hades. Writing in the 1st century AD, Dioscorides recommended henbane as a treatment for insomnia, coughs, mucus, heavy menstrual bleeding, eye pain, gout, and as a general pain reliever, and advised that the herb should be used within a year since it deteriorates quickly.

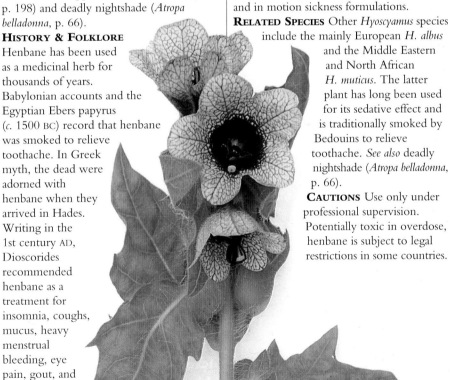

HENBANE has distinctive yellow flowers veined with purple. The plant was used in classical times as a general painkiller.

In the Middle Ages, henbane had the Latin name *dentaria*, denoting its use as a remedy against toothache. Henbane reputedly produces a sensation of lightness, as though one were flying, and it was one of the chief components of witches' "flying ointments."

MEDICINAL ACTIONS & USES Henbane is used extensively in herbal medicine as a sedative and painkiller. It is specifically used for pain affecting the urinary tract, especially pain due to kidney stones, and is also given for abdominal cramping. Its sedative and antispasmodic effect makes it a valuable treatment for the symptoms of Parkinson's disease, relieving tremor and rigidity during the early stages of the illness. Henbane has also been used to treat asthma and bronchitis, usually as a "burning powder" or in the form of a cigarette. Applied externally as an oil, it can relieve painful conditions such as neuralgia, sciatica, and rheumatism. Henbane reduces mucus secretions, as well as saliva and other digestive juices. Like its cousin deadly nightshade, it dilates the pupils. One of henbane's active components, hyoscine, is sometimes used as a substitute for opium (from *Papaver somniferum*, p. 242). Hyoscine is commonly used as a preoperative anesthetic and in motion sickness formulations.

RELATED SPECIES Other *Hyoscyamus* species include the mainly European *H. albus* and the Middle Eastern and North African *H. muticus*. The latter plant has long been used for its sedative effect and is traditionally smoked by Bedouins to relieve toothache. *See also* deadly nightshade (*Atropa belladonna*, p. 66).

CAUTIONS Use only under professional supervision. Potentially toxic in overdose, henbane is subject to legal restrictions in some countries.

OTHER MEDICINAL PLANTS

Hyssopus officinalis
(Labiatae)
HYSSOP

DESCRIPTION Semievergreen shrub growing to 2 ft (60 cm). Has narrow leaves and clusters of blue double-lipped flowers.

HABITAT & CULTIVATION Native to southern Europe, hyssop grows freely in Mediterranean countries, especially in the Balkans and Turkey. It prefers sunny, dry sites and is a common garden herb. The flowering tops are harvested when the plant is in flower in summer.

PARTS USED Flowering tops, essential oil.

CONSTITUENTS Hyssop contains terpenes (including marubiin, a diterpene), a volatile oil (consisting mainly of camphor, pinocamphone, and beta-pinene), flavonoids, hyssopin, tannins, and resin. Marubiin is a strong expectorant. Pinocamphone is toxic, and the volatile oil can cause epileptic seizures.

HISTORY & FOLKLORE In the past, hyssop was so highly esteemed it was regarded as a virtual cure-all. An old saying went, "Whoever rivals hyssop's virtues, knows too much." In the 1st century AD, Dioscorides recommended a recipe containing a mixture of hyssop, figs (*Ficus carica*, p. 209), rue (*Ruta graveolens*, p. 262), honey, and water for treating a range of conditions including pleurisy, tight-chestedness, respiratory congestion, asthma, and chronic coughs. Hyssop is used to flavor some liqueurs, including Chartreuse.

MEDICINAL ACTIONS & USES Currently an undervalued medicinal herb, hyssop is potentially useful since it is both calming and tonic. It has a positive effect when used to treat bronchitis and respiratory infections, especially where there is excessive mucus production. Hyssop appears to encourage the production of a more liquid mucus, and at the same time gently stimulates expectoration. This combined action clears thick and congested phlegm. Hyssop can irritate the mucous membranes, so it is best given after an infection has peaked, when the herb's tonic action encourages a general recovery. As a sedative, hyssop is a useful remedy against asthma in both children and adults, especially where the condition is exacerbated by mucus congestion. Like many herbs with a strong volatile oil, it soothes the digestive tract and can be an effective remedy against indigestion, gas, bloating, and colic.

CAUTIONS Hyssop essential oil can induce epileptic seizures. It should only be used under professional supervision. Hyssop essential oil is subject to legal restrictions in some countries.

Iberis amara
(Cruciferae)
WILD CANDYTUFT

DESCRIPTION Downy annual growing to 1 ft (30 cm). Has deeply toothed leaves and clusters of white or mauve flowers.

HABITAT & CULTIVATION Wild candytuft is native to Europe (especially the Balkans) and North Africa, growing in open areas, arable fields, and vineyards. The aerial parts are gathered in summer; the seeds are gathered after they have matured in autumn.

PARTS USED Aerial parts, seeds.

WILD CANDYTUFT is a traditional remedy for gout.

CONSTITUENTS Contains mustard seed oil glycosides and vitamin C.

MEDICINAL ACTIONS & USES Rarely used in herbal medicine today, wild candytuft is a bitter-tasting tonic, aiding digestion and relieving gas and bloating. It is traditionally taken for gout, rheumatism, and arthritis. It also has a high vitamin C content.

Ilex aquifolium
(Aquifoliaceae)
HOLLY

DESCRIPTION Evergreen bush or tree growing to 15 ft (5 m) with shiny, deep green leaves edged with spines, clusters of small white flowers, and round red berries.

HABITAT & CULTIVATION Holly grows throughout much of Europe, western and central Asia, and North Africa. It is found in woods and hedges, and thrives in gravelly soil or loam. It is also grown as a garden plant. The leaves are gathered in spring, the berries in winter.

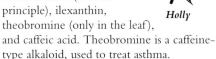

Holly

PARTS USED Leaves, berries.

CONSTITUENTS Holly contains ilicin (a bitter principle), ilexanthin, theobromine (only in the leaf), and caffeic acid. Theobromine is a caffeine-type alkaloid, used to treat asthma.

HISTORY & FOLKLORE Holly has been prominent in Western ritual and religious life for thousands of years. The Druids and other ancient European peoples bedecked their dwellings with holly leaves and berries at the time of the winter solstice. Romans exchanged holly branches during the December festival called *Saturnalia*, a tradition adopted by early Christians. An early Anglo-Saxon herbal, the *Lacnunga*, recommended holly bark boiled with goat's milk to treat a constricted chest. As importantly, the holly tree was considered to protect against witchcraft and spells. In the 19th century, some physicians felt that the bark equalled or surpassed cinchona (*Cinchona* spp., p. 79) as a fever remedy.

MEDICINAL ACTIONS & USES Holly is rarely used today. Its leaves are diuretic, fever-reducing, and laxative, and they have been employed to treat fevers, jaundice, and rheumatism. Holly berries purge the bowels and cause vomiting if taken in large doses.

RELATED SPECIES Many *Ilex* species have been used as purgatives and to lower fevers. *I. vomitoria* was used ceremonially by Native Americans and, as its name suggests, is an emetic herb.

CAUTIONS Take only under professional supervision. Holly berries are toxic, particularly to children.

Ilex paraguariensis
syn. *I. paraguensis*
(Aquifoliaceae)
MATÉ

DESCRIPTION Evergreen shrub or small tree growing to 20 ft (6 m). Has large leaves, white flowers, and small reddish fruit.

HABITAT & CULTIVATION Maté grows wild in northern Argentina, Paraguay, Uruguay, and southern Brazil, and is widely cultivated in Argentina, Spain, and Portugal. The leaves, picked when the berries are ripe, are heated over a wood fire, ground, and then stored in sacks for a year before being sold.

PARTS USED Leaves.

CONSTITUENTS Maté contains xanthine derivatives, including about 1.5% caffeine, about 0.2% theobromine, theophylline, and up to 16% tannins. The high tannin content means that maté should not be consumed with meals, since tannins impair the absorption of nutrients.

MEDICINAL ACTIONS & USES Maté is a traditional South American tea that increases short-term physical and mental energy levels. It is taken as a fortifying beverage in much the same way as tea (*Camellia sinensis*, p. 179) is consumed throughout Asia and Europe. Maté has properties similar to those of tea and coffee (*Coffea arabica*, p. 190). It stimulates the nervous system, and is mildly analgesic and diuretic. As a medicinal herb, maté is used to treat headaches, migraine, neuralgic and rheumatic pain, fatigue, and mild depression. It has also been used in the treatment of diabetes.

RELATED SPECIES *I. guayusa*, from Ecuador, is used in much the same way as maté but is also employed medicinally to treat malaria, liver pain, and syphilis. It is thought to aid

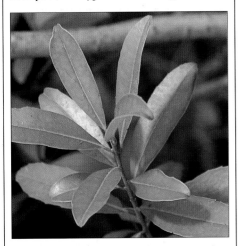

MATÉ makes a pleasant-tasting tea that has a stimulant, mildly analgesic, and diuretic effect.

digestion and cleanse the digestive tract. The Jibaro people and other groups believe that it "calms the nerves" and that it may be beneficial during pregnancy. It is also considered aphrodisiac. *See also* holly (*I. aquifolium*, p. 220).

Illicium verum
(Illiciaceae)
STAR ANISE,
BA JIAO HUI XIAN (CHINESE)

DESCRIPTION Evergreen tree growing to 60 ft (18 m). Has tapering leaves, pale greenish yellow flowers, and star-shaped segmented fruit (seed pods).

HABITAT & CULTIVATION Star anise is native to China, India, and Vietnam. It grows in tropical and subtropical regions,

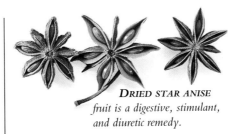

DRIED STAR ANISE
fruit is a digestive, stimulant, and diuretic remedy.

including parts of North America. The fruit is picked when ripe.

PART USED Fruit.

CONSTITUENTS Star anise has a volatile oil containing about 85% anethole, methyl chavicol, and safrole. An extract has antibacterial properties.

HISTORY & FOLKLORE This herb's Chinese name, *ba jiao hui xian*, means "8-horned fennel." Star anise has a similar taste to anise (*Pimpinella anisum*, p. 246) and, like anise, is used mainly as a spice. Though star anise has been used for centuries as a folk medicine, it did not appear in Chinese herbals until the 16th century.

MEDICINAL ACTIONS & USES Used in Chinese herbal medicine as a remedy for rheumatism, back pain, and hernias, star anise has stimulant, diuretic, and digestive properties. It makes an effective remedy for gas and indigestion – especially colic – and can safely be given to children. To treat hernias of the intestine or bladder, star anise is often mixed with fennel (*Foeniculum vulgare*, p. 210). Both herbs help to relax the organ's muscles and relieve spasm. Star anise is also used for toothache.

RELATED SPECIES Japanese star anise (*I. religiosum*) is occasionally used to adulterate star anise, but it is toxic and has a strongly bitter taste. This species is commonly planted around Buddhist temples in Japan. *I. anisatum* is also potentially toxic.

Imperatoria ostruthium
(Umbelliferae)
MASTERWORT

DESCRIPTION Perennial growing to 2 ft (60 cm) with green leaves divided into 3 leaflets with 3 lobes each, white flowers on large umbels, and winged seeds.

HABITAT & CULTIVATION Native to central and southern Europe and Asia, masterwort is most often found in the wild. The root is unearthed in autumn or spring.

PART USED Root.

CONSTITUENTS Masterwort contains a camphoraceous volatile oil (including limonene, phellandrene, alpha-pinene, and a sesquiterpene), peucadanin, oxipeucadanin, and ostrutol.

HISTORY & FOLKLORE From the late Middle Ages onward, masterwort was held

in high regard by herbalists. Pierandrea Matteoli's *Materia Medica* of 1548 explained: "Masterwort powerfully resolves all flatulence in the body, stimulates urine and menstruation, is an admirable remedy for paralysis and cold conditions of the brain… and helps against pestilence and the bites of rabid dogs." A century later, Nicholas Culpeper was no less effusive in recommending masterwort for rheumatic conditions, shortness of breath, kidney and bladder stones, water retention, "falling sickness," and wounds.

MEDICINAL ACTIONS & USES Masterwort is rarely used today, but it may well be an herb that bears further investigation. The root is aromaic, warms central areas of the body, and is a bitter tonic. It has a strong action within the stomach and gut, settling indigestion and relieving gas and cramps. Masterwort is also beneficial for chest conditions, and is used for colds, asthma, and bronchitis. It can also be helpful for menstrual problems.

CAUTION If applied to the skin, masterwort may cause photosensitivity to sunlight.

Inula japonica
syn. *I. britannica* var. *chinensis* (Compositae)
XUAN FU HUA

DESCRIPTION Perennial herb growing to 10 ft (3 m). Has long lance-shaped leaves and yellow daisylike flowers.

HABITAT & CULTIVATION Native to China and Japan, *xuan fu hua* is cultivated throughout China. It is harvested when in flower in late summer.

PARTS USED Flowers, aerial parts.

CONSTITUENTS *Xuan fu hua* contains a volatile oil, flavonoids, phenolic acids, and triterpenes (including taraxasterol).

HISTORY & FOLKLORE *Xuan fu hua* was mentioned in the *Divine Husbandman's Classic* (*Shen'nong Bencaojing*), an herbal written in China in the 1st century AD.

MEDICINAL ACTIONS & USES Used in traditional Chinese medicine as a mildly warming expectorant remedy, *xuan fu hua* is especially suitable when phlegm has accumulated in the chest. The herb is often prescribed for bronchitis, wheezing, chronic coughing, and other chest complaints brought on by "cold conditions." *Xuan fu hua* also has a bitter action, and it helps to strengthen digestive function. It is prescribed to stop vomiting and, on occasions, hiccups. The flowers are normally used in medicinal preparations, but the aerial parts are also taken, generally for less serious conditions.

RELATED SPECIES *See* elecampane (*I. helenium*, p. 105).

Ipomoea purga
syn. *Convolvulus jalapa*
(Convolvulaceae)
JALAP

DESCRIPTION Evergreen vine reaching about 12 ft (4 m). Has heart-shaped leaves and trumpetlike purple flowers.

HABITAT & CULTIVATION Native to Mexico, jalap is cultivated in Central America, the West Indies, and Southeast Asia. The root is unearthed in summer.

PART USED Root.

CONSTITUENTS Jalap contains the resin convolvulin.

HISTORY & FOLKLORE Spanish colonizers learned of jalap's strong purgative effect from Mexican native peoples. Introduced into Europe in 1565, the herb was used for all types of illnesses until the 19th century.

MEDICINAL ACTIONS & USES Jalap is such a powerful cathartic that its medicinal value is questionable. Even in moderate doses it stimulates the elimination of profuse watery stools, and in larger doses it causes vomiting.

RELATED SPECIES *I. turpethum*, native to Asia and Australia, is also a drastic purgative. Other *Ipomoea* species, such as the sweet potato (*I. batatas*, from South America), are important food plants. The seeds of morning glory (*I. violacea*), native to Mexico, contain compounds similar to LSD, and were taken ritually by the Zapotecs and Aztecs.

CAUTION Do not take jalap under any circumstances.

Iris versicolor
(Iridaceae)
BLUE FLAG, WILD IRIS

DESCRIPTION Perennial growing to about 3 ft (1 m). Has erect stems, sword-shaped leaves, and 2–3 resplendent blue to violet flowers per stem.

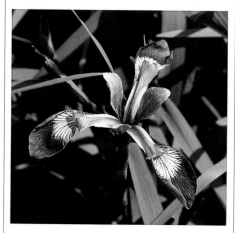

BLUE FLAG was very widely used by Native Americans to treat wounds and sores.

HABITAT & CULTIVATION Blue flag is native to North America. Preferring damp and marshy areas in the wild, it is also widely cultivated as a garden plant. The rhizome is unearthed in autumn.

PART USED Rhizome.

CONSTITUENTS Blue flag contains triterpenoids, salicylic and isophthalic acids, a very small amount of volatile oil, starch, resin, an oleo-resin, and tannins.

HISTORY & FOLKLORE Blue flag was one of the medicinal plants most frequently used by Native Americans. Different tribes made use of it variously as an emetic, cathartic, and diuretic, to treat wounds and sores, and for colds, earache, and cholera. The plant was listed in the *Pharmacopoeia of the United States* from 1820 to 1895. In the Anglo-American Physiomedicalist tradition, blue flag was used as a glandular and liver remedy.

MEDICINAL ACTIONS & USES Blue flag is currently used mainly to detoxify the body. It increases urination and bile production, and has a mild laxative effect. This combination of cleansing actions makes it a useful herb for chronic skin diseases such as acne and eczema, especially where gallbladder problems or constipation contribute to the condition. Blue flag is also given for biliousness and indigestion. In small doses, it relieves nausea and vomiting. However, in large doses blue flag will itself cause vomiting. The traditional use of blue flag for gland problems persists. It is also believed by some to aid weight loss.

CAUTIONS Excessive doses of blue flag cause vomiting. Do not take this plant during pregnancy.

Jasminum grandiflorum
(Oleaceae)
JASMINE

DESCRIPTION Slender evergreen rambler growing to 20 ft (6 m). Has dark green compound leaves and large, sweetly scented tubular white flowers.

HABITAT & CULTIVATION Native to northern India, Pakistan, and the northwestern Himalayas, jasmine is now cultivated as a garden plant and as a source of essential oil.

PARTS USED Flowers, essential oil.

CONSTITUENTS Jasmine's volatile oil contains benzyl alcohol, benzyl acetate, linalol, and linalyl acetate.

HISTORY & FOLKLORE Jasmine was introduced to Europe in the 16th century, and is mainly used as a source of perfume.

MEDICINAL ACTIONS & USES Jasmine flowers make a calming and sedative infusion, taken to relieve tension. The oil is considered antidepressant and relaxing, and is used externally to soothe dry or sensitive skin.

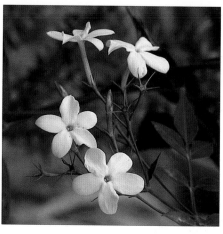

JASMINE flowers are the source of an essential oil that is used to treat stress and depression.

Due to frequent adulteration, the oil is rarely used in aromatherapy.

RELATED SPECIES Arabian jasmine (*J. sambac*), in fact native to Southeast Asia, is used as an eyewash, is added to tea (*Camellia sinensis*, p. 179) to produce jasmine tea, and is used in Buddhist ceremonies.

CAUTION Do not take jasmine essential oil internally.

Juglans cinerea
(Juglandaceae)
BUTTERNUT

DESCRIPTION Deciduous tree growing to 100 ft (30 m). Has gray bark, long leaves with many leaflets, male catkins and female flowers, and an oval-shaped fruit containing a hard dark-colored nut.

HABITAT & CULTIVATION Native to North American forests, butternut is cultivated for its timber in other temperate regions. The bark is collected in autumn.

PART USED Inner bark.

CONSTITUENTS Butternut contains naphthaquinones (including juglone, juglandin, and juglandic acid), a fixed and a volatile oil, and tannins. The naphthaquinones have an approximately similar laxative effect to the anthraquinones found in plants such as senna (*Cassia senna*, p. 72) and Chinese rhubarb (*Rheum palmatum*, p. 124). Juglone is purgative, antimicrobial, antiparasitic, and cancer-inhibiting.

HISTORY & FOLKLORE Butternut bark was employed by Native Americans and New World settlers as a laxative and tonic remedy. Butternut was used to treat a variety of conditions, including rheumatic and arthritic joints, headaches, dysentery, constipation, and wounds.

MEDICINAL ACTIONS & USES Used to this day as a laxative and tonic, butternut is a valuable remedy for chronic constipation, gently encouraging regular bowel movements. It is especially beneficial if combined with a carminative herb, such as ginger (*Zingiber officinale*, p. 153) or angelica (*Angelica archangelica*, p. 166). Butternut also lowers cholesterol levels and promotes the clearance of waste products by the liver. It has a positive reputation in treating intestinal worms, and, being antimicrobial and astringent, it has been prescribed as a treatment for dysentery.

RELATED SPECIES Black walnut (*J. nigra*) is used in the same way as butternut. The bark of the walnut tree (*J. regia*) is used as a gentle purgative, and is also applied to skin afflictions. The nut is used in Chinese herbal medicine as a kidney tonic. The nuts of both varieties are nutritious and have the effect of lowering cholesterol levels.

Juniperus communis
(Cupressaceae)
JUNIPER

DESCRIPTION Coniferous shrub growing to 50 ft (15 m). Has slender twigs with whorls of needlelike leaves, yellow male and blue female flowers on separate plants, and spherical blue-black fruit.

HABITAT & CULTIVATION Juniper is found in Europe, southwestern Asia up to the Himalayas, and North America, where it grows from southern coastal sites to more northerly moorland and mountainous regions. The fruit (berries) is gathered when ripe in autumn.

PARTS USED Fruit, essential oil.

CONSTITUENTS Juniper contains 1–2% volatile oil, consisting of

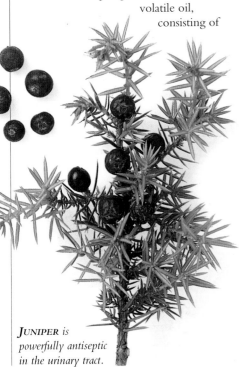

JUNIPER is powerfully antiseptic in the urinary tract.

more than 60 compounds that include myrcene, sabinene, alpha- and beta-pinene, and cineole. Juniper also contains tannins, diterpenes, sugars, resin, and vitamin C.

HISTORY & FOLKLORE In former times, sprigs of juniper flung into the fire were thought to protect against evil spirits. Juniper was also burned to ward off the plague.

MEDICINAL ACTIONS & USES Juniper is tonic, diuretic, and strongly antiseptic within the urinary tract. It is a valuable remedy for cystitis, and helps to relieve fluid retention but should be avoided in cases of kidney disease. In the digestive system, juniper is warming and settling, easing colic and supporting the function of the stomach. Taken internally or applied externally, juniper is helpful for chronic arthritis, gout, and rheumatic conditions. Applied externally as a diluted essential oil, it has a slightly warming effect on the skin and is thought to promote the removal of waste products from underlying tissues. Juniper also stimulates menstruation and increases menstrual flow.

RELATED SPECIES Oil of Cade is produced from *J. oxycedrus* and is applied to skin rashes. Savin (*J. sabina*) is toxic and a powerful abortifacient. The Japanese *J. rigida* is used as a diuretic.

CAUTIONS Do not use juniper during pregnancy or if prone to heavy menstrual bleeding. Do not take if suffering from a kidney infection or kidney disease. Do not take the essential oil internally except under professional supervision.

SELF-HELP USE Urinary infections, p. 314.

Krameria triandra
(Krameriaceae)
RHATANY

DESCRIPTION Dense evergreen shrub growing to 3 ft (90 cm). Has a deep root, oblong leaves, and large red flowers.

HABITAT & CULTIVATION Rhatany is found in Ecuador, Peru, and Bolivia on western slopes of the Andes at altitudes of 3,000–10,000 ft (900–3,000 m). The root is unearthed throughout the year.

PART USED Root.

CONSTITUENTS Rhatany contains 10–20% tannins, including phlobaphene, benzofurans, and n-methyltyrosine.

HISTORY & FOLKLORE A traditional South American remedy, rhatany was used by indigenous people as an astringent and a tooth preservative. Its Spanish name, *raiz para los dientes* (root for the teeth), points to this traditional usage.

MEDICINAL ACTIONS & USES Rhatany is astringent and antimicrobial. It is a useful remedy taken principally for problems affecting the gastrointestinal tract. It is most commonly used for diarrhea and dysentery. Rhatany also makes a good mouthwash and gargle for bleeding and infected gums, canker sores, and sore throats. The plant's astringency makes it effective when used in the form of an ointment, suppository, or wash for treating hemorrhoids. Rhatany may also be applied to wounds to help staunch blood flow, to varicose veins, and over areas of capillary fragility that may be prone to easy bruising.

RELATED SPECIES The Mexican *K. cystisoides* is an astringent remedy used in much the same way as rhatany. Another species native to North and Central America, *K. parvifolia*, was used by the Papago as an eyewash.

Lactuca virosa
(Compositae)
WILD LETTUCE

DESCRIPTION Hollow-stemmed biennial growing to about 4 ft (1.2 m). Has broad spiny leaves and clusters of pale yellow composite flowers. All parts of the plant exude a white milky latex.

HABITAT & CULTIVATION Common throughout Europe, wild lettuce grows in open areas and along roadsides. It is gathered when in flower in late summer.

PARTS USED Leaves, latex.

CONSTITUENTS The latex contains sesquiterpene lactones (including lactucopicrin and lactucerin); the leaves also contain flavonoids and coumarins. The sesquiterpene lactones have a sedative effect.

HISTORY & FOLKLORE In Assyrian herbal medicine, lettuce seeds were reportedly used with cumin (*Cuminum cyminum*, p. 194) as a poultice for the eyes. The physician Dioscorides (1st century AD) wrote that the plant's effect seemed similar to that of the opium poppy (*Papaver somniferum*, p. 242). This view is still widely held – one reason why wild lettuce is still (wrongly) viewed as potentially toxic.

MEDICINAL ACTIONS & USES Wild lettuce is a safe sedative that can be given to adults and children to encourage a sound night's sleep or to calm overactivity or overstimulation. Most commonly, it is recommended for excitability in children. It is also taken to treat coughs, often combined with herbs such as licorice (*Glycyrrhiza glabra*, p. 99). Wild lettuce is thought to lower the libido. It may also be used to relieve pain.

RELATED SPECIES Garden lettuce (*L. sativa*) may be used like wild lettuce but it has a significantly weaker therapeutic action. *L. thunbergii*, native to China and Mongolia, is also used medicinally.

CAUTION If taken in large quantities, wild lettuce may cause drowsiness.

OTHER MEDICINAL PLANTS

Lamium album
(Labiatae)
WHITE DEADNETTLE

DESCRIPTION Perennial growing to 2 ft (60 cm). Has a square stem, toothed oval leaves, and white double-lipped flowers.

HABITAT & CULTIVATION White deadnettle is native to and widespread in Europe and central and northern Asia. It thrives in fields and open areas. It is gathered when in flower in summer.

PARTS USED Flowering tops.

CONSTITUENTS White deadnettle contains a saponin, flavones, mucilage, and tannins.

HISTORY & FOLKLORE Deadnettle is so called because it resembles true nettle (*Urtica dioica*, p. 145), without the stinging hairs. It was also known as archangel, a plant "to make the heart merry, to make a good colour in the face, and to refresh the vital spirits" (John Gerard, *The Herball*, 1597).

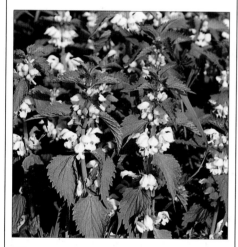

WHITE DEADNETTLE is used to treat gynecological conditions.

MEDICINAL ACTIONS & USES White deadnettle is astringent and demulcent. It is chiefly used as a uterine tonic, to arrest intermenstrual bleeding, and to reduce excessive menstrual flow. It is also a traditional treatment for abnormal vaginal discharge. White deadnettle is sometimes taken to relieve menstrual pain. Its astringency helps to treat diarrhea, and, used externally, it can relieve hemorrhoids and varicose veins.

Larix decidua
syn. *L. europaea*
(Pinaceae)
LARCH

DESCRIPTION Deciduous conifer growing to 160 ft (50 m). Has clusters of needlelike leaves, male and female flowers, and small light brown cones.

HABITAT & CULTIVATION Native to the Alps and the Carpathian mountains of eastern Europe, larch grows to altitudes of 6,500 ft (2,000 m). It is widely cultivated for its timber. The resin is tapped in autumn; the bark is collected when the tree is felled.

PARTS USED Inner bark, resin.

CONSTITUENTS Larch contains lignans, resins, and volatile oil (consisting mainly of alpha- and beta-pinene and limonene).

HISTORY & FOLKLORE Introduced into Britain in 1639, larch has been cultivated there since the early 19th century.

MEDICINAL ACTIONS & USES Larch has astringent, diuretic, and antiseptic properties. The bark may be used to treat bladder and urinary tubule infections such as cystitis and urethritis, and respiratory problems including pharyngitis, tracheitis, and bronchitis. The resin is applied to wounds, where it protects and counters infection. A decoction of the bark is sometimes used to soothe eczema and psoriasis.

CAUTION Do not take if suffering from kidney disease.

Larrea tridentata
(Zygophyllaceae)
CHAPARRAL, CREOSOTE BUSH

DESCRIPTION Thorny shrub growing to 6 ft (2 m), with small finely divided leaves.

HABITAT & CULTIVATION Chaparral is found in large numbers in the deserts of the southwestern US and Mexico.

PARTS USED Aerial parts.

CONSTITUENTS Chaparral contains about 12% resin and nordihydroguaiaretic acid. The latter is reportedly harmful to the lymph glands and the kidneys.

HISTORY & FOLKLORE Widely used by Native Americans, chaparral was taken as a decoction to treat stomach troubles and diarrhea. Young twigs were used for toothache. The leaves were applied as a poultice for respiratory problems and as a wash for skin problems. The plant was listed in the *Pharmacopoeia of the United States* from 1842 to 1942.

MEDICINAL ACTIONS & USES Until recently, chaparral remained in wide use in the US, with an average of 10 tons (9.07 tonnes) consumed each year. It was thought to be a beneficial remedy for rheumatic disease, venereal infections, urinary infections, and certain types of cancer, especially leukemia. Chaparral was also taken internally for skin afflictions such as acne and eczema, and applied as a lotion to sores, wounds, and rashes. Recently, however, its sale was banned in the US, due to concern over its potential toxic effect on the liver.

RELATED SPECIES The South American *L. nitida* is taken to counter indigestion, to induce menstruation, and to treat wounds.

CAUTION Five cases of acute or subacute hepatitis have been reported as being due to ingestion of chaparral. In view of the uncertainty about its safety, the use of chapparal is not recommended and alternative herbs should be employed.

Laurus nobilis
(Lauraceae)
BAY LAUREL

DESCRIPTION Aromatic evergreen shrub or tree growing to a height of 70 ft (20 m). Has leathery dark green leaves, small yellow male and female flowers, and shiny black berries.

HABITAT & CULTIVATION Native to Mediterranean countries, bay laurel prefers damp and shady sites. It is also a popular garden herb, cultivated largely for culinary use. The leaves are picked all year-round.

PARTS USED Leaves, essential oil.

CONSTITUENTS Bay laurel contains up to 3% volatile oil (including 30–50% cineole, linalool, alpha-pinene, alpha-terpineol acetate, mucilage, tannin, and resin).

HISTORY & FOLKLORE In ancient Greece, bay laurel was used in divination by the Delphic Oracle. From ancient Rome comes the tradition that the sudden withering of a bay laurel tree bodes disaster for the household. In ancient Rome, bay laurel leaves were used as a medicine, a spice, and a decorative garland during the December festival of *Saturnalia*. Bay laurel was sacred to the gods Apollo and Aesculapius,

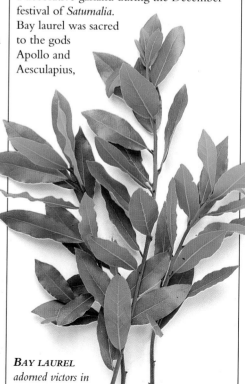

BAY LAUREL adorned victors in ancient Greece.

who together oversaw healing and medicine. The herb was thought to be greatly protective and healing. An infusion of the leaves was taken for its warming and tonic effect on the stomach and bladder, and a plaster made from the leaves was used to relieve wasp and bee stings. The Greek physician Dioscorides (1st century AD) wrote that bay laurel bark "breaks [kidney] stones, and is good for liver infirmities."

MEDICINAL ACTIONS & USES Bay laurel is used mainly to treat upper digestive tract disorders and to ease arthritic aches and pains. It is settling to the stomach and has a tonic effect, stimulating the appetite and the secretion of digestive juices. When used as an ingredient in cooking, bay laurel leaves aid in the digestion and absorption of food. The leaves have much the same positive effect as spearmint (*Mentha spicata*) and rosemary (*Rosmarinus officinalis*, p. 125) in assisting the breakdown of heavy food, especially meat. Bay laurel has also been used to promote the onset of menstruation. The essential oil is chiefly employed as a friction rub, being well diluted in a carrier oil and massaged into aching muscles and joints. A decoction of the leaves may be added to a bath to ease aching limbs.

CAUTIONS Never take bay laurel essential oil internally. An allergic reaction may result from external use; therefore the oil should only be applied in very dilute (2%) concentrations.

Lawsonia inermis syn. *L. alba*
(Lythraceae)
HENNA

DESCRIPTION Heavily scented evergreen shrub or tree growing to 20 ft (6 m). Has narrow pointed leaves, small white or pink flowers, and blue-black berries.

HABITAT & CULTIVATION Native to the Middle East, North Africa, and the Indian subcontinent, henna grows in sunny positions and is widely cultivated for use as a hair restorative and dye. The leaves are picked during the growing season.

PARTS USED Leaves, bark.

CONSTITUENTS Henna contains coumarins, naphthaquinones (including lawsone), flavonoids, sterols, and tannins.

HISTORY & FOLKLORE Henna has been used for thousands of years in North Africa and Asia as a red dye and as a scent. Mummies were wrapped in henna-dyed cloth in ancient Egypt. In Arabia and India, the leaves have traditionally been used to make a pigment for dying intricate linear patterns on the fingers, palms, and feet. The leaves have also been used to dye not only human hair but

the manes and tails of horses. Before meeting Antony, Cleopatra reputedly soaked the sails of her barge in heady henna flower oil.

MEDICINAL ACTIONS & USES Used mainly within Ayurvedic and Unani medicine, henna leaves are commonly taken as a gargle for sore throats, and as an infusion or decoction for diarrhea and dysentery. The leaves are astringent, prevent hemorrhaging, and promote menstrual flow. A decoction of the bark is used to treat liver problems. Applied externally as a plaster, henna also plays a role in the treatment of skin disease – especially fungal infections, acne, and boils.

Leonurus cardiaca
(Labiatae)
MOTHERWORT

DESCRIPTION Perennial herb growing to 5 ft (1.5 m). Has toothed palm-shaped leaves and double-lipped pink flowers growing in clusters.

HABITAT & CULTIVATION Native to central Asia, motherwort is now naturalized in much of Europe and North America. It grows wild in woodlands, open areas, and along roadsides. It is also grown as a garden plant. Motherwort is harvested when in flower in summer.

PARTS USED Aerial parts.

CONSTITUENTS Motherwort contains alkaloids (including L-stachydrine), an iridoid (leonurine), diterpenes, flavonoids, caffeic acid, and tannins.

HISTORY & FOLKLORE As its species name *cardiaca* indicates, motherwort has long been considered a heart remedy. The herbalist Nicholas Culpeper stated that "there is no better herb to drive away melancholy vapours from the heart, to strengthen it and make the mind cheerful" (1652). The Italian physician and herbalist Pierandrea Matteoli held it "useful for palpitations and a pounding heart, spasms and paralysis … [it] thins thick and viscid humours, stimulates urine and menstrual bleeding, and purges stone from the kidneys" (1548).

MEDICINAL ACTIONS & USES A remedy for the heart and nerves and often prescribed for palpitations, motherwort strengthens heart function, especially in conditions where the heart is weak. A gentle sedative and antispasmodic, it promotes relaxation rather than drowsiness. However, it does stimulate the muscles of the uterus, and is especially suitable for delayed menstruation, menstrual pain, and premenstrual tension (especially if shock or distress is a factor). It should not be used if menstrual bleeding is heavy.

RELATED SPECIES Two east Asian species, *L. heterophyllus* (from China) and *L. sibiricus* (from Siberia), are both used therapeutically for the same purposes as motherwort.

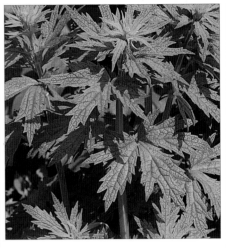

MOTHERWORT has been used to treat palpitations since at least the 16th century.

L. heterophyllus appears to lower blood pressure and to induce menstruation.

CAUTIONS Do not take motherwort during pregnancy. It should also be avoided if there is heavy menstrual bleeding.

SELF-HELP USES Menstrual problems – irregular cycle, p. 315; **Panic attacks**, p. 302.

Lepidium virginicum
(Cruciferae)
VIRGINIA PEPPERGRASS

DESCRIPTION Annual herb growing to about 2 ft (60 cm). Has slender lance-shaped leaves and small white flowers.

HABITAT & CULTIVATION Virginia peppergrass is native to eastern North America and parts of the Caribbean, and is naturalized in Australia. The leaves are mainly gathered in spring.

PARTS USED Leaves, root.

CONSTITUENTS Virginia peppergrass contains high levels of vitamin C.

HISTORY & FOLKLORE The Menominee of eastern North America applied a lotion of Virginia peppergrass (or a bruised fresh plant) to eruptions resulting from contact with poison ivy.

MEDICINAL ACTIONS & USES Virginia peppergrass is nutritious and generally detoxifying. It has been used to treat vitamin C deficiency and diabetes, and to expel intestinal worms. The herb is also diuretic and of benefit in easing rheumatic pain. The root is taken to treat excess mucus within the respiratory tract.

RELATED SPECIES Garden cress (*L. sativum*), native to temperate regions of the northern hemisphere, is cultivated as a salad plant and used occasionally as a "blood-cleanser." *L. oleraceum*, native to New Zealand, is also grown for culinary use.

Leptandra virginica
syn. *Veronicastrum virginicum*
(*Scrophulariaceae*)
BLACK ROOT

DESCRIPTION Perennial herb growing to 3 ft (1 m). Has an erect stem, lance-shaped leaves in whorls, and white flowers.

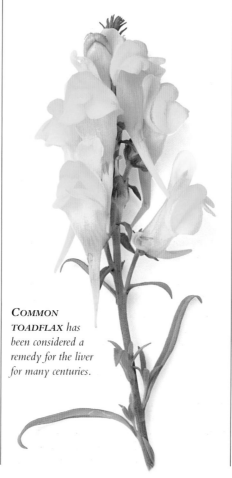

HABITAT & CULTIVATION Black root grows across North America in meadows and woodlands. The root is unearthed in autumn.

PART USED Dried root.

Root

CONSTITUENTS Black root contains a volatile oil, saponins, sugars, and tannins.

HISTORY & FOLKLORE Known to the Native American peoples of Missouri and Delaware as a violent purgative, it was used in moderate doses as a laxative, detoxifier, and a remedy for liver disorders. In the 19th-century Physiomedicalist tradition, black root was taken to stimulate bile production.

MEDICINAL ACTIONS & USES Black root is still used in small doses today as a laxative and a remedy for liver and gallbladder disorders. The herb also treats flatulence and bloating, and eases the discomfort of hemorrhoids and rectal prolapse. It is occasionally given for skin problems if poor liver function is a factor.

CAUTIONS Do not use the fresh root. Do not take during pregnancy.

Levisticum officinale
syn. *Ligusticum levisticum*
(*Umbelliferae*)
LOVAGE

DESCRIPTION Perennial growing to 6 ft (2 m). Has glossy, toothed compound leaves, greenish yellow flowers, and tiny oval seeds.

HABITAT & CULTIVATION Lovage is found in southern Europe and southwestern Asia. It thrives in grassy places on sunny slopes of mountains. The leaves are gathered in spring or early summer, the seeds in late summer, the root in autumn.

PARTS USED Root, seeds, leaves.

CONSTITUENTS Lovage contains a volatile oil (about 70% phthalides), coumarins (including bergapten, psoralen, and umbelliferone), plant acids, beta-sitosterol, resins, and gums. The phthalides are sedative and anticonvulsant.

HISTORY & FOLKLORE The Irish herbalist K'Eogh recorded that lovage "expels flatulence … aids digestion, provokes urination and menstruation, clears the sight, and removes spots, freckles and redness from the face" (1735).

MEDICINAL ACTIONS & USES Lovage is a warming and tonic herb for the digestive and respiratory systems. It treats indigestion, poor appetite, gas and colic, and bronchitis. Lovage is significantly diuretic and antimicrobial, and is commonly taken for urinary tract complaints. It also encourages menstruation and relieves menstrual pain. Its warming nature improves poor circulation.

RELATED SPECIES Scotch lovage (*Ligusticum scotium*) is chiefly regarded as a food. The Chinese *chuan xiong* (*Ligusticum chuanxiong*) is used principally as a means to bring on absent menstruation and to treat menstrual pain. The Chinese *gao ben* (*Ligusticum sinense*) is also used for pain.

CAUTION Do not take during pregnancy.

SELF-HELP USE Heavy menstrual bleeding, p. 315.

Linaria vulgaris
(*Scrophulariaceae*)
COMMON TOADFLAX

DESCRIPTION Upright perennial growing to about 20 in (50 cm). Has linear leaves and yellow double-lipped flowers with long spurs.

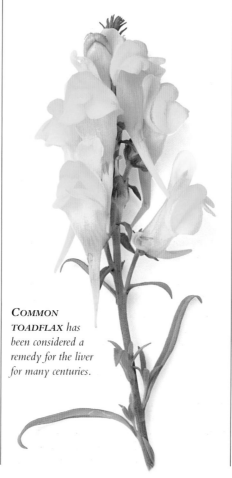

COMMON TOADFLAX has been considered a remedy for the liver for many centuries.

HABITAT & CULTIVATION Common toadflax is native to Europe and Asia, and is naturalized in North America. It flourishes along roadsides and in open areas. It is picked while in flower in summer.

PARTS USED Aerial parts.

CONSTITUENTS Common toadflax contains linarin, sterols, sugars, tannins, and mucilage.

HISTORY & FOLKLORE The herbalist K'Eogh related in 1735 that "An ointment [of toadflax] made with hogs' lard mixed with an egg yolk is excellent for piles."

MEDICINAL ACTIONS & USES Rarely used today, common toadflax is primarily a herb for the liver and digestion. It is helpful in treating jaundice, chronic constipation, and skin diseases. It may be applied externally to soothe sores, skin ulcers, and hemorrhoids.

RELATED SPECIES The southern European ivy-leaved toadflax (*Cymbalaria muralis*) is occasionally crushed and applied to wounds. Fluellin (*Kiksia elatine*), also a European native, is astringent and used to staunch wounds and bleeding. Blue toadflax (*L. canadensis*), native to North America, is used as a diuretic and laxative, and is applied to hemorrhoids.

CAUTIONS Use only under professional supervision. Do not take during pregnancy.

Linum usitatissimum
(*Linaceae*)
LINSEED, FLAX

DESCRIPTION Annual, biennial, or perennial herb growing to 3 ft (1 m). Has a slender stem, lance-shaped leaves, sky-blue flowers, and oily brown seeds.

HABITAT & CULTIVATION Linseed is native to temperate zones of Europe and Asia. It is cultivated worldwide for its fiber, seeds, and seed oil. The seeds are harvested in late summer or early autumn.

PARTS USED Seeds, seed oil.

CONSTITUENTS Linseed contains 30–40% fixed oil (including 36–50% linolenic acid and 23–24% linoleic acid), 6% mucilage, 25% protein, and small amounts of linamarin (a cyanogenic glycoside). Linamarin has a sedative effect on the respiratory system.

HISTORY & FOLKLORE Linseed has been cultivated for at least 7,000 years in the Middle East, and has long been esteemed as a medicinal herb. Pliny (AD 23–79) summed up its many applications by asking, "What department is there to be found of active life in which linseed is not employed? And in what production of the Earth are there greater marvels to us than this?"

MEDICINAL ACTIONS & USES Linseed is rich in mucilage and unsaturated fats, and makes a valuable remedy for many intestinal and chest problems. Taken whole internally,

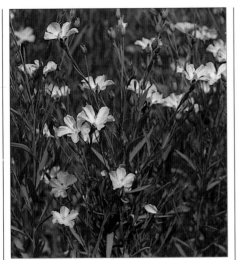

LINSEED has been cultivated since ancient times for its seeds, seed oil, and fiber.

the seeds soothe irritation throughout the digestive tract. They also absorb fluid and swell, drawing in toxins and forming a jellylike mass, which acts as an effective bulk laxative. If the seeds are split before being swallowed, they provide essential fatty acids. To a lesser extent, the seeds benefit the urinary tract. Externally, a poultice of the crushed seeds may be helpful in treating chronic coughs, bronchitis, pleurisy, and emphysema. A poultice of the seeds, or of linseed flour, may be applied to relieve painful boils. A Portuguese recipe recommends linseed oil mixed with red wine to treat wounds.

CAUTION Do not exceed recommended doses. Do not use immature seeds, which may be toxic.

SELF-HELP USE Constipation, p. 317.

Lippia citriodora syn. *Aloysia triphylla* (*Verbenaceae*)
LEMON VERBENA

DESCRIPTION Deciduous shrub growing to 6 ft (2 m). Has strongly scented lance-shaped leaves and clusters of tubular, pale green to mauve flowers.

HABITAT & CULTIVATION Lemon verbena is native to South America. It is cultivated in temperate climates as an aromatic, ornamental plant and for its leaves, which are used to make herbal tea. The leaves are gathered in late summer.

PARTS USED Leaves.

CONSTITUENTS Lemon verbena contains a volatile oil (mainly consisting of citral, cineole, limonene, and geraniole), mucilage, tannins, and flavonoids.

HISTORY & FOLKLORE Lemon verbena was introduced to Europe in 1784. In Spain, France and elsewhere in Europe, the infusion is a popular drink.

MEDICINAL ACTIONS & USES An undervalued medicinal herb, lemon verbena shares qualities with lemon balm (*Melissa officinalis*, p. 111). Both contain a strong lemon-scented volatile oil that has calming and digestive properties. Lemon verbena is gently sedative and has a reputation for soothing abdominal discomfort. Its tonic effect on the nervous system is less pronounced than that of lemon balm, but it nonetheless helps to counter depression.

RELATED SPECIES Yerba dulce (*L. dulcis*), native to Mexico, is used therapeutically as a demulcent and expectorant. In Mexico, many other *Lippia* species are used for their antispasmodic, menstruation-inducing, and stomach-soothing properties. *L. adoensis* is drunk as a tea in West Africa.

SELF-HELP USE Gas & bloating, p. 306.

Liquidambar orientalis (*Hamamelidaceae*)
LEVANT STORAX

DESCRIPTION Deciduous tree growing to a height of 20 ft (6 m). Has purplish-gray bark, lobed leaves, and small single yellow-white flowers.

HABITAT & CULTIVATION Levant storax is found in southwestern Turkey. Storax balsam, a viscid gray-brown liquid, is extracted from the bark, which is prised off the tree in autumn.

PART USED Bark extract.

CONSTITUENTS Levant storax contains cinnamic acid, cinnamyl cinnamate, phenylpropyl cinnamate, triterpene acids, and a volatile oil.

HISTORY & FOLKLORE Levant storax has been the *Liquidambar* species most commonly used medicinally since the 19th century. Levant storax is also employed as a fixative for perfumes.

MEDICINAL ACTIONS & USES Storax balsam has an irritant expectorant effect on the respiratory tract and it is an ingredient of Friar's Balsam, an expectorant mixture that is inhaled to stimulate a productive cough. Levant storax, in the form of balsam, is also applied externally to encourage the healing of skin diseases and problems such as scabies, wounds, and ulcers. Mixed with witch hazel (*Hamamelis virginiana*, p. 100) and rosewater (*Rosa* species), it makes an astringent face lotion. In China, storax balsam is used to clear mucus congestion and to relieve pain and constriction in the chest.

RELATED SPECIES Sweet gum (*L. styraciflua*), which grows mainly in Honduras but is also found farther north, has been used since the time of the Maya for its healing properties.

Liriosma ovata (*Oleaceae*)
MUIRA PUAMA

DESCRIPTION Tree growing to 50 ft (15 m) with a gray trunk, dark brown leaves, white flowers, and orange-yellow fruits.

HABITAT & CULTIVATION Muira puama is native to Brazilian rainforests, especially the Rio Negro and Amazonas regions.

PARTS USED Root, bark, wood.

CONSTITUENTS Muira puama contains esters and plant sterols.

MEDICINAL ACTIONS & USES Muira puama has long been used by indigenous Amazonians as a tonic and aphrodisiac. It is still considered a valuable remedy for impotence. The bark is strongly astringent and may be used as a gargle for sore throats and is taken in the form of an infusion in order to treat diarrhea and dysentery.

Lobaria pulmonaria (*Stictaceae*)
TREE LUNGWORT

DESCRIPTION Gray or light green lichen with forked irregular lobes measuring up to ¾ in (1.5 cm) across.

HABITAT & CULTIVATION Found throughout Europe, tree lungwort grows on trees and rocks in woodland areas. It is gathered throughout the year.

PART USED Lichen.

CONSTITUENTS Tree lungwort contains a variety of plant acids (including stictic and sticinic acid), fatty acids, and mucilage, as well as tannins.

HISTORY & FOLKLORE Tree lungwort has been used since ancient times as a remedy for lung problems. Pierandrea Mattioli (1501–1577), the Italian physician and herbalist, recommended tree lungwort for healing pulmonary ulcers and treating blood-flecked phlegm. It was also used to treat wounds, heal ulcers, reduce menstrual bleeding, relieve dysentery, and halt "choleric vomiting."

MEDICINAL ACTIONS & USES A beneficial but under-used remedy, tree lungwort has expectorant and tonic properties. It aids in clearing congested mucus and helps to increase appetite. In a decoction sweetened with honey, it is appropriate for all conditions that are marked by chronic respiratory mucus, especially coughs and bronchitis. The plant also treats asthma, pleurisy, and emphysema. Being astringent and demulcent, tree lungwort makes a useful treatment for pulmonary ulcers as well as for a variety of gastrointestinal problems. It is a highly suitable herb for treating ailments in children.

Lonicera spp.
(Caprifoliaceae)
HONEYSUCKLE & JIN YIN HUA (CHINESE)

DESCRIPTION A climber growing to 12 ft (4 m) that is deciduous (honeysuckle, *L. caprifolium*) or semievergreen (*jin yin hua*, *L. japonica*). Has paired oval leaves, yellow-orange (honeysuckle) or yellow-white (*jin yin hua*) tubular flowers, and red (honeysuckle) or black (*jin yin hua*) berries.

HABITAT & CULTIVATION Honeysuckle is native to southern Europe and the Caucasus. *Jin yin hua* is native to China and Japan. Both plants are commonly found growing on walls, trees, and in hedges. The flowers and leaves are gathered in summer just before the flowers open.

PARTS USED Flowers, leaves, bark.

CONSTITUENTS Honeysuckle's constituents include a volatile oil, tannins, and salicylic acid. *Jin yin hua* contains a volatile oil (which includes linalool and jasmone), tannins, luteolin, and inositol.

HISTORY & FOLKLORE In Europe, honeysuckle has traditionally been used as a treatment for asthma and other chest conditions. Honeysuckle is one of the Bach Flower Remedies, and in this system of herbal cures it is believed to counter feelings of nostalgia and homesickness. *Jin yin hua* has long been used in Chinese medicine to "clear heat and relieve toxicity."

MEDICINAL ACTIONS & USES Honeysuckle is rarely used in contemporary Western herbal medicine. Traditional usage indicates that different parts of the plant have very different therapeutic benefits. The bark is diuretic and may be taken to relieve gout, kidney stones, and liver problems. The leaves are astringent and make a good gargle and mouthwash for sore throats and canker sores. The flowers, which relieve coughs and are antispasmodic, are traditionally taken as a treatment for asthma. *Jin yin hua* is prescribed for an entirely different range of diseases in Chinese herbal medicine. It is principally employed to counter "hot" infectious disorders such as abscesses, sores, inflammation of the breasts, and dysentery. *Jin yin hua* is also taken to bring down fever.

RESEARCH Chinese research indicates that *jin yin hua* inhibits the tuberculosis bacillus and counters infection. In one trial, *jin yin hua* was combined with *ju hua* (*Chrysanthemum* x *morifolium*, p. 77) and proved to be effective in lowering blood pressure. Given its similarity to *jin yin hua*, honeysuckle could also prove useful against infection.

CAUTION Do not take the berries, which are toxic.

Lophophora williamsii
(Cactaceae)
PEYOTE, MESCAL

DESCRIPTION Cactus growing to 2 in (5 cm). Has a squat gray-green body with tufted hairs, and pink or white flowers.

HABITAT & CULTIVATION Peyote is native to northern Mexico and the southwestern US.

PART USED Whole plant.

CONSTITUENTS Peyote contains alkaloids, principally mescaline, which is a powerful hallucinogen.

HISTORY & FOLKLORE Peyote has been used in Native American religious ceremonies for over 3,000 years. Its use as a hallucinogen was popularized by Aldus Huxley in his book *The Doors of Perception.*

MEDICINAL ACTIONS & USES Peyote is a shamanistic plant, taken in Native American rituals to deepen spiritual understanding. It plays an important part in the emotional and mental state of the community. It is also used to treat fevers, as a painkiller for rheumatism, and to treat paralysis. It is applied as a

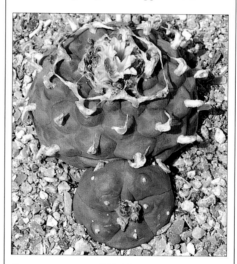

PEYOTE is a powerful hallucinogen. It is used in Native American ceremonies.

poultice for fractures, wounds, and snake bite. Peyote is also used to induce vomiting.

CAUTION The use of peyote and mescaline is illegal in most countries.

Luffa cylindrica
syn. *L. aegyptica*
(Cucurbitaceae)
LOOFAH, SI GUA LUO (CHINESE)

DESCRIPTION Annual vine climbing to 50 ft (15 m). Has large lobed leaves, tendrils, and yellow female flowers producing long, cylindrical, marrowlike fruit.

HABITAT & CULTIVATION Loofah is native

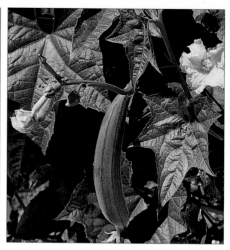

LOOFAH fruit is dried and used in Chinese medicine to treat muscle and joint pain.

to the tropics of Asia and Africa. It is now grown as a fruit in tropical regions around the world. It is harvested when ripe in summer.

PART USED Fruit.

CONSTITUENTS Loofah contains xylan, xylose, and galactan.

HISTORY & FOLKLORE Loofah was brought from India to China in the Tang Dynasty (AD 618–907). It is best known in the West as a bathroom accessory – the dried skeleton of the fruit makes a gentle skin scrubber.

MEDICINAL ACTIONS & USES In Chinese medicine, the inner skeleton of the dried fruit is used to treat pain in the muscles and joints, chest, and abdomen. It is prescribed for chest infections accompanied by fever and pain, and is used to clear congested mucus. Loofah is also given to treat painful or swollen breasts.

RESEARCH Chinese research indicates that the fresh vine has a stronger expectorant effect than the dried fruit.

Lycopodium clavatum
(Lycopodiaceae)
CLUB MOSS

DESCRIPTION Creeping evergreen moss growing to 5 in (12 cm). Has numerous straggling branchlets covered with bright green linear leaves, and scaly spikes bearing yellow spores.

HABITAT & CULTIVATION Club moss is found throughout temperate regions of the northern hemisphere. It is common on mountains and in grassy areas. The plant is gathered in summer.

PARTS USED Moss, spores.

CONSTITUENTS Club moss contains about 0.1–0.2% alkaloids (including lycopodine), polyphenols, flavonoids, and triterpenes.

HISTORY & FOLKLORE Club moss has been used medicinally since at least the Middle

Ages. The whole plant was employed as a diuretic to aid in the flushing out of kidney stones. Being strongly water-resistant, the spores are still used to coat tablets. The spores ignite explosively and have been used in making fireworks.

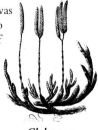

Club moss

MEDICINAL ACTIONS & USES Club moss is diuretic, sedative, and antispasmodic, and it is particularly useful for treating chronic urinary complaints. The herb may also be taken for indigestion and gastritis. The spores may be applied to the skin to relieve and protect itchy or irritated areas.

CAUTION Club moss is potentially toxic in overdose. Use this plant only under professional supervision.

Lycopus virginicus
(Labiatae)
BUGLEWEED

DESCRIPTION Perennial herb growing to a height of 2 ft (60 cm). Has a square stem with lance-shaped leaves and whorls of whitish flowers.

HABITAT & CULTIVATION Bugleweed is common throughout most of North America, thriving close to water. It is harvested in summer when in flower.

PARTS USED Aerial parts.

CONSTITUENTS Bugleweed contains phenolic acids (including derivatives of caffeic, chlorogenic, and ellagic acids).

HISTORY & FOLKLORE In the 19th-century Anglo-American Physiomedicalist tradition, bugleweed was regarded as astringent and calming to the nerves, and was given for loose coughs, internal bleeding, and urinary incontinence. Herbal practitioners once considered the plant to be a mild narcotic.

MEDICINAL ACTIONS & USES Bugleweed has sedative properties and is principally prescribed today to treat an overactive thyroid gland and the racing heartbeat that often accompanies this condition. Bugleweed is also considered an aromatic and tonic astringent that reduces the production of mucus.

RESEARCH Studies indicate that bugleweed and, to some degree, gypsywort (see *Related Species*, below) reduce the activity of the thyroid gland.

RELATED SPECIES Gypsywort (*L. europaeus*), a European native, has astringent and cardiotonic properties. It is taken for palpitations and anxiety, and has been used to lower fever.

CAUTIONS Take only under professional supervision. Do not take during pregnancy.

Lysimachia vulgaris
(Primulaceae)
YELLOW LOOSESTRIFE

DESCRIPTION Attractive perennial growing to 3 ft (1 m) with whorls of broad lance-shaped leaves and bright yellow flowers.

HABITAT & CULTIVATION Native to Europe, yellow loosestrife commonly grows along roadsides and near water. It is also cultivated as a garden plant. It is gathered when in flower in summer.

PARTS USED Aerial parts.

CONSTITUENTS Yellow loosestrife contains a benzoquinone, saponins, flavonoids, and tannins.

HISTORY & FOLKLORE Pliny (AD 23–79) recorded that *lysimachia*, the plant's Latin name, was a tribute to King Lysimachus of Sicily, who was the first to discover its medicinal benefits. The name "loosestrife" refers to the plant's reputed power to prevent conflict, particularly between animals, and to repel insects. The Greek physician Dioscorides (AD 40–90) recommended loosestrife for nosebleeds and to staunch wounds, and noted that its smoke would drive away snakes and flies.

MEDICINAL ACTIONS & USES An astringent herb, yellow loosestrife is principally used to treat gastrointestinal conditions such as diarrhea and dysentery, to stop internal and external bleeding, and to cleanse wounds. It makes a serviceable mouthwash for sore gums and canker sores, and may be used to treat nosebleeds. Yellow loosestrife has also been taken as an expectorant.

RELATED SPECIES The yellow pimpernel (*L. nemorum*), another European native, is also astringent and staunches blood. *Jin qian cao* (*L. christinae*), from China, is a diuretic used to treat urinary pain. A Chinese trial showed that the latter is also effective in treating both kidney stones and gallstones.

Lythrum salicaria
(Lythraceae)
PURPLE LOOSESTRIFE

DESCRIPTION Attractive perennial growing to about 5 ft (1.5 m). Has straight red stems, pointed lance-shaped leaves, and spikes of brilliant purple flowers.

HABITAT & CULTIVATION Purple loosestrife is native to Europe but is now well established in the wild in North America. It thrives in marshes and along rivers and streams, to altitudes of 3,300 ft (1,000 m). It is gathered when in flower in summer.

PARTS USED Aerial parts.

CONSTITUENTS Purple loosestrife contains salicarin, a glycoside (vitexin), tannins, a volatile oil, mucilage, and plant sterols.

HISTORY & FOLKLORE In 1654, the herbalist Nicholas Culpeper praised the herb, writing that "the distilled water is a present remedy for hurts and blows on the eyes, and for blindness … it also cleareth the eyes of dust or any other thing gotten into them, and preserveth the sight." A common plant in Ireland, purple loosestrife was much used there against diarrhea.

MEDICINAL ACTIONS & USES The astringent purple loosestrife is mainly employed as a treatment for diarrhea and dysentery. It can be safely taken by people of all ages; some herbalists recommend it to help arrest diarrhea in breast-feeding babies. The herb may also be used to treat heavy menstrual bleeding and for intermenstrual bleeding. Externally, it is applied as a poultice or lotion to wounds, leg ulcers, and eczema, and used to treat excess vaginal discharge and vaginal itching. Purple loosestrife is now rarely used to treat eye problems, but, as Culpeper's experience suggests, it could be worth further investigation for disorders of the eyes and vision.

RESEARCH The whole plant is reported to be antibiotic, being particularly effective against the micro-organism that causes typhus.

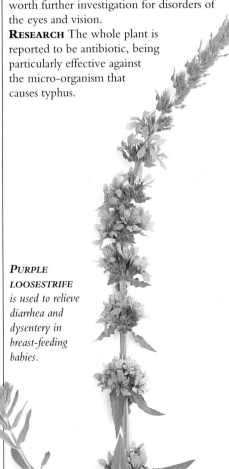

PURPLE LOOSESTRIFE *is used to relieve diarrhea and dysentery in breast-feeding babies.*

Madhuca spp.
(Sapotaceae)
BUTTER TREE

DESCRIPTION Deciduous tree growing to 70 ft (20 m). Has leathery leaves, clusters of scented white flowers, and greenish fruit.

HABITAT & CULTIVATION *Madhuca* species are native to central and northern India. The flowers, leaves, and seeds are gathered in summer.

PARTS USED Flowers, seed oil.

CONSTITUENTS The leaves contain an alkaloid and a saponin; the seeds, a saponin and fixed oil.

HISTORY & FOLKLORE Butter tree has been a source of food and medicine in India for at least 2,000 years. Its flowers are eaten and are fermented to make alcoholic drinks.

MEDICINAL ACTIONS & USES The expectorant flowers are used to treat chest problems such as bronchitis. They are also taken to increase production of breast milk. The leaves are applied as a poultice to relieve eczema. In Indian folk medicine, the leaf ash is mixed with *ghee* (clarified butter) to make a dressing for wounds and burns. The seed oil is laxative, and is taken for constipation and to loosen the stool of hemorrhoid sufferers. The oil is also applied to itchy skin.

Magnolia officinalis
(Magnoliaceae)
HOU PO (CHINESE),
MAGNOLIA

DESCRIPTION Deciduous tree growing to 75 ft (22 m). Has aromatic bark, large leaves, and fragrant creamy white flowers.

HABITAT & CULTIVATION Native to China, *hou po* grows wild in mountainous regions. It is now found in many parts of the world as a garden tree. The bark is stripped in spring.

PART USED Bark.

CONSTITUENTS *Hou po* contains a volatile oil and magnocurarine. Extracts of the plant have a slight muscle-relaxing effect when injected.

HISTORY & FOLKLORE *Hou po* has a long tradition of use as a medicinal herb in China, dating to at least the 1st century AD.

MEDICINAL ACTIONS & USES *Hou po* bark is aromatic, warming, and pungent. It relieves cramping pain and flatulence, and is taken for abdominal distension, indigestion, loss of appetite, vomiting, and diarrhea.

RESEARCH Chinese research suggests that *huo po* is mildly antimicrobial and possibly effective against amebic dysentery.

RELATED SPECIES *Xin yi hua* (*M. liliiflora*), another Chinese species, is principally used

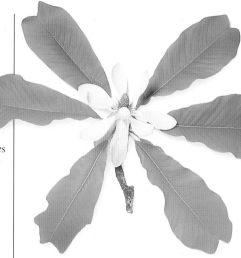

HOU PO is distinguished by its beautiful creamy white flowers.

to treat upper respiratory tract infections and to clear excess mucus.

Malva sylvestris
(Malvaceae)
COMMON MALLOW

DESCRIPTION Biennial growing to about 5 ft (1.5 m). Has a pulpy taproot, erect stem, 5-lobed leaves with scalloped margins, and reddish pink to mauve flowers.

HABITAT & CULTIVATION Common mallow is native to Europe and Asia. It is now naturalized in much of the Americas and Australasia, growing in open areas, along roadsides, and on hedges and fences. The leaves are gathered in spring; the flowers, when in bloom, in summer.

PARTS USED Leaves, flowers, root.

CONSTITUENTS Common mallow contains flavonol glycosides (including gossypin-3-sulfate), mucilage, and tannins. The flowers also contain malvin (an anthocyanin).

HISTORY & FOLKLORE The young leaves and shoots of the common mallow have been eaten since at least the 8th century BC. The plant's many uses gave rise to the Spanish adage, "A kitchen garden and mallow, sufficient medicines for a home."

MEDICINAL ACTIONS & USES Though less useful than marsh mallow (*Althaea officinalis*, p. 163), common mallow is an effective demulcent. The flowers and leaves are emollient and good for sensitive areas of the skin. It is applied as a poultice to reduce swelling and draw out toxins. Taken internally, the leaves reduce gut irritation and have a laxative effect. When common mallow is combined with eucalyptus (*Eucalyptus globulus*, p. 94), it makes a good remedy for coughs and other chest ailments. As with marsh mallow, the root may be given to children to ease teething.

Mandragora officinarum
(Solanaceae)
MANDRAKE

DESCRIPTION Perennial growing to 2 in (5 cm). Has a deep branching root, a rosette of broad floppy leaves, funnel-shaped white to purple flowers, and yellow fruit.

HABITAT & CULTIVATION Native to the Mediterranean region of Europe, mandrake grows on dry riverbeds. Its leaves are picked in summer.

PART USED Root.

CONSTITUENTS Mandrake contains 0.4% tropane alkaloids (hyoscine and hyoscyamine).

HISTORY & FOLKLORE Legend held that the mandrake, on being uprooted, emitted a scream that was so powerful it could kill the person harvesting the plant. Consequently, reported one classical authority, mandrake was pulled up by dogs that had the stems tied to their tails. The fantastic powers attributed to the plant were partly due to the narcotic-like properties of the root. Also influential was the root's shape, which often vaguely resembles the human form. The roots have been carved and used as talismans for thousands of years, especially to aid fertility in women, and as a charm against misfortune. From Roman times onward, mandrake root bark was used as an anesthetic and analgesic, and as a treatment for insanity.

MEDICINAL ACTIONS & USES Mandrake has now largely fallen out of use. It is sometimes used as a poultice or plaster for rheumatic and arthritic pains, or as a decoction for ulcers and other skin disorders.

CAUTIONS Mandrake is toxic. Do not take internally. Use externally only under professional supervision. The plant is subject to legal restrictions in some countries.

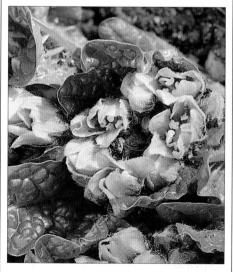

MANDRAKE'S narcotic properties and human-shaped root have inspired much legend and lore.

Manihot esculenta
(Euphorbiaceae)
MANIOC, CASSAVA

DESCRIPTION Shrub growing to 6 ft (2 m). Has fleshy roots, woody stems, large palm-shaped leaves, and green flowers.

HABITAT & CULTIVATION Manioc is native to tropical Central and South America. It grows principally in Brazil and on the eastern side of the Andes. Bitter and sweet varieties are also cultivated as an important food crop in tropical areas around the world. The root is unearthed 8 to 24 months after planting.

PART USED Root.

CONSTITUENTS Manioc contains cyanogenic glycosides (0.02–0.03% in the bitter varieties, 0.007% in the sweet) and starch.

HISTORY & FOLKLORE Bitter manioc has large quantities of highly toxic glycosides,

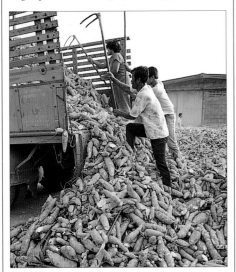

MANIOC is a staple food in many tropical regions of the world.

and must be carefully soaked and cooked before it is safe to eat. (Sweet manioc is safe to eat without such processing.) Tapioca is a native Brazilian name for the processed root, which is used in commercial food preparation as a thickening agent. The Witoto of the Colombian Amazon poison fish with the water used to wash bitter manioc. The Makuna use the wash water to treat scabies.

MEDICINAL ACTIONS & USES Manioc root is easily digestible and makes a suitable, low-protein food for convalescence. The bitter variety may be used to treat scabies, diarrhea, and dysentery. Manioc flour may be used to help dry weeping skin. In China, a poultice is made of manioc, wheat flour, and ginger (*Zingiber officinale*, p. 153) to draw out pus when infection is present.

CAUTION Raw bitter manioc is toxic and has caused many deaths. The root must be carefully soaked and cooked before eating.

Maranta arundinacea
(Marantaceae)
ARROWROOT

DESCRIPTION Perennial growing to 6 ft (2 m). Has a creeping rhizome, many long-stemmed oval leaves, and flowering stems with clusters of creamy white flowers.

HABITAT & CULTIVATION Native to northern South America and the Caribbean islands, arrowroot is cultivated mostly on the island of St. Vincent. The rhizome is unearthed 10 to 11 months after planting.

PART USED Rhizome.

CONSTITUENTS Arrowroot contains 25–27% neutral starch.

HISTORY & FOLKLORE In Central America, the Maya made the root into a poultice for smallpox sores and an infusion for urinary infections. Arrowroot was traditionally used by the Arawak of South America as an antidote to arrow poisons.

MEDICINAL ACTIONS & USES Arrowroot is used in herbal medicine in much the same manner as slippery elm (*Ulmus rubra*, p. 144), as a soothing demulcent and a nutrient of benefit in convalescence. It helps to relieve acidity, indigestion, and colic, and it exerts a mildly laxative action on the large bowel. It may be applied as an ointment or poultice mixed with antiseptic herbs such as myrrh (*Commiphora molmol*, p. 84).

SELF-HELP USE Acidity & indigestion, p. 307.

Marrubium vulgare
(Labiatae)
HOREHOUND

DESCRIPTION Square-stemmed perennial growing to about 20 in (50 cm). Has toothed, downy leaves and double-lipped white flowers.

Dried herb

HABITAT & CULTIVATION Native to Europe, horehound is naturalized in North and South America. It flourishes in in dry, bare, or open areas, and is gathered in spring.

PARTS USED Leaves.

CONSTITUENTS Horehound contains the diterpenes marrubiin (0.3–1.0%) and marrubenol, flavonoids, alkaloids (including betonicine and stachydrine), and 0.6% volatile oil. Marrubiin is strongly expectorant and bitter.

HISTORY & FOLKLORE Horehound has been a remedy for chest problems since ancient times, perhaps most frequently taken as a syrup made with honey or sugar. The Greek physician Dioscorides (AD 40–90) recommended a decoction of the herb for tuberculosis, asthma, and coughs. In 1597, the herbalist John Gerard praised horehound as "a most singular remedy against the cough and wheezing."

MEDICINAL ACTIONS & USES Horehound is a helpful treatment for wheezing, bronchitis, bronchiectasis (a damaged air passage within the lung), bronchial asthma, nonproductive coughs, and whooping cough. The herb apparently causes the secretion of a more fluid mucus, which is more readily cleared by coughing. As a bitter tonic, horehound increases the appetite and supports the function of the stomach. The herb also acts to normalize heart rhythm, improving its regularity. It is less commonly used as a decoction for skin conditions.

Marsdenia condurango
syn. Gonolobus condurango
(Asclepiadaceae)
CONDURANGO

DESCRIPTION Climbing vine growing to 30 ft (10 m). Has heart-shaped leaves and funnel-shaped, whitish green flowers.

HABITAT & CULTIVATION Condurango is native to deciduous forests of the Andes in Peru and Ecuador. The vine is generally found growing at altitudes of between 1,000–2,000 ft (3,300–6,600 m). The bark is collected throughout the year.

PARTS USED Bark, latex.

CONSTITUENTS Condurango bark contains glycosides (based on condurangogenins), a volatile oil, and phytosterols.

HISTORY & FOLKLORE Early in this century, condurango was erroneously yet widely believed to be a remedy for cancer.

MEDICINAL ACTIONS & USES Condurango bark stimulates stomach secretions. Often used in South American folk medicine as a bitter and digestive tonic, it is a specific treatment for nervous indigestion and anorexia nervosa. Its bitterness slowly increases the appetite, as well as the stomach's ability to process increased quantities of food. The herb is also thought to stimulate the liver and pancreas, and may be taken for liver disorders. It also encourages menstruation. The caustic white latex is applied to remove warts.

RESEARCH Condurangogenins in condurango may prove beneficial in countering tumors. The whole plant, however, does not seem to significantly alter cancer development.

RELATED SPECIES *M. zimapanica*, native to Mexico, has been used to poison coyotes.

CAUTION The latex is poisonous and should not be taken internally.

Medicago sativa
(Leguminosae)
ALFALFA, LUCERNE

DESCRIPTION Perennial herb growing to 32 in (80 cm). Has 3-lobed leaves, flowers that range in color from yellow to violet-blue, and spiraling seed pods.

HABITAT & CULTIVATION Native to Asia, Europe, and North Africa, alfalfa is found in meadows and in both open and cultivated areas. Grown in temperate climates as a fodder crop, it is harvested in summer.

PARTS USED Aerial parts, sprouting seeds.

CONSTITUENTS Alfalfa contains isoflavones, coumarins, alkaloids, vitamins, and porphyrins. The isoflavones and coumarins are estrogenic.

HISTORY & FOLKLORE Pliny (AD 23–79) recorded that alfalfa was brought to Greece

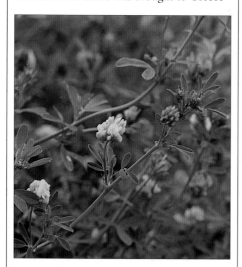

ALFALFA has been cultivated for centuries for its nutritional and medicinal properties.

by Darius, King of Persia (550–486 BC), during his attempt to conquer Athens. The seeds have been eaten for thousands of years.

MEDICINAL ACTIONS & USES Alfalfa is perhaps more therapeutically useful as a food than a medicine. It is given to convalescents who require easily assimilated nutrients. In view of alfalfa's estrogenic activity, it could prove useful in treating problems relating to menstruation and menopause.

CAUTION Do not take if suffering from autoimmune diseases.

Melaleuca leucadendron
(Myrtaceae)
CAJUPUT

DESCRIPTION Aromatic, evergreen tree growing to 130 ft (40 m). Has peeling bark, pale green oval leaves, and clusters of small white flowers on long spikes.

HABITAT & CULTIVATION Native to Southeast Asia, cajuput is cultivated for its essential oil and lumber. The leaves and twigs are gathered throughout the year.

PART USED Essential oil.

CONSTITUENTS The oil contains terpenoids, mainly cineole (50–60%), beta-pinene, alpha-terpineol, and others. Cineole is strongly antiseptic.

MEDICINAL ACTIONS & USES Cajuput is normally combined with other essential oils such as eucalyptus (*Eucalyptus globulus*, p. 94). Its antiseptic properties treat colds, sore throats, coughs, and, especially, chest infections. The diluted oil may either be steam inhaled or applied to the chest or throat to treat laryngitis, tracheitis, and bronchitis. Since cajuput stimulates the circulation and is antispasmodic, it is used as a friction rub for rheumatic joints and neuralgia.

RELATED SPECIES Niaouli (*M. viridiflora*), of New Caledonia, is antiseptic and decongestant, and has properties similar to those of cajuput. *See also* tea tree (*M. alternifolia*, p. 110).

CAUTIONS Take internally only under professional supervision. Do not use during pregnancy. Cajuput essential oil is subject to legal restrictions in some countries.

SELF-HELP USE Chesty coughs & bronchitis, p. 310.

Melilotus officinalis
syn. *M. arvensis*
(Leguminosae)
MELILOT

DESCRIPTION Biennial herb growing to about 3 ft (1 m). Has 3-lobed leaves, spikes of yellow flowers, and brown seed pods.

HABITAT & CULTIVATION Melilot is a plant native to Europe, North Africa, and temperate regions of Asia, and is naturalized in North America. It grows in dry or open areas, and is harvested in late spring.

PARTS USED Aerial parts.

CONSTITUENTS Melilot contains flavonoids, coumarins (including hydroxycoumarin and hydrocoumarin), resin, tannins, and volatile oil. If allowed to spoil, the plant produces dicoumarol, a powerful anticoagulant.

HISTORY & FOLKLORE The Irish herbalist K'Eogh reported in 1735, "a gentlewoman of my acquaintance … had a swelling for a year or more on her right side, which was cured by three or four times rubbing the grieved part with an oil made of this herb."

MEDICINAL ACTIONS & USES As with horse chestnut (*Aesculus hippocastanum*, p. 159), long-term use of melilot – internally or externally – can help varicose veins and hemorrhoids. Melilot also helps reduce the risk of phlebitis and thrombosis. The plant is mildly sedative and antispasmodic, and is given for insomnia (especially in children) and anxiety. It has been used to treat gas and indigestion, bronchitis, problems associated with menopause, and rheumatic pains.

CAUTIONS Do not take melilot if using anticoagulants. If harvested from the wild, melilot should be dried or used immediately, since the spoiled plant is toxic.

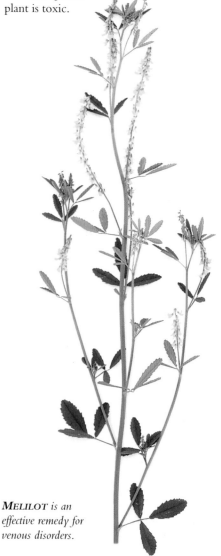

MELILOT is an effective remedy for venous disorders.

Mentha haplocalyx
(Labiatae)
BO HE (CHINESE), CORN MINT

DESCRIPTION Perennial herb growing to 2 ft (60 cm). Has a square stem, toothed oval leaves, and whorls of pale lilac flowers growing from the leaf axils.

HABITAT & CULTIVATION *Bo he* is native to temperate regions of the northern hemisphere and is widely cultivated in China. Harvested 2–3 times a year, the best crops are in early summer and early autumn.

PARTS USED Aerial parts.

CONSTITUENTS *Bo he* contains a volatile oil

comprising mainly menthol (up to 95%) with menthone, menthyl acetate, camphene, limonene, and other terpenoids.

HISTORY & FOLKLORE *Bo he* was first mentioned in *Grandfather Lei's Discussion of Herb Preparation* (c. AD 470). A 15th-century Chinese prescription recommended *bo he* for bloody dysentery.

MEDICINAL ACTIONS & USES In Chinese herbal medicine *bo he* is a popular treatment for colds, sore throats, sore mouth and tongue, and a host of other conditions ranging from toothache to measles. Like peppermint (*M. x piperita*, p. 112), it helps to lower the temperature, has anticongestive properties, and may be taken for dysentery and diarrhea. The juice has also been used to treat earache. *Bo he* is often combined with *ju hua* (*Chrysanthemum x morifolium*, p. 77) to treat headaches and bloodshot or sore eyes.

RELATED SPECIES The Japanese variety of *bo he* (*M. arvensis*) is widely cultivated as a source of menthol. Spearmint (*M. spicata*) is used mainly as a flavoring and culinary herb. *See also* peppermint (*M. x piperita*, p. 112) and pennyroyal (*M. pulegium, see following entry*).

Mentha pulegium
(Labiatae)
PENNYROYAL

DESCRIPTION Powerfully aromatic perennial growing to 16 in (40 cm). Has toothed oval leaves and whorls of lilac flowers arising from the leaf axils.

HABITAT & CULTIVATION Pennyroyal is native to Europe and western Asia, and has become naturalized in the Americas. It thrives in damp areas and is gathered when in flower in summer.

PARTS USED Aerial parts.

CONSTITUENTS Pennyroyal's volatile oil contains pulegone (between 27–92%), isopulegone, menthol, and other terpenoids. Pennyroyal also contains bitters and tannins.

HISTORY & FOLKLORE The Greek natural historian Pliny (AD 23–79) wrote that pennyroyal was considered a better medicinal herb than roses, and that it purified bad water. His contemporary Dioscorides stated that pennyroyal "provokes menstruation and labour." In 1597, John Gerard wrote that "a garland of pennie royal made and worne about the head is of great force against the swimming of the head, and the pains and giddiness thereof." The name *pulegium* derives from the Latin word for flea, referring to pennyroyal's traditional use as a flea repellent.

MEDICINAL ACTIONS & USES Similar in many respects to peppermint (*M. x piperita*, p. 112), pennyroyal is a good digestive tonic. It increases the secretion of digestive juices,

relieves flatulence and colic, and occasionally is used as a treatment for intestinal worms. It makes a good remedy for headaches and for minor respiratory infections, helping to check fever and congestion. Pennyroyal powerfully stimulates the uterine muscles and encourages menstruation. An infusion of pennyroyal is used externally for the treatment of itchiness and formication (a sensation of ants crawling over the body), inflamed skin disorders such as eczema, and rheumatic conditions including gout.

RELATED SPECIES *See* peppermint (*M. x piperita*, p. 112) and *bo he* (*M. haplocalyx, preceding entry*). American pennyroyal (*Hedeoma pulegoides*), while only distantly related, has constituents similar to those of pennyroyal. American pennyroyal is traditionally used as a remedy for colds, headaches, and delayed menstruation.

CAUTIONS Do not use the essential oil, which is highly toxic. Do not take pennyroyal during pregnancy or if menstrual bleeding is heavy.

SELF-HELP USES Digestive headaches & biliousness, p. 309; Nausea with headache, p. 306.

Menyanthes trifoliata
(Menyanthaceae)
BOGBEAN

DESCRIPTION Perennial aquatic plant growing to 9 in (23 cm). Has trefoil leaves and spikes of pink and white flowers with fringed petals.

HABITAT & CULTIVATION Bogbean is native to Europe, Asia, and America. It is found in shallow, fresh water. The leaves are picked in summer.

PARTS USED Leaves.

CONSTITUENTS Bogbean contains iridoid glycosides, flavonol glycosides, coumarins,

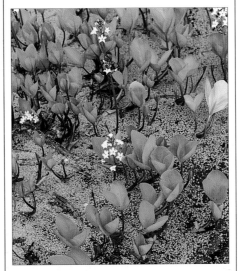

BOGBEAN leaves are gathered in summer, after the plant has come into flower.

phenolic acids, sterols, triterpenoids, tannins, and very small amounts of pyrrolizidine alkaloids. The iridoids are strongly bitter and stimulate digestive secretions.

HISTORY & FOLKLORE Long used as a folk remedy for rheumatism and arthritis, bogbean has also been taken to treat fluid retention, scabies, and fever. In the past, it was used as an adulterant of, or a substitute for, hops (*Humulus lupulus*, p. 102).

MEDICINAL ACTIONS & USES Bogbean is a strongly bitter herb that encourages the appetite and stimulates digestive secretions. It is commonly taken to improve an underactive or weak digestion, particularly if there is abdominal discomfort. This herb is also used as an aid to weight gain. Bogbean is thought to be an effective remedy for rheumatoid arthritis, especially when this condition is associated with weakness, weight loss, and lack of vitality. Bogbean is generally prescribed with other herbs such as celery seed (*Apium graveolens*, p. 61) and white willow (*Salix alba*, p. 128).

CAUTIONS Do not take bogbean if suffering from diarrhea, dysentery, or colitis. Excessive doses may cause vomiting.

Milletta reticulata
(Leguminosae)
JI XUE TENG

DESCRIPTION Low-growing plant with compound leaves and clusters of pea-type flowers producing large bean pods.

HABITAT & CULTIVATION Native to China, *ji xue teng* is cultivated in the southeast of the country.

PARTS USED Root, vine.

CONSTITUENTS Little is known about the active constituents.

HISTORY & FOLKLORE This plant was first recorded in Chinese medical texts in about AD 720.

MEDICINAL ACTIONS & USES In Chinese herbal medicine (*see* pp. 38–41), pain is often thought to be due to poor or obstructed blood flow. In this tradition, *ji xue teng* is classified as an herb that invigorates the blood, and is mainly used to treat menstrual problems. *Ji xue teng* is used to relieve menstrual pain or an irregular or absent cycle, especially where this may be due to blood deficiency such as anemia. It is also prescribed for certain types of arthritic pain, as well as for numbness of the hands and feet.

RESEARCH Limited investigation indicates that *ji xue teng* may be anti-inflammatory and may lower blood pressure.

RELATED SPECIES Various *Milletta* species are used in West Africa, Malaysia, Myanmar (formerly Burma), and India as a means to poison fish.

Mitchella repens
(Rubiaceae)
SQUAW VINE

DESCRIPTION Evergreen herb growing to 1 ft (30 cm) and forming mats on the ground. Has rounded shiny leaves, a flowering stem bearing fragrant white flowers, and small bright red berries.

HABITAT & CULTIVATION Squaw vine is native to the eastern and central US. It grows in dry sites in woodlands, and is harvested in late summer.

PARTS USED Aerial parts, berries.

Aerial parts **CONSTITUENTS** Squaw vine is believed to contain tannins, glycosides, and saponins.

HISTORY & FOLKLORE An infusion of squaw vine was commonly taken by Native American women to hasten childbirth. It was also occasionally used for a variety of other complaints, including insomnia, rheumatic pain, and fluid retention.

MEDICINAL ACTIONS & USES Squaw vine is still extensively used to aid labor and childbirth, and is also considered to have a tonic action on the uterus and the ovaries. It is taken to normalize menstruation and to relieve heavy bleeding and menstrual pain. This herb has also been recommended for stimulating breast-milk production, but other herbs with a similar action, such as fennel (*Foeniculum vulgare*, p. 210), are preferred. The berries, crushed and mixed with tincture of myrrh (*Commiphora molmol*, p. 84), are helpful for sore nipples. An astringent herb, squaw vine has also been prescribed for diarrhea and colitis.

CAUTION Do not take during the first 6 months of pregnancy.

Momordica charantia
(Cucurbitaceae)
CERASEE

DESCRIPTION Annual climber growing to about 6 ft (2 m). Has deeply lobed leaves, yellow flowers, and orange-yellow fruit.

HABITAT & CULTIVATION Native to southern Asia, cerasee is common throughout tropical regions of the world. It is harvested all year long.

PARTS USED Leaves, fruit, seeds, seed oil.

CONSTITUENTS Cerasee contains a fixed oil, an insulin-like peptide, glycosides (mormordin and charantin), and an alkaloid (mormordicine). The peptide is known to lower sugar levels in the blood and urine.

HISTORY & FOLKLORE Cerasee is traditionally taken in Asia, Africa, and the Caribbean to treat the symptoms of diabetes.

MEDICINAL ACTIONS & USES The unripe fruit is used mainly as a treatment for late-onset diabetes. The ripe fruit is a stomach tonic and induces menstruation. In Turkey, the fruit is employed to treat ulcers. The fruit is much used in the West Indies as a cure-all for worms, urinary stones, and fever. The juice of the fruit is used as a purgative. It is also prescribed for colic and gas. A decoction of the leaves is taken for liver problems and colitis, and may be applied to eruptive skin conditions. The seed oil is used on wounds.

RESEARCH Cerasee seeds were investigated in China in the 1980s as a potential contraceptive. Some research suggests that the plant may be harmful to the liver. The fruit demonstrably lowers sugar levels in the blood and urine.

RELATED SPECIES The seeds of the Asian *M. cochinchinensis* are used as a poultice for abscesses, sores, hemorrhoids, and scrofulous conditions. Research shows that a paste of the seeds may help psoriasis and ringworm.

CAUTIONS While cerasee is relatively safe at low dosage, usage longer than 4 weeks is not recommended. Do not take if prone to low blood sugar levels.

Monarda punctata
(Labiatae)
HORSEMINT

DESCRIPTION Aromatic perennial growing to 3 ft (90 cm). Has downy lance-shaped leaves and double-lipped, red-spotted yellow flowers growing in whorls from the leaf axils.

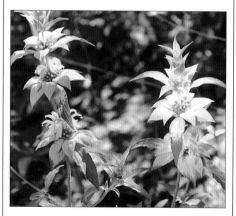

HORSEMINT strongly encourages sweating and the onset of menstruation.

HABITAT & CULTIVATION Native to the eastern and central US, horsemint flourishes in soil that is dry and sandy. The herb is gathered when in flower in summer and autumn.

PARTS USED Aerial parts.

CONSTITUENTS Horsemint's volatile oil has thymol as the main constituent.

HISTORY & FOLKLORE Horsemint's genus name, *Monarda*, was bestowed in honor of Nicolas Monardes, a Spanish physician, whose herbal of 1569 detailed the medicinal uses of a number of New World plants. Horsemint was traditionally taken by Native Americans to treat nausea and vomiting, and to encourage perspiration during colds. It was applied externally as a poultice for swelling and rheumatic pain.

MEDICINAL ACTIONS & USES Having a strong volatile oil, horsemint is primarily used for digestive and upper respiratory problems. It is taken as an infusion to relieve nausea, indigestion, flatulence, and colic. It is also employed to reduce fevers and upper respiratory mucus. The herb has an antiseptic action within the chest. Taken internally or applied externally, horsemint reduces fever by encouraging sweating. It also strongly stimulates menstruation. Applied externally, the plant is a counterirritant. It helps to lessen the pain in arthritic and rheumatic joints by increasing the flow of blood in the affected area, and thereby hastening the flushing out of toxins.

RELATED SPECIES In 19th-century America, oswego tea (*M. didyma*) was considered a tonic for young mothers and was traditionally given to brides. It is thought to be a mild menstrual regulator and an appetite stimulant.

CAUTION Do not take during pregnancy.

Monsonia ovata
(Geraniaceae)
MONSONIA

DESCRIPTION Small, herbaceous plant with multibranched stems, very small oblong leaves, and white solitary, or paired geranium-like flowers.

HABITAT & CULTIVATION Native to South Africa and Namibia, monsonia is found growing in arid conditions. It is gathered when in flower.

PARTS USED Aerial parts.

MEDICINAL ACTIONS & USES Monsonia is used throughout southwestern Africa as a treatment for diarrhea, acute and chronic dysentery, and ulcerative colitis. The plant's astringency tightens and protects the inner linings of the intestines. Given monsonia's long traditional use for intestinal disorders and infections, it is possible – but as yet unsubstantiated by research – that the plant has a direct antimicrobial effect.

RELATED SPECIES Monsonia is a fairly close relative of the *Pelargonium* species. These astringent plants – notably *P. antidysentericum* – are also used to treat stomach ulcers and dysentery.

Montia perfoliata
(Portulacaceae)
MINER'S LETTUCE

DESCRIPTION Annual growing to 4 in (10 cm) with pointed oval leaves (one pair enveloping the stem) and white 5-petaled flowers.

HABITAT & CULTIVATION Miner's lettuce is native to western North America, and has become naturalized in temperate regions around the world, especially in Australia. The plant thrives in acid sandy soils. It is generally gathered from the wild before and during the flowering period. It has also been cultivated as a vegetable.

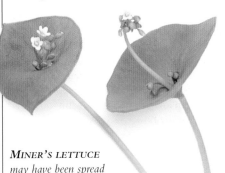

MINER'S LETTUCE may have been spread around the world by itinerant miners.

PARTS USED Aerial parts.

CONSTITUENTS Miner's lettuce is rich in vitamin C.

HISTORY & FOLKLORE Miner's lettuce was a readily available salad vegetable on the west coast of America. It most probably acquired its name during the California gold rush of 1849. Itinerant miners may have later taken the plant with them to Australia, where it is now common.

MEDICINAL ACTIONS & USES Apart from its value as a nourishing vegetable, miner's lettuce, like its relative purslane (*Portulaca oleracea*, p. 253), may be taken as a spring tonic and an effective diuretic.

Morinda officinalis
(Rubiaceae)
BA JI TIAN

DESCRIPTION Deciduous plant with white flowers and a root that yields a yellow dye.

HABITAT & CULTIVATION *Ba ji tian* is native to China. It is cultivated in Guangdong, Guangxi, and Fujian provinces. The root is unearthed in early spring.

PART USED Root.

CONSTITUENTS *Ba ji tian* contains morindin and vitamin C.

HISTORY & FOLKLORE The earliest written record of *ba ji tian's* use is in the *Divine Husbandman's Classic (Shen'nong Bencaojing)* of the 1st century AD.

MEDICINAL ACTIONS & USES The pungent, sweet-tasting *ba ji tian* is an important Chinese herb. It is a kidney tonic, and therefore strengthens the *yang*. It is also used as a sexual tonic, treating impotence and premature ejaculation in men, infertility in both men and women, and a range of other, often hormonally linked conditions, such as an irregular menstrual cycle. *Ba ji tian* is also prescribed for conditions affecting the lower back or pelvic region, including pain, cold, and urinary weakness – especially frequent urination or incontinence.

Morus alba
(Moraceae)
WHITE MULBERRY,
SANG YE (CHINESE)

DESCRIPTION Deciduous tree growing to about 50 ft (15 m). Has toothed leaves, flowers in catkins, and white berries.

HABITAT & CULTIVATION White mulberry is native to China. It is grown worldwide as a garden ornamental. The leaves are gathered in late autumn, the twigs in early summer, and the berries when ripe in summer. The root is dug up in winter.

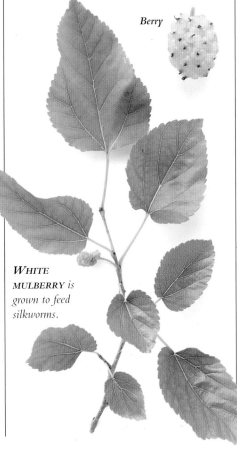

Berry

WHITE MULBERRY is grown to feed silkworms.

PARTS USED Leaves, twigs, fruit, root bark.

CONSTITUENTS The leaves contain flavonoids, anthocyanins, and artocapin. The fruit contains the vitamins A, B_1, B_2, and C.

HISTORY & FOLKLORE White mulberry has been cultivated for over 5,000 years for its leaves (*sang ye*), the preferred food of the silkworm. The silkworm's feces are used in Chinese medicine to treat vomiting.

MEDICINAL ACTIONS & USES White mulberry leaves are expectorant, encouraging the loosening and coughing up of mucus, and are prescribed in China as a treatment for coughs. The leaves are also taken to treat fever, sore and inflamed eyes, sore throats, headaches, dizziness, and vertigo. The fruit juice is cleansing and tonic, and has often been used as a gargle and mouthwash. The root bark may be used for toothache, and it is considered laxative. An extract of the leaves has been given by injection for elephantiasis. The twigs are used to combat excess fluid retention and joint pain. The fruit is taken to prevent premature graying of the hair, and to treat dizziness, ringing in the ears, blurred vision, and insomnia.

RELATED SPECIES The black mulberry (*M. nigra*), native to Iran, is cultivated for its sweet, deep red fruit.

Murraya koenigii
(Rutaceae)
CURRY PATTA

DESCRIPTION Aromatic, deciduous shrub or tree growing to about 20 ft (6 m). Has strongly scented leaves, clusters of small white flowers, and black berries.

HABITAT & CULTIVATION Curry patta is native to subtropical forests in much of southern Asia. It is widely cultivated in India for its leaves.

PARTS USED Leaves, berries.

CONSTITUENTS Curry patta contains a glycoside (koenigin), volatile oil, and tannins.

HISTORY & FOLKLORE Curry patta is a common flavoring in Indian food.

MEDICINAL ACTIONS & USES Curry patta leaves increase digestive secretions and relieve nausea, indigestion, and vomiting. They also treat diarrhea and dysentery. The leaves are considered a hair tonic in India and are thought to prevent graying. They may also be used as a poultice to help heal burns and wounds. Juice from the berries may be mixed with lime juice (*Citrus aurantiifolia*) and applied to soothe insect bites and stings.

RELATED SPECIES The very bitter leaves of cosmetic bark (*M. paniculata*) are taken to treat congestion and to reduce fevers by increasing sweating. In China, they have been used to help speed childbirth.

Musa spp.
(Musaceae)
BANANA, PLANTAIN

DESCRIPTION Evergreen, palmlike perennials growing to 28 ft (9 m). Have large shiny green leaves, hanging flowering stems, and bunches of elongated green fruit that turn yellow on ripening.

HABITAT & CULTIVATION *Musa* species are native to India and Southeast Asia, and are extensively cultivated in tropical and subtropical regions. The fruit is generally picked when immature and then allowed to ripen. The leaves are gathered as required.

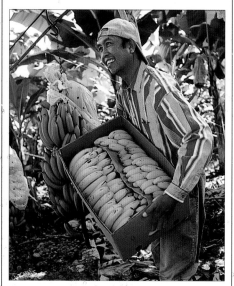

BANANAS are picked before they fully ripen. They are a useful remedy for diarrhea.

PARTS USED Fruit, leaves, root.

HISTORY & FOLKLORE The delicious and highly nutritious banana fruit is the yield of careful horticulture, which had its origins with wild plants in prehistoric times.

MEDICINAL ACTIONS & USES Unripe bananas and plantains are astringent and are used to treat diarrhea. Plantain leaves, dried and made into a syrup, are used widely in Cuba to treat coughs and chest conditions such as bronchitis. The root is strongly astringent and has been given to arrest the coughing up of blood.

Myrica cerifera
(Myricaceae)
BAYBERRY

DESCRIPTION Evergreen shrub or small tree growing to 30 ft (10 m). Has narrow leaves, small yellow flowers in catkins, and gray waxy berries.

HABITAT & CULTIVATION Bayberry is found in coastal regions of the eastern and southern US as far west as Texas. The root bark is collected in autumn or spring.

PART USED Root bark.

CONSTITUENTS Bayberry contains triterpenes (including taraxerol, taraxerone, and myricadiol), flavonoids, tannins, phenols, resins, and gums. Myricadiol has a mild effect on potassium and sodium levels. Myricitrin is antibacterial.

HISTORY & FOLKLORE European settlers in North America believed that bayberry plants had many medicinal benefits. A 1737 account stated that the plants "expel wind and ease all manner of pains proceeding from cold, therefore are good in colic, palsies, convulsions, epilepsies, and many other disorders." The root bark was listed in the *US National Formulary* from 1916 to 1936.

MEDICINAL ACTIONS & USES Bayberry is commonly used to increase circulation, stimulate perspiration, and keep bacterial infections in check. Colds, flu, coughs, and sore throats benefit from treatment with this herb. It helps to strengthen local resistance to infection and to tighten and dry mucous membranes. An infusion is helpful for strengthening spongy gums, and a gargle is used for sore throat. Bayberry's astringency helps intestinal disorders such as irritable bowel syndrome and mucous colitis. An infusion can also help treat excess vaginal discharge. A paste of the powdered root bark may be applied onto ulcers and sores.

CAUTION Do not take during pregnancy.

Myroxylon pereirae syn. *M. balsamum* var. *pereirae*
(Leguminosae)
PERUVIAN BALSAM

DESCRIPTION Evergreen tree growing to 50 ft (15 m). Has gray bark, compound leaves dotted with oil glands, white pealike flowers, and yellow seed pods.

HABITAT & CULTIVATION Native to Central America, Peruvian balsam grows wild in tropical forests. It is cultivated in Central and South America and India. A thick, reddish brown oleo-resin (balsam) exudes from incisions made in the bark.

PART USED Oleo-resin.

CONSTITUENTS The oleo-resin contains 50–65% volatile oil (mainly benzyl benzoate and benzyl cinnamate) and resins.

MEDICINAL ACTIONS & USES Peruvian balsam is strongly antiseptic and stimulates repair of damaged tissue. It is usually taken internally as an expectorant and decongestant to treat emphysema, bronchitis, and bronchial asthma. It may also be taken to treat sore throats and diarrhea. Externally, the balsam is applied to skin afflictions.

RELATED SPECIES The balsam from similar species growing in Peru was used by the Inca to relieve fevers and colds.

CAUTION Peruvian balsam may cause allergic skin reactions.

Myrtus communis
(Myrtaceae)
MYRTLE

DESCRIPTION Evergreen shrub growing to 10 ft (3 m). Has dark green leaves, white flowers, and purple-black berries.

HABITAT & CULTIVATION Myrtle is native to the Mediterranean region and is grown for its essential oil. The leaves are picked in spring.

PARTS USED Leaves, essential oil.

CONSTITUENTS Myrtle contains tannins, flavonoids, and a volatile oil (mainly alpha-pinene, cineole, and myrtenol).

HISTORY & FOLKLORE In ancient Greece, myrtle was dedicated to Aphrodite, the goddess of love, and brides bedecked themselves with myrtle leaves.

MEDICINAL ACTIONS & USES Myrtle leaves are astringent, tonic, and antiseptic. They may be used externally to heal wounds, or internally to remedy digestive and urinary disorders. The essential oil is antiseptic and decongestant, and is used for chest problems such as bronchitis.

CAUTION Do not take the essential oil internally except with professional advice.

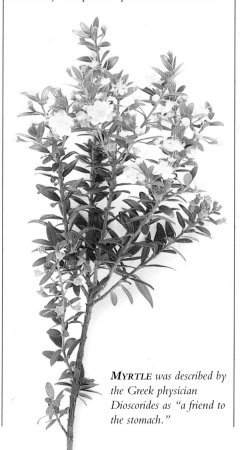

MYRTLE was described by the Greek physician Dioscorides as "a friend to the stomach."

Nasturtium officinale
(Cruciferae)
WATERCRESS

DESCRIPTION Creeping perennial growing to 2 ft (60 cm), with compound leaves, spikes of white 4-petaled flowers, and small sickle-shaped pods.

HABITAT & CULTIVATION Found in temperate regions throughout the world, watercress thrives along or in fresh running water. Although commonly found in the wild, it is also widely cultivated as a salad herb. Watercress is best gathered before it flowers in summer.

PARTS USED Aerial parts.

CONSTITUENTS Watercress contains vitamins A, B$_1$, B$_2$, C, and E, and minerals (especially iodine, iron, and phosphorus).

HISTORY & FOLKLORE Watercress has long been valued as a food and medicinal plant. It is said that the ancient Greeks admonished the witless to "eat cress," since the herb was thought to help remedy disorders of the brain. Xenophon, a Greek general in the 5th century BC, attributed other virtues to it, recommending the Persians to feed it to their children to build up their strength. In European folk medicine, watercress is considered a "blood-cleanser" and was formerly used as a spring tonic.

MEDICINAL ACTIONS & USES Watercress is a valuable source of vitamins and a good detoxifying herb. Its high content of vitamin C and minerals makes it a remedy that is particularly valuable for chronic illnesses. The plant is thought to stimulate the appetite and to relieve indigestion, to help in cases of chronic bronchitis (especially where there is excessive mucus production), to be generally stimulating, and to act as a powerful diuretic.

Nepeta cataria
(Labiatae)
CATNIP

DESCRIPTION Downy, aromatic perennial growing to 3 ft (1 m). Has heart-shaped, gray-green leaves and whorls of white flowers with purple spots.

HABITAT & CULTIVATION Catnip is native to Europe and naturalized in North America. It grows in dry roadside places and in mountainous regions up to altitudes of 5,000 ft (1,500 m). Catnip is gathered when in flower in summer and autumn.

PARTS USED Aerial parts.

CONSTITUENTS Catnip contains iridoids, tannins, and volatile oil (mainly comprising alpha- and beta-nepetalactone, citronellol, and geraniol).

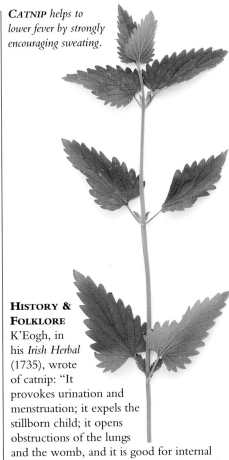

CATNIP helps to lower fever by strongly encouraging sweating.

HISTORY & FOLKLORE K'Eogh, in his *Irish Herbal* (1735), wrote of catnip: "It provokes urination and menstruation; it expels the stillborn child; it opens obstructions of the lungs and the womb, and it is good for internal bruises and shortness of breath. Drunk with salt and honey, it expels worms from the body." Best known for its appeal to felines, catnip can be difficult to grow if there are cats in the neighborhood.

MEDICINAL ACTIONS & USES Catnip is settling to the stomach, sedative, and, since it powerfully stimulates sweating, fever reducing. Its pleasant taste and gentle action make it suitable for colds, flu, and fever in children, especially when it is mixed with elderflower (*Sambucus nigra*, p. 131) and honey. Catnip is markedly antiflatulent, settling indigestion and colic, and is also useful in treating headaches related to digestive problems. A tincture makes a good friction rub for rheumatic and arthritic joints, and, as an ointment, treats hemorrhoids.

SELF-HELP USE Digestive infections, p. 305.

Nicotiana tabacum
(Solanaceae)
TOBACCO

DESCRIPTION Annual or biennial plant growing to a height of 3 ft (1 m). Has an erect stem, large oval leaves, and pink or white flowers.

HABITAT & CULTIVATION Tobacco is native to tropical America and now grown worldwide, chiefly to produce smoking tobacco but also as the source of an insecticide. Leaves for smoking are gathered, dried, and cured.

PARTS USED Leaves.

CONSTITUENTS Tobacco contains alkaloids (notably nicotine) and a volatile oil. Nicotine is stimulant and addictive.

HISTORY & FOLKLORE Even in 17th-century England, opinions on smoking were sharply divided. King James I unsuccessfully tried to ban "a custome loathsome to the eye, hatefull to the nose, harmfull to the braine [and] dangerous to the lungs." In Central America, tobacco was prescribed by the Maya for asthma, convulsions, and skin disease. Tobacco has been used ritually in many Native American cultures.

MEDICINAL ACTIONS & USES Tobacco is no longer used medicinally. The dried leaves make a good insecticide, but external application should be avoided since nicotine is readily absorbed through the skin.

CAUTION Tobacco should not be taken in any form.

Nigella sativa
(Ranunculaceae)
BLACK CUMIN

DESCRIPTION Annual herb growing to 1 ft (30 cm). Has an upright branching stem, fine deeply cut leaves, gray-blue flowers, and toothed seed pods.

HABITAT & CULTIVATION Native to western Asia, black cumin is grown throughout much of Asia and the Mediterranean region for its seeds and as a garden plant. The seeds are gathered once they are ripe.

PARTS USED Seeds.

CONSTITUENTS The seeds contain 40% fixed oil, a saponin (melantin), and up to 1.4% volatile oil.

HISTORY & FOLKLORE Black cumin was found in the tomb of Tutankhamun, but its role in ancient Egypt, medicinal or otherwise, is unknown. Dioscorides, a Greek physician of the 1st century AD, recorded that black cumin seeds were taken to treat headaches, nasal congestion, toothache, and intestinal worms, and, in large quantities, as a diuretic, a promoter of menstruation, and to increase breast-milk production.

MEDICINAL ACTIONS & USES Like many culinary herbs, black cumin seeds benefit the digestive system, soothing stomach pain and and easing gas and colic. The seeds are also antiseptic and are used to treat intestinal worms, especially in children. The seeds are much used in India to increase breast milk.

CAUTION Love-in-a-mist (*N. damascena*) should not be used as a substitute for black cumin seeds.

Notopterygium incisium
(Umbelliferae)
QIANG HUO

DESCRIPTION Carrot-family member with an upright ridged stem, deeply cut leaves, and flowers in dense clusters.

HABITAT & CULTIVATION *Qiang huo* is native to central and western China. The root is unearthed in spring or autumn.

PART USED Root.

CONSTITUENTS *Qiang huo* contains a volatile oil, including angelical.

HISTORY & FOLKLORE *Qiang huo* has been used in China since at least the 2nd century BC, and is listed in the *Divine Husbandman's Classic* (*Shen'nong Bencaojing*, 1st century AD).

MEDICINAL ACTIONS & USES *Qiang huo* is taken mainly for colds and chills, fevers, headaches, general aches and pains, and malaise. The herb is warming and pungent, and promotes sweating. It is also prescribed for neck and back pain.

CAUTION At high dosage *qiang huo* may cause vomiting.

Nymphaea alba
(Nymphaceae)
WHITE WATER LILY

DESCRIPTION Perennial aquatic plant with deep roots, plate-shaped leaves on long cylindrical stems, and large-petaled white flowers occasionally tinged with pink.

HABITAT & CULTIVATION Native to Europe, white water lily is found in ponds and in still water in lakes, rivers, and canals. The rhizome is gathered in autumn.

PARTS USED Rhizome, flowers.

CONSTITUENTS The rhizome contains alkaloids (nymphaeine and nupharine), resin, glycosides, and tannins.

HISTORY & FOLKLORE According to the 17th-century herbalist Nicholas Culpeper, "The leaves do cool all inflammations, and so doth the flowers also, either by the syrup or the conserve: the syrup helpeth much to procure rest, and to settle the brains of frantic persons, by cooling the hot distemperature of the head."

MEDICINAL ACTIONS & USES The rhizome of the white water lily is astringent and antiseptic. A decoction treats dysentery or diarrhea due to irritable bowel syndrome. White water lily has also been employed to treat bronchial congestion and kidney pain, and taken as a gargle for sore throats. The rhizome may be used to make a douche for vaginal soreness and discharge, or to make a poultice – often in combination with slippery elm (*Ulmus rubra*, p. 144) or linseed (*Linum usitatissimum*, p. 226) – for boils and

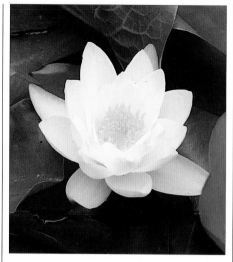

WHITE WATER LILY flowers have a sedative effect, calming nervous tension and anxiety.

abscesses. White water lily flowers have long been reputed to reduce sexual drive. Their generally calming and sedative effect on the nervous system makes them useful in the treatment of insomnia, anxiety, and other disorders where nervous agitation is a factor.

RESEARCH Studies suggest that white water lily may, as has been claimed, diminish sexual drive. The plant has been found to lower blood pressure in animals.

RELATED SPECIES The white pond lily (*N. odorata*) is a close American relative used for much the same purposes. The rhizome of the white lotus (*N. lotus*), native to tropical Africa and Asia, has been used medicinally since the earliest times, and is taken for gastrointestinal problems.

Ocimum basilicum
(Labiatae)
SWEET BASIL, BASIL

DESCRIPTION Strongly aromatic annual growing to 20 in (50 cm). Has shiny oval leaves, a square stem, and small white flowers in whorls.

HABITAT & CULTIVATION Sweet basil, also known as basil, is probably native to India. Over 150 varieties are now grown around the world for their distinctive flavor and essential oil. The leaves and flowering tops are gathered as the plant comes into flower.

PARTS USED Leaves, flowering tops, essential oil.

CONSTITUENTS Sweet basil contains a volatile oil (about 1%), which consists principally of linalool and methyl chavicol, along with small quantities of methyl cinnamate, cineole, and other terpenes.

HISTORY & FOLKLORE In his 1st-century

AD *Materia Medica*, the Greek physician Dioscorides described the African belief that eating sweet basil checks the pain of a scorpion's sting. Ancient Romans used the herb to relieve gas, to counteract poisoning, as a diuretic, and to stimulate breast-milk production. The 17th-century herbalist Nicholas Culpeper again evoked scorpions with his tale of a man who, after smelling basil, grew one of the beasts in his brain.

MEDICINAL ACTIONS & USES Sweet basil acts principally on the digestive and nervous systems, easing flatulence, stomach cramps, colic, and indigestion. It can be used to prevent or relieve nausea and vomiting, and helps to kill intestinal worms. Sweet basil has a mildly sedative action, proving useful in treating nervous irritability, tiredness, depression, anxiety, and insomnia. It may also be taken for epilepsy, migraine, and whooping cough. The herb has been traditionally taken to increase breast-milk production. Applied externally, basil leaves act as an insect repellent. The juice from the leaves brings relief to insect bites. Sweet basil has an established antibacterial action.

RELATED SPECIES See also holy basil (*O. sanctum*, p. 114). Bush basil (*O. basilicum* var. *minimum*) has a much milder action than basil, and is occasionally used to relieve cramps and flatulence.

CAUTION The essential oil should not be taken internally.

SELF-HELP USE Minor bites, stings & swellings, p. 303.

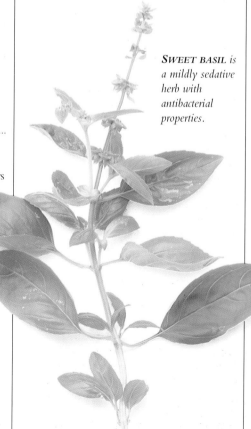

SWEET BASIL is a mildly sedative herb with antibacterial properties.

Oenothera biennis
(Onagraceae)
EVENING PRIMROSE

DESCRIPTION Biennial herb growing to 8 in (20 cm). Has red blotches on stem, crinkled lance-shaped leaves, 4-petaled yellow flowers, and elongated seed capsules.

HABITAT & CULTIVATION Native to North America, evening primrose is now commonly found in many temperate zones around the world. It thrives in open areas, especially in dunes and sandy soil. It is grown commercially for its seed oil.

PARTS USED Leaves, stem bark, flowers, seed oil.

CONSTITUENTS Evening primrose oil is rich in essential fatty acids – cis-linoleic (about 70%) and cis-gammalinolenic acid (about 9%) in particular. Its action mostly depends on the gammalinolenic acid (GLA), a precursor of prostaglandin E_1. The oil is often combined with vitamin E to prevent oxidation.

Evening primrose

MEDICINAL ACTIONS & USES The flowers, leaves, and stem bark of evening primrose have astringent and sedative properties. All three parts have been employed in the treatment of whooping cough. Evening primrose has also been taken for digestive problems and asthma, and used as a poultice to ease the discomfort of rheumatic disorders. The oil, applied externally, is beneficial in the treatment of eczema, certain other itchy skin conditions, and breast tenderness. Taken internally, the oil has an effect in lowering blood pressure and in preventing the clumping of platelets. The oil is now commonly taken for premenstrual problems, including tension and abdominal bloating. Multiple sclerosis may benefit from internal treatment with the oil, as may rheumatoid arthritis, intermittent claudication (a cramplike pain in the leg), and other problems relating to the circulation.

CAUTION Do not take evening primrose oil if suffering from epilepsy.

Olea europaea
(Oleaceae)
OLIVE

DESCRIPTION Evergreen tree growing to 30 ft (10 m). Has a deeply grooved, gray trunk, small leathery leaves, clusters of small greenish white flowers, and a green fruit ripening to black.

HABITAT & CULTIVATION Olive trees grow wild in the Mediterranean region and are cultivated in Mediterranean countries and in regions with a similar climate in the Americas. The leaves may be gathered throughout the year, the fruit in late summer. The leaves of wild trees are believed to contain a higher concentration of active principles.

PARTS USED Leaves, oil.

CONSTITUENTS Olive leaves contain oleoropine, oleasterol, and leine. Olive oil contains about 75% oleic acid, a mono-unsaturated fatty acid.

HISTORY & FOLKLORE The olive was probably first cultivated in Crete in about 3500 BC. The tree has many symbolic associations: the branch is an emblem of peace, and the leaves were worn in a crown by victors in the ancient Olympic games. The leaves have been employed since at least those times as a means to clean wounds. The oil has been used for ritual anointing in some religions.

MEDICINAL ACTIONS & USES Olive leaves lower blood pressure and help to improve the function of the circulatory system. They are also mildly diuretic and may be used to treat conditions such as cystitis. Possessing some ability to lower blood sugar levels, the leaves have been taken for diabetes. The oil is nourishing and improves the balance of fats within the blood. It is traditionally taken with lemon juice in teaspoonful doses to treat gallstones. The oil has a generally protective action on the digestive tract and is useful for dry skin. Externally, it is a good, although sticky, carrier oil for essential oils.

RESEARCH Clinical trials have shown that olive leaves lower blood pressure.

SELF-HELP USES Cradle cap, p. 318; Stretch marks, p. 317.

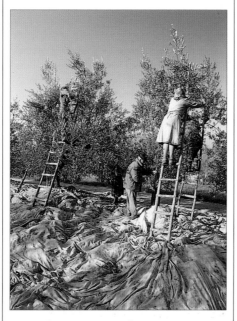

OLIVE *harvesting is carried out in many groves much as it was centuries ago.*

Ononis spinosa
(Leguminosae)
SPINY RESTHARROW

DESCRIPTION Spiny perennial with 3 small leaflets per leaf, bright pink pealike flowers, and small seed pods.

HABITAT & CULTIVATION A relatively common European plant, spiny restharrow thrives in dry grassland and along roadsides.

PART USED Root.

CONSTITUENTS Spiny restharrow root contains phenols, lectins, triterpenoids, and a volatile oil (comprising mainly trans-anethole). The volatile oil is diuretic; the other constituents are antidiuretic. A decoction of the root is antidiuretic, since the volatile oil is lost in the steam during preparation. For a diuretic action, the root is made into an infusion.

HISTORY & FOLKLORE Spiny restharrow's diuretic properties were well known in ancient Greece.

MEDICINAL ACTIONS & USES The root is used as a diuretic and to prevent kidney and bladder stones. It is also of value in treating gout and cystitis. For excess fluid retention, spiny restharrow is best taken as a short-term treatment, in the form of an infusion.

Operculina turpethum
(Convolvulaceae)
TURPETH

DESCRIPTION Twining climber with white tuberous roots, oval leaves, clusters of white funnel-shaped flowers, and round fruit.

HABITAT & CULTIVATION Native to tropical India, turpeth is now found in tropical regions around the world. The root is unearthed throughout the year.

PART USED Root.

CONSTITUENTS Turpeth root contains turpethin resin (approximately 4%) and a volatile oil.

HISTORY & FOLKLORE Turpeth has been used for several thousand years as a purgative in Ayurvedic medicine.

MEDICINAL ACTIONS & USES Turpeth root is chiefly used in small to moderate doses to clear the bowels. Sometimes known as "Indian jalap," it is used in much the same way as this plant (*Ipomoea purga*, p. 222), though its action is less drastic. Turpeth should be taken with care and combined with herbs that ease cramps and flatulence, such as ginger (*Zingiber officinale*, p. 153). In Ayurvedic medicine, turpeth is often prescribed with picrorrhiza (*Picrorrhiza kurroa*, p. 246) to treat jaundice.

CAUTIONS Take only under professional supervision. Do not take during pregnancy.

Opuntia ficus-indica
(Cactaceae)
PRICKLY PEAR

DESCRIPTION Perennial cactus growing to 10 ft (3 m). Has large spatula-shaped stems covered in clusters of spines, brilliant yellow flowers, and roundish purple fruit.

HABITAT & CULTIVATION Prickly pear is native to Mexico and naturalized in semi-tropical regions around the world. The fruit is harvested when ripe; the stems when required.

PARTS USED Flowers, fruit, stems.

CONSTITUENTS The fruit of prickly pear contains mucilage, sugars, vitamin C, and other fruit acids. The flowers contain a flavonoid.

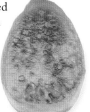

Prickly pear fruit

HISTORY & FOLKLORE Prickly pear fruit is used to make conserves and an alcoholic drink in Mexico. The split stems have been bound around injured limbs as a first-aid measure.

MEDICINAL ACTIONS & USES Prickly pear flowers are astringent and reduce bleeding, and are used for problems affecting the gastrointestinal tract – particularly diarrhea, colitis, and irritable bowel syndrome. They are also taken to treat an enlarged prostate gland. The fruit is nutritious.

Orchis mascula
(Orchidaceae)
PURPLE ORCHID, SALEP

DESCRIPTION Perennial herb growing to 2 ft (60 cm). Narrow leaves often have purple-black blotches. Flowering stem bears purple or purple-pink flowers. It has two tuberous roots, one larger than the other.

HABITAT & CULTIVATION Purple orchid is native to Europe, the Middle East, and North Africa. It is commonly found in clearings in woodland, scrubland, and grassland. Salep – the tuber of purple orchid and other orchid species – is gathered and dried in autumn.

PART USED Tuber.

CONSTITUENTS Purple orchid contains about 48% mucilage.

HISTORY & FOLKLORE Various species of orchid have been used medicinally since antiquity. Purple orchid was mentioned by the physician Dioscorides in the 1st century AD. Its two tuberous roots have been eaten as a vegetable. Folk wisdom maintained that a pregnant woman eating the larger of the two tubers would give birth to a boy. In Thessaly in Greece, women ate the tubers to increase their sexual appetite.

MEDICINAL ACTIONS & USES Once believed to have aphrodisiac powers, purple orchid is now seen as a nourishing vegetable somewhat similar to the potato (*Solanum tuberosum*, p. 269). Its current medicinal use is generally confined to the treatment of diarrhea and irritated gastrointestinal tracts in children.

Origanum majorana
syn. *Majorana hortensis*
(Labiatae)
SWEET MARJORAM

DESCRIPTION Woody perennial herb growing to 20 in (50 cm). Has aromatic oval leaves and pinkish white flowers emerging from the upper leaf axils.

HABITAT & CULTIVATION Sweet marjoram is native to countries bordering the Mediterranean. It is much cultivated as a culinary herb and for its essential oil.

PARTS USED Aerial parts, essential oil.

CONSTITUENTS Sweet marjoram contains about 3% volatile oil (comprising sabinene hydrate, sabinene, linalool, carvacrol, and other terpenes), flavonoids, caffeic and rosmarinic acid, and triterpenoids.

HISTORY & FOLKLORE In 1597, the herbalist John Gerard made this assessment: "Sweet marjoram is a remedy against cold diseases of the braine and head, being taken anyway to your best liking; put up into the nostrils it provokes sneesing, and draweth forth much baggage flegme; it easeth the toothache being chewed in the mouth."

MEDICINAL ACTIONS & USES While used mainly as a culinary herb, sweet marjoram is also medicinally valuable due to its stimulant and antispasmodic properties. Like oregano (*O. vulgare, see following entry*), it treats flatulence, colic, and respiratory problems. Sweet marjoram appears to have a stronger effect on the nervous system than its cousin oregano. Sweet marjoram is a good general tonic, helping to relieve anxiety, headaches, and insomnia. The herb is also thought to lower sexual drive.

CAUTIONS Do not take as a medicine during pregnancy. Do not take essential oil internally.

Origanum vulgare
(Labiatae)
OREGANO

DESCRIPTION Upright perennial herb growing to about 32 in (80 cm). Has square red stems, elliptical leaves, and clusters of deep pink flowers.

HABITAT & CULTIVATION Oregano is native to Europe and naturalized in the Middle East. The plant thrives in chalky soils close to the sea. It is gathered when in flower in summer.

PARTS USED Aerial parts, essential oil.

CONSTITUENTS Oregano contains a volatile oil (comprising carvacrol, thymol, beta-bisabolene, caryophyllene, linalool, and borneol), tannins, resin, sterols, and flavonoids. Both carvacrol and thymol are antibacterial and antifungal.

HISTORY & FOLKLORE Much used by the ancient Greeks, oregano has had a more significant role in medicine than sweet marjoram (*O. majorana, see preceding entry*). The 18th-century herbalist K'Eogh described oregano as having "a hot dry nature. It is good against pains of the stomach and heart and also useful for coughs, pleurisy and obstructions of the lungs and womb, and it also comforts the head and nerves."

MEDICINAL ACTIONS & USES Oregano helps to settle flatulence and stimulates the flow of bile. Strongly antiseptic, oregano may be taken to treat respiratory conditions such as coughs, tonsillitis, bronchitis, and asthma. It is also considered to be a useful promoter of menstruation. The diluted oil can be applied externally to toothache or painful joints.

CAUTIONS Do not take as a medicine during pregnancy. External use may cause irritation of the skin. Do not take essential oil internally.

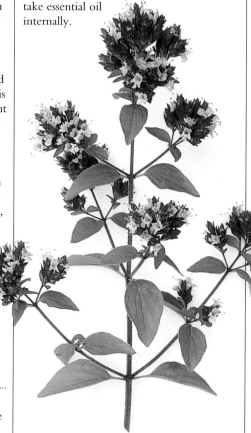

OREGANO'S essential oil, well diluted, is a traditional remedy for toothache.

Orthosiphon aristata
(Labiatae)
JAVA TEA

DESCRIPTION Shrub growing to about 3 ft (1 m). Has pointed leaves and lilac-colored flowers with very long stamens.

HABITAT & CULTIVATION Java tea is native to Southeast Asia and Australia. Now cultivated as a medicinal plant, it is picked as required throughout the year.

PARTS USED Leaves.

CONSTITUENTS Java tea contains flavones (including sinensetin), a glycoside (orthosiphonin), a volatile oil, and large amounts of potassium.

HISTORY & FOLKLORE The plant's Dutch Indonesian name, *koemis koetjing* (cat's whiskers), probably derives from its long whiskery stamens.

MEDICINAL ACTIONS & USES Java tea is listed in the French, Indonesian, Dutch, and Swiss pharmacopoeias. The herb is thought to increase the kidneys' ability to eliminate nitrogen-containing compounds. It is often used as a diuretic and as a treatment for kidney infections, stones, and poor renal function resulting from chronic nephritis. It is also used to treat cystitis and urethritis.

RELATED SPECIES *O. stamineus*, also from Java, is a very similar species.

Paeonia officinalis
(Paeoniaceae)
PEONY

DESCRIPTION Perennial growing to 2 ft (60 cm). Has a tuberous root, upright stems, oval to lance-shaped leaflets, and attractive large red, red-purple, or white flowers.

HABITAT & CULTIVATION Peony is native to southern Europe and the Mediterranean region. It is found in mountain woodlands and is widely cultivated as a garden plant. The root is unearthed in autumn.

PART USED Root.

CONSTITUENTS Peony is thought to contain paeonine, a volatile oil, tannins, and resin.

HISTORY & FOLKLORE Since the time of Hippocrates (470–377 BC), peony has been used to treat epilepsy. Ibn el Beitar, a medieval Arab physician, recommended a necklace of peony seeds to ward off epilepsy in children. The Greek physician Dioscorides (AD 40–90) wrote that the root provokes menstruation and may be used to expel the placenta after childbirth. Mrs. Grieve, the author of *A Modern Herbal* (1931), recounted how "in ancient times, peony was thought to be of divine origin, an emanation from the moon, and to shine during the night protecting the shepherds and their flocks."

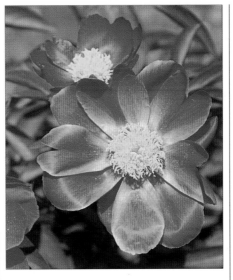

PEONY is named after Paeon, the physician of the Greek gods.

MEDICINAL ACTIONS & USES While it is rarely used in contemporary European herbal medicine, peony is thought to be antispasmodic and sedative. The root may be employed to treat whooping cough and nervous irritation, and suppositories are sometimes made of the root to relieve anal and intestinal spasms.

RELATED SPECIES Chinese peony (*Paeonia lactiflora*, p. 115) is often used in Chinese herbal medicine.

CAUTIONS Take peony only under professional supervision. Do not take during pregnancy.

Panax notoginseng
(Araliaceae)
SAN QI

DESCRIPTION Deciduous perennial with an erect stem growing to 3 ft (1 m), compound leaves, small greenish flowers, and small berrylike fruit.

HABITAT & CULTIVATION Native to China, *san qi* is now rare in the wild. It is cultivated commercially in southern and central China. The root is unearthed before flowering or after the fruit has ripened.

PART USED Root.

CONSTITUENTS *San qi* contains steroidal saponins (including arasaponin A and arasaponin B) and a flavonoid (dencichine).

HISTORY & FOLKLORE Despite its importance as a tonic, *san qi* was only recorded in Chinese herbal medicine in 1578, in the *Compendium of Materia Medica* by Li Shizen. He described the root as being "more valuable than gold."

MEDICINAL ACTIONS & USES Like ginseng (*P. ginseng*, p. 116), *san qi* is a tonic that supports the function of the adrenal glands, in particular the production of corticosteroids and male sex hormones. *San qi* also helps to improve blood flow through the coronary arteries, thus finding use as a treatment for arteriosclerosis, high blood pressure, and angina. *San qi* treats internal bleeding of almost any kind. It may also be applied externally as a poultice to help heal wounds and bruises.

RESEARCH Studies have confirmed *San qi's* longstanding reputation as a means to stop bleeding. A Chinese trial indicated that the herb hastens blood clotting. Another clinical trial, again in China, associated the herb with positive improvements in the coronary circulation, in lessening the symptoms of angina, and in the reduction of blood pressure levels.

CAUTION Do not take during pregnancy.

Panax quinquefolium
(Araliaceae)
AMERICAN GINSENG

DESCRIPTION Deciduous perennial growing to about 1 ft (30 cm). Has a smooth stem, leaves with oblong to oval leaflets, small greenish flowers, and kidney-shaped scarlet berries.

HABITAT & CULTIVATION American ginseng is native to North America and the Himalayas. A woodland plant, it is rarely seen in the wild due to overharvesting. It is cultivated in Wisconsin, and in China and France. The root is gathered in autumn.

PART USED Root.

CONSTITUENTS American ginseng contains steroidal saponins, including panaquilon.

HISTORY & FOLKLORE Native American people may have considered this herb a means to increase female fertility. From the mid-18th century, the collection of the herb for export to China became a virtual goldrush, with so many Native Americans out collecting the herb that settlers reported finding villages almost deserted. The Ojibwa people always planted a seed to replace the herb, but this was not universal practice. American ginseng became rare toward the end of the 19th century.

MEDICINAL ACTIONS & USES The action of this herb is presumed to be similar to, but milder than, that of its Chinese cousin, *P. ginseng* (p. 116). American ginseng increases tolerance to stress of all kinds. In traditional Chinese medicine, the herb is employed as a *yin* tonic, treating weakness, fever, wheezing, and coughs.

RELATED SPECIES See ginseng (*P. ginseng*, p. 116), san qi (*P. notoginseng*, preceding entry), and Siberian ginseng (*Eleutherococcus senticosus*, p. 92).

CAUTION Do not take during pregnancy.

Papaver rhoeas
(Papaveraceae)

CORN POPPY

DESCRIPTION Delicate hairy-stemmed annual growing to 3 ft (90 cm). Has lance-shaped basal leaves, deeply incised stem leaves, red 4-petaled flowers with black anthers, and small rounded seed capsules.

HABITAT & CULTIVATION Corn poppy is native to Europe, North Africa, and temperate regions of Asia, and is naturalized in North and South America. It thrives on cultivated land and along roadsides. The flowers are picked in summer.

PARTS USED Flowers.

CONSTITUENTS Corn poppy contains alkaloids (including papaverine, rhoeadine, isorhoeadine, and many others), meconic acid, mekocyanin, mucilage, and tannin. The alkaloids are similar to those in the opium poppy (*P. somniferum, following entry*), but are much milder.

HISTORY & FOLKLORE The Irish herbalist K'Eogh stated in 1735 that this poppy "has a cooling and refreshing nature. By drinking a decoction of five or six heads in wine, pain is alleviated and sleep is induced … the bruised leaves of the green heads can be applied to boils, hot ulcers, and burning fevers." The herb was listed in the *British Pharmacopoeia Codex* (1949).

MEDICINAL ACTIONS & USES Corn poppy flowers are mildly analgesic and sedative, and have long been used in European herbal medicine, particularly for ailments in children and the elderly. Used chiefly as a mild pain reliever and as a treatment for irritable coughs, corn poppy also reduces nervous overactivity. The herb may also be used for insomnia, nervous irritability, coughs – especially paroxysmal coughs – and asthma, and is usually given as a syrup.

RELATED SPECIES See also opium poppy (*P. somniferum, following entry*), Mexican poppy (*Argemone mexicana*, p. 169), California poppy (*Eschscholzia californica*, p. 205), and greater celandine (*Chelidonium majus*, p. 185).

CAUTIONS Use only under professional supervision. All parts of this species except the seeds are potentially toxic if eaten.

Papaver somniferum
(Papaveraceae)

OPIUM POPPY

DESCRIPTION Thick-stemmed annual growing to about 3 ft (1 m). Has numerous, broadly oval, dull green leaves, delicate, solitary, pink to purple or white flowers, and globe-shaped seed capsules.

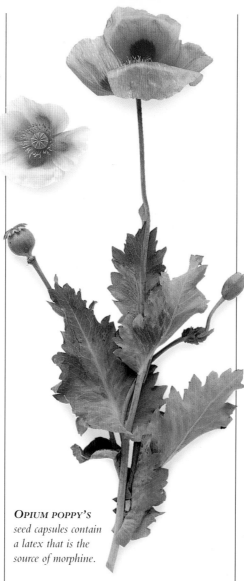

OPIUM POPPY'S seed capsules contain a latex that is the source of morphine.

HABITAT & CULTIVATION Native to western Asia, opium poppy is now cultivated commercially around the world as the source of morphine and codeine, and as an illegal crop for the production of opium and heroin. During the summer, the seed capsules are cut, and the white latex that exudes is gathered the next day and dried.

PART USED Latex.

CONSTITUENTS Opium poppy contains over 40 opium alkaloids, including morphine (up to 20%), narcotine (about 5%), codeine (about 1%), and papaverine (about 1%). It also contains meconic acid, albumin, mucilage, sugars, resin, and wax. Many of the opium poppy's alkaloids have a well-established therapeutic action. Morphine is one of the most powerful analgesics of all, used extensively in conventional medicine to relieve pain, especially in terminal illness. Codeine is a milder analgesic used for headaches and other pain, and in the symptomatic treatment of diarrhea. Opium's strongly addictive nature is well established.

HISTORY & FOLKLORE Cultivated for its medicinal properties for at least 4,000 years, the opium poppy was introduced to Greece about 3,000 years ago, and from there spread throughout Europe. It was unknown in China until the 7th century AD, and in Japan until the 15th century. It is mentioned in the Assyrian herbals (*c.* 1700 BC), and the Greek physician Dioscorides (AD 40–90) wrote that "a decoction of the leaves and flowerheads if drunk and bathed on the head is unrivalled in inducing sleep. The mashed heads, mixed with flour, make a useful plaster for treating inflammations and St. Anthony's fire [erysipelas, a bacterial infection of the skin]."

MEDICINAL ACTIONS & USES Opium (the dried latex) is a potent narcotic, analgesic, and antispasmodic, and has been taken to relieve pain of all kinds. In all the main herbal traditions it is regarded as a powerful "cold" remedy, reducing physical function and sedating or suppressing nervous activity, pain, and coughs. In view of its addictive nature, opium is mainly used after other less powerful analgesics have failed to bring relief. It is also a remedy for acute diarrhea and severe coughs.

RESEARCH Much research into opium poppy has been done, confirming most of the uses listed above.

RELATED SPECIES See also corn poppy (*P. rhoeas, preceding entry*), Mexican poppy (*Argemone mexicana*, p. 169), California poppy (*Eschscholzia californica*, p. 205), and greater celandine (*Chelidonium majus*, p. 185).

CAUTIONS Use opium poppy only under professional supervision. It is subject to legal restrictions in most countries.

Parietaria judaica
syn. *P. diffusa*
(Urticaceae)

PELLITORY-OF-THE-WALL

DESCRIPTION Annual growing to 28 in (70 cm). Has deep green leaves, greenish flowers, and small dark seeds.

HABITAT & CULTIVATION Native to Europe, this plant is commonplace in southern countries, where it is found on walls and in dry stony sites. It is gathered in summer when in flower.

PARTS USED Aerial parts.

CONSTITUENTS & ACTIONS Pellitory-of-the-wall contains flavonoids and tannins.

HISTORY & FOLKLORE For more than 2,000 years, pellitory-of-the-wall has been valued as a diuretic, a soother of chronic coughs, and a balm for wounds and burns.

MEDICINAL ACTIONS & USES Pellitory-of-the-wall is chiefly employed as a diuretic, demulcent, and stone-preventing herb. In European herbal medicine, it is regarded as having a restorative action on the kidneys, supporting and strengthening their function. It has been prescribed for nephritis, pyelitis (inflammation of the kidney), kidney stones, renal colic (pain caused by kidney stones), cystitis, and edema (fluid retention). It is also occasionally taken as a laxative.

CAUTION Do not take pellitory-of-the-wall if suffering from hay fever or other allergies.

Paullinia cupana
syn. *P. sorbilis*
(Sapindaceae)
GUARANA

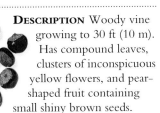
Seeds

DESCRIPTION Woody vine growing to 30 ft (10 m). Has compound leaves, clusters of inconspicuous yellow flowers, and pear-shaped fruit containing small shiny brown seeds.

HABITAT & CULTIVATION Guarana is native to tropical forests of the Brazilian Amazon and is also cultivated in Brazil. The seeds are gathered when ripe.

PARTS USED Seeds.

CONSTITUENTS Guarana contains xanthine derivatives (including up to 7% caffeine, together with theobromine and theophylline), tannins, and saponins. The xanthines are stimulant, diuretic, and reduce fatigue over the short term.

HISTORY & FOLKLORE In Brazil, guarana is traditionally prepared by roasting, crushing, and drying the seeds. The resulting "cakes" are made into a tea, taken to counter fatigue or to treat diarrhea. Guarana has recently become a popular alternative to coffee.

MEDICINAL ACTIONS & USES Guarana's medicinal uses are largely the same as those of coffee (*Coffea arabica*, p.190) – it is taken for headache and migraine, for mild depressive states, and to boost energy levels. The problems that apply to long-term or excessive coffee consumption also apply to guarana – both stimulate over the short term but tend to inhibit the body's natural restorative processes over the longer term. In view of guarana's significant tannin content, long-term use is even less advisable, because tannins impair the intestines' ability to absorb nutrients. Nevertheless, guarana is a useful short-term remedy for boosting energy levels or for a tension headache that cannot be treated with rest. Guarana's astringency also treats chronic diarrhea.

RELATED SPECIES *P. yoco*, native to the Colombian Amazon, is used by indigenous peoples to reduce fevers, as a stimulant, and as a postmalarial treatment.

CAUTION Do not take if suffering from cardiovascular disease or high blood pressure.

Pausinystalia yohimbe
syn. *Corynanthe yohimbe*
(Rubiaceae)
YOHIMBE

DESCRIPTION Evergreen tree growing to 100 ft (30 m). Has reddish brown bark, oblong or elliptical leaves, and clusters of small yellow flowers.

HABITAT & CULTIVATION Yohimbe is native to the forests of western Africa, especially Cameroon, Zaire, and Gabon. The bark is gathered at any time of year.

PART USED Bark.

CONSTITUENTS Yohimbe contains about 6% indole alkaloids (including yohimbine), pigments, and tannins. The alkaloids have a cerebral stimulant action at moderate doses but are highly toxic in large doses. Yohimbine has been used in conventional medicine to treat impotence.

HISTORY & FOLKLORE Yohimbe has an ancient reputation in western Africa, especially among the Bantu people, as a male aphrodisiac and mild hallucinogen.

MEDICINAL ACTIONS & USES Yohimbe is not used much in herbal medicine because of its potential toxicity. In western Africa, it is often employed as a stimulant and as a means to counter impotence.

CAUTIONS Take only under professional supervision. The herb is subject to legal restrictions in many countries.

Peganum harmala
(Zygophyllaceae)
HARMALA, AFRICAN RUE

DESCRIPTION Multibranched, shrubby perennial growing to 20 in (50 cm). Has deeply cleft linear leaves, white 5-petaled flowers, and rounded 3-celled seed capsules.

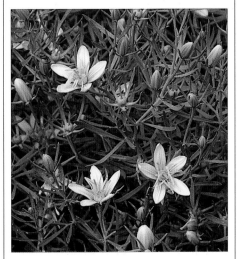

HARMALA, *which thrives in dry conditions, has been used as an intoxicant in the Middle East.*

HABITAT & CULTIVATION Native to the Middle East, North Africa, and southern Europe, harmala is naturalized in other subtropical regions, including Australia. It thrives in saline soil in semidesert areas. The seeds are gathered in summer.

PARTS USED Seeds, root.

CONSTITUENTS Harmala contains up to 4% indole alkaloids (including harmine, harmaline, and harmalol) which are similar in action to the alkaloids found in ayahuasca (*Banisteriopsis caapi*, p. 174), yohimbe (*Pausinystalia yohimbe*, preceding entry), and passion flower (*Passiflora incarnata*, p. 117). Harmine has been used to help alleviate the tremors of Parkinsonism.

HISTORY & FOLKLORE Since the earliest times, harmala has been used in the Middle East as a means to induce intoxication. Known to the Greek physician Dioscorides (AD 40–90), Galen (AD 131–200), and Avicenna (AD 980–1037), harmala was also used to expel intestinal worms and to promote the onset of menstrual flow.

MEDICINAL ACTIONS & USES Despite its long history as a euphoric and purported aphrodisiac, harmala is rarely used in contemporary herbal medicine due to its potential toxicity. The seeds have been taken to treat eye disorders and to stimulate breast-milk production. In central Asia, harmala root is a popular medicinal remedy, used in the treatment of rheumatism and nervous conditions.

CAUTION This plant is toxic and should not be used under any circumstances.

Pergularia extensa
(Asclepiadaceae)
PERGULARIA

DESCRIPTION Perennial climber with broad oval leaves and small greenish white flowers.

HABITAT & CULTIVATION Pergularia is native to India. Its aerial parts are gathered throughout the year.

PARTS USED Aerial parts.

CONSTITUENTS Pergularia contains a resin, bitter principles, and plant sterols.

MEDICINAL ACTIONS & USES Pergularia is thought to have bitter, expectorant, diuretic, and laxative properties, and is employed in several ways in Indian herbal medicine. It is prescribed as a treatment for bronchitis and asthma, and as a means to curtail heavy menstrual or nonmenstrual uterine bleeding. Juice from the leaves may be applied to relieve the pain and swelling of cysts and rheumatic joints. The juice may also be taken internally for rheumatism, generally in combination with ginger (*Zingiber officinale*, p. 153).

Petasites hybridus
(Compositae)
BUTTERBUR

DESCRIPTION Downy perennial growing to 3 ft (1 m). Has very large heart-shaped leaves, and lilac-pink flowers growing in large spikes.

HABITAT & CULTIVATION Butterbur flourishes throughout Europe. It prefers damp or moist sites, along roadsides and the banks of streams. The aerial parts are gathered in summer; the root, in spring or autumn.

PARTS USED Aerial parts, root.

CONSTITUENTS Butterbur contains pyrrolizidine alkaloids (notably senecione), sesquiterpene lactones, a volatile oil, pectin, mucilage, and inulin (in the root). In isolation, pyrrolizidine alkaloids are toxic to the liver.

HISTORY & FOLKLORE The genus name *Petasites* comes from the Latin *petasus* – a hat worn by travelers (butterbur's leaves were used for this purpose by country folk). Nicholas Culpeper wrote in his *English Physitian* (1652) that butterbur root was "very available against the plague, and pestilential fevers, by provoking sweat."

MEDICINAL ACTIONS & USES Butterbur has tonic and expectorant properties, and is antispasmodic and analgesic, acting specifically on the stomach, bile ducts, and duodenum. It has been used mainly to treat chest problems such as bronchitis, asthma,

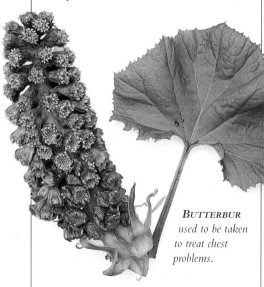

BUTTERBUR used to be taken to treat chest problems.

and whooping cough. Butterbur helps to strengthen digestion, in particular where indigestion results from obstructed bile flow. This herb has also been given for inflammation of the urinary tract, and it has been used externally as a poultice to treat wounds and skin eruptions.

CAUTIONS In view of its toxic alkaloid content, do not take butterbur internally. The use of alternative herbs is advised.

Petroselinum crispum
(Umbelliferae)
PARSLEY

DESCRIPTION Annual herb growing to 1 ft (30 cm). Has an erect stem, bright green compound smooth or crinkled leaves, umbels of small white flowers, and tiny ribbed seeds.

HABITAT & CULTIVATION Parsley is native to Europe and the eastern Mediterranean. Today it is rarely found in the wild, but is cultivated throughout the world as a nutritious salad herb. The leaves may be picked from spring to autumn, and the seeds are gathered when just ripe.

PARTS USED Leaves, root, seeds.

CONSTITUENTS Parsley contains a volatile oil (including about 20% myristicin, about 18% apiole, and many other terpenes), flavonoids, phthalides, coumarins (including bergapten), vitamins A, C, and E, and high levels of iron. The flavonoids are anti-inflammatory and antioxidant. Myristicin and apiole have diuretic properties. The volatile oil relieves cramps and flatulence, and is a strong uterine stimulant.

HISTORY & FOLKLORE Parsley was known in ancient Greece and Rome – but more as a diuretic, digestive tonic and stimulant of menstrual flow than as a salad herb. In Rome, parsley was associated with the goddess Persephone, queen of the underworld, and was used in funeral ceremonies. Parsley was introduced into Britain in 1548. Parsley has the unusual ability of masking strong odors, that of garlic in particular (which is one reason for the herb's popularity as a garnish in cooking).

MEDICINAL ACTIONS & USES The fresh leaves are highly nutritious and can be considered a natural vitamin and mineral supplement in their own right. The seeds have a much stronger diuretic action than the leaves, and may be substituted for celery seeds (*Apium graveolens*, p. 61) in the treatment of gout, rheumatism, and arthritis. Both plants act by encouraging the flushing out of waste products from the inflamed joints and the waste's subsequent elimination via the kidneys. Parsley root is more commonly prescribed than the seeds or leaves in herbal medicine. It is taken as a treatment for flatulence, cystitis, and rheumatic conditions. Parsley is also valued as a promoter of menstruation, being helpful both in stimulating a delayed period and in relieving menstrual pain.

CAUTIONS Parsley is a safe herb at normal dosage and consumption levels, but excessive quantities of the seeds are toxic. Do not take the seeds during pregnancy or if suffering from kidney disease.

Peumus boldus
(Umbelliferae)
BOLDO

DESCRIPTION Strongly aromatic multibranched evergreen shrub or tree growing to 20 ft (6 m). Has egg-shaped leathery leaves with a lemony scent, clusters of white or yellow bell-shaped flowers, and small yellow berries.

Dried leaves

HABITAT & CULTIVATION Boldo is native to Chile and Peru, and naturalized in the Mediterranean region and the west coast of North America. It grows on dry sunny slopes and in mountain pastures in the Andes, where it is much cultivated. The leaves are gathered throughout the year.

PARTS USED Leaves.

CONSTITUENTS Boldo contains 0.7% isoquinoline alkaloids (including boldine), as well as a volatile oil and flavonoids.

HISTORY & FOLKLORE Boldo is a traditional remedy used by the Araucanian people in Chile as a tonic. The berries were also eaten as a food.

MEDICINAL ACTIONS & USES Boldo stimulates liver activity and bile flow and is chiefly valued as a remedy for gallstones and liver or gallbladder pain. It is normally taken for a few weeks at a time, either as a tincture or infusion. Boldo is also a mild urinary antiseptic and demulcent, and may be taken for infections such as cystitis. In the Anglo-American tradition, boldo is combined with barberry (*Berberis vulgaris*, p. 175) and fringe tree (*Chionanthus virginicus*, p. 186) in the treatment of gallstones.

CAUTIONS Do not take this herb during pregnancy. Boldo is subject to legal restrictions in some countries.

Phaseolus vulgaris
(Leguminosae)
FRENCH BEAN, HARICOT BEAN

DESCRIPTION Slender-stemmed, annual climber growing to 12 ft (4 m). Has pointed oval leaflets, curly tendrils, clusters of white or lilac flowers, and a bean pod containing kidney-shaped seeds.

HABITAT & CULTIVATION French bean is thought to originate from South America. Varieties are cultivated all over the world. The ripe beans are gathered in summer.

PARTS USED Bean pods, beans.

CONSTITUENTS French beans contain allantoin, sugars, leucine, tyrosine, arginine, and inositol.

HISTORY & FOLKLORE French beans have

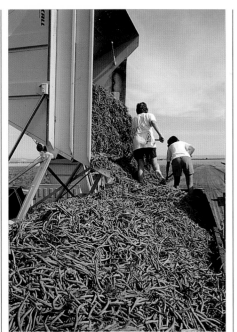

FRENCH BEANS are intensively cultivated all over the world.

been used since ancient times in the treatment of diabetes. In her book *A Modern Herbal* (1931), Mrs. Grieve recorded that "because of the seed's close resemblance to a male testicle … [ancient Egyptians] made it an object of sacred worship and forbade its use as a food."

MEDICINAL ACTIONS & USES As well as being an important food in many parts of the world, French beans have two main medicinal uses. The pods are a medium-strength diuretic, stimulating urine flow and the flushing of toxins from the body. Powdered or infused, they are also hypoglycemic, reducing blood glucose levels in the treatment of diabetes. Powdered beans may be dusted on areas of weeping eczema to relieve itching and help dry the skin.

Phellodendron amurense
(Rutaceae)
HUANG BAI

DESCRIPTION Deciduous tree growing to 40 ft (12 m). Has compound leaves with 7 lance-shaped leaflets, clusters of green flowers, and round berries.

HABITAT & CULTIVATION *Huang bai* is native to China, Japan, and Korea, and is cultivated in northeastern China. The bark of 10-year-old trees is collected in spring.

PART USED Bark.

CONSTITUENTS *Huang bai* contains isoquinoline alkaloids (including berberine), sesquiterpene lactones, and plant sterols. Due to its alkaloid content, *huang bai* is antimicrobial and antibiotic.

HISTORY & FOLKLORE Listed in the *Divine Husbandman's Classic (Shen'nong Bencaojing)*, of the 1st century AD, *huang bai* was regarded as an herb to be used with care.

MEDICINAL ACTIONS & USES A strongly bitter remedy, *huang bai* is used within Chinese herbal medicine to "drain damp heat." It is prescribed for conditions such as acute diarrhea and dysentery, jaundice, vaginal infection (including trichomonas), and certain skin conditions. It is also given for urinary system disorders such as frequent urination, pain, and infection.

RESEARCH Clinical trials in China indicate that the bark is useful in the treatment of meningitis and conjunctivitis.

RELATED SPECIES *P. chinense*, also native to China, is used in a similar manner.

CAUTIONS Take *huang bai* only under professional supervision. Do not take *huang bai* during pregnancy.

Physalis alkekengi
syn. *P. franchetti*
(Solanaceae)
WINTER CHERRY,
CAPE GOOSEBERRY

DESCRIPTION Perennial herb growing to 32 in (80 cm). Has oval- to diamond-shaped leaves, long-stemmed white flowers, and a papery sheath surrounding an orange-red fruit.

HABITAT & CULTIVATION Winter cherry is native to central and southern Europe and China. It grows wild along damp roadsides. It is widely cultivated in warm temperate and subtropical regions, including North and South America and South Africa. The fruit is gathered once it has ripened in summer.

PARTS USED Fruit.

CONSTITUENTS Winter cherry contains flavonoids, plant sterols, vitamins A (carotene) and C, and, in the roots, tropane-type alkaloids.

HISTORY & FOLKLORE The Greek physician Dioscorides (1st century AD) considered winter cherry to be beneficial as a diuretic and a treatment for jaundice. In Spain, a therapeutic wine made with the fruit was taken to treat excess fluid retention and problems of the bladder and urinary tubules.

MEDICINAL ACTIONS & USES Though commonly eaten as a fruit, winter cherry is also a useful diuretic, and helpful in a variety of urinary and arthritic problems. The fruit is traditionally used within European herbal medicine to treat kidney and bladder stones, fluid retention, and gout. It has also been taken to reduce fever.

CAUTION The foliage and unripe fruit are harmful if eaten.

Phytolacca decandra
(Phytolaccaceae)
POKEWEED

DESCRIPTION Herbaceous perennial growing to 10 ft (3 m). Has alternate lance-shaped leaves, greenish white flowers growing in spikes, and clusters of fleshy, deep purple berries.

HABITAT & CULTIVATION Native to North America, pokeweed is now naturalized in the Mediterranean region. It thrives in damp woodland and in open areas. The root is unearthed in late autumn.

PART USED Root.

CONSTITUENTS Pokeweed contains triterpenoid saponins, lectins, proteins, resin, and mucilage. The triterpenoid saponins are strongly anti-inflammatory, the proteins antiviral, and the lectins mitogenic (break up chromosomes).

HISTORY & FOLKLORE Pokeweed was widely used by Native Americans and European settlers as a poultice for skin diseases, sores, ulcers, and tumors. It was also given internally to relieve pain and to induce vomiting. The berries yield a strong red dye, which in the past was added to confectionery and alcoholic drinks – including port wine.

MEDICINAL ACTIONS & USES Pokeweed is taken internally as a tincture in small amounts to treat rheumatic and arthritic conditions. The root has also been used to treat respiratory tract infections, such as sore throats and tonsillitis, as well as swollen glands and chronic infections. The herb is sometimes prescribed for pain and infection of the ovaries or testes, and as a lymphatic "decongestant," stimulating the clearance of waste products. As a poultice or ointment, it is applied to sore and infected nipples and breasts, acne, folliculitis, fungal infections, and scabies.

CAUTIONS The plant is highly toxic in overdose. Use only under professional supervision. Do not take during pregnancy.

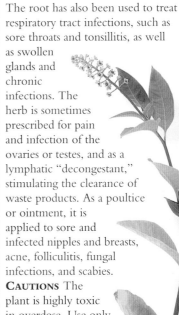

POKEWEED contains proteins that act against viral infection.

OTHER MEDICINAL PLANTS

Picrasma excelsa
syn. *Picraenia excelsa*
(Simaroubaceae)

QUASSIA

DESCRIPTION Deciduous tree growing to 100 ft (30 m). Has smooth gray bark, compound leaves, small yellow flowers, and pea-sized black fruit.

HABITAT & CULTIVATION Native to tropical America and the Caribbean, quassia grows in forests and near water. It is cultivated mainly for medicinal use. The bark is harvested throughout the year.

PART USED Bark.

CONSTITUENTS Quassia contains quassinoid bitter principles (including quassin), alkaloids, a coumarin (scopoletin), and vitamin B_1. Some of the quassinoids have cytotoxic (cell-killing) and antileukemic actions.

HISTORY & FOLKLORE Quassia bark was first introduced into Europe from Surinam in 1756. The herb is named after Quassi, a native healer, who told Europeans of its therapeutic value.

MEDICINAL ACTIONS & USES The strongly bitter quassia supports and strengthens weak digestive systems. It increases bile flow, the secretion of salivary juices and stomach acid production, and improves the digestive process as a whole. Quassia is commonly used to stimulate a weak appetite, especially in the treatment of anorexia. The herb's bitterness has led to its being used as a treatment for malaria and other fevers, and in the Caribbean it is given for dysentery. The bark has been used in the form of an enema to expel threadworms and other parasites. A decoction of the bark may be employed as an insect repellent.

CAUTION Excessive doses of quassia bark may cause irritation of the digestive tract and vomiting.

Picrorrhiza kurroa
(Scrophulariaceae)

PICRORRHIZA

DESCRIPTION Hairy perennial with serrated elliptical leaves and spikes of white or lilac flowers.

HABITAT & CULTIVATION Picrorrhiza is native to the mountains of India, Nepal, and Tibet. The rhizome is gathered in autumn.

PART USED Rhizome.

CONSTITUENTS Picrorrhiza contains the bitter glycoside kutkin (composed of picrosides I to III and kutkoside), cucurbitacins, and apocynin. Apocynin is powerfully anti-inflammatory and reduces platelet aggregation.

HISTORY & FOLKLORE Picrorrhiza has been used in Ayurvedic medicine since the earliest times as a laxative, bile-inducing, and bitter tonic herb, given for conditions as varied as snake bite and hepatitis.

MEDICINAL ACTIONS & USES In India, picrorrhiza is used as a bitter tonic, equivalent in many respects to gentian (*Gentiana lutea*, p. 97), and given for a wide range of digestive and liver troubles, including insufficient stomach acid secretion, indigestion, jaundice, hepatitis, liver cirrhosis, and constipation. In China, picrorrhiza is chiefly employed to treat chronic diarrhea and dysentery. Picrorrhiza also helps treat asthma, acute and chronic infections, conditions where the immune system is compromised, and autoimmune diseases, including psoriasis and vitiligo. Its traditional use for liver disorders is well founded, and picrorrhiza may play an important part in helping to treat serious liver disease.

RESEARCH In 1992 Indian trials, extracts of the herb were shown to boost immunity to infection and to have a specific action against *Leishmania donovani*, which causes the tropical parasitic disease leishmaniasis. Indian research also indicates that picrorrhiza has therapeutic value in the treatment of autoimmune disease and of cases of lowered immune activity.

RELATED SPECIES *P. scrophulariaeflora* is used interchangeably with picrorrhiza in Chinese herbal medicine.

CAUTION Take picrorrhiza only under professional supervision.

Pimenta officinalis
(Myrtaceae)

ALLSPICE

DESCRIPTION Aromatic evergreen tree growing to 40 ft (12 m). Has leathery oblong leaves, clusters of small white flowers, and tiny green berries that turn brown as they mature.

HABITAT & CULTIVATION Allspice is native to the Caribbean and to Central and South America, and is extensively cultivated in Jamaica and other parts of the region. The berries are gathered before they are fully ripe because the volatile oil content reduces as they mature.

PARTS USED Berries, essential oil.

CONSTITUENTS Allspice contains about 4% volatile oil (comprising up to 80% eugenol), proteins, lipids, the vitamins A, C, B_1, B_2, and minerals.

HISTORY & FOLKLORE Used as a spice in the Caribbean before the arrival of Europeans, allspice is now an ingredient in many well-known sauces, chutneys, and condiments.

MEDICINAL ACTIONS & USES A digestive stimulant, allspice is taken to relieve flatulence and indigestion. It is also taken to treat diarrhea. Allspice is often combined with herbs that have a tonic or laxative effect. The herb has an action similar to that of cloves (*Eugenia caryophyllata*, p. 95); both are stimulant, stomach-settling, and antiseptic. The essential oil is also stomach-settling.

CAUTIONS Do not take the essential oil internally without professional guidance. Do not take allspice as a medicine during pregnancy.

Pimpinella anisum
(Umbelliferae)

ANISE

DESCRIPTION Erect annual growing to 2 ft (60 cm), with feathery leaves, umbels of yellow flowers, and ridged gray-green seeds.

HABITAT & CULTIVATION Anise is native to the eastern Mediterranean, western Asia, and North Africa. It is widely cultivated for its seeds, which are used both medicinally and as a flavoring agent in cooking.

PARTS USED Seeds, essential oil.

ANISE SEEDS, which benefit the digestion, are harvested when ripe in autumn.

CONSTITUENTS Anise contains a volatile oil (comprising 70–90% anethole, together with methyl chavicol and other terpenes), furanocoumarins, flavonoids, fatty acids, phenylpropanoids, sterols, and proteins. Anethole has an observed estrogenic effect, and the seeds as a whole are mildly estrogenic. This effect may substantiate the herb's use as a stimulant of sexual drive and of breast-milk production.

HISTORY & FOLKLORE Anise has been cultivated in Egypt for at least 4,000 years. Pharaonic medical texts indicate that the seeds were used as a diuretic, to treat digestive problems, and to relieve toothache. The plant was also well known to the ancient Greeks. Dioscorides (1st century AD) wrote that anise "warms, dries and dissolves; facilitates breathing, relieves pain, provokes urine and eases thirst." In his *A New Herball* of 1551, William Turner recorded that "Anyse maketh the breth sweter and swageth payne."

MEDICINAL ACTIONS & USES Anise seeds are well known for their ability to reduce gas and bloating, and to settle the digestion. They are commonly given to infants and children to relieve colic, and to people of all ages to relieve nausea and indigestion. Anise seeds' antispasmodic properties make them helpful in countering menstrual pain, asthma, whooping cough, and other spasmodic coughs, and bronchitis. Their expectorant action justifies their use for these respiratory ailments. Anise seeds are thought to increase breast-milk production, and may be beneficial in treating impotence and frigidity. Anise essential oil is used for similar complaints, and is also used externally for lice and scabies.

CAUTIONS Do not take the essential oil internally except under professional supervision. Do not take anise during pregnancy, except in amounts normally used in cooking.

SELF-HELP USES Acidity & indigestion, p. 307; Digestive upsets, gas, & colic, p. 318; Gas & bloating, p. 306; Stomach spasm, p. 305.

Pinguicula vulgaris
(Lentibulariaceae)
BUTTERWORT

DESCRIPTION Insectivorous perennial growing to 4 in (10 cm). Has fleshy leaves in a basal rosette and double-lipped, purple-blue flowers.

HABITAT & CULTIVATION Native to northern and western Europe, butterwort is found growing in moorland and on mountains. The leaves are gathered from the wild in midsummer.

PARTS USED Leaves.

CONSTITUENTS Butterwort contains mucilage, tannins, benzoic acid, cinnamic acid, and valeric acid. Cinnamic acid has antispasmodic properties.

HISTORY & FOLKLORE Butterwort was often used in Welsh herbal medicine as a purgative. In Lapland, the plant has been used to curdle reindeer milk.

MEDICINAL ACTIONS & USES Butterwort is rarely employed in European herbal medicine today. Its main use is as a cough remedy, with properties similar to those of sundew (*Drosera rotundifolia*, p. 200), another insect-eating plant. Butterwort may be used to treat chronic and convulsive coughs.

RELATED SPECIES The similar *P. grandiflora*, native to the Pyrenees, has been used to treat spasmodic coughs.

CAUTION Take butterwort only under professional supervision.

Pinus sylvestris
(Pinaceae)
SCOTS PINE

DESCRIPTION Coniferous tree growing to 100 ft (30 m). Has reddish brown bark, fine linear needlelike leaves, yellowish buds in winter, and oval to conical cones.

HABITAT & CULTIVATION Native to mountainous regions of Europe and north and west Asia, Scots pine is now widely distributed throughout the northern hemisphere. The leaves are gathered in summer. The stems are usually harvested when the tree is felled.

PARTS USED Leaves, branches, stems, seeds, essential oil.

CONSTITUENTS The leaves of Scots pine contain a volatile oil (consisting mainly of alpha-pinene, but also including beta-pinene, delta-limonene, and other constituents).

HISTORY & FOLKLORE Scots pine essential oil is frequently added to disinfectants and other preparations. The distilled resin produces turpentine.

MEDICINAL ACTIONS & USES The leaves of Scots pine, taken internally, have a mildly antiseptic effect within the chest, and may also be used for arthritic and rheumatic problems. Essential oil from the leaves may be taken for asthma, respiratory infections, and digestive disorders such as gas. Scots pine branches and stems yield a thick resin, which is also antiseptic within the respiratory tract. The seeds yield an essential oil with diuretic and respiratory-stimulant properties. The seeds are used for bronchitis, tuberculosis, and bladder infections. A decoction of the seeds may be applied to suppress excessive vaginal discharge.

CAUTIONS Do not use if prone to allergic skin reactions. Take essential oil internally only under professional supervision.

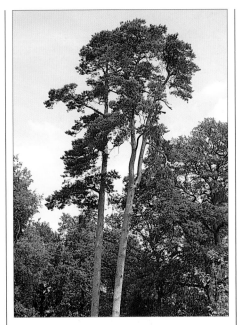

SCOTS PINE leaves, seeds, and oil have a mildly antiseptic effect in the respiratory and urinary tracts.

Piper angustifolia
(Piperaceae)
MATICO

DESCRIPTION Perennial shrub reaching 10 ft (3 m). Has deeply veined, aromatic lance-shaped leaves, spikes of tiny yellow flowers, and small black fruit.

HABITAT & CULTIVATION Matico is native to mountainous regions of Bolivia, Peru, and Ecuador. It is found in the wild and is widely cultivated in these and other countries in tropical South America. The leaves are gathered throughout the year.

PARTS USED Leaves.

CONSTITUENTS Matico contains a volatile oil (including camphor, borneol, and azulene), tannins, mucilage, and resins.

HISTORY & FOLKLORE Matico was and is used by Andean people as a wound-healing remedy and urinary antiseptic. European settlers learned of it in the 19th century, and it became an official drug in some South American pharmacopoeias.

MEDICINAL ACTIONS & USES Matico is an aromatic stimulant, diuretic, and astringent used extensively for gastric and intestinal problems, including peptic ulcers, diarrhea, and dysentery. It is commonly used in South American herbal medicine for internal bleeding, particularly within the digestive tract – for example, rectal bleeding and hemorrhoids. It is also taken for bleeding in the urinary tract. Applied externally, a decoction of matico makes a valuable remedy for minor wounds, insect stings, and inflamed skin, and it may also be used either as a mouthwash or a douche.

OTHER MEDICINAL PLANTS

Piper betle
(Piperaceae)
BETEL

DESCRIPTION Slender, climbing vine growing to 15 ft (5 m). Has heart-shaped leaves, tiny yellow-green flowers, and small spherical fruit.

HABITAT & CULTIVATION Betel is native to Malaysia and southern India. It is widely cultivated in much of southern Asia, East Africa and Madagascar, and the Caribbean. The leaves are gathered throughout the year and dried for extracts or to use whole.

PARTS USED Leaves, root, fruit.

CONSTITUENTS Betel leaves contain up to 1% volatile oil (including cadinene, chavicol, chavibetol, and cineole). As with many volatile oils, the percentages are variable. Malaysian samples have been shown to contain up to 69% chavibetol.

HISTORY & FOLKLORE Betel leaves, wrapped around areca nut (*Areca catechu*) and lime (*Citrus aurantiifolia*), are known to have been chewed in India and Southeast Asia for several thousand years. Betel leaves are described in the *Mahavasama*, the most ancient Sri Lankan text. Chewing betel eventually blackens the teeth. Long-term use of the herb is thought to increase the incidence of cancer of the mouth and tongue. Ironically the habit of chewing betel is now being replaced in many regions with cigarette smoking.

MEDICINAL ACTIONS & USES Betel leaves are chiefly used as a gentle stimulant, apparently inducing a mild sensation of well-being. They also affect the digestive system, stimulating salivary secretions, relieving gas, and preventing worm infestation. In many Asian traditions, including Ayurvedic medicine, betel leaves are thought to have aphrodisiac and nerve tonic properties. In Chinese herbal medicine, betel root, leaves, and fruit are sometimes

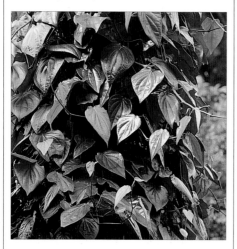

BETEL leaves, traditionally chewed with areca nut and lime, give a mild sensation of well-being.

used as a mild tonic and stomach-settling herb. The root has been used with black pepper (*P. nigrum, see below*) or jequirity (*Abrus precatorius*, p. 156) to produce sterility in women.

CAUTION The observed increase in the occurrence of oral cancers in regular users makes it unwise to chew betel.

Piper cubeba
(Piperaceae)
CUBEB

DESCRIPTION Climbing perennial growing to 20 ft (6 m). Has oval to oblong evergreen leaves, small flowers forming spikes, and round brown fruit.

HABITAT & CULTIVATION Native to Indonesia, cubeb is cultivated in much of tropical Asia, especially in the shade of coffee bushes (*Coffea arabica*, p. 190). The fruit is gathered when immature.

PART USED Fruit.

CONSTITUENTS Cubeb contains a volatile oil (up to 20%), a bitter principle (cubebin), an alkaloid (piperidine), resin, and fixed oil.

MEDICINAL ACTIONS & USES Like other members of the pepper family, cubeb has a significant antiflatulent and antiseptic action. In addition, the fruit is used to counter infections of the urinary tract, and has been taken in the past as a treatment for gonorrhea. Cubeb is helpful in relieving digestive problems such as flatulence and bloating, and its expectorant properties have been brought to bear in the treatment of chronic bronchitis.

CAUTION Cubeb should be not be taken by people suffering from inflammatory conditions of the digestive tract.

Piper nigrum
(Piperaceae)
PEPPER

DESCRIPTION Perennial woody climber growing to about 15 ft (5 m). Has large oval leaves, spikes of small white flowers, and clusters of small round fruits, which ripen from green to red.

HABITAT & CULTIVATION Native to southwestern India, pepper is now cultivated in tropical areas around the world. The fruit is harvested from plants at least 3 years old. Green peppercorns are picked unripe and pickled, black peppercorns are picked unripe and dried, red peppercorns are picked ripe and dried, and white peppercorns are picked ripe and soaked in water for 8 days before drying.

PARTS USED Fruit, essential oil.

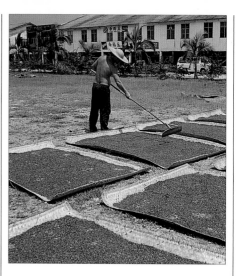

DRYING PEPPER, a spice that is still highly valued both medicinally and in cooking.

CONSTITUENTS Pepper contains a volatile oil (including beta-bisabolene, camphene, beta-caryophyllene, and many other terpenes and sesquiterpenes), up to 9% alkaloids (especially piperine, largely responsible for the herb's acrid taste), about 11% proteins, and small amounts of minerals. White pepper contains very little volatile oil.

HISTORY & FOLKLORE Cultivated as a spice and a medicine since ancient times, pepper was a vital commodity in world trade for thousands of years. Attila the Hun is reputed to have demanded 3,000 lb of pepper as ransom during his siege of the city of Rome (AD 408).

MEDICINAL ACTIONS & USES The familiar sharp taste of pepper reflects the stimulant effect it has on the digestive tract and the circulatory system. Pepper is commonly taken, either alone or in combination with other herbs and spices, to warm the body, or to improve digestive function in cases of nausea, stomachache, flatulence, bloating, constipation, or lack of appetite. The essential oil eases rheumatic pain and toothache. It is antiseptic and antibacterial, and reduces fever.

CAUTION Do not take the essential oil internally without professional supervision.

SELF-HELP USE Back pain, p. 313.

Piscidia erythrina
(Leguminosae)
JAMAICA DOGWOOD

DESCRIPTION Deciduous tree or shrub growing to 50 ft (15 m). Has compound leaves, blue to white flowers with red stripes, and winged seed pods.

HABITAT & CULTIVATION Jamaica dogwood is native to the southern US, Central America, northern South America, and the Caribbean. It is grown mainly for its wood, which is used in boat-building. The root bark is stripped when the tree is felled.

PART USED Root bark.

CONSTITUENTS Jamaica dogwood contains isoflavones (including lisetin, jamaicin, and icthyone), organic acids (such as piscidic acid), beta-sitosterol, and tannins.

HISTORY & FOLKLORE The pounded bark and twigs have been used by Native Caribs and Afro-Caribbeans to stupefy fish.

MEDICINAL ACTIONS & USES Jamaica dogwood is a useful and undervalued remedy that acts as a sedative and painkiller. It is chiefly employed in the treatment of insomnia and overexcitability, since it calms mental activity. It is also prescribed for nerve pain, toothache, and menstrual pain. As an antispasmodic, it is useful for treating muscle spasms, especially in the back, and spasmodic respiratory ailments such as asthma and whooping cough.

CAUTIONS Do not take Jamaica dogwood during pregnancy or if suffering from heart problems.

Pistacia lentiscus
(Anacardiaceae)
MASTIC TREE

DESCRIPTION Multibranched perennial growing to 10 ft (3 m). Has small elliptical leathery leaves, clusters of reddish flowers, and round scarlet fruit that ripens to black.

HABITAT & CULTIVATION Mastic tree is native to the Mediterranean region. It grows wild in scrub and in open areas. Besides growing wild, it is also cultivated for its resin, which is collected from incisions made in the bark in summer and autumn.

PART USED Resin.

CONSTITUENTS The resin contains alpha- and beta-masticoresins, a volatile oil (comprising mainly alpha-pinene), tannins, masticin, and mastic acid. Pinenes are strongly antiseptic.

HISTORY & FOLKLORE Mastic resin was used by the ancient Egyptians for embalming the dead.

MEDICINAL ACTIONS & USES Mastic resin is rarely used today, though it could be employed as an expectorant for bronchial troubles and coughs, and as a treatment for diarrhea. It has also been used to treat a range of skin conditions, including boils and ulcers. The resin has been mixed with other compounds as a temporary filling for decayed teeth.

RELATED SPECIES The pistachio nut is produced by *P. vera*, which is also native to the Mediterranean region.

Plantago major
(Plantaginaceae)
COMMON PLANTAIN

DESCRIPTION Perennial plant growing to 10 in (25 cm). Has a basal rosette of broad, deeply veined leaves and dense clusters of tiny green flowers on spikes.

HABITAT & CULTIVATION Common plantain is native to Europe and temperate regions of Asia. Rarely cultivated, it is normally picked from the wild. The leaves are gathered throughout the summer.

PARTS USED Leaves.

CONSTITUENTS Common plantain contains iridoids (such as aucubin, also found in *Euphrasia* species), flavonoids (including apigenin), tannins, plant acids, and mucilage. Aucubin increases uric acid excretion by the kidneys; apigenin is anti-inflammatory.

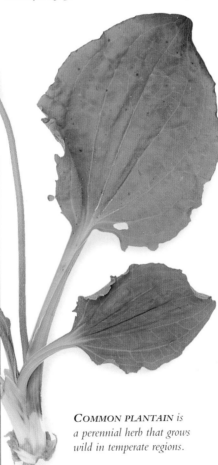

COMMON PLANTAIN is a perennial herb that grows wild in temperate regions.

HISTORY & FOLKLORE In Gaelic, this herb is known as "the healing plant" because it was used in Ireland to treat wounds and bruises. It is a plant that has accompanied European colonization around the world – some Native Americans called it "Englishman's foot" because it seemed to spring up in the footsteps of white settlers.

MEDICINAL ACTIONS & USES Common plantain quickly staunches blood flow and encourages the repair of damaged tissue. It

may be used instead of comfrey (*Symphytum officinale*, p. 136) in treating bruises and broken bones. An ointment or lotion may be used to treat hemorrhoids, fistulae (abnormal passages in the skin), and ulcers. Taken internally, common plantain is diuretic, expectorant, and decongestant. It is commonly prescribed for gastritis, peptic ulcers, diarrhea, dysentery, irritable bowel syndrome, respiratory congestion, loss of voice, and urinary tract bleeding.

RELATED SPECIES Ribwort plaintain (*P. lanceolata*) is used in the same way as common plaintain. *Che qian cao* (*P. asiatica*) is used in Chinese medicine as a diuretic and to counter mucus.

SELF-HELP USES Allergic rhinitis with mucus, p. 300; **Diarrhea**, p. 318.

Plumbago zeylanica
(Plumbaginaceae)
CEYLON LEADWORT

DESCRIPTION Evergreen shrub, often a climber, growing to 6 ft (2 m). Has oval pointed leaves, spikes of 5-petaled white flowers, and angled seed capsules.

HABITAT & CULTIVATION Ceylon leadwort is native to southern India and Malaysia, and is now naturalized in much of Southeast Asia and in Africa. The leaves and root are gathered throughout the year.

PARTS USED Leaves, root.

CONSTITUENTS Ceylon leadwort contains plumbagin, which stimulates sweating.

HISTORY & FOLKLORE In Africa, the juice of Ceylon leadwort is used as a tattoo dye.

MEDICINAL ACTIONS & USES Ceylon leadwort root is acrid and stimulates sweating. In West Africa, the root is traditionally mixed with okra (*Hibiscus esculentus*) to treat leprosy. In Nepal, a decoction of the root is used to treat baldness. In Indian herbal medicine, the leaves and root are used to treat infections and digestive problems such as dysentery. Externally, a paste of the leaves and root is applied to painful rheumatic areas or to chronic and itchy skin problems. The paste acts as a counterirritant. By raising blisters and increasing circulation, it speeds the clearing of toxins from the affected area.

RELATED SPECIES European leadwort (*P. europaea*) root is also irritant when applied externally. It has been used to treat toothache, and, in the form of a poultice or plaster, back pain and sciatica. The Caribbean *P. scandens* is used in a similar manner to treat rheumatic aches and pains and skin problems.

CAUTIONS Use only under professional supervision. Taken internally, the root is potentially toxic and may induce abortion. Do not use Ceylon leadwort during pregnancy.

Podophyllum peltatum
(Berberidaceae)
AMERICAN MANDRAKE

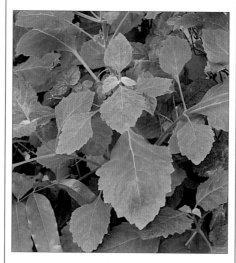

DESCRIPTION Perennial plant growing to 16 in (40 cm). Has a forked stem, two deeply lobed, umbrella-like leaves, white flowers, and small yellow fruit.

American mandrake

HABITAT & CULTIVATION American mandrake is native to northeastern North America. It is commonly found in damp woodland and pastureland. The rhizome is unearthed in autumn.

PART USED Rhizome.

CONSTITUENTS The rhizome of American mandrake contains lignans (especially podophyllotoxin), flavonoids, resin, and gums. The lignans are responsible for the rhizome's purgative action.

HISTORY & FOLKLORE American mandrake was commonly used as a purgative, emetic, and worm-expelling herb by Native Americans. In the US in the 19th century, both herbal and conventional medical practitioners regarded the plant as the safest and most readily available purge.

MEDICINAL ACTIONS & USES Despite 19th-century beliefs in its safety, American mandrake is no longer taken internally because of its cytotoxic (cell-killing) action. However, applied externally as a poultice, lotion, or ointment, the root can be an effective treatment for all kinds of warts.

RESEARCH The lignans in American mandrake – podophyllotoxin in particular – act against tumors and have been extensively researched for their anticancer potential. Semisynthetic derivatives of podophyllotoxin appear to be the most promising, having minimal toxicity.

RELATED SPECIES The Himalayan *P. hexandrum* may have similar actions.

CAUTIONS Do not take American mandrake internally. The plant is subject to legal restrictions in most countries.

Pogostemon cablin
syn. *P. patchouli*
(Labiatae)
PATCHOULI

DESCRIPTION Aromatic perennial growing to 3 ft (1 m). Has square stems, oval leaves, and spikes bearing whorls of white to light purple flowers.

HABITAT & CULTIVATION Native to Malaysia and the Philippines, patchouli is now cultivated in tropical and subtropical regions around the world. The shoots and leaves may be picked either 2 or 3 times a year, depending on the soil and climate.

PARTS USED Young leaves and shoots, essential oil.

CONSTITUENTS Patchouli contains a volatile oil comprising mainly the sesquiterpenes patchoulol (35%) and bulnesene.

HISTORY & FOLKLORE Patchouli has been used extensively in Asian medicine, featuring in the Chinese, Indian, and Arabic traditions. Its most common use has been as an aphrodisiac. The oil is extensively employed in India today as a fragrance and as an insect repellent.

PATCHOULI is the source of an essential oil.

MEDICINAL ACTIONS & USES Patchouli is used in herbal medicine in Asia as an aphrodisiac, antidepressant, and antiseptic. It is also employed for headaches and fever. Patchouli essential oil is used in aromatherapy to treat skin complaints. It is thought to have a regenerative effect on skin tone and to help clear conditions such as eczema and acne. The oil may also be used for varicose veins and hemorrhoids.

CAUTION Do not take essential oil internally.

Polygala senega
(Polygalaceae)
SENECA SNAKEROOT

DESCRIPTION Perennial growing to about 16 in (40 cm). Has narrow lance-shaped leaves with toothed edges and spikes of whitish pink flowers.

HABITAT & CULTIVATION Seneca snakeroot is native to North America, and found in dry, stony, open ground and woodland. It is cultivated in western Canada. The root is unearthed in autumn.

PART USED Root.

CONSTITUENTS Seneca snakeroot contains triterpenoid saponins (including sengins), phenolic acids, methyl salicylate, polygalitol, and plant sterols. The triterpenoid saponins promote the clearing of mucus from the bronchial tubes.

HISTORY & FOLKLORE This plant's name refers to the Seneca tribe of North America, which employed the root to treat snake bite. Seneca snakeroot was highly valued by both Native Americans and European settlers. In 1768, Dr. Alexander Garden of Charleston wrote that "The Seneka is the most powerful and efficacious antiphlogistic [fever- and inflammation-reducing substance] attenuant among the Galenical medicines."

MEDICINAL ACTIONS & USES In North American and European herbal medicine, Seneca snakeroot is used as an expectorant to treat bronchial asthma, chronic bronchitis, and whooping cough. The root has a stimulant action on the bronchial mucous membranes, promoting the coughing up of mucus from the chest and thereby easing wheezing. In large doses, the root is emetic. It is also thought to promote sweating and to stimulate saliva secretion.

RELATED SPECIES *Yuan zhi* (*P. tenuifolia*), native to China and Japan, has similar constituents. *Yuan zhi* is taken to treat congestion in the chest and to "calm the spirit and quieten the heart." *See also* milkwort (*P. vulgaris, following entry*).

CAUTION In excessive doses, Seneca snakeroot causes diarrhea and vomiting.

Polygala vulgaris
(Polygalaceae)
MILKWORT

DESCRIPTION Short perennial with pointed, lance-shaped leaves and spikes of small, blue, mauve, or white flowers.

HABITAT & CULTIVATION Milkwort is common in grassy and moorland areas in much of western and northern Europe. It is gathered from the wild when the plant is in flower in summer.

PARTS USED Aerial parts, root.

CONSTITUENTS Milkwort contains triterpenoid saponins, a volatile oil, gaultherin, and mucilage.

HISTORY & FOLKLORE Milkwort has been most often used to treat chest problems such as pleurisy and dry coughs. In larger doses, the plant acts as an emetic. In his *Irish Herbal* (1735), K'Eogh stated that "it has a hot dry nature, and it encourages the production of milk in nursing mothers."

MEDICINAL ACTIONS & USES The bitter-tasting milkwort still has a reputation for increasing milk production in nursing mothers, but this attribute is in fact unfounded. Although milkwort is infrequently used in European herbal medicine today, it – like Seneca snakeroot

(*P. senega, see preceding entry*) – is a valuable herb for the treatment of respiratory troubles such as chronic bronchitis, bronchial asthma, and convulsive coughs, including whooping cough. Milkwort is also considered to have sweat-inducing and diuretic properties.

Polygonatum multiflorum
(Liliaceae)
SOLOMON'S SEAL

DESCRIPTION Perennial growing to about 20 in (50 cm). Has arching stems, alternate elliptical leaves, delicate greenish white, bell-shaped flowers, and blue-black fruit.

HABITAT & CULTIVATION Native to Europe and to temperate regions of Asia and North America, Solomon's seal is quite rare in the wild. However, it is a common ornamental garden plant. The rhizome is unearthed in autumn.

PART USED Rhizome.

CONSTITUENTS Solomon's seal contains saponins (similar to diosgenin), flavonoids, and vitamin A.

HISTORY & FOLKLORE Solomon's seal has been used in Western herbal medicine since classical times, and was described by Dioscorides, Pliny, and Galen. The herbalist John Gerard, writing in 1597, explained its name: "The root is white and thicke, full of knobs or joints, in some places resembling the mark of a seale, whereof I think it tooke the name *Sigillum Solomonis*." In China, the herb's first recorded use goes back to the *Divine Husbandman's Classic (Shen'nong Bencaojing)* of the 1st century AD. In North America, the plant was known to various Native American tribes. The Penobscot used it as part of a formula for treating gonorrhea.

MEDICINAL ACTIONS & USES Like arnica (*Arnica montana*, p. 170), Solomon's seal is believed to prevent excessive bruising and to stimulate tissue repair. Used mainly in the form of a poultice, the rhizome has astringent and demulcent actions that undoubtedly contribute to its ability to accelerate healing. Solomon's seal has also been recommended as a treatment for tuberculosis, as a remedy for menstrual problems, and as a tonic. In Chinese herbal medicine, it is considered a *yin* tonic, and is thought to be particularly applicable to problems affecting the respiratory system – sore throats, dry and irritable coughs, bronchial congestion, and chest pain.

RELATED SPECIES Angular or scented Solomon's seal (*P. odoratum*) is used in much the same way as *P. multiflorum*.

CAUTION Do not take internally except under professional advice. The aerial parts, especially the berries, are harmful if eaten.

Polygonum aviculare
(Polygonaceae)
KNOTGRASS, BIAN XU
(CHINESE)

DESCRIPTION Annual creeper growing to 20 in (50 cm). Has lance-shaped leaves and clusters of small pink or white flowers.

HABITAT & CULTIVATION Knotgrass is found in temperate regions throughout the world. It thrives in open areas and along shorelines. The plant is gathered throughout the summer.

PARTS USED Aerial parts.

CONSTITUENTS Knotgrass contains tannins, flavonoids, polyphenols, silicic acid (about 1%), and mucilage.

HISTORY & FOLKLORE Knotgrass has been used as a diuretic in Chinese herbal medicine for over 2,000 years. In the Western tradition, the 1st-century AD physician Dioscorides likewise considered the herb a diuretic, as well as a remedy for heavy menstrual bleeding and snake bite.

MEDICINAL ACTIONS & USES A herb with astringent and diuretic properties, knotgrass is used in European herbal medicine to treat diarrhea and hemorrhoids, to expel worms, to staunch bleeding wounds, to reduce heavy menstrual flow, and to stop nosebleeds. Knotgrass is also taken for pulmonary complaints since its silicic acid content helps strengthen connective tissue within the lungs. In the Chinese tradition, knotgrass is given for intestinal worms, to treat diarrhea and dysentery, and as a diuretic, particularly in cases of painful urination.

RESEARCH Chinese research indicates that the plant is a useful medicine for bacillary dysentery. Of 108 people with this disease treated with a paste of knotgrass (taken internally), 104 recovered within 5 days.

RELATED SPECIES *See also* bistort (*P. bistorta, following entry*), and *he shou wu* (*P. multiflorum*, p. 121).

Polygonum bistorta
(Polygonaceae)
BISTORT

DESCRIPTION Perennial growing to 12 in (30 cm). Has long basal leaves, dense spikes of small pink flowers, and dark nutlets.

HABITAT & CULTIVATION Native to Europe, Asia, and North America, bistort prefers damp conditions. The leaves are gathered in spring, the rhizome in autumn.

PARTS USED Leaves, rhizome.

CONSTITUENTS Bistort contains polyphenols (including ellagic acid), tannins (15–20%),

phlobaphene, flavonoids, and a trace of the anthraquinone emodin.

HISTORY & FOLKLORE Bistort rhizomes have long been employed for their astringency. As the rhizomes also contain large amounts of starch, they have also been roasted and eaten as a vegetable in Russia and North America.

MEDICINAL ACTIONS & USES One of the most strongly astringent of all herbs, bistort is used to contract tissues and staunch blood flow. It makes a valuable mouthwash and gargle for treating spongy gums, canker sores, and sore throats, and is also useful as a wash for small burns and wounds, a douche for excessive vaginal discharge, and an ointment for hemorrhoids and anal fissures. Internally, bistort may be taken to treat peptic ulcers, ulcerative colitis, and conditions such as dysentery and irritable bowel syndrome that give rise to diarrhea. Bistort is occasionally used in cases of urinary problems such as cystitis and for upper respiratory congestion.

RELATED SPECIES *P. hydropiper*, which is native to Europe, may be used to relieve heavy menstrual bleeding. *See also* knotgrass (*P. aviculare*, *preceding entry*).

CAUTION Use bistort internally for no more than 3–4 weeks at a time.

SELF-HELP USE Diarrhea, p. 307.

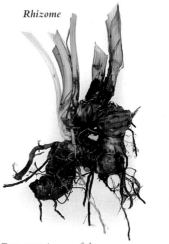

Rhizome

BISTORT *is one of the most astringent of all medicinal plants.*

Polymnia uvedalia
(Compositae)
BEARSFOOT

DESCRIPTION Perennial herb growing to 6 ft (2 m) with large 3-lobed leaves and yellow flowers.

HABITAT & CULTIVATION Bearsfoot is native to the eastern US. It grows from New York southward, preferring rich soil. The root is unearthed in autumn.

PART USED Root.

HISTORY & FOLKLORE Bearsfoot root was used by Native Americans as a stimulant and laxative remedy. In the 19th century, it became a widely popular healing herb in North America, having a specific use as a treatment for mastitis (inflammation of the breast tissue).

MEDICINAL ACTIONS & USES Bearsfoot is perhaps best known for its use as a hair tonic, having traditionally been a popular ingredient in hair lotions. It is still used in this way, but today the root is more often taken internally as a treatment for non-malignant swollen glands and especially for mastitis. The root is thought to have a beneficial effect on the stomach, liver, and spleen, and may be taken to relieve indigestion and liver malfunction. The herb has laxative properties, and it may also act to relieve pain.

Polypodium vulgare
(Polypodiaceae)
POLYPODY

DESCRIPTION Delicate perennial fern growing to a height of 1 ft (30 cm). Has slender knotty rhizomes and curving fronds that are dotted with brown spores (sori) on their lower surface.

HABITAT & CULTIVATION Native to Europe and northern Asia, polypody is commonly found growing in damp woodland and thickets, and on walls. The rhizome is unearthed in autumn.

PART USED Rhizome.

CONSTITUENTS Polypody rhizome contains saponins (based on polypodosapogenin), ecdysteroids, phloroglucins, volatile oil, fixed oil, and tannins.

HISTORY & FOLKLORE Polypody has been used medicinally in Europe since ancient times. Like mistletoe (*Viscum album*, p. 281), polypody often grows on host trees, for example, oak (*Quercus robur*, p. 258). This was thought to impart great medicinal value to the plant. The Greek physician Dioscorides, writing in the 1st century AD, noted that polypody was used to purge mucus and was an ingredient of a plaster

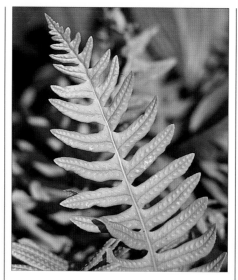

POLYPODY is often seen growing in damp woodland in Europe and northern Asia.

applied to dislocated fingers and to sores that occur between the fingers.

MEDICINAL ACTIONS & USES Polypody stimulates bile secretion and is a gentle laxative. Traditionally, it has been used in European herbal medicine as a treatment for hepatitis and jaundice, and as a remedy for indigestion and loss of appetite. Polypody makes a safe treatment for constipation in children. The rhizome is also expectorant, having a supportive and mildly stimulating effect on the respiratory system. It may be taken for the relief of congestion, bronchitis, pleurisy, and dry irritable coughs. The rhizome combines well with marsh mallow (*Althaea officinalis*, p. 163).

CAUTION Polypody may cause a skin rash when applied externally.

Pomaderris elliptica
(Rhamnaceae)
KUMARHOU

DESCRIPTION Branching tree growing to about 10 ft (3 m). Has shiny leaves and clusters of yellow-white flowers.

HABITAT & CULTIVATION Kumarhou is native to New Zealand.

PARTS USED Aerial parts.

MEDICINAL ACTIONS & USES Kumarhou is a traditional Maori remedy that has been used to treat a wide range of illnesses. Its most common use is as a remedy for problems of the respiratory tract, such as asthma and bronchitis. However, it has also been used in the treatment of indigestion and heartburn, diabetes, and kidney problems. Kumarhou is considered to be a detoxifier and "blood cleansing" plant, and is used to treat skin rashes and sores, including lesions produced by skin cancer.

Populus x *candicans*
syn. *P.* x *gileadensis*
(Salicaceae)
BALM OF GILEAD

DESCRIPTION Deciduous tree growing to 80 ft (25 m). Has heart-shaped leaves, buds producing a sticky resin, and female catkins.

HABITAT & CULTIVATION Naturalized in northern temperate regions, balm of Gilead is also cultivated as an ornamental tree. The buds and bark from young branches are collected in spring.

PARTS USED Buds, stem bark.

CONSTITUENTS Balm of Gilead buds contain flavonoids, phenolic glycosides (including salicin), and fatty acids. Salicin's analgesic, anti-inflammatory, and fever-reducing actions resemble those of aspirin.

HISTORY & FOLKLORE Balm of Gilead has been used for several thousand years to soothe inflamed or irritated skin. The 17th-century herbalist Nicholas Culpeper recorded that "The oyntment called populeon, which is much of this poplar, is singular for all heat and inflammation in any part of the body and tempereth the heat of wounds: It is much use to dry up the milk in women's breasts, when they have weaned their children."

MEDICINAL ACTIONS & USES Balm of Gilead is a common ingredient of cough mixtures. Its expectorant, antiseptic, and analgesic properties make it an excellent remedy for sore throats, dry irritable coughs, bronchitis, and other respiratory ailments. In France and Germany, balm of Gilead is applied as a salve to scrapes, small wounds, chapped and itchy skin, sunburn, chilblains, and hemorrhoids. A preparation of balm of Gilead, applied externally, may also help relieve the pain of rheumatic joints and strained muscles. As Culpeper noted, the plant is also thought to reduce breast-milk production.

RESEARCH Studies have demonstrated that balm of Gilead buds have significant expectorant, antibacterial, antifungal, and anti-inflammatory properties. Research undertaken into the bud resin of this and other poplar species has been largely prompted by the resin's chemical

Balm of Gilead

similarity to propolis, a naturally antibiotic resin that is gathered by bees and used in the construction of hives.

CAUTIONS Although balm of Gilead has not been proven to reduce the production of breast milk, breast-feeding mothers should not take this herb internally. Do not take if allergic to aspirin.

SELF-HELP USE Coughs, p. 310.

Populus tremuloides
(Salicaceae)
QUAKING ASPEN

DESCRIPTION Deciduous, spreading tree growing to 70 ft (20 m). Has oval, slightly sticky buds and round, finely toothed leaves that quiver in the wind.

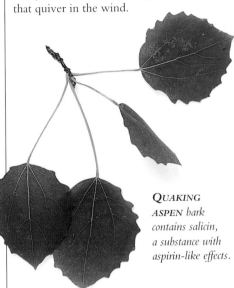

QUAKING ASPEN bark contains salicin, a substance with aspirin-like effects.

HABITAT & CULTIVATION Native to North America, quaking aspen prefers damp and moist areas, and is commonly found growing alongside rivers and in valleys, along roadsides, and in groves. It is also widely cultivated in temperate regions. The bark is collected in early spring.

PART USED Bark.

CONSTITUENTS The bark contains phenolic glycosides (including salicin and populin) and tannins. Salicin and populin are salicylates, substances that have fever-reducing, pain-relieving, and anti-inflammatory properties that are similar to those of aspirin.

HISTORY & FOLKLORE The Ojibwa people used an oily compound made from bear fat and quaking aspen to treat earache. Other Native Americans used the bark for diverse purposes, including as a wash for sore eyes.

MEDICINAL ACTIONS & USES Like willow bark (*Salix alba*, p. 128), quaking aspen bark has widely recognized anti-inflammatory and pain-relieving properties. It is often taken to treat arthritic and rheumatic aches and pains. It is also used to lower fever, especially when this condition is associated with rheumatoid arthritis. Being a stimulant, quaking aspen bark acts as a tonic remedy in the treatment of anorexia and other debilitated states. The bark's significant astringent and antiseptic qualities make it useful for treating diarrhea and the symptoms of irritable bowel syndrome. It is also used to treat urinary tract infections.

CAUTION Do not take quaking aspen if allergic to aspirin.

Poria cocos
syn. *Sclerotium cocos*
(Polyporaceae)
FU LING, INDIAN BREAD

DESCRIPTION Subterranean fungus growing to 1 ft (30 cm) across. Has a wrinkled brown mantle and a white interior.

HABITAT & CULTIVATION *Fu ling* grows in northern India, central China, and North America. Commonly found on the roots of fir trees, it is harvested from midsummer to early spring.

PART USED Inner mass of the fungus.

CONSTITUENTS *Fu ling* contains beta-pachyman, beta-pachymanase, and pachymic acid.

HISTORY & FOLKLORE *Fu ling* has been used in Chinese herbal medicine for well over 2,000 years. It has formed a part of many traditional tonic formulas, notably the "Decoction of the four rulers" in which it is mixed with ginseng (*Panax ginseng*, p. 116), *bai zhu* (*Atractylodes macrocephala*, p. 172), and *gan cao* (*Glycyrrhiza uralensis*, p. 215). This decoction was prescribed by the physician Wang Ji (1463–1539) as part of a regimen to treat syphilis.

MEDICINAL ACTIONS & USES *Fu ling* is much used as a diuretic and tonic in Chinese herbal medicine, being classified as an herb that "drains dampness" (*see* pp. 38–42). It is prescribed for a variety of conditions affecting the urinary system, including fluid retention and difficulty in passing urine. *Fu ling* has a soothing and tranquilizing effect on the nervous system, and can be most helpful in treating stress-related problems such as anxiety, tension headaches, palpitations, and difficulty in sleeping. In common with many other tonic herbs, *fu ling* plays a useful role in supporting convalescence after long-term illness.

RESEARCH Traditionally, *fu ling* is reputed to be a diuretic, but research in China involving both laboratory animals and humans failed to show a diuretic action for the herb.

Portulaca oleracea
(Portulacaceae)
PURSLANE

DESCRIPTION Annual plant growing to 6 in (15 cm). Has small rounded leaves and clusters of small yellow flowers.

HABITAT & CULTIVATION Native to Europe and Asia, purslane is now one of the most widely distributed of plants, growing from Australia and China to the Americas. Often found growing near water, it is gathered throughout the summer.

PARTS USED Aerial parts.

CONSTITUENTS Purslane contains mucilage, plant acids, sugars, vitamins A, B$_1$, and C, and calcium. Chinese research (unconfirmed in the West) also lists noradrenaline and dopamine as constituents.

HISTORY & FOLKLORE Purslane's use as a medicinal herb in Europe, Iran, and India dates back at least 2,000 years, and it was probably eaten as a vegetable well before then. In ancient Rome, purslane was used to treat headaches, stomachache and dysentery, intestinal worms, and lizard bite.

MEDICINAL ACTIONS & USES Purslane has long been considered valuable in the treatment of urinary and digestive problems. The diuretic effect of the juice makes it useful in the alleviation of bladder ailments – for example, difficulty in passing urine. The plant's mucilaginous properties also make it a soothing remedy for gastrointestinal problems such as dysentery and diarrhea. In Chinese herbal medicine, purslane is employed for similar problems and, additionally, for appendicitis. The Chinese also use the plant as an antidote for wasp stings and snake bite. Used as an external wash, the juice or a decoction relieves skin ailments such as boils and carbuncles, and also helps to reduce fever.

RESEARCH Clinical trials in China indicate that purslane has a mild antibiotic effect. In one study, the juice was shown to be effective in treating hookworms. Other studies suggest that it is valuable against bacillary dysentery. When injected, extracts of the herb induce powerful contractions of the uterus. Taken orally, purslane juice weakens uterine contractions.

CAUTION Do not take purslane as a medicine during pregnancy.

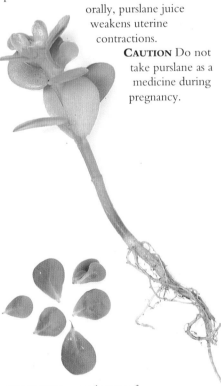

PURSLANE is a good source of vitamins and calcium. It also has antibiotic properties.

Potentilla anserina
(Rosaceae)
SILVERWEED

DESCRIPTION Perennial plant growing to 16 in (40 cm). Has toothed compound leaves that are silvery on the underside, and 5-petaled yellow flowers.

HABITAT & CULTIVATION Silverweed is found in Europe, Asia, and North America, where it flourishes in dry, grassy places. The aerial parts are collected in late summer, the root at the same time or in autumn.

PARTS USED Aerial parts, root.

CONSTITUENTS Silverweed contains 2–10% ellagitannins, flavonoids, choline, and bitters.

HISTORY & FOLKLORE William Withering, the 18th-century doctor who discovered the cardiotonic effects of foxglove (*Digitalis purpurea*, p. 199), recommended a teaspoon of dried leaves to be taken at 3-hour intervals to assuage bouts of malarial fever. Silverweed was once considered antispasmodic and was taken to ease colic and menstrual pain, but this property is now subject to doubt.

MEDICINAL ACTIONS & USES Contemporary medical herbalists believe that silverweed's main medicinal value lies in its astringency. Silverweed makes an effective gargle for sore throats and is a helpful remedy for diarrhea. It is less astringent than its close relative tormentil (*P. erecta, see following entry*), but it also has a gentler action within the gastrointestinal tract. It is used externally as a lotion or ointment for bleeding hemorrhoids.

Potentilla erecta
syn. *P. tormentilla*
(Rosaceae)
TORMENTIL

DESCRIPTION Downy, creeping perennial growing to 4 in (10 cm). Has leaves bearing 5 leaflets and numerous 4-petaled yellow flowers.

HABITAT & CULTIVATION Native to temperate regions of Asia and Europe, tormentil thrives in grassy sites and on heaths and moorland. The aerial parts are harvested in summer, the root in autumn.

PARTS USED Aerial parts, root.

CONSTITUENTS Tormentil contains 15–20% tannins, catechins, ellagitannins, and a phlobaphene.

HISTORY & FOLKLORE According to the 17th-century herbalist Nicholas Culpeper, the anatomist Andreas Vesalius (1514–1564) was "of the opinion that a decoction of this root is no less effectual to cure the French pox [syphilis] than guaiacum [*Guaiacum*

officinale, p. 216] or china [*Cinchona pubescens*, p. 79]." He also claimed the herb "is most excellent to stay all kinds of fluxes of blood or humours in man or woman, whether it be at nose, mouth, belly, or any wound in the veins or elsewhere."

MEDICINAL ACTIONS & USES Containing even more tannins than oak bark (*Quercus robur*, p. 258), all parts of tormentil are strongly astringent, finding use wherever this action is required. The plant makes a beneficial gargle for throat infections, and an effective mouthwash for treating canker sores and infected gums. Tormentil may be taken for conditions that give rise to diarrhea, such as irritable bowel syndrome, colitis, ulcerative colitis, and dysentery, and for rectal bleeding. Applied externally as a lotion or ointment, tormentil helps relieve hemorrhoids (especially those that are bleeding). In the form of a lotion, tormentil is used to help staunch wounds and protect areas of damaged or burned skin.

Primula veris
(Primulaceae)
COWSLIP

DESCRIPTION Hairy perennial growing to 4 in (10 cm). Has a basal rosette of slightly rough oblong leaves. Stems bear clusters of bright yellow bell-shaped flowers.

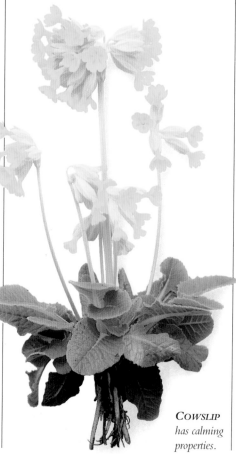

COWSLIP
has calming properties.

HABITAT & CULTIVATION Cowslip grows in Europe and western Asia, preferring fields and pastures with chalky soils. The flowers and leaves are gathered in spring and summer, the root in autumn. This increasingly rare plant should not be picked from the wild.

PARTS USED Flowers, leaves, root.

CONSTITUENTS Cowslip contains triterpenoid saponins, flavonoids, phenols, tannins, and a trace of volatile oil. The flavonoids, mainly in the flowers, are antioxidant, anti-inflammatory, and antispasmodic. The triterpenoid saponins, which are concentrated in the root (5–10%), are strongly expectorant.

HISTORY & FOLKLORE This plant is so closely associated with springtime that it is known as *primavera* (spring) in Spanish and Italian. Cowslip has long been reputed to preserve beauty. The 16th-century herbalist William Turner wrote: "Some weomen … sprinkle ye floures of cowslip with whyte wine and after … wash their faces with that water to … make them fayre in the eyes of the worlde rather than in the eyes of God, whom they are not afryd to offend."

MEDICINAL ACTIONS & USES Cowslip is an underused but valuable plant. The root is strongly expectorant, stimulating a more liquid mucus and thus easing the clearance of phlegm. It is given for chronic coughs, especially those associated with chronic bronchitis and mucous congestion. The root is also thought to be mildly diuretic and antirheumatic, and to slow blood clotting. The leaves have similar properties to the root but are weaker in action. The flowers are believed to be sedative, and are recommended for overactivity and sleeplessness, particularly in children. Cowslip flowers' antispasmodic and anti-inflammatory properties make them potentially useful in the treatment of asthma and other allergic conditions.

CAUTIONS Do not take cowslip during pregnancy, if allergic to aspirin, or if taking anticoagulant medication. Excessive doses can cause vomiting and diarrhea.

Prunus armeniaca
(Rosaceae)
APRICOT

DESCRIPTION Sturdy, deciduous tree growing to 30 ft (10 m). Has finely serrated oval leaves, clusters of white (or, rarely, pink) 5-petaled flowers, and lightly freckled pale yellow to deep purple fruits.

HABITAT & CULTIVATION Native to China and Japan, apricot is now cultivated in Asia, North Africa, and California. The fruit is collected when ripe in late summer.

PARTS USED Fruit, seeds, bark.

CONSTITUENTS Apricot fruit contains fruit sugars, vitamins, and iron. The kernels contain up to 8% amygdalin, the cyanogenic glycoside that yields laetrile and hydrocyanic (prussic) acid. The bark contains tannins.

HISTORY & FOLKLORE In India and China, the apricot has been appreciated for well over 2,000 years. Dong Feng, a physician who practiced at the end of the 2nd century AD, is said to have asked for his payment in apricot trees.

MEDICINAL ACTIONS & USES Apricot fruit is nutritious, cleansing, and mildly laxative. A decoction of the astringent bark soothes inflamed and irritated skin. Although the kernels contain highly toxic prussic acid, they are prescribed in small amounts in the Chinese tradition as a treatment for coughs, asthma, and wheezing, and for excessive mucus and constipation. An extract from the kernels, laetrile, has been used in Western medicine as a highly controversial treatment for cancer. The kernels also yield a fixed oil, similar to almond oil (from *P. amygdalus*), that is often used in the formulation of cosmetics.

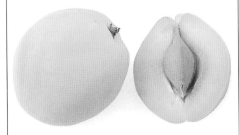

APRICOT kernels yield laetrile, which has been used as a controversial treatment for cancer.

RESEARCH Chinese trials show that apricot kernel paste helps combat vaginal infection.

CAUTION Apricot kernels are highly toxic in all but the smallest amounts and should not be consumed.

Prunus avium
(Rosaceae)
SWEET CHERRY

DESCRIPTION Deciduous shrub or tree growing to 25 ft (8 m). Has reddish brown bark, oval to elliptical leaves, clusters of 2–6 white flowers, and almost spherical, red fruit.

HABITAT & CULTIVATION Native to southwestern Asia, sweet cherry is naturalized in Europe and cultivated in temperate regions around the world. The stems and ripe fruit are collected in summer.

PARTS USED Stems, fruit.

CONSTITUENTS The stems of sweet cherry contain phenols, including salicylic acid, and tannins. Cherry fruit contains small amounts

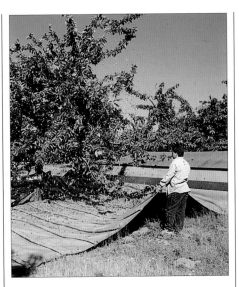

SWEET CHERRY fruit and stems have been harvested for medicinal use since classical times.

of salicylates and cyanogenic glycosides, and vitamins A, B$_1$, and C. The seeds also contain amygdalin, a cyanogenic glycoside.

HISTORY & FOLKLORE Dioscorides, a 1st-century AD physician, claimed that cherries relieve gas. The 16th-century herbalist John Gerard recorded the French custom of hanging cherries in houses to ward off fever.

MEDICINAL ACTIONS & USES In European herbal medicine, cherry stems have long been used for their diuretic and astringent properties. They have been prescribed for cystitis, nephritis, urinary retention, and for arthritic problems, notably gout. Cherries can be a helpful part of an overall regimen treating arthritic problems. Cherries' high sugar content makes them mildly laxative.

CAUTION The seeds are toxic and should not be consumed.

Prunus mume
(Rosaceae)
WU MEI, JAPANESE APRICOT

DESCRIPTION Deciduous tree growing to 30 ft (10 m). Has pointed oval to elliptical leaves, white flowers, and yellow fruit.

HABITAT & CULTIVATION Native to China, *wu mei* grows wild and is planted in the southern and eastern provinces. The fruit is picked in late spring.

PART USED Fruit.

CONSTITUENTS *Wu mei* contains fruit acids and sugars, vitamin C, and plant sterols.

MEDICINAL ACTIONS & USES The sour-tasting astringent *wu mei* is used in Chinese medicine to counter diarrhea and dysentery, to stop bleeding, and to ease coughs. It may also be effective in expelling hookworms. Externally, a plaster of the fruit is applied to

the sites of removed corns and warts to speed healing and the formation of new skin.

RESEARCH Laboratory research undertaken in China indicates that *wu mei* fruit has antibiotic properties.

Prunus serotina
(Rosaceae)
BLACK CHERRY

DESCRIPTION Deciduous tree growing to 100 ft (30 m). Has elliptical to oblong leaves, white flowers, and purple-black fruit.

HABITAT & CULTIVATION Native to North America, black cherry grows throughout much of the US. It is cultivated in central Europe for its lumber. The bark is collected in late summer and early autumn.

PART USED Inner bark.

CONSTITUENTS Black cherry contains prunasin (a cyanogenic glycoside that yields hydrocyanic acid), benzaldehyde, eudesmic acid, coumarins, and tannins. Prunasin reduces the cough reflex.

HISTORY & FOLKLORE Cherokee women traditionally took black cherry bark to ease labor pain. Other Native Americans used it in the treatment of coughs and colds, hemorrhoids, and diarrhea. European settlers learned of the bark's medicinal properties, and in the 19th century it became a widely used remedy.

MEDICINAL ACTIONS & USES Figuring in official pharmacopoeias and much used in the Anglo-American tradition, black cherry bark effectively counters chronic dry and irritable coughs. Combined with coltsfoot (*Tussilago farfara*, p. 277), it treats asthma and whooping cough. The astringent bark also eases indigestion and the symptoms of irritable bowel syndrome, especially when these conditions are of nervous origin.

CAUTION Black cherry bark is highly toxic in excessive doses.

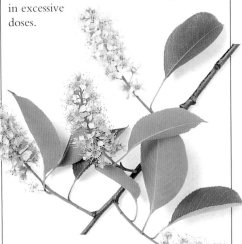

BLACK CHERRY bears long spikes of white flowers, followed by fleshy blue-black fruit.

255

Psoralea corylifolia
(Leguminosae)
BU GU ZHI, SCURF PEA

DESCRIPTION Perennial growing to 3 ft (90 cm). Has oval leaves, yellow cloverlike flowers, and black seed pods containing yellow-black seeds.

HABITAT & CULTIVATION *Bu gu zhi* is native to southern and southeastern Asia and cultivated in China. The fruit is gathered when ripe in autumn.

PARTS USED Seeds.

CONSTITUENTS *Bu gu zhi* contains psoraline, isopsorlin, and bavachin.

HISTORY & FOLKLORE In the Chinese tradition, *bu gu zhi* has long been considered a tonic remedy. It was first documented in *Grandfather Lei's Discussion of Herb Preparations*, written in about AD 490.

MEDICINAL ACTIONS & USES Valued as a *yang* tonic, *bu gu zhi* is taken in China to treat impotence and premature ejaculation and to improve vitality. The seeds are also used to counter debility and other problems reflecting "kidney *yang* deficiency," such as lower back pain, frequent urination, and incontinence. *Bu gu zhi* is used externally to treat skin conditions such as psoriasis, alopecia (loss of hair), and vitiligo (loss of skin pigmentation). In Vietnam, a tincture of the seeds is used to treat rheumatism.

RESEARCH Studies in China indicate that this herb is of value in the treatment of skin disorders, including vitiligo.

CAUTION Applied externally, this herb may sensitize the skin, resulting in an allergic reaction to sunlight.

Pterocarpus marsupium
(Leguminosae)
KINO

DESCRIPTION Handsome deciduous tree growing to 52 ft (16 m). Has leaves with 5–7 oval, leathery leaflets and numerous small yellow or white flowers.

HABITAT & CULTIVATION Native to Sri Lanka, India, Malaysia, and the Philippines, kino grows in tropical rainforests. The tree is cultivated for its lumber and for the sap ("kino") that exudes from cuts made in the trunk. The sap is collected year-round.

PART USED Sap.

CONSTITUENTS Kino contains tannins, flavonoids, and marsupsin.

MEDICINAL ACTIONS & USES The strongly astringent kino tightens the mucous membranes of the gastrointestinal tract. It can treat chronic diarrhea and relieve the irritation caused by intestinal infection and colitis. Although its taste is unpleasant, this herb makes a good mouthwash and gargle. It is widely used in Asia as a douche for excessive vaginal discharge.

Pueraria lobata
syn. *P. thunbergiana*
(Leguminosae)
GE GEN (CHINESE), KUDZU

DESCRIPTION Deciduous climber growing to 100 ft (30 m). Has leaves with 3 broadly oval leaflets, curling tendrils, and spikes of pea-type purple flowers.

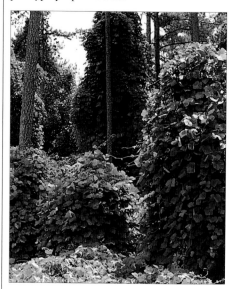

GE GEN is used in China to treat alcoholism and is an ingredient in a remedy for hangovers.

HABITAT & CULTIVATION Native to China, Japan, and eastern Asia, *ge gen* is naturalized in the US. It is cultivated in the central and eastern provinces of China. The root is unearthed in spring or autumn.

PART USED Root.

CONSTITUENTS *Ge gen* contains isoflavonoids, puerarin, daidzein, and plant sterols. Daidzein is estrogenic.

HISTORY & FOLKLORE From the 6th century BC onward, Chinese herbalists have considered *ge gen* to be a remedy for muscular pain and a treatment for measles. The authority known as the "Sage of Medicine," Zhang Zhongjing (AD 150–c. 219), recommended *ge gen* if the patient "has a stiff back and muscles, does not breathe easily, and is susceptible to gas."

MEDICINAL ACTIONS & USES In China, *ge gen* is frequently used as a remedy for measles, often in combination with *sheng ma* (*Cimicifuga foetida*). *Ge gen* is also given for muscle aches and pains, especially when they are linked with fever or are affecting the neck and upper back. The root may be taken to treat headache, dizziness, or numbness caused by high blood pressure. *Ge gen* also treats diarrhea and dysentery. The root is prescribed with *ju hua* (*Chrysanthemum* x *morifolium*, p. 77) to treat alcohol intoxication, hangovers, and alcoholism.

RESEARCH Chinese studies indicate that *ge gen* increases cerebral blood flow in patients with arteriosclerosis, and eases neck pain and stiffness. US research indicates that *ge gen* may suppress the desire for alcohol.

RELATED SPECIES The closely related *P. mirifica* and *P. tuberosa* have been investigated for their contraceptive effect.

Pulmonaria officinalis
(Boraginaceae)
LUNGWORT

DESCRIPTION Perennial growing to 1 ft (30 cm). Has broad oval basal leaves, smaller upper leaves mottled with white spots, and clusters of pink-purple flowers.

HABITAT & CULTIVATION Lungwort is native to Europe and the Caucasus. It flourishes in mountain pastures and in damp sites. The leaves are gathered in late spring.

PARTS USED Leaves.

CONSTITUENTS Lungwort contains allantoin, flavonoids, tannins, mucilage, saponin, and vitamin C. Unlike many of its relatives in the borage family, it does not contain pyrrolizidine alkaloids.

HISTORY & FOLKLORE According to the medieval Doctrine of Signatures, which held that a plant's appearance pointed to the ailment it treated, lungwort was effective for chest ailments because its leaves resemble lung tissue.

MEDICINAL ACTIONS & USES Given its high mucilage content, lungwort is indeed a useful remedy for chest conditions, and it is particularly beneficial in cases of chronic bronchitis. It combines well with herbs such as coltsfoot (*Tussilago farfara*, p. 277) as a

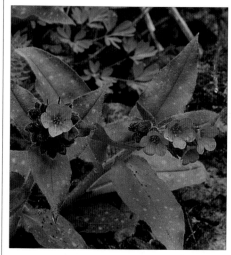

LUNGWORT'S speckled leaves were once considered a sign of its ability to cure lung problems.

treatment for chronic coughs (including whooping cough), and it can be taken for asthma. Lungwort can also be used as a treatment for sore throat and congestion. In the past, lungwort was given for the coughing up of blood arising from tubercular infection. Lungwort leaves are astringent and have been applied externally to stop bleeding.

CAUTION Lungwort is subject to legal restrictions in some countries.

Pulsatilla chinensis
(Ranunculaceae)
CHINESE ANEMONE,
BAI TOU WENG (CHINESE)

DESCRIPTION Perennial herb growing to 10 in (25 cm). Has erect downy stems, compound leaves, bell-shaped flowers, and feathery seed heads.

HABITAT & CULTIVATION Chinese anemone is native to eastern Asia, and is found in Mongolia, China, and Japan. The root is unearthed either before the plant comes into flower in spring, or in autumn.

PART USED Root.

CONSTITUENTS Chinese anemone contains lactones (including protoanemonin and anemonin), pulsatoside, and anemonol. Protoanemonin is antibacterial and irritant. It is absent from the dried root.

HISTORY & FOLKLORE Chinese anemone root was first documented in Chinese medicine in the *Divine Husbandman's Classic (Shen'nong Bencaojing)*, an herbal written in the 1st century AD.

MEDICINAL ACTIONS & USES Chinese anemone root is thought to clear toxicity and to lower fever. It is most commonly taken as a decoction to counter infection within the gastrointestinal tract. The root is also used to treat malarial fever and vaginal infections.

RESEARCH Chinese studies have shown the root to be potentially valuable as a treatment for amebic dysentery.

RELATED SPECIES *See* pulsatilla (*Anemone pulsatilla*, p. 165).

CAUTION Take Chinese anemone only under professional supervision.

Punica granatum
(Lythraceae)
POMEGRANATE

DESCRIPTION Deciduous shrub or tree growing to 20 ft (6 m). Has branches tipped with spines, whorls of lance-shaped leaves, scarlet flowers, and leathery-rinded round fruit containing many pulp-covered seeds.

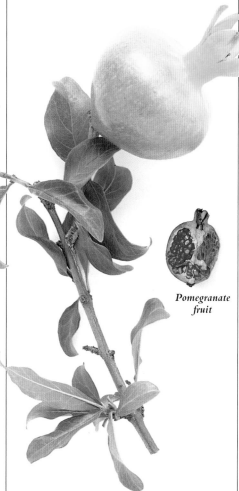

Pomegranate fruit

POMEGRANATE'S leathery fruit and jewel-toned seeds appear in ancient Greek mythology.

HABITAT & CULTIVATION Native to southwestern Asia, pomegranate has become naturalized in Europe. The tree is widely cultivated for its fruit, which is gathered in autumn when it is ripe. The bark is also gathered in autumn.

PARTS USED Rind, bark, fruit pulp.

CONSTITUENTS Pomegranate fruit rind (*shi liu pi*) and bark contain pelletierene alkaloids, elligatannins (up to 25%), and triterpenoids. The alkaloids are highly toxic.

HISTORY & FOLKLORE In 1500 BC, the pharaoh Tuthmosis reputedly brought back pomegranate to Egypt from Asia. Prized as a fruit, it was also sought after as a means to rid the body of worms. The Greek physician Dioscorides, in the 1st century AD, knew of the herb's ability to expel worms, but this attribute was subsequently forgotten in Europe for nearly 1,800 years. In the early 19th century, after an Indian herbalist used pomegranate to cure an Englishman of tapeworms, English doctors in India became interested in pomegranate, and its medicinal properties were investigated.

MEDICINAL ACTIONS & USES Both the rind and bark of the pomegranate are considered to be specific remedies for tapeworm infestation. The alkaloids present in the rind and bark cause the worm to release its grip on the intestinal wall. If a decoction of pomegranate rind or bark is immediately followed by a dose of a strong laxative or purgative, the worm will be voided. The rind and bark are also strongly astringent and occasionally have been used to treat diarrhea. In Spain, the juice of pomegranate fruit pulp is taken to comfort an upset stomach and as a remedy to relieve gas and flatulence.

CAUTIONS Pelletierene alkaloids are highly toxic. Do not use the rind or bark unless under professional supervision. This plant, and especially its bark extracts, is subject to legal restrictions in some countries.

Pygeum africanum
(Boraginaceae)
PYGEUM

DESCRIPTION Evergreen tree growing to 120 ft (35 m). Has oblong leaves, white flowers, and red berries.

HABITAT & CULTIVATION Pygeum is native to Africa. It is still harvested from the wild, but severe shortages have led to the establishment of commercial farming.

PART USED Bark.

CONSTITUENTS Pygeum contains phytosterols (beta-sitosterol), triterpenes (ursolic and oleanolic acids), long-chain alcohols (n-tetracosanol), and tannins.

HISTORY & FOLKLORE Pygeum has been valued in Africa for its hard wood, often used to make wagons, and for its bark, which is taken to treat urinary disorders.

MEDICINAL ACTIONS & USES In conventional medicine in France, the fat-soluble extract of pygeum bark has become the primary treatment for an enlarged prostate gland. A decoction of the bark may reduce the severity of chronic prostate inflammation, and it may also help reverse male sterility when this is due to insufficient prostate secretions. In combination with other plants, pygeum may be valuable in the treatment of prostatic cancer.

RESEARCH Trials carried out in France in the 1960s established that pygeum extract has positive effects on the prostate gland. Specifically, the extract increases glandular secretions and reduces levels of cholesterol within the organ. In most Western countries, surgery is the main option for enlarged prostates, but in France pygeum is prescribed in 81% of cases.

RELATED SPECIES The fruit kernels of the Asian *P. gardneri* are used to poison fish.

CAUTION Take pygeum only under professional supervision.

257

Quercus robur
(Fagaceae)
ENGLISH OAK

DESCRIPTION Slow-growing, long-lived, deciduous tree reaching 150 ft (45 m). Has deeply lobed leaves, long catkins, and green to brown fruit (acorns).

HABITAT & CULTIVATION English oak grows throughout Europe, in woods, forests, and along roadsides. The tree is also cultivated for its lumber, which is extremely durable. The bark is collected in spring and the fruit in autumn.

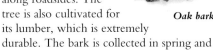

Oak bark

PARTS USED Bark, galls (growths produced by insects or fungi).

CONSTITUENTS English oak bark contains 15–20% tannins (including phlobatannin, ellagitannins, and gallic acid). Oak galls contain about 50% tannins.

HISTORY & FOLKLORE Sacred to the Druids, the oak tree has been esteemed in European herbal medicine for its astringent bark, leaves, and acorns. The bark has also been used to tan leather and to smoke fish. Oak lumber was formerly used to build the naval fleets of European nations, and whole forests were cleared in order to meet the shipbuilders' needs.

MEDICINAL ACTIONS & USES English oak bark, prepared as a decoction, is used as a gargle to treat sore throats and tonsillitis. It may also be applied as a wash, lotion, or ointment to treat hemorrhoids, anal fissures, small burns, and other skin problems. Less commonly, a decoction of the bark is taken in small doses to treat diarrhea, dysentery, and rectal bleeding. Powdered oak bark may be sniffed to treat nasal polyps, or sprinkled on eczema to dry the affected area. Oak galls are very astringent. They are used, in small quantities, in place of bark.

CAUTION Do not take common oak bark internally for more than 4 weeks at a time.

SELF-HELP USE Hemorrhoids, p. 302.

Quillaja saponaria
(Rosaceae)
SOAP BARK

DESCRIPTION Evergreen tree growing to 70 ft (20 m). Has glossy oval leaves, white flowers, and star-shaped fruit.

HABITAT & CULTIVATION Soap bark is native to Chile and Peru, and is now cultivated in California and India for medicinal and industrial use. The bark is gathered throughout the year.

PART USED Inner bark.

CONSTITUENTS Soap bark contains up to 10% triterpenoid saponins, calcium oxalate, and tannins. The saponins are strongly expectorant and can cause inflammation of the digestive tract.

HISTORY & FOLKLORE In Peru and Chile, soap bark has traditionally been used by Andean peoples as an alternative to soap for bathing and for washing clothes. The bark has been used medicinally by these peoples as an expectorant.

MEDICINAL ACTIONS & USES Soap bark has a long tradition of use as a treatment for chest problems. Its strong expectorant effect is beneficial in the treatment of bronchitis, especially in the early stages of the illness. Like other medicinal plants that contain saponins, soap bark stimulates the production of a more fluid mucus in the airways, facilitating the clearing of phlegm through coughing. Soap bark is useful for treating any condition featuring congested mucus within the chest, but it should not be used for dry, irritable coughs. Soap bark is also used externally, appearing in the formulations of dandruff shampoos.

CAUTIONS Use only under professional supervision. Given soap bark's irritant effect on the digestive tract, internal use must be carefully monitored.

Ranunculus ficaria
(Ranunculaceae)
LESSER CELANDINE,
PILEWORT

DESCRIPTION Mat-forming perennial growing to 6 in (15 cm). Has small tubers, fleshy heart-shaped leaves, and shiny-petaled, brilliant yellow flowers.

HABITAT & CULTIVATION Lesser celandine is native to western Asia, North Africa, and Europe. Commonly found in woods, along roadsides, and in bare, open spaces, it is collected when it comes into flower in spring.

PARTS USED Aerial parts.

CONSTITUENTS Lesser celandine contains saponins, protoanemonin and anemonin, tannins, and vitamin C. Protoanemonin is antibacterial and irritant; it is absent from the dried herb.

HISTORY & FOLKLORE Lesser celandine has been used from the earliest times as a medicine for the relief of hemorrhoids and ulcers. The Greek physician Dioscorides, writing in the 1st century AD, noted that the plant blisters the skin, treats scabies and infected nails, and has a "watery virtue." In 1652, the herbalist Nicholas Culpeper recounted the medieval belief that simply carrying lesser celandine on one's person was sufficient to cure hemorrhoids.

MEDICINAL ACTIONS & USES Lesser celandine makes a useful ointment or suppository for treating hemorrhoids.

RELATED SPECIES Various other *Ranunculus* species have been used in herbal medicine, even though all are toxic and irritant to a greater or lesser degree. In North America, the Meskawi people used the flowers and stigma of the yellow water crowfoot (*R. delphinifolius*) as a snuff to provoke sneezing, and mixed it with other herbs to treat respiratory conditions such as mucus and nasal congestion.

CAUTION Do not take lesser celandine orally.

SELF-HELP USE Hemorrhoids, p. 302.

LESSER CELANDINE is used fresh in ointments and suppositories to treat hemorrhoids.

Raphanus sativus
(Cruciferae)
RADISH

DESCRIPTION Bristly annual growing to about 3 ft (1 m). Has a swollen tap root, deeply cut compound leaves, pale violet to lilac flowers, and cylindrical seed pods.

HABITAT & CULTIVATION Radish is believed to be native to southern Asia. Cultivated varieties are grown around the world as vegetables and for medicinal use. The root is unearthed in autumn.

PART USED Root.

CONSTITUENTS Radish contains glucosilinates, which yield a volatile oil, raphanin, and vitamin C. Raphanin has antibiotic properties.

HISTORY & FOLKLORE Herodotus (*c.* 485–*c.* 425 BC) wrote that the builders of the pyramids in ancient Egypt were paid in radishes, onions, and garlic. In Egypt, the plant was used as a vegetable and a medicine. In ancient Rome, radish oil was applied to treat skin diseases. In China, radish was listed in the *Tang Materia Medica* (AD 659) as a digestive stimulant.

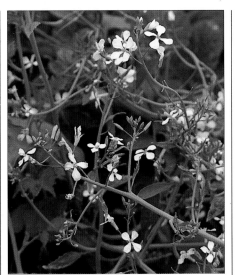

RADISH has been used since at least the 7th century to aid digestion.

MEDICINAL ACTIONS & USES Radish stimulates the appetite and digestion. The common red radish is eaten as a salad vegetable and an appetizer. The juice of the black radish is drunk to counter gassy indigestion and constipation. Black radish juice has a tonic and laxative action on the intestines and indirectly stimulates the flow of bile. Consuming radish generally results in improved digestion, but some people are sensitive to its acridity and robust action. In China, radish is eaten to relieve abdominal distension. The root is also prepared "dry-fried" to treat chest problems.

CAUTIONS Some people may suffer indigestion after consuming radish or its juice. Radish should not be taken by people suffering from gastritis, peptic ulcer, or thyroid conditions, and it should not be taken for more than 3–4 weeks at a time.

Rauvolfia serpentina
(Apocynaceae)

INDIAN SNAKEROOT,
SARPAGANDHA (HINDI)

DESCRIPTION Evergreen shrub growing to 3 ft (1 m). Has whorls of elliptical leaves, tiny pink and white tubular flowers, and glossy red berries.

HABITAT & CULTIVATION Indian snakeroot is native to much of southern and southeastern Asia, including India, Malaysia, and Indonesia. It is widely cultivated for medicinal use, notably in India and the Philippines. The root of plants at least 18 months old is unearthed in late winter.

PART USED Root.

CONSTITUENTS Indian snakeroot contains a complex mixture of indole alkaloids,

including reserpine, rescinnamine, ajmaline, and yohimbine. Ajmaline has been used to regulate heartbeat.

HISTORY & FOLKLORE Indian snakeroot is listed in the *Charaka Samhita*, the earliest Ayurvedic medical text (*c.* 700 BC). The plant has been used since at least that time to treat mental illness and insomnia. Indian snakeroot's status as a healing plant was first recorded in Europe in 1785, but it was not until 1946 that conventional Western medicine recognized the herb's efficacy. After that date, the whole plant, and its reserpine extract in particular, were widely used in conventional medicine to lower high blood pressure and lessen the symptoms of mental illness.

MEDICINAL ACTIONS & USES Indian snakeroot is useful in the treatment of high blood pressure and anxiety. The root has a pronounced sedative and depressant effect on the sympathetic nervous system. By reducing the system's activity, the herb brings about the lowering of blood pressure. It may also be used to treat anxiety and insomnia, as well as more serious mental health problems such as psychosis. Indian snakeroot is a slow-acting remedy, and it takes some time for its effect to become fully established.

RESEARCH Indian snakeroot and its alkaloids have been extensively researched since the 1930s. Despite concerns raised in the medical journal *The Lancet* in 1974, there is little evidence to show that the root has serious side effects at normal dosage.

RELATED SPECIES The West African species *R. vomitoria* is used as a sedative, aphrodisiac, and anticonvulsant in traditional African medicine.

CAUTIONS Take only under professional supervision. Indian snakeroot is subject to legal restrictions in some countries.

Rhamnus frangula
syn. *Frangula alnus*
(Rhamnaceae)

ALDER BUCKTHORN

DESCRIPTION Deciduous shrub or small tree growing to 15 ft (5 m). Has smooth brown bark, oval to elliptical leaves, white flowers, and small round berries ripening from yellow to black.

HABITAT & CULTIVATION Alder buckthorn grows in the northeastern parts of the US and in Europe (except for the Mediterranean region and the extreme north). It prefers marshy woodland. The bark of trees at least 3–4 years old is collected in late spring and early summer, and is dried and stored for at least 1 year before use.

PART USED Bark.

CONSTITUENTS Alder buckthorn contains

3–7% anthraquinones (including frangulin and emodin), anthrones, anthranols, an alkaloid (armepavine), tannins, and flavonoids. The anthrones and anthranols induce vomiting, but the severity of their effect lessens after long-term storage. The anthraquinones found in alder buckthorn and closely related species act on the wall of the colon, stimulating a bowel movement approximately 8–12 hours after ingestion.

HISTORY & FOLKLORE Common buckthorn (*R. catharticus*), a related plant with similar medicinal properties, "purgeth downwards both choler and flegm, and the watery humors of such as have the dropsie, and strengtheneth the inward parts again by binding," according to the 17th-century herbalist Nicholas Culpeper.

MEDICINAL ACTIONS & USES Alder buckthorn is a laxative and a cathartic, and is most commonly taken as a treatment for chronic constipation. Once dried and stored, it is significantly milder than senna (*Cassia senna*, p. 72) or common buckthorn (*R. catharticus*) and may be safely used over the long term to treat constipation and to encourage the return of regular bowel movements. Alder buckthorn is a particularly beneficial remedy if the muscles of the colon are weak and if there is poor bile flow. However, the plant should not be used to treat constipation resulting from excessive tension in the colon wall.

RELATED SPECIES Cascara sagrada (*R. purshiana*), which is native to Pacific North America, is used much like alder buckthorn. Common buckthorn, a European native, is today used mainly in veterinary medicine.

CAUTIONS Use only dried bark that has been stored for at least a year, since the fresh bark is violently purgative. The berries may also be harmful if eaten.

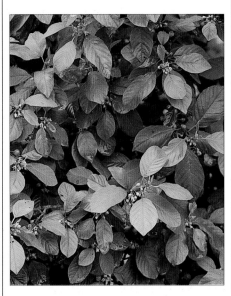

ALDER BUCKTHORN bark is toxic when fresh but is safe to use once dried and stored for a year.

Rhus glabra
(Anacardiaceae)
SMOOTH SUMAC

DESCRIPTION Deciduous shrub growing to a height of about 6 ft (2 m). Has straggling branches, compound leaves in pairs, large clusters of greenish-red flowers and downy deep red berries.

HABITAT & CULTIVATION Native to North America, smooth sumac is found on the borders of woods, along fences and roadsides and in neglected sites. The root bark is collected in autumn, the berries when ripe in late summer.

PARTS USED Root bark, berries.

CONSTITUENTS Smooth sumac contains tannins. Its other constituents are unknown.

HISTORY & FOLKLORE Indigenous peoples across North America used smooth sumac and closely related species to treat hemorrhoids, rectal bleeding, dysentery, venereal disease, and bleeding after childbirth. John Josselyn, a 17th-century New England naturalist, observed: "The English use to boyl [the plant] in beer, and drink it for colds; and so do the Indians, from whom the English had the medicine."

MEDICINAL ACTIONS & USES The astringent root bark of smooth sumac is often used as a decoction. It is taken to alleviate diarrhea and dysentery, applied externally to treat excessive vaginal discharge and skin eruptions, and used as a gargle for sore throats. The berries are diuretic, help reduce fever, and may be of use in late-onset diabetes. The berries are also astringent and can be used as a gargle for mouth and throat complaints.

RELATED SPECIES Sweet sumac (*R. aromatica*) has a similar range of uses. Poison ivy (*R. toxicodendron*) was formerly used in herbal medicine as a treatment for rheumatism, paralysis, and certain skin disorders. It is itself highly irritant to the skin and causes severe dermatitis.

Ribes nigrum
(Grossulariaceae)
BLACKCURRANT

DESCRIPTION Erect deciduous shrub growing to 5 ft (1.5 m). Has serrated, palm-shaped lobed leaves, small greenish white flowers and clusters of black berries.

HABITAT & CULTIVATION Blackcurrant is native to the temperate regions of Europe, western and central Asia, and the Himalayas. It is cultivated for its sour-sweet fruit. The leaves are gathered in early summer, the berries when ripe in mid- to late summer.

PARTS USED Leaves, berries.

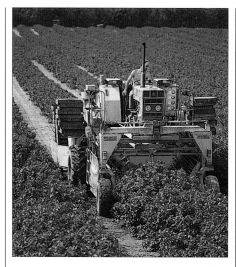

BLACKCURRANT fruit is harvested in summer. The juice is extremely rich in vitamin C.

CONSTITUENTS Blackcurrant leaves contain a volatile oil, tannins, and vitamin C; the berries contain anthocyanosides (about 0.3%), flavonoids, pectin, tannins, vitamin C, and potassium.

MEDICINAL ACTIONS & USES In Europe, blackcurrant leaves are used for their diuretic effect. By encouraging the elimination of fluid, the leaves help to reduce blood volume and thereby to lower blood pressure. The leaves are also used as a gargle for sore throats and canker sores. According to French investigators, blackcurrant leaves increase the secretion of cortisol by the adrenal glands, and thus stimulate the activity of the sympathetic nervous system. This action may prove useful in the treatment of stress-related conditions. Blackcurrant berries and their juice are high in vitamin C. They help improve resistance to infection and make a valuable remedy for treating colds and flu. According to the herbal authority R. F. Weiss, the juice is "as good as, if not better than, lemon juice (*Citrus limon*) for patients with pneumonia, influenza, etc." The juice also helps to stem diarrhea, and calms indigestion. Juice that is fresh or vacuum-sealed is more effective than concentrate.

Ricinus communis
(Euphorbiaceae)
CASTOR BEAN PLANT

DESCRIPTION Evergreen shrub growing to about 30 ft (10 m) in its natural state, but a much smaller annual when cultivated. Has large, palm-shaped leaves, green female flowers, and prickly red seed capsules.

HABITAT & CULTIVATION Castor bean plant is probably native to eastern Africa. It is cultivated in hot climates around the world, especially in Africa and southern Asia. The seed capsules are gathered throughout the year when nearly ripe and are then put out in the sun to mature.

PARTS USED Seed oil, seeds.

CONSTITUENTS The seeds contain 45–55% fixed oil, which consists mainly of glycerides of ricinoleic acid, ricin (a highly toxic protein), ricinine (an alkaloid), and lectins. The seeds are highly poisonous – 2 are sufficient to kill an adult – but the toxins do not pass into the expressed oil.

HISTORY & FOLKLORE Castor oil has been used medicinally for about 4,000 years. Until recently, it was given regularly to children "to help keep the system clear". Because to its unpleasant taste, castor oil is remembered as the bane of many childhoods.

MEDICINAL ACTIONS & USES Castor oil is well known for its strongly laxative (and, in higher doses, purgative) action, prompting a bowel movement about 3–5 hours after ingestion. The oil is so effective that it is regularly used to clear the digestive tract in cases of poisoning. Castor oil is well tolerated by the skin, and it is sometimes used as a vehicle for medicinal and cosmetic preparations. In India, the oil is massaged into the breasts after childbirth to stimulate milk flow. Indian herbalism uses a poultice of castor oil seeds to relieve swollen and tender joints. In China, the crushed seeds are used to treat facial palsy.

CAUTIONS Do not ingest the seeds, which are extremely poisonous. Do not take castor oil during pregnancy or more often than once every few weeks as a treatment for constipation.

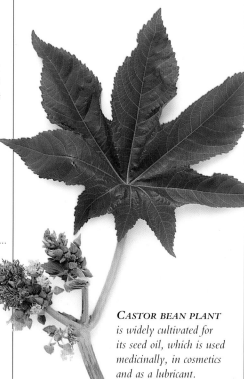

CASTOR BEAN PLANT *is widely cultivated for its seed oil, which is used medicinally, in cosmetics and as a lubricant.*

Rosa canina
(Rosaceae)
DOG ROSE

DESCRIPTION Climbing perennial growing to 10 ft (3 m). Has curved thorns, leaves with 2–3 pairs of toothed leaflets, pink or white flowers, and scarlet fruit (called "hips").

HABITAT & CULTIVATION Native to Europe, temperate areas of Asia, and North Africa, dog rose grows in hedgerows and in thickets and open areas. The fruit is picked in autumn.

PART USED Hips.

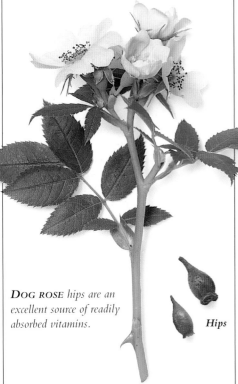

DOG ROSE hips are an excellent source of readily absorbed vitamins.

Hips

CONSTITUENTS Dog rose hips contain vitamins C (up to 1.25%), A, B_1, B_2, B_3 and K, flavonoids, tannins (2–3%), invert sugar, pectin, plant acids, polyphenols, carotenoids, volatile oil and vanillin.

HISTORY & FOLKLORE The hips of the dog rose were a popular sweetmeat in the Middle Ages. The plants were not esteemed to the same degree as were cultivated roses (*see R. gallica, following entry*), but dog rose was valued as the source of a widely used folk remedy for chest problems.

MEDICINAL ACTIONS & USES Dog rose hips have extremely high levels of vitamins. When consumed fresh, they provide vitamins and other nutrients in a form that is readily absorbed by the body. They are used to make rose hip syrup, a nourishing drink for young children. The tannin content of rose hips makes them a gentle remedy for diarrhea. The hips are mildly diuretic. Additionally, dog rose hips reduce thirst and alleviate gastric inflammation.

Rosa gallica
(Rosaceae)
ROSE

DESCRIPTION Deciduous shrub growing to about 5 ft (1.5 m). Has a smooth stem, sharp thorns, serrated leaves with 2–3 pairs of leaflets, semidouble deep pink or red flowers and scarlet hips.

HABITAT & CULTIVATION Native to the Middle East, the rose is not now found in the wild except as a garden escape. It has been cultivated for at least 3,000 years. The flowers are gathered in summer.

PARTS USED Flowers, essential oil.

CONSTITUENTS Rose contains a volatile oil consisting of geraniol, nerol, citronellol, geranic acid and other terpenes, and many other substances.

HISTORY & FOLKLORE The rose comes originally from Iran and has been cultivated there since antiquity. Sappho, the 6th-century BC Greek poet, described the red rose as the "queen of flowers". In Rome, it was much used in festivities, and the petals were consumed as food. Rosewater was prepared by the Arab physician Avicenna (AD 980–1037). During the Middle Ages and the Renaissance, the rose was esteemed as a remedy for depression.

MEDICINAL ACTIONS & USES The rose is not currently used in herbal medicine, but it is probably time for a re-evaluation of its medicinal benefits. The essential oil, called "attar of rose", is used in aromatherapy as a mildly sedative, antidepressant and anti-inflammatory remedy. Rose petals and their preparations have a similar action. They also help reduce high cholesterol levels. Rosewater is mildly astringent and makes a valuable lotion for inflamed and sore eyes.

CAUTION Do not take the essential oil internally without professional supervision.

Rubia tinctorum
(Rubiaceae)
MADDER

DESCRIPTION Evergreen perennial growing to 3 ft (1 m). Has whorls of finely toothed lance-shaped leaves, greenish white flowers and black berries containing 2 seeds.

HABITAT & CULTIVATION Madder is native to southern Europe, western Asia and North Africa. It flourishes in open areas, along roadsides, and amid rubble. The root is unearthed in autumn.

PART USED Root.

CONSTITUENTS Madder contains anthraquinone derivatives (including ruberythric acid, alizarin, and purpurin), an iridoid (asperuloside), resin, and calcium.

HISTORY & FOLKLORE Throughout history, madder has been used principally as a dye – its fermented root yields a strong red pigment that has been used to color fabric. In the ancient world, madder root was taken medicinally to treat jaundice, sciatica, and paralysis, and it was also used as a diuretic. The 18th-century Irish herbalist K'Eogh indicated that the herb was used in his day for a similar range of conditions: "The roots open obstructions of the liver and spleen, kidneys and womb … and provoke urine". When ingested, madder imparts its distinctive color to bones, milk, and urine. There can be little doubt that it owed much of its reputation as a diuretic to this property.

MEDICINAL ACTIONS & USES Madder fell largely out of use in the 19th century, and is now only rarely employed to treat kidney and bladder stones.

Rubus fruticosus
(Rosaceae)
BLACKBERRY

DESCRIPTION Sprawling, prickly shrub growing to 12 ft (4 m). Has palm-shaped leaves with 3–5 lobes, white to pale pink flowers, and clusters of black berries.

HABITAT & CULTIVATION *Fruit*
Native to temperate areas of Europe, blackberry is naturalized in the Americas and in Australia. It grows along roads, in open areas, and in woodland. The leaves are picked in summer, the berries in summer and autumn.

PARTS USED Leaves, berries.

CONSTITUENTS Blackberry leaves contain tannins, flavonoids, and gallic acid. The fruit contains anthocyanins, pectin, fruit acids, and vitamin C.

HISTORY & FOLKLORE In the 1st century AD, the physician Dioscorides recommended ripe blackberries in a gargle for sore throat. In European folk medicine, blackberry leaves have long been used for washing and staunching wounds. Arching blackberry runners that had rooted at both ends were credited with magical properties – in parts of England, children with hernias were pushed under arched runners for a magical cure.

MEDICINAL ACTIONS & USES Blackberry leaves are strongly astringent and may be used as a mouthwash to strengthen spongy gums and ease mouth ulcers, as a gargle for sore throats, and as a decoction to relieve diarrhea and hemorrhoids. The berries make a pleasant gargle for swallowing.

RELATED SPECIES See raspberry (*R. idaeus, following entry*).

Rubus idaeus
(Rosaceae)
RASPBERRY

DESCRIPTION Deciduous shrub growing to 6 ft (2 m). Has woody stems with prickles, pale green leaves with 3–7 leaflets, white flowers, and red berries.

HABITAT & CULTIVATION Native to Europe and Asia, raspberry now grows wild and is cultivated in many temperate regions. The leaves are collected in early summer, the fruit when ripe in summer.

PARTS USED Leaves, fruit.

CONSTITUENTS Raspberry leaves contain polypeptides, flavonoids, and tannins. The fruit contains pectin, fruit sugars, fruit acids, and vitamins A, B$_1$, and C.

HISTORY & FOLKLORE In 1735, the Irish herbalist K'Eogh described uses for raspberry flowers and fruit: "An application of the flowers bruised with honey is beneficial for inflammations of the eyes, burning fever and boils… The fruit is good for the heart and diseases of the mouth." Raspberry leaves have also been taken for centuries, often in the form of a tea, to help speed childbirth.

MEDICINAL ACTIONS & USES Raspberry leaves are still used to encourage easy labor. Although the specific mode of action is unknown, the leaves are thought to strengthen the longitudinal muscles of the uterus, increasing the force of contractions and thereby hastening childbirth. A decoction of raspberry leaves may be used to relieve diarrhea. The leaves also find use as an astringent external remedy – as an eyewash for conjunctivitis, a mouthwash for mouth problems, or a lotion for ulcers, wounds, or excessive vaginal discharge. The fruit is nutritious and mildly astringent.

CAUTION Do not take medicinally during the early stages of pregnancy.

SELF-HELP USE Preparing for childbirth, p. 317.

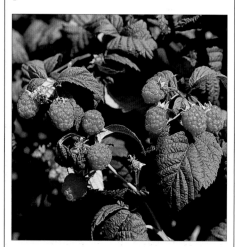

RASPBERRY leaves and fruit have been used since classical times as an astringent remedy.

Rumex acetosella
(Polygonaceae)
SHEEP'S SORREL

DESCRIPTION Slender, low-growing perennial. Has arrow-shaped leaves and terminal spikes bearing small green flowers that turn red as their seeds ripen.

HABITAT & CULTIVATION Sheep's sorrel is found in most temperate regions of the world. It grows in open areas and meadows, and is gathered in early summer.

PARTS USED Aerial parts.

CONSTITUENTS Sheep's sorrel contains oxalates and anthraquinones (including chrysophanol, emodin, and physcion). In isolation, the anthraquinones are irritant and have a laxative effect.

HISTORY & FOLKLORE Apart from its role as a salad vegetable, sheep's sorrel is an ingredient of an anticancer remedy known as essiac. A Native American formula, essiac also includes burdock (*Arctium lappa*, p. 62), slippery elm (*Ulmus rubra*, p. 144), and Chinese rhubarb (*Rheum palmatum*, p. 124). Western herbalists learned of it earlier in this century, after a Canadian nurse observed the recovery from breast cancer of a patient who had taken the formula. Essiac has since had a checkered history. Despite attempts to initiate proper clinical trials, none has yet been undertaken.

MEDICINAL ACTIONS & USES Sheep's sorrel is a detoxifying herb, the fresh juice having a pronounced diuretic effect. Like other members of the dock family, it is mildly laxative and holds out potential as a long-term treatment for chronic disease, in particular that of the gastrointestinal tract.

RELATED SPECIES Sorrel (*R. acetosa*) is a European relative that is also taken for its detoxifying effect. *See also* yellow dock (*R. crispus*, p. 126) and Chinese rhubarb (*Rheum palmatum*, p. 124).

CAUTION Sheep's sorrel should not be taken by people who tend to develop kidney stones.

Ruscus aculeatus
(Liliaceae)
BUTCHER'S BROOM

DESCRIPTION Bushy evergreen perennial growing to 3 ft (1 m). Has leaflike leathery branches with a terminal spine, greenish white flowers, and shiny red berries.

HABITAT & CULTIVATION Butcher's broom is found throughout much of Europe, western Asia, and North Africa. It is a protected species, growing wild in woodland and on uncultivated ground. Cultivated plants are gathered in autumn, when in fruit.

PARTS USED Aerial parts, rhizome.

CONSTITUENTS Butcher's broom contains saponin glycosides, including ruscogenin and neoruscogenin. These constituents have a structure similar to that of diosgenin, found in wild yam (*Dioscorea villosa*, p. 89). They are anti-inflammatory and cause the contraction of blood vessels, especially veins.

HISTORY & FOLKLORE Much used in antiquity, butcher's broom was described by the 1st-century AD Greek physician Dioscorides as having the ability to promote urine flow and menstrual bleeding. He also considered the herb useful for treating bladder stones, jaundice, and headache. The plant's name comes from its use as a broom in butchers' shops in Europe up until the 20th century.

MEDICINAL ACTIONS & USES Butcher's broom is not used much today, but, in view of its positive effect on varicose veins and hemorrhoids, it could be due for a revival. In the European tradition, both the aerial parts and the rhizome are considered to be diuretic and mildly laxative.

CAUTION Do not take butcher's broom if suffering from high blood pressure.

Ruta graveolens
(Rutaceae)
RUE

DESCRIPTION Strongly aromatic, evergreen perennial growing to 3 ft (1 m). Has fleshy 3-lobed leaves, yellow-green 5-petaled flowers, and round seed capsules.

HABITAT & CULTIVATION Rue grows in the Mediterranean region, preferring open, sunny sites. It is also cultivated in many parts of the world as both a garden ornamental and a medicinal plant. The aerial parts are gathered in summer.

PARTS USED Aerial parts.

CONSTITUENTS Rue contains about 0.5% volatile oil (including 50–90% 2-undecanone), flavonoids (including rutin), furanocoumarins (including bergapten), about 1.4% furoquinoline alkaloids (including fagarine, skimmianine, arborinine, and others). Rutin has the effect of supporting and strengthening the inner lining of blood vessels and reducing blood pressure.

HISTORY & FOLKLORE In ancient Greece and Egypt, rue was employed to stimulate menstrual bleeding, to induce abortion, and to strengthen the eyesight.

MEDICINAL ACTIONS & USES Rue is chiefly used to encourage the onset of menstruation. It stimulates the muscles of the uterus and promotes menstrual blood flow. In European herbal medicine, rue has also been taken to treat conditions as varied as hysteria, epilepsy, vertigo, colic, intestinal worms, poisoning,

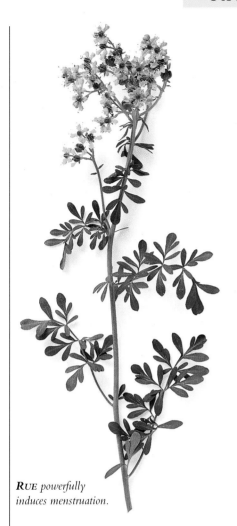

RUE powerfully induces menstruation.

and eye problems. The latter use is well founded since an infusion used as an eyewash brings quick relief to strained and tired eyes, and reputedly improves the eyesight. Rue has been used to treat many other conditions, including multiple sclerosis and Bell's palsy.

RELATED SPECIES The related species, *R. chalepensis*, which is also native to the Mediterranean region, is used to expel worms, to promote menstrual flow, and to soothe sore eyes.

CAUTIONS Rue is toxic if taken to excess. Never take during pregnancy. The fresh plant frequently causes dermatitis, so wear gloves while handling it. Taken internally, rue may cause an allergic skin reaction to sunlight.

Salvia sclarea
(Labiatae)
CLARY SAGE

DESCRIPTION Square-stemmed biennial growing to 3 ft (1 m). Has hairy wrinkled leaves and whorls of pale blue flowers.

HABITAT & CULTIVATION Native to southern Europe and the Middle East, clary sage is now cultivated in France and Russia for its essential oil. It prefers sunny conditions and dry soil. It is gathered in summer, usually in its second year.

PARTS USED Aerial parts, seeds, essential oil.

CONSTITUENTS Clary sage contains 0.1% volatile oil (consisting mainly of linalyl acetate and linalool), diterpenes, and tannins.

HISTORY & FOLKLORE Clary sage has been perceived both as a weaker version of its close relative, sage (*S. officinalis*, p. 130), and as a significant herb in its own right. Since the seeds were once commonly used to treat eye problems, it was also known as "clear eye." In 1652, the herbalist Nicholas Culpeper recommended a decoction of the seeds to draw out splinters and thorns.

MEDICINAL ACTIONS & USES An antispasmodic and aromatic plant, clary sage is used today mainly to treat digestive problems such as gas and indigestion. It is also regarded as a tonic, calming herb that helps relieve menstrual pain and premenstrual problems. Because of its estrogen-stimulating action, clary sage is most effective when levels of this hormone are low. The plant can therefore be a valuable remedy for complaints associated with menopause, particularly hot flashes.

CAUTIONS Do not take the essential oil internally. Do not use clary sage during pregnancy.

Sanguinaria canadensis
(Papaveraceae)
BLOODROOT

DESCRIPTION Perennial plant growing to 6 in (15 cm). Has palm-shaped leaves and solitary flower stems bearing attractive white flowers with 8–12 petals.

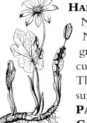

Bloodroot

HABITAT & CULTIVATION Native to northeastern North America, bloodroot grows in shady woods. It is cultivated as a garden plant. The rhizome is unearthed in summer or autumn.

PART USED Rhizome.

CONSTITUENTS Bloodroot contains isoquinoline alkaloids, notably sanguinarine (1%), and many others, including berberine. Sanguinarine is a strongly expectorant substance that also has antiseptic and local anesthetic properties.

HISTORY & FOLKLORE Bloodroot was a traditional remedy of Native Americans, who used it to treat fevers and rheumatism, to induce vomiting, and as an element in divination. The rhizome's bright red juice has been used as a rouge. From 1820 to 1926, bloodroot was listed as an expectorant in the *Pharmacopoeia of the United States*.

MEDICINAL ACTIONS & USES In contemporary herbal medicine, bloodroot is chiefly employed as an expectorant, promoting coughing and the clearing of mucus from the respiratory tract. The plant is prescribed for chronic bronchitis and – since it also has an antispasmodic effect – for asthma and whooping cough. Bloodroot may also be used as a gargle for sore throats, and as a wash or ointment for fungal and viral skin conditions such as athlete's foot and warts. Prepared as a powder, bloodroot may be sniffed to treat nasal polyps.

CAUTIONS Take only under professional supervision and do not exceed the dose. Bloodroot induces vomiting in all but very small doses, and in excessive doses it is toxic. Do not take during pregnancy, while breast-feeding, or if suffering from glaucoma.

Sanguisorba officinalis syn. *Poterium officinalis*
(Rosaceae)
GREATER BURNET

DESCRIPTION Perennial herb growing to 2 ft (60 cm). Has long-stalked compound leaves with 13 leaflets and purple flowers.

HABITAT & CULTIVATION Native to Europe, North Africa, and temperate regions of Asia, greater burnet flourishes in damp pastures, especially in mountainous regions. It is cultivated as a fodder crop and as a salad vegetable, and is gathered in summer.

PARTS USED Aerial parts, root.

CONSTITUENTS Greater burnet contains tannins, including sanguisorbic acid, dilactone (a phenolic acid), and gum.

HISTORY & FOLKLORE In Europe, greater burnet has long been used as a fodder for animals and as an ingredient in beer-making. As its Latin name implies, it has also been used as a wound healer: *sanguis* means "blood"; *sorbeo* means "I staunch." In Chinese medicine the herb has been used to staunch bleeding.

MEDICINAL ACTIONS & USES Greater burnet is still used to slow or arrest blood flow. In both the Chinese and European traditions, it is taken internally to treat heavy periods and uterine hemorrhage. Externally, a lotion or ointment may be used for hemorrhoids, burns, wounds, and eczema. Greater burnet is also a valuable astringent and is employed for a variety of gastro-intestinal problems, including diarrhea, dysentery, and ulcerative colitis, particularly if accompanied by bleeding.

RESEARCH Chinese research indicates that the whole herb heals burns more effectively than the extracted tannins. Patients suffering from eczema showed marked improvement when treated with an ointment made from greater burnet root and petroleum jelly.

Sanicula europaea
(Umbelliferae)
SANICLE

DESCRIPTION Perennial growing to 16 in (40 cm). Has long-stalked, palm-shaped, shiny leaves, with clusters of pale pink to greenish white flowers.

HABITAT & CULTIVATION Found throughout most of Europe and western and central Asia, sanicle is common in woodland areas, particularly in damp, shady sites. It is collected in summer.

PARTS USED Aerial parts.

CONSTITUENTS Sanicle contains up to 13% saponins, allantoin, a volatile oil, tannins, chlorogenic and rosmarinic acid, mucilage, and vitamin C. Allantoin increases the healing rate of damaged tissue. Rosmarinic acid is anti-inflammatory.

HISTORY & FOLKLORE Hildegard of Bingen (1098–1179) wrote the earliest extant description of sanicle's use in healing wounds. During the 15th and 16th centuries sanicle became a popular herbal medicine. The 17th-century English herbalist Nicholas Culpeper wrote of sanicle's ability "to heal all green wounds speedily, or any ulcer, imposthumes, or bleedings inwardly," and compared its benefits to those of comfrey (*Symphytum officinale*, p. 136) and self-heal (*Prunella vulgaris*, p. 122).

MEDICINAL ACTIONS & USES With its longstanding reputation for healing wounds and treating internal bleeding, sanicle is a potentially valuable plant, but it is not used much in contemporary herbal medicine. Sanicle may be used to treat bleeding within the stomach or intestines, the coughing up of blood, and nosebleeds. It may also be of use in treating diarrhea and dysentery, bronchial and congestive problems, and sore throats. This herb is traditionally thought to be detoxifying and has also been taken internally for skin problems. Externally, sanicle may be applied as a poultice or ointment for wounds, burns, chilblains, hemorrhoids, and inflamed skin.

Santalum album
(Santalaceae)
SANDALWOOD, CHANDAN

DESCRIPTION Semiparasitic, evergreen tree growing to 30 ft (10 m). Has lance-shaped leaves, clusters of pale yellow to purple flowers, and small, nearly black fruit.

HABITAT & CULTIVATION Native to eastern India, sandalwood is cultivated in Southeast Asia for its wood and essential oil. The trees are felled throughout the year.

PARTS USED Wood, essential oil.

CONSTITUENTS Sandalwood contains 3–6% volatile oil (which consists predominantly of the sesquiterpenols alpha- and beta-santalol), resin, and tannins.

HISTORY & FOLKLORE Sandalwood's aroma has been highly esteemed in China and India for thousands of years. The wood is frequently burned as incense and plays a part in Hindu ritual. The heartwood is most often used in perfumery, but has been taken as a remedy in China since about AD 500.

Sandalwood

MEDICINAL ACTIONS & USES Sandalwood and its essential oil are used for their antiseptic properties in treating genitourinary conditions such as cystitis and gonorrhea. In Ayurvedic medicine, a paste of the wood is used to soothe rashes and itchy skin. In China, sandalwood is held to be useful for chest and abdominal pain.

CAUTION Do not take sandalwood essential oil internally.

Saponaria officinalis
(Caryophyllaceae)
SOAPWORT

DESCRIPTION Perennial growing to a height of 3 ft (1 m). Has lance-shaped leaves and clusters of delicate

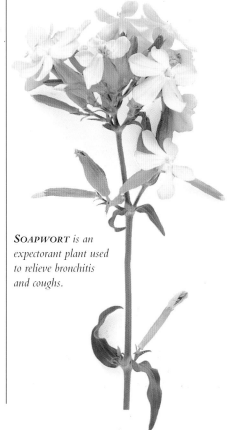

SOAPWORT is an expectorant plant used to relieve bronchitis and coughs.

5-petaled tubular pink flowers.

HABITAT & CULTIVATION Native to temperate regions of Europe, Asia, and North America, soapwort thrives in open woodland areas and on railroad embankments. It has been widely cultivated as a garden plant. The herb is gathered while in flower in summer, and the root is unearthed in autumn.

PARTS USED Root, aerial parts.

CONSTITUENTS All parts of soapwort contain saponins (around 5%), resin, and a small quantity of volatile oil.

HISTORY & FOLKLORE Soapwort has mostly been used as a substitute for soap, especially in washing clothes. The 1st-century AD Greek physician Dioscorides may have had soapwort in mind when he described a plant used for washing wool. He claimed that the plant's roots were diuretic and expectorant, and that it was taken to treat coughs, asthma, and "passions of the liver." Boerhaave (1668–1738), a Dutch physician, recommended soapwort as a treatment for jaundice.

MEDICINAL ACTIONS & USES Soapwort's main internal use is as an expectorant. Its strongly irritant action within the gut is thought to stimulate the cough reflex and increase the production of a more fluid mucus within the respiratory passages. Consequently, the plant is prescribed for the treatment of bronchitis, coughs, and some cases of asthma. Soapwort may be taken for other problems, including rheumatic and arthritic pain. A decoction of the root and, to a lesser extent, an infusion of the aerial parts of the herb make soothing washes for eczema and other itchy skin conditions.

CAUTIONS Soapwort is potentially toxic. Take internally only under professional supervision.

Sargassum fusiforme
(Sargassaceae)
HAI ZAO

DESCRIPTION Brown seaweed (alga) with long, thin fronds.

HABITAT & CULTIVATION *Hai zao* is found along the coastlines of China and Japan, where it is often seen floating in large masses. It is gathered from the sea and shore throughout the year.

PART USED Whole plant.

CONSTITUENTS *Hai zao* contains alginic acid, mannitol, potassium, and iodine.

HISTORY & FOLKLORE Wang Tao, an 8th-century Chinese physician, recommended *hai zao* for goiter (an enlargement of the thyroid gland due to iodine deficiency). *Hai zao* is eaten as a vegetable in Chinese and Japanese cuisine.

MEDICINAL ACTIONS & USES *Hai zao* is

used in a similar way to its European counterpart, kelp (*Fucus vesiculosus*, p. 211). In Chinese medicine, it is given principally to treat thyroid problems caused by low iodine levels within the body. The herb also helps to combat other thyroid conditions that produce enlargement of the gland, for example Hashimoto's thyroiditis. *Hai zao* is prescribed to treat cases of scrofula (enlargement of the lymph glands in the neck due to tubercular infection) and edema (fluid retention).

RESEARCH Chinese research indicates that *hai zao* has antifungal and moderately anticoagulant actions.

RELATED SPECIES In Chinese medicine, *S. fusiforme* is used interchangeably with *S. pallidum*.

CAUTION Do not take *hai zao* for thyroid problems except under professional supervision.

Sarothamnus scoparius syn. *Cytisus scoparius*
(Leguminosae)
BROOM

DESCRIPTION Tall deciduous shrub growing to a height of 6 ft (2 m). Has narrow ridged stems, small trefoil leaves, and bright yellow

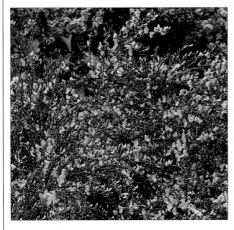

BROOM, taken under professional guidance, helps to regulate an overly rapid heartbeat.

flowers in leafy terminal spikes.

HABITAT & CULTIVATION Native to Europe, broom is commonly found on heaths, along roadsides, and in open woodland. It is naturalized in many temperate regions, including in the US. The flowering tops are gathered from spring to autumn.

PARTS USED Flowering tops.

CONSTITUENTS Broom contains quinolizidine alkaloids (particularly sparteine and lupanine), phenethylamines, isoflavones, flavonoids, a volatile oil, caffeic and p-coumaric acids, tannins, and pigments. Sparteine reduces the heart rate, and the

isoflavones are estrogenic.

HISTORY & FOLKLORE Both the common and species names of this plant indicate its usefulness as a sweeper (*scopa* means "broom" in Latin). Broom's medicinal value is not mentioned in classical writings, but it does appear in medieval herbals. The 12th-century *Physicians of Myddfai* recommended broom as a means to treat suppressed urine: "Seek broom seed, and grind into fine powder, mix with drink and let it be drank. Do this till you are quite well." The Plantagenet kings of England are so named because of their adoption of a sprig of broom (in Latin, *planta genista*) as a heraldic device. Broom tops have been pickled and used as a condiment similar to capers (*Capparis spinosa*, p. 180).

MEDICINAL ACTIONS & USES Broom is used mainly as a remedy for an irregular, fast heartbeat. The plant acts on the electrical conductivity of the heart, slowing and regulating the transmission of the impulses. Broom is also strongly diuretic, stimulating urine production and thus countering fluid retention. Since broom causes the muscles of the uterus to contract, it has been used to prevent blood loss after childbirth.

CAUTIONS Take broom internally only under professional supervision. Do not take during pregnancy or if suffering from high blood pressure. The plant is subject to legal restrictions in some countries.

Satureja montana
(Labiatae)
WINTER SAVORY

DESCRIPTION Semievergreen aromatic herb growing to 16 in (40 cm). Has lance-shaped leaves and clusters of white-pink flowers.

HABITAT & CULTIVATION Native to southern Europe, winter savory thrives in sunny, well-drained sites. It is commonly cultivated as a garden herb. The flowering tops are collected in summer.

PARTS USED Flowering tops, essential oil.

CONSTITUENTS Winter savory contains about 1.6% volatile oil, composed mainly of carvacrol, p-cymene, linalool, and thymol.

HISTORY & FOLKLORE Winter savory was classified as "heating and drying" by the classical physicians Dioscorides and Galen, and was thought to have therapeutic benefits similar to those of thyme (*Thymus vulgaris*, p. 142).

MEDICINAL ACTIONS & USES Winter savory is most often used in cookery, but it also has marked medicinal benefits. It settles gas and stimulates the digestion, helping to alleviate flatulence and colic. It is warming and has been taken as a remedy for chest

infections and bronchitis. The essential oil is strongly antibacterial and may be used to treat candidiasis and other fungal conditions.

RELATED SPECIES Summer savory (*S. hortensis*) is a similar annual herb that has a milder essential oil. Calamint (*Calamintha ascendens*, p. 179) is another close relative.

CAUTIONS Do not take the essential oil internally without professional supervision. Do not take winter savory during pregnancy.

WINTER SAVORY helps to alleviate flatulence, indigestion, and colic.

Saussurea lappa syn. *S. costus*
(Compositae)
KUTH

DESCRIPTION Upright perennial herb growing to 10 ft (3 m). Has heart-shaped leaves and blue-black flower heads.

HABITAT & CULTIVATION Native to the Indian subcontinent, kuth is most commonly found in mountainous areas of Kashmir. The root is gathered in autumn.

PARTS USED Root, essential oil.

CONSTITUENTS Kuth contains a volatile oil (consisting of terpenes, sesquiterpenes, and aplotaxene), an alkaloid (saussarine), and a resin. Saussarine depresses the parasympathetic nervous system.

HISTORY & FOLKLORE Kuth root has been used in Indian medicine for at least 2,500 years. It has also been exported to China and the Middle East. The fragrant root is often used in perfumery. In India, it is valued as an aphrodisiac and for its reputed ability to prevent gray hair.

MEDICINAL ACTIONS & USES Kuth is used in the Ayurvedic and Unani Tibb traditions in India for its tonic, stimulant, and antiseptic properties. The root is commonly taken, with other herbs, for respiratory system problems such as bronchitis, asthma, and coughs. It is also used to treat cholera.

CAUTION Do not take kuth essential oil internally.

OTHER MEDICINAL PLANTS

Schizonepeta tenuifolia
(Labiatae)
JING JIE

DESCRIPTION Perennial plant growing to 25 ft (8 m) with upright square stems, lance-shaped leaves, and whorls of small flowers.

HABITAT & CULTIVATION Native to the Far East, *jing jie* is widely cultivated in eastern China. The aerial parts of the plant are gathered in autumn.

PARTS USED Aerial parts.

CONSTITUENTS *Jing jie* contains a volatile oil, the main constituents of which are menthone and limonene.

MEDICINAL ACTIONS & USES In the Chinese tradition, *jing jie* is valued as an aromatic and warming herb. It is taken to alleviate skin conditions such as boils and itchiness. *Jing jie* also induces sweating and is used to treat fever and chills and as a remedy for measles. It is often combined with *bo he* (*Mentha haplocalyx*, p. 232).

RESEARCH Chinese studies have confirmed *jing jie's* ability to increase blood flow in the vessels just beneath the skin.

Scolopendrium vulgare
(Polypodiaceae)
HARTSTONGUE

DESCRIPTION Evergreen fern growing to 2 ft (60 cm). Has long tongue-shaped fronds with twin rows of spores on the underside.

HABITAT & CULTIVATION Hartstongue is found throughout much of Europe, North Africa, East Asia, and North America. It prefers shaded sites in woodland and on banks and walls. The fronds are gathered throughout the summer.

PARTS USED Fronds.

CONSTITUENTS Hartstongue contains

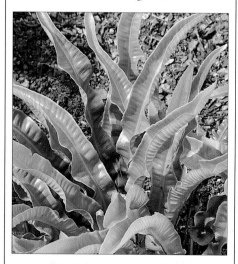

HARTSTONGUE is found growing in shady woodland sites across the northern hemisphere.

tannins, mucilage, and flavonoids (including leucodelphidin).

HISTORY & FOLKLORE Hartstongue has been prescribed as a treatment for diarrhea and dysentery for at least 2,000 years. In Wales and the Scottish Highlands, it was traditionally used as a poultice for wounds, scalds, and burns, and as an ointment for hemorrhoids. In Japan, the fronds were smoked by the Ainu people.

MEDICINAL ACTIONS & USES Hartstongue was valued in the past for its ability to heal wounds, but today it is employed chiefly as a mild astringent. It is sometimes used in the treatment of diarrhea and mucous colitis, and it may be of benefit to the liver and spleen. Hartstongue appears to have expectorant properties, and it is also mildly diuretic.

Scrophularia nodosa
(Scrophulariaceae)
FIGWORT

DESCRIPTION Upright perennial herb growing to 3 ft (1 m). Has a square stem, oval leaves, small round brown flowers in clusters, and green seed capsules.

HABITAT & CULTIVATION Native to Europe, Central Asia, and North America, figwort thrives in wet or damp places, in open woodland, on riverbanks, and along ditches. The herb is gathered in the summer while in flower.

PARTS USED Aerial parts.

CONSTITUENTS Figwort contains iridoids (including aucubin, harpagoside, and acetyl harpagide), flavonoids, cardioactive glycosides, and phenolic acids. Harpagoside and harpagide are thought to account for its antiarthritic activity.

HISTORY & FOLKLORE Figwort's genus name, *Scrophularia*, alludes to the plant's age-old use as a treatment for scrofula. In this condition, the lymph nodes of the neck, infected with tuberculosis, swell to form hard, protruding lumps beneath the skin. Figwort root resembles these swollen glands, and therefore, according to the Doctrine of Signatures (which holds that a plant's appearance indicates the ailments it treats), the herb was considered to be an appropriate remedy for treating scrofula. Indeed, in the 16th and 17th centuries, figwort was esteemed as the best medicinal plant for relieving all kinds of swellings and tumors.

MEDICINAL ACTIONS & USES Figwort is an herb that supports detoxification of the body and may be used as a treatment for various types of skin conditions. Taken internally as an infusion or applied externally, figwort is of value in treating chronic skin diseases such as eczema and psoriasis. Applied externally, it will also help speed

the healing of burns, wounds, hemorrhoids, and ulcers. Figwort's traditional use as a treatment for swellings and tumors continues in Europe to this day. The herb is also mildly diuretic, and it is reputed to be effective when used to expel worms.

RELATED SPECIES Water figwort (*S. aquatica*), another plant that is native to Europe, has similar properties, as does the American *S. marylandica*. In China, *S. ningopoensis* is used to treat infections and to clear toxicity.

CAUTION Do not take figwort if suffering from a heart condition.

Selenicereus grandiflorus
(Cactaceae)
NIGHT-BLOOMING CEREUS

DESCRIPTION Climbing multibranched perennial cactus with upright cylindrical stems and aerial roots. Produces large flower buds opening into night-blooming white flowers that grow to 8 in (20 cm) across, and red oval fruit.

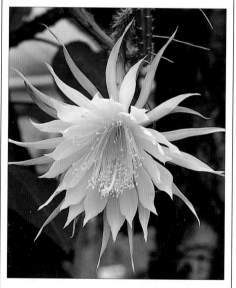

NIGHT-BLOOMING CEREUS has spectacular flowers that open at dusk and close at dawn.

HABITAT & CULTIVATION Native to Mexico and Central America, night-blooming cereus is now rarely found in the wild. It is cultivated both as an ornamental and a medicinal plant. The flowers and young stems are gathered in summer.

PARTS USED Flowers, young stems.

CONSTITUENTS Night-blooming cereus contains alkaloids (including cactine), flavonoids (isorhamnetin), and a pigment. Cactine's cardiotonic effect is considered similar to that of cardiac glycosides (see foxglove, *Digitalis* species, p. 199).

MEDICINAL ACTIONS & USES Since it is in short supply, night-blooming cereus is not used much at present, but it is a valuable remedy for the heart. It stimulates the action of the heart, increasing the strength of contractions while slowing heart rate. It is prescribed for various conditions, including angina and low blood pressure, and is often given as a tonic during recovery from a heart attack. In the Caribbean, the juice of the whole plant is used to expel worms, and the stems and flowers are used in the treatment of rheumatism.

CAUTIONS Take only under professional supervision. Excessive doses may cause stomach upset and hallucinations.

Sempervivum tectorum
(Crassulaceae)
HEN-AND-CHICKS,
HOUSELEEK

DESCRIPTION Succulent perennial growing to 4 in (10 cm). Has round rosettes of leaves and flowering stems bearing clusters of bell-shaped red flowers.

HABITAT & CULTIVATION This plant is native to central and southern Europe and now grows wild in northern Europe, North Africa, and western Asia, preferring sandy, dry soil. It is widely cultivated as a garden plant. The leaves are picked in summer.

PARTS USED Leaves, leaf juice.

CONSTITUENTS Hen-and-chicks contains tannins, mucilage, and malic and formic acid.

HISTORY & FOLKLORE The Frankish King Charlemagne (AD 742–814) told his subjects to plant hen-and-chicks on their roofs since the plant reputedly warded off lightning and fire. The plant's genus name, *Sempervivum* (forever living), refers to its hardiness.

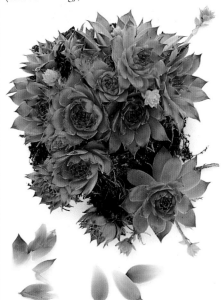

HEN-AND-CHICKS' succulent leaves contain tannins and mucilage, both soothing to the skin.

MEDICINAL ACTIONS & USES Hen-and-chicks leaves and their juice are used for their cooling and astringent effect, being applied externally to soothe many skin conditions, including burns, wounds, boils, and corns. Traditionally, the leaves have been chewed to relieve toothache, and the juice has been sniffed to stop nosebleeds. Hen-and-chicks is still used externally, but internal use is not advised because in large doses it induces vomiting.

CAUTION Do not take this plant internally.

Senecio aureus
(Compositae)
LIFEROOT, SQUAW WEED

DESCRIPTION Upright perennial growing to 3 ft (1 m). Has lance-shaped leaves and clusters of yellow daisy-type flowers.

HABITAT & CULTIVATION Native to eastern North America, liferoot is found in marshes, on damp ground, and on riverbanks. The aerial parts are gathered in summer.

PARTS USED Aerial parts.

CONSTITUENTS Liferoot contains a volatile oil, pyrrolizidine alkaloids (including senecine, senecionine, and otosenine), tannins, and resin. In isolation, the pyrrolizidine alkaloids are highly toxic to the liver.

HISTORY & FOLKLORE The North American Catawba people used liferoot to treat gynecological problems in general and to relieve labor pains in particular.

MEDICINAL ACTIONS & USES Until recently, liferoot was employed in Anglo-American herbalism much as it was in earlier times – as a means to induce menstrual periods and to bring relief to menopausal complaints. Today, the plant is recommended only for external use as a douche for excessive vaginal discharge.

RELATED SPECIES *See* ragwort (*S. jacobaea, following entry*).

CAUTIONS Do not take liferoot internally. The plant is subject to legal restrictions in some countries.

Senecio jacobaea
(Compositae)
RAGWORT

DESCRIPTION Biennial or perennial plant growing to about 3 ft (1 m). Has lobed compound leaves and dense clusters of bright yellow daisy-type flowers.

HABITAT & CULTIVATION Ragwort is native to much of Asia, Europe, and North Africa, and is naturalized in North America

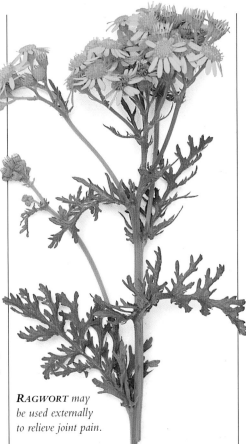

RAGWORT may be used externally to relieve joint pain.

and Australia. It thrives in open grassland, meadows, and along roadsides. It is considered a noxious weed in many parts of the world. The aerial parts of the plant are collected in summer.

PARTS USED Aerial parts.

CONSTITUENTS Ragwort contains a volatile oil, pyrrolizidine alkaloids (including seneciphylline, senecionine, and jacoline), tannins, and resin. In isolation, pyrrolizidine alkaloids are highly toxic to the liver.

HISTORY & FOLKLORE Ragwort is highly poisonous to cattle and sheep, and is normally left alone by grazing animals. In the past, it was prescribed to help lower fever by inducing sweating.

MEDICINAL ACTIONS & USES Although no longer taken internally, ragwort still finds use as a poultice, ointment, or lotion applied to relieve pain and inflammation. Conditions treated by ragwort include rheumatism and rheumatoid arthritis, and neuralgic conditions such as sciatica.

RESEARCH Dutch research in 1994 showed that ragwort plants grown with reduced levels of light produce significantly lower levels of toxic pyrrolizidine alkaloids.

RELATED SPECIES Dusty miller (*S. cineraria*), a related species native to the Caribbean, is traditionally used as a treatment for cataracts. *See also* liferoot (*S. aureus, preceding entry*).

CAUTIONS Use only under professional supervision. Ragwort should not be taken internally nor applied to broken skin.

Sesamum indicum
(Pedaliaceae)
SESAME, HEI ZHI MA

DESCRIPTION Erect annual growing to 6 ft (2 m). Has lance-shaped to oval leaves, white, pink, or mauve flowers, and oblong seed capsules bearing many small gray seeds.

HABITAT & CULTIVATION Native to Africa, sesame is cultivated in tropical and subtropical areas around the world. The root is unearthed in summer; the seeds are collected after the seed capsules have turned brown-black.

PARTS USED Seeds, seed oil, root.

CONSTITUENTS The seeds are highly nutritious and contain 55% oil, comprising mainly unsaturated fats (about 43% each of oleic and linoleic acids), 26% protein, vitamins B_3 and E, folic acid, and minerals (especially calcium).

HISTORY & FOLKLORE Sesame was one of the plants found in the tomb of Tutankhamun (1370–1352 BC). In ancient Egypt, the seeds were eaten and also pressed to yield oil, which was burned in lamps and used to make ointments. Sesame has also been eaten and used in India and China for thousands of years.

MEDICINAL ACTIONS & USES Sesame is principally used as a food and flavoring agent in China, but it is also taken to redress "states of deficiency," especially those affecting the liver and kidneys. The seeds are prescribed for problems such as dizziness, tinnitus (ringing in the ears), and blurred vision (when due to anemia). Because of their lubricating effect within the digestive tract, the seeds are also considered a remedy for "dry" constipation. The seeds have a marked ability to stimulate breast-milk production. Sesame seed oil benefits the skin and is used as a base for cosmetics. A decoction of the root is used in various traditions to treat coughs and asthma.

RESEARCH In experiments undertaken using laboratory animals, sesame seeds have been shown to lower blood sugar levels and also to raise the levels of stored carbohydrates (glycogen).

Smilax spp.
(Liliaceae)
SARSAPARILLA

DESCRIPTION Perennial woody climber growing to 15 ft (5 m). Has broadly ovate leaves, tendrils, and small greenish flowers.

HABITAT & CULTIVATION Sarsaparilla species are found in tropical rainforests and in temperate regions in Asia and Australia. The root is gathered throughout the year.

PART USED Root.

CONSTITUENTS Sarsaparilla contains 1–3% steroidal saponins, phytosterols (including beta- and e-sitosterol), about 50% starch, resin, sarsapic acid, and minerals.

HISTORY & FOLKLORE Brought from the New World to Spain in 1563, sarsaparilla was heralded as a cure for syphilis, reportedly having been used in the Caribbean with some success. The claims, however, were grossly inflated, and the herb's popularity soon waned. In Mexico, the herb has traditionally been used to treat a variety of skin problems. Before it was replaced by artificial agents, sarsaparilla root was the original flavoring for root beer.

MEDICINAL ACTIONS & USES Sarsaparilla is anti-inflammatory and cleansing, and can bring relief to skin problems such as eczema, psoriasis, and itchiness, and help treat rheumatism, rheumatoid arthritis, and gout. It has a tonic and specifically testosterogenic action on the body, leading to increased muscle bulk, and it has a potential use for impotence. Sarsaparilla also has a progesterogenic action, making it beneficial in premenstrual problems, and debility and depression associated with menopause. In Mexico, the root is still frequently consumed for its reputed tonic and aphrodisiac properties. Native Amazonian peoples take sarsaparilla to improve virility and to treat menopausal problems.

RESEARCH Chinese tests indicate that sarsaparilla holds potential against leptospirosis, a rare disease transmitted to humans by rats. The root, in combination with five other herbs, was also tested as a treatment for syphilis. Reportedly, 90% of the acute cases subsequently cleared.

Solanum dulcamara
(Solanaceae)
COMMON NIGHTSHADE

DESCRIPTION Slender-stemmed, woody climber growing to 12 ft (4 m). Has deeply lobed oval leaves, dark purple flowers with yellow anthers, and scarlet oval berries.

HABITAT & CULTIVATION Native to Europe, North Africa, and northern Asia, this herb has been naturalized in North America. A common wayside plant, it flourishes in open areas. The twigs are collected in spring or autumn, and the root bark in autumn.

PARTS USED Twigs, root bark.

CONSTITUENTS Common nightshade contains steroidal alkaloids (including solasodine and soldulcamaridine), steroidal saponins, and about 10% tannins.

HISTORY & FOLKLORE In 1735, the Irish herbalist K'Eogh summarized its uses: "It has a hot, dry nature. A decoction in wine … opens obstructions of the liver and spleen, and is therefore good for jaundice. It also heals all internal wounds, bruises and ruptures, for it dissolves congealed blood, causing it to be passed by the urine." The Swedish botanist Carolus Linnaeus (1707–1778) considered common nightshade to be a valuable remedy for fever and also for inflammatory disorders.

MEDICINAL ACTIONS & USES This plant has stimulant, expectorant, diuretic, and detoxifying properties.

COMMON NIGHTSHADE treats skin problems.

It appears to be most effective taken internally to treat skin problems such as eczema, itchiness, psoriasis, and warts. A decoction of the twigs, applied as a wash, may also help to lessen the severity of these conditions. The herb may also be taken to relieve asthma, chronic bronchitis, and rheumatic conditions, including gout.

CAUTION Common nightshade is toxic in excess. Take only under professional care.

Solanum melongena
(Solanaceae)
EGGPLANT

DESCRIPTION An erect, herbaceous perennial growing to 28 in (70 cm). Has slightly wooly leaves, violet flowers, and large purple fruit.

HABITAT & CULTIVATION Native to India and Southeast Asia, the eggplant is now cultivated in many tropical areas and also grown under glass in cooler climates. The ripe fruit is gathered in summer or autumn.

PARTS USED Fruit, fruit juice, leaves.

CONSTITUENTS Eggplant contains proteins, carbohydrates, and vitamins A, B_1, B_2, and C.

HISTORY & FOLKLORE Eggplants have been cultivated as a food in southern and eastern Asia since ancient times.

MEDICINAL ACTIONS & USES Eggplant fruit lowers blood cholesterol levels, and it is suitable as part of a diet to help regulate high blood pressure. Although the fruit can be applied fresh as a poultice for hemorrhoids, it is more commonly used in the form of an oil or ointment. The fruit and its juice are effective diuretics. A soothing, emollient poultice for burns, abscesses, cold sores, and similar conditions can be made from eggplant leaves.

CAUTION Eggplant leaves are toxic and should only be used externally.

Solanum tuberosum
(Solanaceae)
POTATO

DESCRIPTION Perennial growing to 3 ft (1 m). Has branching stems with compound leaves, white or purple flowers, green berries, and swollen tubers (potatoes).

HABITAT & CULTIVATION Native to Chile, Bolivia, and Peru, the potato plant with its many varieties is cultivated around the world. The tuber is normally unearthed from autumn to early spring.

PART USED Tuber.

CONSTITUENTS Potato contains starch, large amounts of vitamins A, B_1, B_2, C, and K, minerals (especially potassium), and very small quantities of atropine alkaloids. One property of these alkaloids is the reduction of digestive secretions, including acids produced in the stomach.

HISTORY & FOLKLORE Many different potato species and varieties were cultivated by the Quechua and Aymara peoples of the central Andes. In the early 16th century, the potato was introduced into Europe by Spanish voyagers returning from the New World. It was not until the 18th century that the potato became a staple ingredient in the European diet. Although potato cooking water has no established medicinal benefit, it is reputedly good for cleaning silver.

MEDICINAL ACTIONS & USES Taken in moderation, potato juice can be helpful in the treatment of peptic ulcers, bringing relief from pain and acidity. The juice or the mashed pulp may be used externally to soothe painful joints, headache, backache, skin rashes, and hemorrhoids. Potato skins are used in India to treat swollen gums and to heal burns.

RELATED SPECIES The root of the Brazilian *S. insidiosum* is used as a diuretic and stomach-supporting remedy.

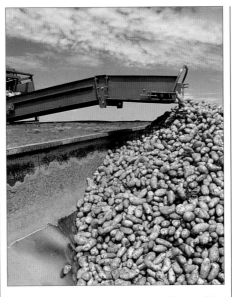

POTATO can be helpful in relieving the painful symptoms of a gastric ulcer.

CAUTIONS All parts of the plant except the tuber are poisonous. Excessive doses of potato juice are toxic. Do not drink the juice of more than one large potato per day.

Solanum xanthocarpum
(Solanaceae)
KANTAKARI

DESCRIPTION Prickly perennial growing to 3 ft (1 m) with many branches. Has oval leaves, purple flowers, and yellow fruit.

HABITAT & CULTIVATION Native to tropical Asia, kantakari prefers open areas. The leaves and root are gathered as needed; the seeds are gathered when mature.

PARTS USED Leaves, seeds, root.

CONSTITUENTS Kantakari contains steroidal alkaloids (including solanocarpine).

MEDICINAL ACTIONS & USES In the Ayurvedic tradition, kantakari leaves are taken to treat gas and constipation, and are made into a gargle for throat and gum disorders. The expectorant, anticongestive seeds may be taken to relieve asthma and to clear bronchial mucus. The root is used to treat snake and scorpion bites.

CAUTION Use kantakari only under professional supervision.

Solidago virgaurea
(Compositae)
GOLDENROD

DESCRIPTION Perennial plant growing to 28 in (70 cm). Has toothed leaves and branched spikes of golden yellow flowers.

HABITAT & CULTIVATION Native to Europe and Asia and naturalized in North America, goldenrod prefers open areas and hillsides. The plant is gathered in summer while in flower.

PARTS USED Aerial parts.

CONSTITUENTS Goldenrod contains saponins, diterpenes, phenolic glucosides, acetylenes, cinnamates, flavonoids, tannins, hydroxybenzoates, and inulin. The saponins are antifungal.

HISTORY & FOLKLORE The herbalist John Gerard wrote in 1597 that "goldenrod is extolled above all other herbes for the stopping of bloud in bleeding wounds."

MEDICINAL ACTIONS & USES Antioxidant, diuretic, and astringent, goldenrod is a valuable remedy for urinary tract disorders. It is used both for serious ailments such as nephritis and for more common problems like cystitis. The herb also reputedly helps flush out kidney and bladder stones. Goldenrod's saponins act specifically against the *Candida* fungus, the cause of yeast infections and oral thrush. The herb can also be taken for sore throats, chronic nasal congestion, and diarrhea. Due to its mild action, goldenrod is appropriate for treating gastroenteritis in children. It may be used as a mouthwash or douche for yeast infections.

RELATED SPECIES Canadian goldenrod (*S. canadensis*) has similar properties.

SELF-HELP USES Allergic rhinitis with mucus, p. 300; Urinary infections, p. 314.

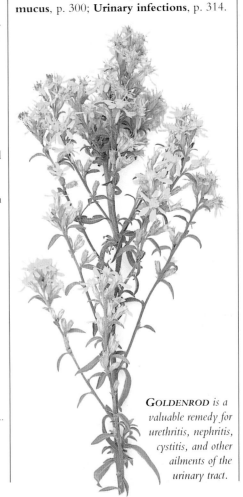

GOLDENROD is a valuable remedy for urethritis, nephritis, cystitis, and other ailments of the urinary tract.

Sorbus aucuparia
(Rosaceae)

EASTERN MOUNTAIN ASH, ROWAN

DESCRIPTION Deciduous tree growing to 40 ft (12 m). Has reddish bark, compound leaves, clusters of small white flowers, and clusters of round red-orange fruit (berries).

Mountain ash berries

HABITAT & CULTIVATION Mountain ash grows throughout the northern hemisphere, where it is found in woodland. It is also cultivated as an ornamental tree.

PART USED Fruit.

CONSTITUENTS The fruit contains tannins, sorbitol, malic and sorbic acids, sugars, and vitamin C. The seeds contain cyanogenic glycosides, which, in a reaction upon contact with water, produce the extremely poisonous prussic acid.

HISTORY & FOLKLORE In the Scottish Highlands, this tree was believed to be a reliable antidote to witchcraft. Highlanders planted it near their houses, and cowherds believed that by using an ash switch to drive their cattle, they could protect them from evil influences. The fruit has long been used to make preserves and alcoholic drinks.

MEDICINAL ACTIONS & USES The astringent berries are taken as a jam or an infusion to treat diarrhea and hemorrhoids. Infusions may also be used as a gargle for sore throats and as a wash for hemorrhoids and excessive vaginal discharge.

CAUTION Remove the toxic seeds prior to using the fruit as a medicine or a food.

Spigelia marilandica
(Loganiaceae)

PINKROOT

DESCRIPTION Perennial plant with oval to lance-shaped leaves, spikes of brilliant red-pink flowers, and a double seed capsule.

HABITAT & CULTIVATION Native to the southern regions of the US, pinkroot grows in dry, rich soil in woodland clearings and borders. The root is unearthed in autumn.

PART USED Root.

CONSTITUENTS Pinkroot contains alkaloids (mainly spigeleine), a volatile oil, tannin, and resin. Spigeleine is emetic and irritant to the stomach.

HISTORY & FOLKLORE Pinkroot was used extensively by Native Americans as a worm-expelling herb. It was gathered for trade with white settlers by the Creek and Cherokee

peoples. From the late 18th century onward, pinkroot became a major deworming herb in North America and Europe.

MEDICINAL ACTIONS & USES Pinkroot is used today solely to expel intestinal worms – particularly tapeworms and roundworms. It is prescribed with other herbs such as senna (*Cassia senna*, p. 72) and fennel (*Foeniculum vulgare*, p. 210) to ensure the elimination of both the worms and the root itself, which is potentially toxic if it is absorbed through the gut.

RELATED SPECIES Several *Spigelia* species act as worm-expelling herbs, for example *S. flemmingania*, native to Brazil, and *S. anthelmia*, native to the Caribbean, Venezuela, and Colombia. *S. anthelmia* also contains isoquinoline alkaloids and is used in the treatment of heart disease.

CAUTION Use pinkroot only under professional supervision.

Stachys officinalis
syn. *S. betonica*
(Labiatae)

BETONY

DESCRIPTION Mat-forming perennial growing to 2 ft (60 cm). Has toothed elliptical leaves and spikes of pink or white flowers.

HABITAT & CULTIVATION Betony grows throughout most of Europe and occurs in Asia as far east as the Caucasus. It prefers meadows, heathland, and hilly areas. The aerial parts are collected when the plant is in flower in early summer.

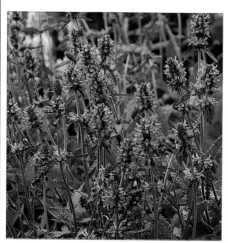

BETONY *is an age-old headache remedy. Its name may derive from the Celtic for "good head."*

PARTS USED Aerial parts.

CONSTITUENTS Betony contains alkaloids (including stachydrine, and betonicine), as well as betaine, choline, and tannins.

HISTORY & FOLKLORE Betony has been regarded as a panacea since classical times.

Antonius Musa, the physician to Emperor Augustus (63 BC–AD 14), claimed that betony would cure 47 different illnesses. The herb has always been particularly valued as a remedy for headaches.

MEDICINAL ACTIONS & USES No longer regarded as a panacea, betony nevertheless has real value as a remedy for headaches and facial pain. The plant is also mildly sedative, relieving nervous stress and tension. In British herbal medicine, betony is thought to improve nervous function and to counter overactivity. It is taken to treat "frayed nerves," premenstrual complaints, poor memory, and tension. The plant has astringent properties, and in combination with other herbs, such as comfrey (*Symphytum officinale*, p. 136) and linden flowers (*Tilia* species, p. 275), it is effective against sinus headaches and congestion. Betony may be taken alone or with yarrow (*Achillea millefolium*, p. 54) to help staunch nosebleeds. Betony is also mildly bitter. It stimulates the digestive system and the liver, and has an overall tonic effect on the body.

CAUTION Do not take betony during pregnancy.

Stellaria media
(Caryophyllaceae)

CHICKWEED

DESCRIPTION Sprawling perennial growing to about 6 in (15 cm). Has hairy stems, oval leaves, and starlike white flowers.

HABITAT & CULTIVATION Native to Europe and Asia, chickweed is now found in most regions of the world. It grows easily in open areas and is generally regarded as a troublesome weed. The plant is harvested in summer.

PARTS USED Aerial parts.

CONSTITUENTS Chickweed contains triterpenoid saponins, coumarins, flavonoids, carboxylic acids, and vitamin C. The saponins may account for the herb's ability to reduce itchiness.

HISTORY & FOLKLORE Dioscorides, a Greek physician writing in the 1st century AD, described chickweed's applications as follows: "It [chickweed] may usefully be applied with cornmeal for inflammation of the eyes. The juice may also be introduced into the ear in earache." Apart from its medicinal uses, chickweed is a tasty and nutritious vegetable.

MEDICINAL ACTIONS & USES Chickweed is chiefly used to treat irritated skin, being applied as juice, poultice, ointment, or cream. Chickweed may soothe severe itchiness where all other remedies have failed. It is often used to relieve eczema, varicose veins, and nettle rash (urticaria). An infusion of the fresh or dried plant may be added to a bath,

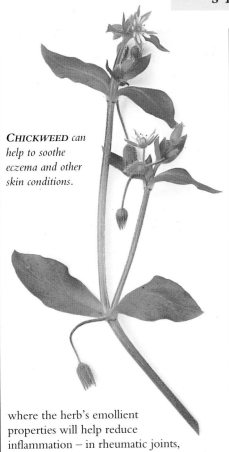

CHICKWEED can help to soothe eczema and other skin conditions.

where the herb's emollient properties will help reduce inflammation – in rheumatic joints, for example – and encourage tissue repair. Chickweed may also be taken internally to treat chest ailments. In small quantities, this herb also aids digestion.

CAUTIONS If taken in excessive doses, chickweed may cause diarrhea and vomiting. Do not take during pregnancy.

SELF-HELP USES Diaper rash & inflamed skin rashes, p. 318; **Eczema**, p. 300; **Nettle rash**, p. 303.

Stillingia sylvatica
(Euphorbiaceae)
QUEEN'S DELIGHT

DESCRIPTION Perennial growing to 4 ft (1.2 m). Has leathery leaves, yellow flowers without petals, and 3-lobed fruit.

HABITAT & CULTIVATION Queen's delight is native to the southeastern US, where it prefers sandy soils. The root is unearthed in autumn.

PART USED Root.

CONSTITUENTS Queen's delight contains alkaloids, diterpene esters, fixed oil, volatile oil, resin, and tannins. The fresh root is considered most active.

HISTORY & FOLKLORE Queen's delight was used by Native Americans as a purgative, a treatment for skin eruptions, and a remedy for venereal disease. Greek women who had just given birth took a decoction of the root or were bathed with an infusion. Queen's delight was included in the *Pharmacopoeia of*

the United States from 1831 to 1926.

MEDICINAL ACTIONS & USES Queen's delight appears to promote general detoxification. It is taken internally to help clear constipation, boils, weeping eczema, and scrofula (tubercular infection of the lymph glands of the neck). The fresh root is also taken for the treatment of bronchitis, laryngitis, and throat infection. Externally, it is applied in the form of a lotion to hemorrhoids and to itchy skin conditions such as eczema and psoriasis.

CAUTIONS Use only under professional supervision. Queen's delight is emetic and purgative in large doses.

Strophanthus kombe
(Apocynaceae)
STROPHANTHUS

DESCRIPTION Woody vine climbing to 30 ft (10 m). Has elliptical leaves, large yellow to white bell-shaped flowers, and long slender seed pods.

HABITAT & CULTIVATION Strophanthus is native to eastern Africa. It grows wild in rainforests and is commercially cultivated. The seeds are gathered when the pod is ripe.

PARTS USED Seeds.

CONSTITUENTS Strophanthus contains up to 10% cardiac glycosides. These slow the heart rate and improve the heart's efficiency. *See* foxglove (*Digitalis* species, p. 199).

HISTORY & FOLKLORE Strophanthus is a swift, sure poison, even in small doses. It has long been used as an arrow toxin in Africa.

MEDICINAL ACTIONS & USES Strophanthus may be prescribed like foxglove to treat heart disease, but strophanthus' active constituents are less well absorbed. One authority recommended it as a gentle heart tonic, of particular benefit when combined with valerian (*Valeriana officinalis*, p. 146) and deadly nightshade (*Atropa belladonna*, p. 66). Like most herbs containing cardiac glycosides, strophanthus is strongly diuretic.

RELATED SPECIES Two west African species, *S. gratus* and *S. hispidus*, have been used in Nigeria to treat snake bite. Both herbs have been investigated and have been shown to delay blood clotting.

CAUTION Strophanthus is potentially toxic. Use only under professional supervision.

Strychnos nux-vomica
(Loganiaceae)
NUX VOMICA

DESCRIPTION Evergreen tree growing to 50 ft (15 m). Has glossy oval leaves, tubular white flowers, and yellow fruit containing

5–8 disk-shaped seeds.

HABITAT & CULTIVATION Nux vomica is native to southeastern Asia. It grows wild and is cultivated commercially. The seeds are gathered when mature.

PARTS USED Seeds.

CONSTITUENTS Nux vomica contains 3% indole alkaloids (predominantly strychnine, with many others), loganin, chlorgenic acid, and fixed oil. Strychnine is a lethal poison, producing intense muscle spasms.

HISTORY & FOLKLORE Nux vomica seeds were first brought to Europe in the 15th century, probably as a poison for game and rodents. In 1640, the seeds were first used in European medicine, as a stimulant.

MEDICINAL ACTIONS & USES Though rarely used internally due to its toxicity, nux vomica can be an effective nervous system stimulant, particularly in the elderly. In Chinese herbal medicine the seeds are used externally to relieve pain, to treat various types of tumors, and to relieve paralysis, including Bell's palsy (facial paralysis). Nux vomica is a common homeopathic remedy prescribed mainly for digestive problems, sensitivity to cold, and irritability.

RESEARCH In a Chinese clinical trial, a paste made from nux vomica seeds was applied to 15,000 patients with Bell's palsy. The success rate more than 80% of the cases.

RELATED SPECIES Many *Strychnos* species are equally potent and have been used as arrow poisons – for example, *S. malaccensis* from Southeast Asia. A few others either produce edible fruits, like *S. unguacha*, native to tropical Africa, or are used medicinally – for instance, *S. ligustria*, native to Indonesia, which is used to treat fever, intestinal worms, and snake bite.

CAUTIONS Nux vomica and strychnine are subject to legal restrictions in most countries. Take nux vomica only in homeopathic preparations.

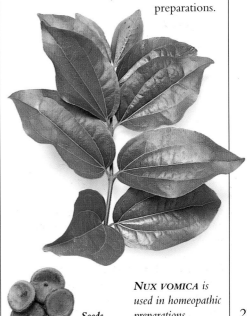

NUX VOMICA is used in homeopathic preparations.

Seeds

OTHER MEDICINAL PLANTS

Styrax benzoin
(Styraceae)
BENZOIN GUM

DESCRIPTION Shrubby deciduous tree growing to 28 ft (9 m). Has pointed oval leaves and clusters of fragrant bell-shaped white flowers.

HABITAT & CULTIVATION Native to Southeast Asia, benzoin grows in tropical rainforests. It is also cultivated for its gum, which exudes from incisions made in the bark of trees that are at least 7 years old.

PART USED Gum.

CONSTITUENTS Benzoin gum contains variable quantities of cinnamic, benzoic and sumaresinolic acid esters, free acids (such as benzoic acid), benzaldehyde, and vanillin.

MEDICINAL ACTIONS & USES Benzoin gum is strongly antiseptic and astringent. It may be used externally on wounds and ulcers to tighten and disinfect the affected tissue. When taken internally, benzoin gum acts to settle cramps, to stimulate coughing, and to disinfect the urinary tract. Benzoin gum is an ingredient of Friar's Balsam, an antiseptic and expectorant steam inhalation for sore throats, head and chest colds, asthma, and bronchitis.

Symplocarpus foetidus
(Araceae)
SKUNK CABBAGE

DESCRIPTION Unpleasant-smelling perennial plant growing to 30 in (75 cm). Has a thick tuberous rootstock, cabbagelike leaves, and numerous small purple flowers on a hooded spike.

HABITAT & CULTIVATION Native to northern North America, skunk cabbage thrives in meadows, swamps, and marshes. The root and rhizome are collected in autumn or early spring.

PARTS USED Root, rhizome.

CONSTITUENTS Skunk cabbage contains a volatile oil, serotonin (5HT), and resins.

HISTORY & FOLKLORE The Winnebago and Dakota peoples used the expectorant and antispasmodic skunk cabbage root to treat asthma and bronchitis. The root was also employed as a poultice to draw out splinters and thorns, to heal wounds, and to relieve headaches. It was commonly used in America in the 19th century.

MEDICINAL ACTIONS & USES Skunk cabbage is still used primarily as an expectorant, treating cases of whooping cough, asthma, and bronchitis. It is also taken for upper respiratory problems such as nasal congestion and hay fever. Less commonly, skunk cabbage is used as a

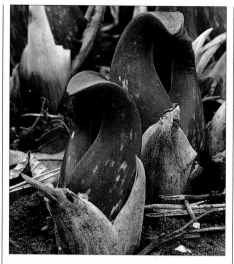

SKUNK CABBAGE is a foul-smelling plant with a powerful expectorant action.

treatment for epilepsy, headaches, vertigo, and rheumatic problems, and as a means to stop bleeding.

CAUTIONS Handling fresh skunk cabbage may cause the skin to blister. Excessive doses can induce nausea, headaches, and dizziness.

Tamarindus indica
(Leguminosae)
TAMARIND

DESCRIPTION Evergreen tree growing to 80 ft (25 m). Has fine compound leaves, clusters of orange-yellow flowers, and brittle gray-brown seed pods (fruit) containing up to 12 round seeds.

HABITAT & CULTIVATION Native to Madagascar, the tamarind is now cultivated in many tropical regions, including the Caribbean, India, Southeast Asia, and China.

PART USED Fruit.

CONSTITUENTS Tamarind contains 16–18% plant acids (including nicotinic acid – vitamin B_3), a volatile oil (with geranial, geraniol, and limonene), sugars, pectin, 0.8% potassium, and fats. Vitamin C was formerly believed to be among the constituents of tamarind, but this is now disputed.

Fruit

HISTORY & FOLKLORE Sailors ate tamarind fruit as a nourishing complement to their otherwise starchy diet in the belief that eating the fruit would prevent scurvy. However, it appears that tamarind does not in fact contain vitamin C. Tamarind is a major ingredient in many chutneys and condiments, notably Worcestershire sauce.

MEDICINAL ACTIONS & USES Tamarind is a wholesome and cleansing fruit that improves digestion, relieves gas, soothes sore throats, and acts as a mild laxative. In Ayurvedic medicine, it is given to improve the appetite and to strengthen the stomach. It is also used to relieve constipation. However, mixed with cumin and sugar, tamarind is also prescribed as a treatment for dysentery. In southern India, tamarind soup is taken to treat colds and other ailments that cause the production of excessive mucus. In Chinese medicine, tamarind is considered a cooling herb, appropriate for treating the condition known as "summer heat." The fruit is also given for loss of appetite and vomiting in pregnancy.

SELF-HELP USE Sore throats, p. 311.

Tanacetum vulgare
(Compositae)
TANSY

DESCRIPTION Strongly aromatic perennial growing to 3 ft (1 m). Has an erect stem, feathery compound leaves, and clusters of yellow disk-shaped flower heads.

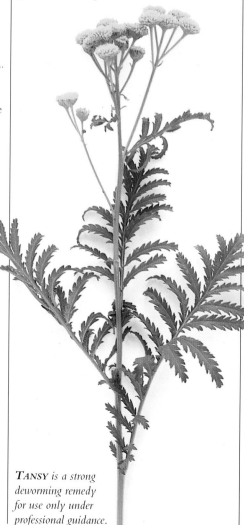

TANSY is a strong deworming remedy for use only under professional guidance.

HABITAT & CULTIVATION Found throughout temperate zones in the northern hemisphere, tansy grows in open areas, along roadsides, and close to water. The flowering tops are collected as the flowers open in summer.

PARTS USED Flowering tops.

CONSTITUENTS Tansy contains a volatile oil, which includes significant levels of thujone and camphor, sesquiterpene lactones, flavonoids, and resin. The volatile oil strongly induces menstruation.

HISTORY & FOLKLORE Although it is not mentioned in surviving classical texts, tansy was described by medieval herbalists, notably Hildegard of Bingen (12th century). Ever since that time, tansy has been used most commonly as a worm-expelling plant. In England, tansy puddings were consumed during Lent. The 16th-century herbalist John Gerard described the puddings as being "pleasant in taste and good for the stomach."

MEDICINAL ACTIONS & USES Tansy has been used in the past as a carminative to aid digestion. However it is not used much today because of its potential toxicity. When the plant is taken, it is chiefly in order to expel intestinal worms and to help stimulate menstrual bleeding. Tansy may be used externally to kill scabies, fleas, and lice, but even external application of tansy preparations carries the risk of toxicity.

CAUTIONS Use only under professional supervision. Tansy is possibly unsafe for internal and external use, and should never be taken during pregnancy. The plant, and especially its essential oil, are subject to legal restrictions in some countries.

Taxus baccata
(*Taxaceae*)
YEW

DESCRIPTION Slow-growing evergreen tree reaching 80 ft (25 m) in height. Has rust-red bark and flattened, dark green, needlelike leaves. The female trees produce fleshy, red, cuplike fruit.

HABITAT & CULTIVATION Yew grows throughout northern temperate zones. More often found in cultivation than in the wild, it prefers lime-rich soil. The leaves are gathered in spring.

PARTS USED Leaves.

CONSTITUENTS Yew contains a mixture of alkaloids known as taxine, and also diterpenes (including taxol in some varieties), lignans, tannin, and resin.

HISTORY & FOLKLORE The yew tree was sacred to the Druids, who are believed to have considered it an emblem of immortality. The Druids planted yews in holy sites, a practice that continued with the coming of

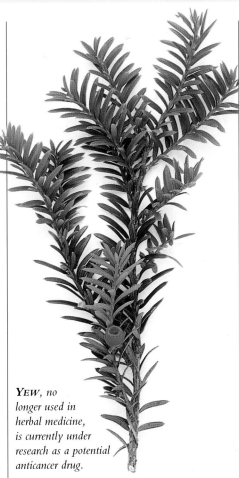

YEW, no longer used in herbal medicine, is currently under research as a potential anticancer drug.

Christianity. Many medieval churchyards contain ancient yews, some thought to be over 1,000 years old. In the Middle Ages, the best longbows were made from yew wood, as were "magic wands."

MEDICINAL ACTIONS & USES Though yew has been used in small doses to treat rheumatic and urinary problems, its extreme toxicity makes it an unsafe medicinal plant.

RESEARCH Taxol inhibits cell division and has been extensively researched for its potential as an anticancer drug. Taxol is most commonly found in the Pacific yew (*T. brevifolia*), though some varieties of *T. baccata* also contain the substance. Studies have been conducted since the 1980s in search for potential cancer treatments.

CAUTION Yew is extremely toxic. Do not take under any circumstances.

Terminalia belerica
(*Combretaceae*)
BELERIC MYROBALAN

DESCRIPTION Evergreen tree with clusters of oval leaves, spikes of small, greenish, unpleasant-smelling flowers, and hairy brown fruit.

HABITAT & CULTIVATION Beleric myrobalan is native to India, Malaysia, and

the Philippines. It is found in forests and is cultivated for its astringent fruit, which is gathered both immature and ripe.

PART USED Fruit.

CONSTITUENTS The fruit contains tannins and anthraquinones.

MEDICINAL ACTIONS & USES Beleric myrobalan fruit is astringent, tonic, and laxative. It is principally employed as a treatment for digestive and respiratory problems. In Indian herbal medicine, the ripe fruit is taken for diarrhea and indigestion, and the unripe fruit is used as a laxative for chronic constipation. Beleric myrobalan is also often used to treat upper respiratory tract infections that cause symptoms of sore throats, hoarseness, and coughs. Externally, the fruit is applied as a lotion for sore eyes.

RELATED SPECIES Many *Terminalia* species are used to make astringent remedies and also for their lumber. *See* chebulic myrobalan (*T. chebula, following entry*).

CAUTION Do not take beleric myrobalan during pregnancy.

Terminalia chebula
(*Combretaceae*)
CHEBULIC MYROBALAN

DESCRIPTION Evergreen tree growing to 70 ft (20 m). Has egg-shaped leaves, white flowers in terminal spikes, and small 5-ribbed fruit.

HABITAT & CULTIVATION Native to Central Asia and India, chebulic myrobalan is found throughout Iran, Pakistan, and India. The fruit is collected when ripe.

PART USED Fruit.

CONSTITUENTS Chebulic myrobalan contains anthraquinones, tannins, chebulic acid, resin, and a fixed oil.

HISTORY & FOLKLORE Chebulic myrobalan has been used in Indian medicine for several thousand years, and has long been considered a prime remedy for all manner of digestive problems.

MEDICINAL ACTIONS & USES Laxative and astringent, the fruit gently improves bowel regularity without excessively irritating the colon. Like Chinese rhubarb (*Rheum palmatum*, p. 124), chebulic myrobalan may be used as a treatment for diarrhea and dysentery. The fruit's tannins protect the gut wall from irritation and infection, and tend to reduce intestinal secretions. Likewise, the fruit helps to counter acidic indigestion and heartburn. A decoction of chebulic myrobalan may be used as a gargle and mouthwash, as a lotion for sore and inflamed eyes, and as a douche for vaginitis and excessive vaginal discharge.

CAUTION Do not take chebulic myrobalan during pregnancy.

Teucrium chamaedrys
(Labiatae)

WALL GERMANDER

DESCRIPTION Perennial herb growing to 10 in (24 cm). Has a woody root, toothed, dark green, oval leaves, and spikes of pink tubular flowers.

HABITAT & CULTIVATION Native to Europe, North Africa, and western Asia, wall germander is commonly found growing on dry, stony ground. The aerial parts are gathered in summer.

PARTS USED Aerial parts.

CONSTITUENTS Wall germander contains iridoid glycosides (including harpagide), diterpenes, a volatile oil (60% caryophyllene), tannins, and polyphenols.

HISTORY & FOLKLORE The Greek physician Dioscorides, writing in the 1st century AD, noted that wall germander was a popular medicinal plant in northern Italy, that the fresh leaves were eaten to stave off plague, and that the plant was also used to relieve coughs and asthma.

MEDICINAL ACTIONS & USES Infusions of wall germander have long been used to treat gout, rheumatism, stomach problems, fever, and congestion. The plant has also been taken to aid weight loss and is a common ingredient in tonic wines. Wall germander has been used as a mouthwash for sore gums and as a lotion to help heal wounds.

RELATED SPECIES The related *T. capense*, which is native to South Africa, is a soothing remedy for hemorrhoids. A European species, *T. marum*, treats gallbladder and stomach problems. Wood sage (*T. scorodonia*), another European plant, has uses similar to those of wall germander.

CAUTION Wall germander's safety is not clearly established; use over the long term may damage the liver. French practitioners have imposed a voluntary ban on its use. Until its safety has been confirmed, use of alternative herbs is advised.

Theobroma cacao
(Sterculiaceae)

CACAO, COCOA

DESCRIPTION Evergreen tree growing to 25 ft (8 m). Has pale brown bark, glossy oval leaves, clusters of small yellow flowers, and large pear-shaped red-yellow seed pods.

HABITAT & CULTIVATION Native to Mexico and Central America, cacao is now a major crop throughout the tropics. The seed pods are collected twice yearly.

PARTS USED Seeds.

CONSTITUENTS The seed pulp contains xanthines, a fixed oil, and many constituents responsible for its flavor. The seeds contain very small amounts of endorphins, which are powerful painkillers that occur naturally within the body.

HISTORY & FOLKLORE The word "chocolate" derives from *chócolatl*, the name given to this tree by the Aztecs. In 1720, Cotton Mather, an American preacher and natural historian, praised cacao, writing that the plant "supplies the Indian with bread, water, wine, vinegar, brandy, milk, oil, honey, sugar, needles, thread, linen, clothes, caps, spoons, besoms, baskets, paper, and nails; timber, coverings for their houses; masts, sails, cordage for their vessels; and medicine for their diseases; and what can be desired more?"

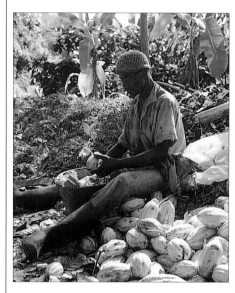

CACAO is cultivated in tropical regions around the world. The seed pulp is the source of cocoa.

MEDICINAL ACTIONS & USES Although cacao is most often used as a food, it also has therapeutic value as a nervous system stimulant. In Central America and the Caribbean, the seeds are taken as a heart and kidney tonic. The plant may be used to treat angina and as a diuretic. Cacao butter makes a good lip salve, and is often used as a base for suppositories.

RESEARCH In 1994, Argentinian researchers showed that cacao extracts counter the bacteria responsible for boils and septicemia.

Thuja occidentalis
(Cupressaceae)

ARBOR VITAE

DESCRIPTION Evergreen tree growing to 30 ft (10 m). Has scalelike leaves, male and female flowers, and small egg-shaped cones.

HABITAT & CULTIVATION Native to the northeastern US, arbor vitae flourishes in wet, marshy ground and along riverbanks. It has become a popular ornamental tree in Europe. The leaves are gathered in summer.

PARTS USED Leaves.

CONSTITUENTS Arbor vitae contains a volatile oil (with up to 60% thujone), flavonoids, wax, mucilage, and tannins.

HISTORY & FOLKLORE Many Native American peoples prized arbor vitae as a medicine for fever, headaches, coughs, swollen hands, and rheumatic problems. It was burned as a smudge (smoky fire) for its scent and to ward off evil spirits. The 19th-century Eclectic herbalists used arbor vitae as a remedy for bronchitis, rheumatism, and uterine cancer. It has also been used to treat the side effects of the smallpox vaccination.

Arbor vitae twig

MEDICINAL ACTIONS & USES Arbor vitae has an established antiviral activity. It is most often used to treat warts and polyps, being prescribed both internally and externally for these conditions. It is also used as part of a regime for treating cancer – especially cancer of the uterus. Arbor vitae makes an effective expectorant and decongestant remedy, and may be used to treat acute bronchitis and other respiratory infections. It induces menstruation and can be taken to bring on delayed periods, although this use is inadvisable if menstrual pain is severe. Arbor vitae is diuretic, and is used to treat acute cystitis and bed-wetting in children. Extracts may be painted on painful joints or muscles as a counter-irritant, improving local blood supply and easing pain and stiffness.

CAUTIONS Take only under professional supervision. Do not take arbor vitae during pregnancy or while breast-feeding.

SELF-HELP USE Warts, p. 304.

Thymus serpyllum
(Labiatae)

WILD THYME

DESCRIPTION Tuft-forming evergreen herb growing to a height of 3 in (7 cm). Has square stems, small aromatic oval leaves, and spikes of bright mauve flowers.

HABITAT & CULTIVATION Native to Europe, thyme prefers heaths, moorland, and barren places. The herb is collected when in flower in summer.

PARTS USED Flowering tops.

CONSTITUENTS Wild thyme contains volatile oil (with thymol, carvacrol, and linalool), flavonoids, caffeic acid, tannins, and resin. The volatile oil's properties are similar to, but less potent than, those of thyme oil (from *Thymus vulgaris*, p. 142).

HISTORY & FOLKLORE The 17th-century herbalist Nicholas Culpeper advised taking wild thyme to treat internal bleeding, coughing, and vomiting. He noted that "it comforts and strengthens the head, stomach, reins [ureters] and womb, expels wind and breaks the stone." Carolus Linnaeus, the 18th-century Swedish botanist, used the plant to treat headaches and hangovers.

MEDICINAL ACTIONS & USES Like its close relative thyme (*Thymus vulgaris*, p. 142), wild thyme is strongly antiseptic and antifungal. It may be taken as an infusion or syrup to treat flu and colds, sore throats, coughs, whooping cough, chest infections, and bronchitis. Wild thyme has decongestant properties and helps clear a stuffy nose, sinusitis, ear congestion, and related complaints. It has been used to expel threadworms and roundworms in children, and is used to settle gas and colic. Wild thyme's antispasmodic action makes it useful in relieving period pain. Externally, it may be applied as a poultice to treat mastitis (inflammation of the breast), and an infusion may be used as a wash to help heal wounds and ulcers. Wild thyme is also used in herbal baths and pillows.

RELATED SPECIES See thyme (*T. vulgaris*, p. 142).

CAUTION For worms in children, use only under professional supervision.

Tilia spp.
(Tiliaceae)
LINDEN, LIME

DESCRIPTION Deciduous tree growing to 100 ft (30 m), with smooth gray bark, heart-shaped leaves, and clusters of pale yellow flowers with winglike bracts.

HABITAT & CULTIVATION Native to Europe, linden is found in the wild, but is also often planted in gardens and along roads. The flowers are collected in summer.

PARTS USED Flowers.

CONSTITUENTS Linden contains flavonoids (especially quercetin and kaempferol), caffeic and other acids, mucilage (about 3%), tannins, volatile oil (0.02-0.1%), and traces of benzodiazepine-like compounds. The flavonoids improve circulation.

HISTORY & FOLKLORE Greek myth recounts how Philyra, a nymph, was raped by the god Saturn in the guise of a horse, and eventually gave birth to the famed centaur, Cheiron. Philyra was so devastated that she begged the gods not to leave her among mortals. The gods granted her wish by transforming her into a linden tree.

MEDICINAL ACTIONS & USES Linden is an antispasmodic, sweat-inducing, and sedative remedy. It relieves tensions and sinus headaches, helping to calm the mind and allow easy sleep. Linden is an excellent remedy for stress and panic, and is used specifically to treat nervous palpitations. The flowers bring relief to colds and flu by reducing nasal congestion and soothing fever. Linden flowers are commonly taken to lower high blood pressure, particularly when emotional factors are involved. The flowers are used over the long term to treat high systolic blood pressure associated with arteriosclerosis. Because of their emollient quality, linden flowers are used in France to make a lotion for itchy skin.

LINDEN flowers treat many complaints, from nervous palpitations to itchy skin.

Tragopogon pratensis
(Compositae)
GOAT'S BEARD

DESCRIPTION Erect annual or perennial growing to 2 ft (60 cm). Has narrow leaves and solitary yellow flowers succeeded by handsome dandelion-like flower heads.

HABITAT & CULTIVATION Native to Europe, goat's beard is found in dry, grassy sites. The root is unearthed in autumn.

PART USED Root.

CONSTITUENTS The root contains inulin, inositol, mannitol, and plant sterols.

HISTORY & FOLKLORE Goat's beard has long been eaten as a vegetable, and was praised by John Gerard in 1597 as "a most pleasant tasting and wholesome meate."

MEDICINAL ACTIONS & USES Like its cousin dandelion (*Taraxacum officinale*, p. 140), goat's beard is considered a useful remedy for the liver and gallbladder. It appears to have a detoxifying action, and may stimulate the appetite and digestion. Its high inulin content makes this herb a useful food for diabetics. Inulin is a nutrient made of fructose rather than glucose units, and therefore does not raise blood glucose levels.

RELATED SPECIES Salsify (*T. porrifolius*) is a common winter food in southern Europe. It is also a cleansing plant, and is used to treat arteriosclerosis and high blood pressure.

Trifolium pratense
(Leguminosae)
RED CLOVER

DESCRIPTION Perennial herb growing to 16 in (40 cm). Has a hairy upright stem, leaves with 3 (or, rarely, 4) oval leaflets with a white crescent marking, and pink to purple egg-shaped flower heads.

HABITAT & CULTIVATION Native to Europe and Asia, and naturalized in North America and Australia, red clover is widely cultivated for hay and as a nitrogen-fixing crop. The flower heads are collected when newly opened in summer.

PARTS USED Flower heads.

CONSTITUENTS Red clover contains flavonoids, phenolic acids (such as salicylic acid), volatile oil (including methyl salicylate and benzyl alcohol), sitosterol, starch, and fatty acids. Flavonoids in the flowers and leaves are estrogenic.

HISTORY & FOLKLORE The crescent markings across clover leaflets were once viewed as a sign that the plant would help cataracts (in accordance with the Doctrine of Signatures, which held that a plant's appearance indicated the ailments it treated). This herb has been used to treat breast cancer. A concentrated decoction was applied to the tumor site, which apparently encouraged the tumor to grow outward and eventually clear the body.

MEDICINAL ACTIONS & USES Red clover is used to treat skin conditions, normally in combination with other purifying herbs such as burdock (*Arctium lappa*, p. 62) and yellow dock (*Rumex crispus*, p. 126). It is also expectorant and may be used for spasmodic coughs. Red clover's estrogenic effect may be of use in treating menopausal complaints.

RESEARCH There has been little research into red clover's medicinal actions, but it is known that the herb has a contraceptive effect in sheep.

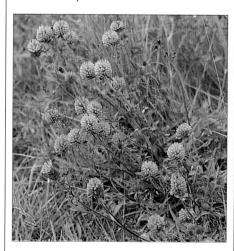

RED CLOVER is a common wayside plant, but it is also cultivated as a fodder crop.

Trigonella foenum-graecum
(*Leguminosae*)
FENUGREEK

DESCRIPTION Strongly aromatic annual growing to about 32 in (80 cm). Has trifoliate leaves, yellowish white pealike flowers, and sickle-shaped pods.

HABITAT & CULTIVATION Native to North Africa and countries bordering the eastern Mediterranean, fenugreek grows in open areas and is widely cultivated, notably in India. The seeds are collected during the autumn.

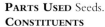

PARTS USED Seeds.

CONSTITUENTS *Fenugreek seeds*
Fenugreek contains a volatile oil, alkaloids (including trigonelline), saponins (based on diosgenin), flavonoids, mucilage (about 27%), protein (about 25%), fixed oil (approximately 8%), vitamins A, B$_1$, and C, and minerals.

HISTORY & FOLKLORE The Egyptian Ebers papyrus (*c.* 1500 BC) records a prescription for burns that includes fenugreek. The seeds were also used in ancient Egypt to induce childbirth. In the 5th century BC, the Greek physician Hippocrates considered fenugreek a valuable soothing herb. His countryman Dioscorides, writing in the 1st century AD, recommended fenugreek as a remedy for all types of gynecological problems, including infection of the uterus and inflammation of the vagina and vulva.

MEDICINAL ACTIONS & USES Fenugreek is often used in herbal medicine in North Africa, the Middle East, and India, being esteemed as a remedy for a wide variety of conditions. The nourishing seeds are given during convalescence and to encourage weight gain, especially in anorexia. They are also helpful in lowering fever, with some authorities comparing their ability to that of quinine. The seeds' soothing effect makes them of value in treating gastritis and gastric ulcers. They are used to induce childbirth and to increase breast-milk production. Fenugreek is also thought to be antidiabetic and to lower blood cholesterol levels. Externally, the seeds may be applied as a paste to treat abscesses, boils, ulcers, and burns, or used as a douche for excessive vaginal discharge. The seeds also freshen bad breath and help restore a dulled sense of taste. In China, fenugreek is used as a pessary to treat cervical cancer.

RESEARCH In animal experiments, fenugreek has been shown to inhibit liver cancer, stimulate uterine contractions, and to have an antidiabetic action.

CAUTION Do not take fenugreek seeds during pregnancy.

Trillium erectum
(*Liliaceae*)
BETHROOT

DESCRIPTION Attractive perennial with an erect stem growing to 16 in (40 cm). Has 3 wavy leaves and an unpleasant-smelling, 3-petaled, red to yellow flower.

HABITAT & CULTIVATION Native to North America, bethroot grows in shady positions in woodlands. The rhizome is usually unearthed after the leaves have fallen in autumn.

PART USED Rhizome.

CONSTITUENTS Bethroot contains saponins (such as trillin), tannin, resin, fixed oil, and a trace of volatile oil.

HISTORY & FOLKLORE Various *Trillium* species were used by Native Americans to aid childbirth, to treat irregular menstrual periods, menstrual pain, and excessive vaginal discharge, and as a poultice to soothe sore nipples.

MEDICINAL ACTIONS & USES
Bethroot is a valuable remedy for heavy menstrual or intermenstrual bleeding, helping to reduce blood flow. It is also used to treat bleeding associated with uterine fibroids. Bethroot may also be taken for bleeding within the urinary tubules and, less often, for the coughing up of blood. It remains a valuable herb in facilitating childbirth. A douche of bethroot is useful for excessive vaginal discharge and yeast infections.

CAUTION Do not take during pregnancy except under professional supervision.

Tropaeolum majus
(*Tropaeolaceae*)
NASTURTIUM

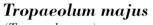

DESCRIPTION Climbing annual growing to 10 ft (3 m). Has straggling stems, rounded leaves, and orange to yellow trumpet-shaped flowers with a long spur.

HABITAT & CULTIVATION Native to Peru, nasturtiums flourish in sunny sites. They are grown as an ornamental and as a salad herb. All parts of the plant are harvested in summer.

PARTS USED Flowers, leaves, seeds.

CONSTITUENTS Nasturtiums contain glucocyanates (including glycotropeoline), spilanthol, myrosin (an enzyme), oxalic acid, and vitamin C.

HISTORY & FOLKLORE The nasturtium has long been used in Andean herbal medicine as a disinfectant and wound healing herb, and as an expectorant to relieve chest conditions.

MEDICINAL ACTIONS & USES All parts of the nasturtium appear to be antibiotic, but

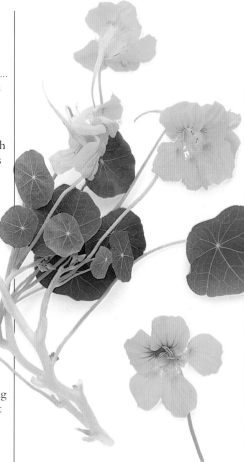

NASTURTIUM flowers have antibiotic properties and may be used to heal wounds.

the constituents responsible are unknown. An infusion of the leaves may be used to increase resistance to bacterial infections and to clear nasal and bronchial congestion – apparently the remedy both reduces the formation of mucus and stimulates the clearing and coughing up of phlegm. In addition, nasturtiums make an effective antiseptic wash for external use. The juice of the plant has been taken internally for the treatment of scrofula (tubercular infection of the lymph nodes). The piquant-tasting leaves and flowers (and juice) are high in vitamin C and make an excellent salad vegetable, while the ground seeds have purgative properties.

Tsuga canadensis
(*Pinaceae*)
CANADA HEMLOCK

DESCRIPTION Evergreen tree growing to 100 ft (30 m). Has reddish brown bark, short narrow needlelike leaves, and small male and female cones.

HABITAT & CULTIVATION Canada hemlock is native to eastern parts of North America, growing in woodland and marshy sites. The bark is collected from mature trees throughout the year.

PART USED Bark.

CONSTITUENTS Canada hemlock contains volatile oil (which incorporates alpha-pinene, bornyl acetate, and cadinene), 10–14% tannins, and resin.

HISTORY & FOLKLORE Native Americans may have given Canada hemlock to the explorer Jacques Cartier in 1535. He and his crew, exploring the St. Lawrence River, had fallen sick with scurvy, but all made a quick recovery upon taking a decoction of leaves and bark. Many Native American people used the bark to treat wounds.

MEDICINAL ACTIONS & USES The bark of Canada hemlock is astringent and antiseptic. A decoction may be taken to treat diarrhea, colitis, diverticulitis, and cystitis. Externally, Canada hemlock can be used as a douche to treat excessive vaginal discharge, yeast infections, and a prolapsed uterus; as a mouthwash and gargle for gingivitis and sore throats; or as a wash to cleanse wounds.

Tussilago farfara
(Compositae)
COLTSFOOT

DESCRIPTION Perennial herb growing to 12 in (30 cm). Has flowering stems with purple scales, yellow-gold flowers, and heart-shaped leaves.

HABITAT & CULTIVATION Indigenous to Europe and northern Asia, and naturalized in North America, coltsfoot is a common plant often found along roadsides and in open areas. The flowers are gathered in late winter, the leaves in summer.

PARTS USED Leaves, flowers.

CONSTITUENTS Coltsfoot contains flavonoids, about 8% mucilage (consisting of polysaccharides), 10% tannins, pyrrolizidine alkaloids, vitamin C, and zinc. The pyrrolizidine alkaloids may have a toxic effect on the liver, but are largely destroyed when the parts are boiled to make a decoction. The polysaccharides are anti-inflammatory and immunostimulant. The flavonoids are anti-inflammatory and antispasmodic.

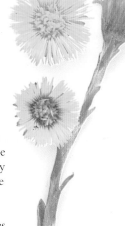

COLTSFOOT has long been used as a remedy for coughs.

HISTORY & FOLKLORE For at least 2,500 years, coltsfoot has been taken as a cough remedy and smoked as a means to ease breathing. Dioscorides, a Greek physician of the 1st century AD, recommended it for dry coughs, and "for those who are unable to breathe except standing upright."

MEDICINAL ACTIONS & USES An effective demulcent and expectorant herb, coltsfoot is one of the most popular European remedies for treating chest problems. In Europe, the leaves are preferred to the flowers (which contain higher amounts of pyrrolizidine alkaloids), but in China the flowers are preferred. Both parts are taken as a decoction for chest conditions. When used as a syrup or a medicinal cigarette, coltsfoot also relieves asthma. This herb is used as a specific treatment for spasmodic coughs. It combines well with licorice (*Glycyrrhiza glabra*, p. 99), thyme (*Thymus vulgaris*, p. 142), and black cherry (*Prunus serotina*, p. 255). In China, coltsfoot is classified as a "warming" herb that helps relieve coughing and wheezing.

RESEARCH Extracts of the whole plant have been shown to increase immune resistance. In a Chinese trial involving 36 patients suffering from bronchial asthma, 75% showed some improvement after treatment, but the antiasthmatic effect was short-lived.

CAUTIONS Do not use coltsfoot flowers. Do not take the leaves for more than 3–4 weeks at a time. Do not take coltsfoot during pregnancy or while breast-feeding. The herb is not suitable for children under age 6. Coltsfoot is subject to legal restrictions in some countries.

Tylophora asmatica
(Asclepidaceae)
ASMATICA, INDIAN LOBELIA

DESCRIPTION Perennial, twining climber with lance-shaped leaves and greenish flowers producing many flat seeds.

HABITAT & CULTIVATION Native to the Indian subcontinent, asmatica grows wild on the plains of India. The leaves are gathered when the plant is in flower.

PARTS USED Leaves.

CONSTITUENTS Asmatica contains alkaloids (including tylophorine), flavonoids, sterols, and tannins. Tylophorine has anti-inflammatory and antitumor properties.

HISTORY & FOLKLORE Asmatica has long been used in Ayurvedic medicine to induce vomiting and expectoration, and to treat dysentery and rheumatic conditions.

MEDICINAL ACTIONS & USES Considered a specific remedy for asthma, asmatica may relieve symptoms for up to 3 months. It is also beneficial in cases of hay fever, and is prescribed for acute allergic problems such as eczema and nettle rash. The plant holds potential as a treatment for chronic fatigue syndrome and other immune system disorders. Asmatica may relieve rheumatoid arthritis and may also be of value in the treatment of cancer.

RESEARCH Extensive laboratory and clinical research in India has established that asmatica is an effective remedy for asthma. In the 1970s, a number of clinical trials showed that a majority of asthmatic patients taking the herb for just 6 days gained relief from asthma for up to a further 12 weeks. However, the leaves do produce side effects. The plant's alternative name, Indian lobelia, alludes not only to its value in treating asthma but also to its irritating effect on the digestive tract – properties that are shared by *Lobelia* species (see *L. inflata*, p. 108).

CAUTION Take asmatica only under professional supervision.

Typha angustifolia
(Typhaceae)
PU HUANG, CATTAIL

DESCRIPTION Stout upright plant growing to 6 ft (2 m). Has long flat narrow leaves rising parallel to the stem, a distinctive brown cylindrical head of female flowers, and straw-colored male flowers immediately above.

HABITAT & CULTIVATION *Pu huang* flourishes in marshes, swamps, and other freshwater sites in both temperate and tropical zones, and is cultivated. The pollen is shaken off the blooming plant.

PART USED Pollen.

CONSTITUENTS *Pu huang* contains isorhamnetin, pentacosane, and plant sterols.

HISTORY & FOLKLORE Coopers in Europe traditionally placed the leaves of this plant between the staves of barrels to render them watertight. The pollen is highly flammable and has been used as a combustible agent in fireworks. The root has been eaten as a vegetable in times of famine.

MEDICINAL ACTIONS & USES In Chinese herbal medicine, the astringent *pu huang* pollen has been employed chiefly to stop internal or external bleeding. The pollen may be mixed with honey and applied to wounds and sores, or taken orally to reduce internal bleeding of almost any kind – for example, nosebleeds, uterine bleeding, or blood in the urine. The pollen is now also used in the treatment of angina (pain in the chest or arm due to lack of oxygen to the heart muscle). *Pu huang* does not appear to have been used as a medicine in the European herbal tradition.

CAUTION Do not take during pregnancy.

Uncaria rhyncophylla
(Rubiaceae)
GOU TENG

DESCRIPTION Climbing perennial growing to 30 ft (10 m). Has opposite lance-shaped leaves, thorns, and composite flower heads.

HABITAT & CULTIVATION Native to China and Southeast Asia, *gou teng* is cultivated in the southern and eastern provinces of China. The stems and thorns are collected in autumn and winter.

PARTS USED Stems, thorns.

CONSTITUENTS *Gou teng* contains alkaloids (including rhyncophylline and corynoxeine, isorhyncophylline, and hirsutine) and nicotinic acid.

HISTORY & FOLKLORE The first recorded use of *gou teng* in Chinese medicine is in the *Miscellaneous Records* (*c.* AD 500).

MEDICINAL ACTIONS & USES *Gou teng* is a sedative and antispasmodic, and is mainly used to ease symptoms such as tremors, seizure, spasms, headache, and dizziness. It is also prescribed for infantile convulsions. In Chinese herbal medicine it "extinguishes [internal] wind and stops tremors." It is also used by the Chinese to reduce high blood pressure and excess liver "fire."

RESEARCH Chinese tests on laboratory animals indicate that *gou teng* lowers blood pressure and has a significant sedative action.

RELATED SPECIES Like *gou teng*, pale catechu (*U. gambier*) contains a constituent that lowers blood pressure. It also contains catechin, a substance that powerfully protects the liver from infection. Pale catechu is used as an astringent remedy.

CAUTION Take *gou teng* only under professional supervision.

Urginea maritima
syn. *Drimia maritima*
(Liliaceae)
SQUILL

DESCRIPTION Perennial growing to 5 ft (1.5 m) from a large white or red bulb. Has a single flowering stem, a rosette of large basal leaves, and a dense spike of white flowers.

HABITAT & CULTIVATION Native to southern Spain, the Canary Islands, and South Africa, squill is cultivated in the Mediterranean region. The bulb of the white (but not the red) variety is unearthed in late summer.

PART USED Bulb.

CONSTITUENTS Squill contains cardiac glycosides (0.15-2.4% bufadienolides, including scillaren A), flavonoids, anthocyanidins, and mucilage. The cardiac glycosides are strongly diuretic and relatively

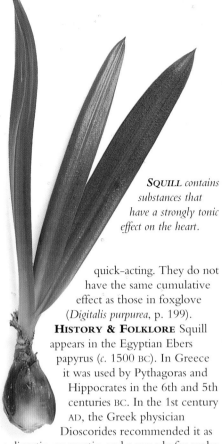

SQUILL contains substances that have a strongly tonic effect on the heart.

quick-acting. They do not have the same cumulative effect as those in foxglove (*Digitalis purpurea*, p. 199).

HISTORY & FOLKLORE Squill appears in the Egyptian Ebers papyrus (*c.* 1500 BC). In Greece it was used by Pythagoras and Hippocrates in the 6th and 5th centuries BC. In the 1st century AD, the Greek physician Dioscorides recommended it as a diuretic, an emetic, and a remedy for snake bite and asthma. The white bulb has been most used, but the red bulb was preferred by the medieval medical school in Salerno, Italy.

MEDICINAL ACTIONS & USES Squill is a diuretic, emetic, cardiotonic, and expectorant plant that finds use in a wide range of conditions. It makes a good diuretic in cases of water retention. Since its active constituents do not accumulate to a great degree within the body, it is a potential substitute for foxglove in aiding a failing heart. At low dosage, squill is an effective expectorant. At higher doses, it acts as an emetic. Squill is also used in homeopathic preparations.

CAUTION Use only under professional supervision. Squill is toxic in excessive doses.

Vaccinium myrtillus
(Ericaceae)
BILBERRY

DESCRIPTION Deciduous shrub growing to about 16 in (40 cm). Has erect multi-branched stems, pointed oval leaves, small white or pink flowers, and spherical berries that ripen to purple-black.

HABITAT & CULTIVATION Bilberry is native to Europe and North America. It thrives in heathland, on moors, and in moist undergrowth. The fruit and leaves are collected in summer.

PARTS USED Fruit, leaves.

CONSTITUENTS The fruit contains about 0.5% anthocyanosides, vitamins B_1 and C, pro–vitamin A, 7% tannins, and plant acids. The anthocyanosides have a tonic effect on the blood vessels.

HISTORY & FOLKLORE Bilberries have been eaten as a fruit since prehistoric times.

MEDICINAL ACTIONS & USES Ripe bilberries are mildly laxative due to their fruit sugar content. The dried fruit, however, is markedly binding and has an antibacterial action. A decoction of the dried fruit is useful for treating diarrhea in children. Bilberry's high anthocyanin content makes it a potentially valuable treatment for varicose veins, hemorrhoids, and capillary fragility. A decoction of the fruit is used as a mouthwash. The leaves may be helpful in prediabetic states but are not an alternative to conventional treatment. They may be taken for urinary tract infections.

RELATED SPECIES Cowberry (*V. vitis-idaea*), cranberry (*V. macrocarpon*), and uva-ursi (*Arctostaphylos uva-ursi*, p. 168) are all urinary antiseptics.

CAUTION Do not use the leaves for longer than 3 weeks at a time.

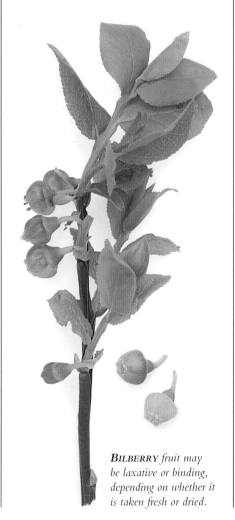

BILBERRY fruit may be laxative or binding, depending on whether it is taken fresh or dried.

Veratrum viride
(Liliaceae)

AMERICAN HELLEBORE

DESCRIPTION Perennial growing to 8 ft (2.5 m). Has oval to linear leaves and green flowers on short stalks.

HABITAT & CULTIVATION American hellebore is found growing throughout northern North America west of the Rocky Mountains. It grows in damp, low-lying sites, marshes, and swamps. The rootstock is unearthed in autumn.

PART USED Rootstock.

CONSTITUENTS American hellebore contains steroidal and other alkaloids, and chelidonic acid. Some of the alkaloids lower blood pressure and dilate the peripheral blood vessels. They have been used in conventional medicine to treat high blood pressure and rapid heartbeat.

HISTORY & FOLKLORE American hellebore was used by the Iroquois to treat congestion, by the Cherokee to ease rheumatic pain, and by European settlers as a delousing agent. The plant has also been used to treat pneumonia, gout, rheumatism, and fever.

MEDICINAL ACTIONS & USES American hellebore is a highly toxic plant that is rarely used in herbal medicine today. It is an effective insecticide, but it can cause side effects, even when applied to unbroken skin. The plant is used in homeopathic preparations to slow heart rate.

RELATED SPECIES False hellebore (*V. californicum*), native to the west coast of America, was used by the Shoshone and other Native Americans as a female contraceptive – a decoction of the root was taken daily for 3 weeks to produce permanent sterility. The white false hellebore (*V. album*), a European plant, has constituents and uses similar to those of American hellebore, and is also highly toxic. Chinese species, including *V. nigrum*, are used as emetics and expectorants, and externally as insecticides.

CAUTION False hellebore is highly toxic. Use only under professional supervision.

Verbascum thapsus
(Scrophulariaceae)

MULLEIN

DESCRIPTION Upright biennial growing to 6 ft (2 m). Has slightly hairy, gray-green oval to lance-shaped leaves, and spikes of bright yellow flowers.

HABITAT & CULTIVATION Mullein is native to central and southern Europe and western Asia. It is now also naturalized in many other temperate regions. Mullein grows on open uncultivated land and along roadsides. The

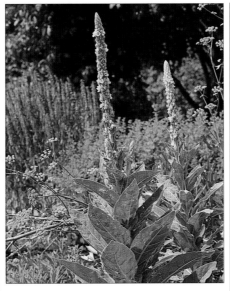

MULLEIN is a good expectorant remedy for coughs and other chest problems.

leaves and flowers are collected during the summer.

PARTS USED Leaves, flowers.

CONSTITUENTS Mullein contains mucilage, flavonoids, triterpenoid saponins, volatile oil, and tannins.

HISTORY & FOLKLORE Mullein was once credited with magical as well as medicinal virtues. John Gerard, a 16th-century herbalist, expressed doubts about the former: "there be some who think that this herbe being carryed aboute one, doth help the falling sickness … which thing is vaine and superstitious." However, he did affirm mullein's value as a cough medicine.

MEDICINAL ACTIONS & USES Mullein is a valuable herb for coughs and congestion, and is a specific treatment for tracheitis and bronchitis. The leaves and the flowers may be used as an infusion to reduce mucus formation and stimulate the coughing up of phlegm. Mullein combines well with other expectorants such as coltsfoot (*Tussilago farfara*, p. 277) and thyme (*Thymus vulgaris*, p. 142). Applied externally, mullein is emollient and makes a good wound healer. In Germany, the flowers are steeped in olive oil, and the resulting fixed oil is used as a remedy for ear infections and hemorrhoids.

Veronica officinalis
(Scrophulariaceae)

SPEEDWELL

DESCRIPTION Creeping hairy perennial growing to 20 in (50 cm). Has oval leaves and darkly veined, lilac flowers.

HABITAT & CULTIVATION A common wild plant in Europe and North America, speedwell is most often found on heaths and in dry, grassy places. It is picked in summer.

PARTS USED Aerial parts.

CONSTITUENTS Speedwell contains iridoid glycosides (including aucubin), acetopenone glucosides, and flavonoids (including apigenin and scutellarin).

HISTORY & FOLKLORE Speedwell was formerly considered a useful diuretic and expectorant. It was commonly used to treat congestion, coughs, and chronic skin conditions. It was also given to counter nervous exhaustion due to excessive mental activity or concentration. However, in 1935, the French medicinal plant therapist Leclerc stated that "the infusion has no more virtue than the hot water used to prepare it."

MEDICINAL ACTIONS & USES Speedwell is now considered to have only a slight therapeutic effect. It is rarely used today.

Viburnum prunifolium
(Caprifoliaceae)

BLACK HAW

DESCRIPTION Deciduous shrub growing to 15 ft (5 m). Has serrated oval leaves, clusters of white flowers, and blue-black berries.

HABITAT & CULTIVATION Native to central and southern North America, black haw grows in woodland. The branch bark is stripped in the spring or autumn, the root bark in the autumn only.

PARTS USED Bark, root bark.

CONSTITUENTS Black haw contains coumarins (including scopoletin and aesculetin), salicin, 1-methyl-2,3-dibutyl hemimellitate, viburnin, plant acids, a trace of volatile oil, and tannin.

HISTORY & FOLKLORE The Catawba people used black haw bark to treat dysentery. In the 19th century, the bark was considered to be a uterine tonic, and a decoction was commonly used to help arrest hemorrhage of the uterus.

MEDICINAL ACTIONS & USES Black haw is antispasmodic and astringent, and is regarded as a specific treatment for menstrual pain. Echoing its 19th-century applications, the bark is also used to treat other gynecological conditions, such as prolapse of the uterus, heavy menopausal bleeding, morning sickness, and threatened miscarriage. Black haw's antispasmodic property makes it of value in cases where colic or other cramping pain affects the bile ducts, the digestive tract, or the urinary tract.

RELATED SPECIES The closely related *V. rufidulum* was used by the Menominee people to treat cramps and colic. *See also* cramp bark (*Viburnum opulus*, p. 148).

CAUTION People who are allergic to aspirin should not take black haw.

SELF-HELP USE Menstrual pain, p. 315.

Vinca minor
(Apocynaceae)
LESSER PERIWINKLE

DESCRIPTION A mainly ground-hugging, evergreen shrub arching to 18 in (45 cm). Has rooting stems, shiny elliptical leaves, and 5-petaled violet-blue flowers.

HABITAT & CULTIVATION Native to Europe, lesser periwinkle grows along roadsides and woodland borders. It is also cultivated as a garden plant. The leaves are gathered in spring.

PARTS USED Leaves.

CONSTITUENTS Lesser periwinkle contains about 7% indole alkaloids (including vincamine, vincine, and vincaminine), a bisindol alkaloid (vincarubine), and tannins. Vincamine increases blood flow and oxygen supply to the brain.

HISTORY & FOLKLORE In his *Herbarium*, the 2nd-century AD Roman writer Apuleius described lesser periwinkle's virtues "against the devil sickness and demoniacal possessions and against snakes and wild beasts." He also specifies the rituals used in harvesting the herb: "This wort thou shalt pluck thus, saying, 'I pray thee, *vinca pervinca*, thee that art to be had for thy many useful qualities … outfit me so that I be shielded and ever prosperous and undamaged by poisons and by water.' When thou shalt pluck this wort, thou shalt be clean of every uncleanness, and thou shalt pick it when the moon is nine nights old."

MEDICINAL ACTIONS & USES Lesser periwinkle is employed as an astringent and blood-staunching herb. Its astringency makes it a useful mouthwash for sore throats, gingivitis, and canker sores. Its staunching ability is effective against internal bleeding, heavy menstrual bleeding, and nosebleeds. Since vincamine was discovered in the leaves, lesser periwinkle has been used to treat arteriosclerosis and for dementia due to insufficient blood flow to the brain.

RELATED SPECIES Greater periwinkle (*V. major*) also has similar astringent activity. *See also* Madagascar periwinkle (*V. rosea*, following entry).

CAUTION Do not take during pregnancy.

Vinca rosea
(Apocynaceae)
MADAGASCAR PERIWINKLE

DESCRIPTION Fleshy perennial growing to 32 in (80 cm). Has glossy oval leaves and bright, white to red, 5-petaled flowers.

HABITAT & CULTIVATION Thought to be a native of Madagascar, this herb is now common in many tropical and subtropical regions worldwide. It is cultivated commercially as a garden ornamental. The herb and root are gathered in summer.

PARTS USED Aerial parts, root.

CONSTITUENTS Madagascar periwinkle contains over 70 different indole alkaloids, including vinblastine, vincristine, alstonine, ajmalicine, leurocristine, and reserpine.

MEDICINAL ACTIONS & USES This plant is used in folk medicine in the Philippines as a remedy for diabetes. In the Caribbean, the flowers are used as a soothing eyewash.

RESEARCH Madagascar periwinkle's traditional use as a treatment for diabetes has led to extensive investigation into its properties. Vincristine and vinblastine are powerful anticancer agents, and are two of the most important medicinal compounds found in plants in the last 40 years. Vincristine is a standard treatment for Hodgkin's disease, and vinblastine for childhood leukemia. Although extracts from Madagascar periwinkle have been shown to lower blood sugar levels, simple preparations of the whole plant may not be effective.

CAUTION Take Madagascar periwinkle only under professional supervision.

Viola odorata
(Violaceae)
SWEET VIOLET

DESCRIPTION Creeping perennial growing to 6 in (15 cm). Has toothed, oval leaves, and very attractive, violet-blue or white flowers with a 5-petaled corolla.

HABITAT & CULTIVATION Native to much of Europe and Asia, sweet violet is a common wayside plant also found along roadsides and in woodland. The flowers and leaves are collected in spring, the root in autumn.

PARTS USED Flowers, leaves, root.

CONSTITUENTS Sweet violet contains phenolic glycosides (including gaultherin), saponins (myrosin and violin), flavonoids, an alkaloid (odoratine), and mucilage.

HISTORY & FOLKLORE In classical myth, sweet violet was associated with death, but classical physicians also knew it as an effective emetic and cough remedy. The 17th-century herbalist Nicholas Culpeper stated that: "All the violets are cold and moist while they are fresh and green, and are used to cool any heat or distemperature of the body either inwardly or outwardly."

MEDICINAL ACTIONS & USES Sweet violet flowers and leaves have a gentle expectorant and demulcent action, and they induce light sweating. They are often used as an infusion or syrup for treating coughs, chest colds, and congestion. The flowers and leaves are used in British herbal medicine to treat breast and stomach cancer. The root is a much stronger expectorant and, at higher doses, is emetic.

RELATED SPECIES The related dog violet (*V. canina*) has approximately the same uses as sweet violet. The Chinese *V. yedoens* is prescribed in that country's herbal tradition for hot swellings and tumors, mumps, and abscesses. *See also* heartsease (*V. tricolor*, following entry).

Viola tricolor
(Violaceae)
HEARTSEASE

DESCRIPTION Annual, biennial, or perennial plant growing to 15 in (38 cm). Has lobed oval leaves and handsome violet, yellow, and white pansy-type flowers.

HABITAT & CULTIVATION Heartsease is native to Europe, North Africa, and temperate regions of Asia, and has become naturalized in the Americas. It thrives in many habitats, from grassy mountainous areas to coastal sites, and is cultivated as a garden plant. The aerial parts are gathered in summer.

PARTS USED Aerial parts.

CONSTITUENTS Heartsease contains flavonoids, methyl salicylate, mucilage, gums, resin, and a saponin.

HISTORY & FOLKLORE K'Eogh wrote in his 1735 *Irish Herbal* that heartsease flowers "cure convulsions in children, cleanse the lungs and breast and are very good for fevers, internal inflammations and wounds."

MEDICINAL ACTIONS & USES In Western herbal medicine, heartsease is used as a

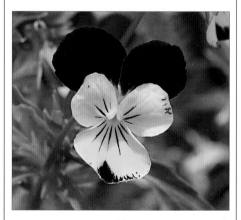

HEARTSEASE grows wild in temperate areas and is widely cultivated as a garden plant.

purifying herb and is taken for skin conditions such as eczema. An infusion also makes a useful wash for itchiness. Being expectorant, heartsease is used to treat bronchitis and whooping cough. The plant has a diuretic action and can be used to treat rheumatism, cystitis, and difficulty in passing urine.

SELF-HELP USE Nettle rash, p. 303.

Viscum album
(Loranthaceae)

EUROPEAN MISTLETOE

DESCRIPTION Parasitic evergreen shrub that forms bunches up to 10 ft (3 m) across on host trees. Has narrow leathery leaves, yellowish flowers in clusters of 3, and sticky, round white berries.

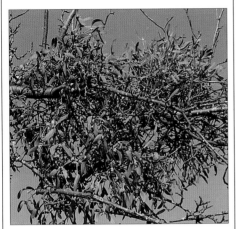

EUROPEAN MISTLETOE was the "golden" bough that saved the legendary Aeneas from the underworld.

HABITAT & CULTIVATION Native to Europe and northern Asia, European mistletoe grows on host trees, especially apple trees. It is harvested in autumn.

PARTS USED Leaves, branches, berries.

CONSTITUENTS European mistletoe contains glycoproteins, polypeptides (viscotoxins), flavonoids, caffeic and other acids, lignans, acetylcholine, and, in the berries, polysaccharides. Viscotoxins inhibit tumors and stimulate immune resistance.

HISTORY & FOLKLORE In Norse mythology, a mistletoe bough was used to slay Balder, the god of peace. The plant was subsequently entrusted to the goddess of love, and kissing under it became obligatory.

MEDICINAL ACTIONS & USES European mistletoe is chiefly used to lower blood pressure and heart rate, ease anxiety, and promote sleep. In low doses it also relieves panic attacks, headaches, and improves concentration. European mistletoe is also prescribed for tinnitus and epilepsy. In anthroposophical medicine, extracts of the berries are injected to treat cancer.

RESEARCH European mistletoe's efficacy as an anticancer treatment has been subject to a significant amount of research. There is no doubt that certain constituents, especially the viscotoxins, exhibit an anticancer activity, but the value of the whole plant in cancer treatment is not fully accepted.

CAUTION European mistletoe, and especially the berries, are highly toxic. Take only under professional supervision.

Vitis vinifera
(Vitaceae)

GRAPE

DESCRIPTION Deciduous climber with erect rambling stems, tendrils, palm-shaped leaves, clusters of small pale green flowers, and bunches of fruit (grapes) that vary in color from green to black.

HABITAT & CULTIVATION Native to southern Europe and western Asia, grapes are cultivated in warm temperate regions throughout the world for their fruit and to produce wine. The leaves are collected in summer, the fruit in autumn.

PARTS USED Leaves, fruit, sap.

CONSTITUENTS Grapes contain flavonoids, tannins, tartrates, inositol, carotenes, choline, and sugars. The fruit contains tartaric and malic acids, sugars, pectin, tannin, flavone glycosides, anthocyanins (in red leaves and red grapes), vitamins A, B_1, B_2, and C, and minerals. The anthocyanins reduce capillary permeability.

HISTORY & FOLKLORE Nicholas Culpeper in 1652 recommended grapes as a mouthwash, writing that "the ashes of the burnt branches will make teeth that are as black as a cole to be as white as snow; if you do but every morning rub them with it. It is a most gallant tree of the sun very sympathetical to the body of man, and that's the reason spirit of wine is the greatest cordial amongst all vegetables."

MEDICINAL ACTIONS & USES Grape leaves, especially the red leaves, are astringent and anti-inflammatory. They are taken as an infusion to treat diarrhea, heavy menstrual bleeding, and uterine hemorrhage, as a wash for canker sores, and as a douche for vaginal discharge. Red leaves and grapes are helpful in the treatment of varicose veins, hemorrhoids, and capillary fragility. The sap from the branches is used as an eyewash. Grapes are nourishing and mildly laxative, and they support the body through illness, especially of the gastrointestinal tract and liver. Because the nutrient content of grapes is close to that of blood plasma, grape fasts are recommended for detoxification. The dried fruit (raisins or sultanas) is mildly expectorant and emollient, with a slight effect in easing coughs. Wine vinegar is astringent, cooling, and soothing to the skin.

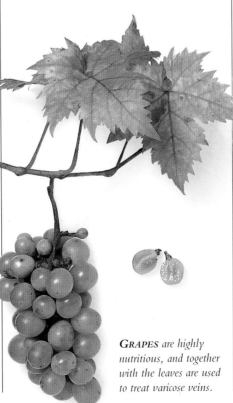

GRAPES are highly nutritious, and together with the leaves are used to treat varicose veins.

Ziziphus jujuba
(Rhamnaceae)

JUJUBE, DA ZAO (CHINESE)

DESCRIPTION Spiny deciduous tree growing to approximately 25 ft (8 m). Has oblong, bluntly toothed leaves, clusters of small greenish yellow flowers, and reddish brown or black, oval fruit.

HABITAT & CULTIVATION Native to China, Japan, and Southeast Asia, the jujube is widely cultivated in tropical and subtropical regions of Asia and the Mediterranean. The fruit is collected in early autumn.

PART USED Fruit.

CONSTITUENTS Jujube contains saponins, flavonoids, sugars, mucilage, vitamins A, B_2, and C, and calcium, phosphorus, and iron.

HISTORY & FOLKLORE Used in Chinese herbal medicine for at least 2,500 years, jujube has a pleasant, sweet taste and high nutritional value. It is mentioned in the *Classic of Odes*, a 6th-century BC anthology of Chinese poetry.

MEDICINAL ACTIONS & USES Jujube is both a delicious fruit and an effective herbal remedy. It aids weight gain, improves muscular strength, and increases stamina. In Chinese medicine, jujube is prescribed as a *qi* tonic to strengthen liver function. Mildly sedative and antiallergenic, it is given to reduce irritability and restlessness. It is also used to improve the taste of unpalatable prescriptions.

RESEARCH In Japan, jujube has been shown to increase immune-system resistance. In China, laboratory animals fed a jujube decoction gained weight and showed improved endurance. In one clinical study, 12 patients with liver ailments were given jujube, peanuts, and brown sugar nightly. In 4 weeks, their liver function had improved.

RELATED SPECIES The sedative *Z. spinosa* is used in Chinese medicine to "nourish the heart and quieten the spirit."

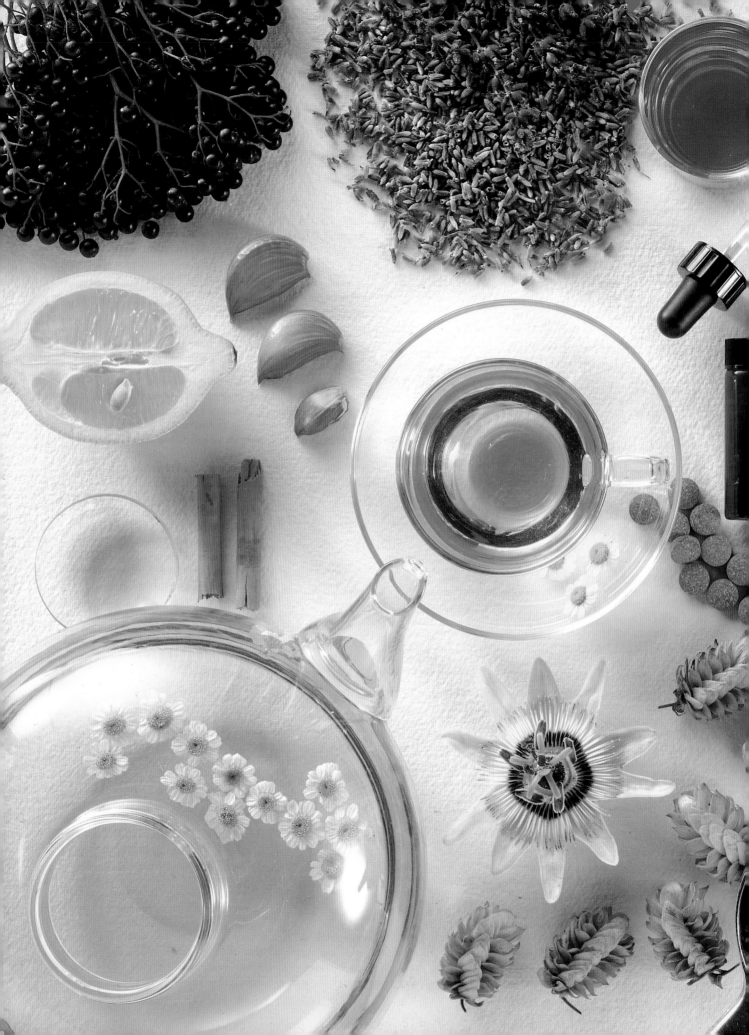

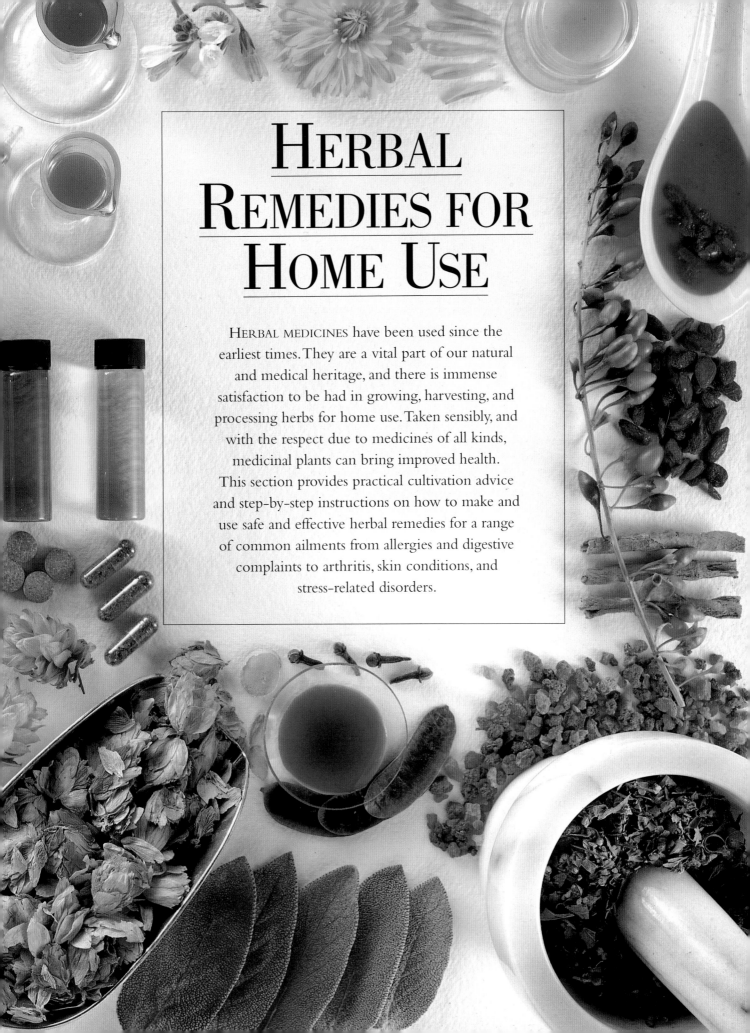

HERBAL REMEDIES FOR HOME USE

HERBAL MEDICINES have been used since the earliest times. They are a vital part of our natural and medical heritage, and there is immense satisfaction to be had in growing, harvesting, and processing herbs for home use. Taken sensibly, and with the respect due to medicines of all kinds, medicinal plants can bring improved health. This section provides practical cultivation advice and step-by-step instructions on how to make and use safe and effective herbal remedies for a range of common ailments from allergies and digestive complaints to arthritis, skin conditions, and stress-related disorders.

GROWING MEDICINAL PLANTS

GROWING MEDICINAL PLANTS may be more time-consuming than buying them, but it brings with it the unique pleasure of producing your own herbal remedies. Many medicinal herbs are easy to grow and will flourish indoors, on a windowsill, or in the garden, providing a year-round supply of fresh, sweet-smelling natural medicines.

THE MEDICINAL HERB GARDEN

Planning an herb garden depends on a range of factors, including the space available, exposure, soil, conditions, and climate. As a starting point, details of 10 of the most common and useful medicinal plants for growing in temperate climates are given in the chart below. Some of them, such as thyme (*Thymus vulgaris*, p. 142) and sage (*Salvia officinalis*, p. 130), may be grown indoors. A number of other medicinal herbs, including German chamomile (*Chamomilla recutita*, p. 76), lady's mantle (*Alchemilla vulgaris*, p. 161), and lavender (*Lavandula officinalis*, p. 107), also grow well in a temperate climate. If in doubt about how to care for plants or what will grow well in your garden, consult a nursery.

OUTDOOR GARDENS

Choose a range of hardy herbs to grow in your garden that will establish themselves easily and produce plenty of foliage that can be harvested. Plant exotic or less hardy herbs in sheltered sunny sites or in containers.

CONTAINER GARDENS

Many medicinal plants, such as peppermint (*Mentha* x *piperita*, p. 112) or bay laurel (*Laurus nobilis*, p. 224), can be grown in pots, hanging baskets, or window boxes. Care must be taken to prevent them from drying out or becoming pot bound (where the plant becomes too large for the container). Less hardy plants should be moved to sheltered sites or indoors during the winter.

GROWING PLANTS UNDER COVER

Sheltered gardening offers the opportunity to grow more unusual plants. Use the greenhouse to cultivate exotic plants, such as lemon grass (*Cymbopogon citratus*, p. 196), for medicinal and culinary use, as well as for growing seedlings to be planted outdoors. Tender plants, such as holy basil (*Ocimum sanctum*, p. 114), thrive indoors, and some indoor plants, such as aloe vera (*Aloe vera*, p. 57), have the added advantage of absorbing polluting chemicals from the air.

BUYING MEDICINAL HERBS

Reputable herb nurseries are the best place to buy herbs when particular varieties or species are required. Be clear about what plants you want before visiting the nursery. When buying for medicinal use, purchase the standard medicinal, rather than an improved or ornamental variety.

CULTIVATION

Bear in mind the following points when planning the garden and choosing herbs.

SITE

The majority of medicinal plants prefer a sunny aspect and moderately well-drained soil. It is possible to improve a site – for example, by planting hedges as windbreaks. Choose sheltered sunny corners for delicate herbs, and avoid planting on land formerly used for industrial purposes, which may be contaminated.

TEMPERATURE

Some plants can tolerate only very specific temperature ranges and will not survive exposure to deep or long periods of frost. These include many herbs – for example, rosemary (*Rosmarinus officinalis*, p. 125). Protect frost-tender plants from the wind to avoid the wind chill factor. Spring is the best time to plant most herbs. Wintering plants in a green-house or cool indoor site is often the only way to keep subtropical plants in cool temperate climates, while other herbs will thrive indoors all year round in a warm sunny position.

SOIL

Soils vary greatly depending on the proportions of sand, silt, and clay content. Sandy soils drain easily and need feeding, while clay soils can become waterlogged and require drainage.

PRUNING

Pruning is used to remove dead wood and improve the shape, size, and quality of growth. It is an important garden activity and needs to be done correctly for different woody plants to benefit – check the best time of year for each plant. Deadheading plants, especially shrubs, encourages fresh growth. Pruning and

USEFUL HERBS TO GROW

PLANT	WHEN TO PLANT	CULTIVATION METHOD	CONDITIONS & CARE	MEDICINAL USES
Aloe vera (*Aloe vera*, p. 57)	spring/autumn	offsets	■ sunny site indoors; pot as needed; do not overwater	■ fresh plant gel for minor burns and wounds
Comfrey (*Symphytum officinale*, p. 136)	spring/autumn	seed/division	■ warm sunny site; moist soil	■ ointment or poultice for sprains and bruises (use the leaf only)
Feverfew (*Tanacetum parthenium*, p. 139)	autumn/spring	seed/cutting/division	■ well-drained or dry stony soil in sun	■ fresh leaf or tincture for headaches and migraine
Lemon balm (*Melissa officinalis*, p. 111)	spring/autumn	seed/cutting/division	■ moist soil in sun; cut back after flowering	■ infusion for anxiety, poor sleep, and nervous indigestion; lotion for cold sores
Calendula (*Calendula officinalis*, p. 69)	spring/autumn	seed	■ well-drained soil; full sun; remove dead flower heads	■ cream for cuts, scrapes, inflamed skin; infusion for fungal infections
Peppermint (*Mentha* x *piperita*, p. 112)	spring/autumn	cutting/division	■ sunny but moist site; do not allow to dry out	■ infusion for indigestion and headaches; lotion for itchy skin
Rosemary (*Rosmarinus officinalis*, p. 125)	spring/autumn	seed/cutting	■ sunny sheltered site; protect with burlap in winter	■ infusion as a stimulating nerve tonic and to aid a weak digestion
Sage (*Salvia officinalis*, p. 130)	autumn/spring	seed/cutting/layering	■ well-drained or dry, sunny, sheltered site	■ infusion for sore throats, canker sores, and diarrhea
St. John's wort (*Hypericum perforatum*, p. 104)	spring/autumn	seed/division	■ well-drained to dry soil with sun or partial shade	■ tincture for depression and menopause; infused oil is antiseptic and heals wounds
Thyme (*Thymus vulgaris*, p. 142)	spring/summer	seed/cutting/division	■ well-drained soil; may need a layer of gravel; sunny site	■ infusion for coughs, colds, and chest infections; lotion for fungal infections

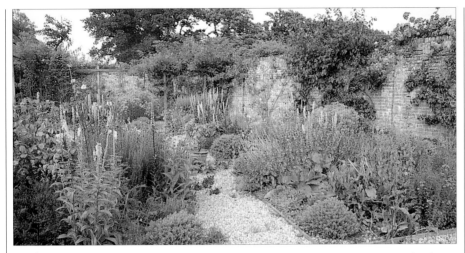

Cultivated herb gardens can create a colorful aromatic area with the added benefit of providing a ready supply of fresh herbs to use both medicinally and in cooking.

tidying the garden regularly also reduces pests and diseases.

WATERING

Water well after planting and then, if needed, once a week (rather than a little each day) in the morning or early evening. Do not overwater since many herbs produce medicinally active constituents in dry conditions. Water dry potted plants thoroughly before planting.

WEEDING & FERTILIZING

Weeding is necessary since weeds compete with other plants for nutrients and water. Keep beds and containers as free from weeds as possible. Most medicinal herbs should not be fertilized or mulched since this tends to reduce their therapeutic strength. However, sandy soils should be fed with a good-quality fertilizer to maintain the nutrients in the soil.

PESTS & DISEASES

Use only organic methods to treat pests, diseases, and insect infestation. Aphids can be eradicated using soapy water or water in which garlic skins have been soaked for 2 days. Separate any infected plants to counter further contamination.

PROPAGATION METHODS

There is a wide variety of propagation methods. Choose the one most suited to the plant. When planting, prepare the ground in advance, taking into account the requirements of the individual plant, and the soil, site, and time of year as well as the anticipated size of the mature plant.

SEED

Seeds can be sown either in containers or in prepared soil in open ground. It is important to time the sowing of seeds to enable seedlings to be planted outside when weather and soil become sufficiently warm. Annuals and biennials can be grown with ease from seed and will grow vigorously throughout the summer. Check the germination requirements of perennials before buying seeds since some varieties germinate easily while others, such as Siberian ginseng (*Eleutherococcus senticosus*, p. 92), can be far more difficult.

CUTTINGS

This is one of the most popular methods of propagation. It is suitable for woody perennial herbs. Cuttings are usually taken from the stem, although some plants may also be propagated from roots. Choose young healthy plants, and take the cutting just below a leaf and stem joint using a clean, sharp knife. Strip off the lowest leaves and dip the stem in hormone rooting powder before inserting it in suitable soil mix. Some plants are very difficult to propagate this way, so check before attempting this method.

ROOT DIVISION

This is an easy way to propagate plants that form clumps. Divide spring-flowering herbaceous plants in autumn, and autumn-flowering herbaceous plants in spring. Carefully lift a mature plant, divide it into smaller sections, and replant both the new and the mature plant.

PLANTS FROM PRODUCE

Purchase pots of culinary herbs from a grocery or supermarket, split the seedlings into 3 to 4 small clumps, and pot them separately. Fresh roots, such as ginger (*Zingiber officinale*, p. 153), or bulblets, such as garlic (*Allium sativum*, p. 56), can be planted in pots or in prepared ground outside, if the temperature allows.

LAYERING

Layering involves encouraging a shoot or stem to form roots by making a small slit in its underside and burying it, with the growing tip above ground. When the layer roots emerge, remove and pot. The practice of "mound layering"

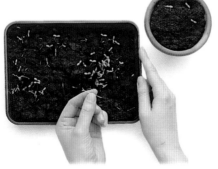

Fresh ginger root rapidly produces many new shoots if planted in moist soil mix in warm conditions above 70°F (21°C).

is suitable for woody herbs such as sage (*Salvia officinalis*, p. 130). Pile free-draining soil over the base of the plant and when the layered stems have formed new roots, remove and pot.

OFFSETS

Offsets are produced from most herbs that grow from a bulb or corm, such as garlic (*Allium sativum*, p. 56). These can be detached during dormancy and replanted.

SOWING SEEDS IN CONTAINERS

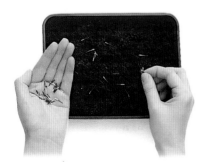

1 *Fill a seed tray with seed soil mix and water well. Sprinkle on the seeds, covering large seeds with a fine layer of compost. Cover the tray with glass or place in a plastic bag and store in a warm place (up to 70°F/21°C).*

2 *Once the seeds have germinated, fill a number of pots with soil mix. Gently lift up a seedling, insert it in a small hole in the soil mix, and pack the soil around it. Water thoroughly and do not allow to dry out.*

HARVESTING & PROCESSING

ALTHOUGH SOME HERBS may be collected all year, most have a particular growing season and must be harvested and either used immediately or preserved for use in the following year. See the individual herb entries on pp. 54–281 for harvesting times. Herbs need to be processed quickly to prevent deterioration and retain their healing action. Gather only healthy plants, free from disease, insect damage, or pollution.

HARVESTING FROM THE WILD

Wild plants offer a free and natural source of herbal remedies and give the satisfaction of collecting herbs in the traditional way. Furthermore, active constituents are often more highly concentrated in wild plants since the herb is likely to be growing in its preferred environment.

IDENTIFICATION
Proper identification of wild plants is essential. Use a field or wild flower guide to help you, since many plants look similar. If in doubt, do not pick the plant, because poisoning can result from misidentification.

ECOLOGICAL & LEGAL FACTORS
While common species, such as nettle (*Urtica dioica*, p. 145), may be readily harvested from the wild, many rarer species are under great pressure due to the lack of a suitable habitat. In many countries it is illegal to uproot any wild plant, and certain species may be protected. Although gathering medicinal plants such as helonias (*Chamaelirium luteum*, p. 75) or gentian (*Gentiana lutea*, p. 97) may be legal in some

countries, it will only reduce their future chances of survival in the wild. *Never pick rare or uncommon plants from the wild, even if they are locally plentiful, and do not collect more than you will use. Do not harvest bark from the wild.*

Before harvesting, consider where the plant is growing and whether it could be contaminated by pollution. Do not collect from roadsides, close to factories, or in areas where crop spraying has occurred. Ideally, you will be familiar with the site from which you are harvesting herbs and knowledgeable about local pollution risks.

HARVESTING FROM YOUR GARDEN

Cultivated herbs provide a ready supply of fresh material in a controlled environment. Harvesting garden plants can be combined with pruning the plant, removing unwanted shoots, and encouraging bushiness. Cut perennials carefully so that plants can quickly regrow. Some medicinal plants, such as lemon balm (*Melissa officinalis*, p. 111), provide two or more crops per year.

GENERAL ADVICE

Harvesting medicinal herbs requires careful planning to make sure that the parts are processed in peak condition and fast enough to retain their active ingredients.

EQUIPMENT
If possible, use a wooden tray or an open basket for collecting medicinal herbs. This prevents crushing and deterioration of the plant. In the wild, a non-nylon rucksack or canvas sack may be more appropriate. Take a field or wildflower guide with you to aid in identification. Always make cuts with a sharp knife or scissors to minimize damage to the plant, and in general try to handle plants as little as possible. Wear gloves if gathering prickly or allergenic plants, such as rue (*Ruta graveolens*, p. 262), to avoid an allergic reaction.

WHAT TO LOOK FOR
Collect material from healthy plants that are free from disease, insect damage, and, in the case of wild plants, pollution. It is important to discard any damaged plants since they can lead to disease or decay in dried plant material. Do not mix cut plant material to avoid mistakes in identification.

WHEN TO HARVEST
Gather herbs in dry weather, preferably on a sunny morning after the dew has evaporated. Picking in the right weather conditions, when the plant is at its peak of maturity, ensures that it will have a high concentration of active constituents. Unless otherwise stated in the individual plant entries on pp. 54–281, leaves are best collected as they open during the spring or summer months, flowers as they start to bloom, fruit and berries just as they become ripe, and roots in the autumn once the plant has drawn its vitality back below the ground. Bark must be gathered with great care if the shrub or tree is to survive – in most cases, harvest it in spring or autumn.

THE CORRECT MEDICINAL PART
In many cases, different parts of the same plant – for example, the leaves and seeds – can have quite different actions and uses. Make sure that you harvest the correct medicinal part of the plant for your purposes.

PROCESSING QUICKLY
Only collect plant material that you will be able to either use or process immediately after harvesting. This is important because fresh plant material, especially tender flowers and leaves, deteriorates very quickly, and the medicinally active constituents are often the first to be affected. In particular, aromatic herbs, which leave their scent in the air or on your skin, can lose their volatile oils within hours. Salad leaves and culinary herbs are best eaten right away to make the most of their nutrients, although they can be stored for a few days in a plastic bag filled with air in a refrigerator.

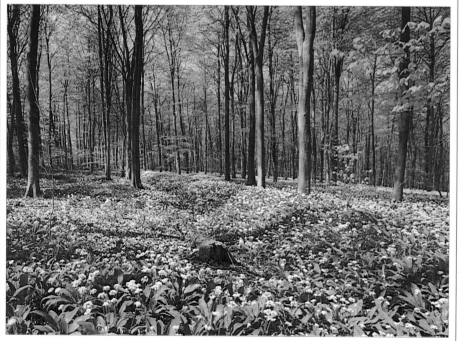

Ramsons *can be found carpeting shady sites in damp woods. The bulb and aerial parts are harvested in early summer for their antibiotic healing properties.*

PROCESSING

Herbs can be preserved in a number of ways, the most common and simple method being air or oven drying. A warm dry place is ideal for this purpose. Always use plain paper for drying herbs, never printed newspaper. Dried herbs can be stored for many months in a dark glass jar or a brown paper bag (*see* p. 288).

AERIAL PARTS

These include all the parts of the plant growing above ground – stems, leaves, flowers, berries, and seeds. The stems are normally cut 2–4 in (5–10 cm) above ground shortly after the plant has begun to flower, when it is putting the most effort into growth. Perennials may be cut higher above ground to encourage further crops. Remove and dry large flowers and leaves separately; smaller ones can be dried on the stem.

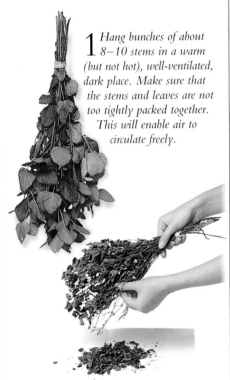

1 *Hang bunches of about 8–10 stems in a warm (but not hot), well-ventilated, dark place. Make sure that the stems and leaves are not too tightly packed together. This will enable air to circulate freely.*

2 *Once brittle but not bone dry, separate small stems, leaves, flowers, and seeds from the stems by carefully rubbing the bunches over a large sheet of plain paper.*

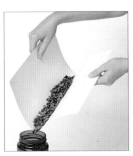

3 *Carefully pour the dried material from the paper into a dark glass jar with a screw top or a brown paper bag.*

LARGE FLOWERS

In most cases, flowers are picked just after they have opened, usually during the spring or summer. Sometimes only specific parts of the flower are used, such as the petals of calendula (*Calendula officinalis*, p. 69), while other flowers are used whole.

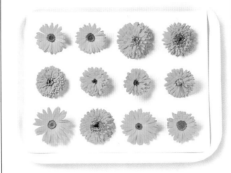

1 *Separate large flower heads from stems and remove any insects or dirt. Place the flowers on absorbent paper in a dry place, allowing sufficient room between them for air to circulate.*

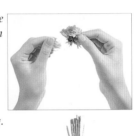

2 *Once dry, store flower heads in a brown paper bag or dark glass jar. Remove calendula petals from the central part of the flower before storing.*

SMALL FLOWERS

Small blooms can be picked with the stalk attached and separated later. Hang small flowers, such as lavender (*Lavandula officinalis*, p. 107), upside down in a paper bag, or suspended over a tray (*see* Seeds below). If the stems are fleshy, dry as for large flowers, above.

FRUIT & BERRIES

Harvest fruit and berries in early autumn when ripe but still firm. If allowed to become overripe, they may not dry properly. They can be picked individually or in bunches.

Place berries or fruit on absorbent paper on trays. Put in a warmed oven (turned off) with the door ajar for 3–4 hours. Move to a dry, warm, dark site, and turn occasionally. Discard any moldy berries or fruit.

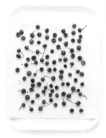

ROOTS, RHIZOMES, TUBERS & BULBS

The underground parts of the plant are usually gathered in autumn after the aerial parts have withered or become inactive and before the soil is waterlogged or frozen. Many roots may also be collected in early spring before the root loses its vitality to aerial growth. Dig deeply around the root, lifting it carefully out of the ground. Some tap roots are very difficult to uproot completely. Remove the required amount and replant the remaining underground part.

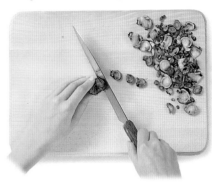

1 *Shake off any soil clinging to the root parts, and thoroughly wash and clean them in warm water, removing any small unwanted side roots or damaged soft spots. Chop into small slices or pieces with a sharp knife.*

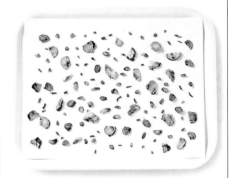

2 *Spread out the root pieces on absorbent paper on a tray and place in a warmed oven (turned off) with the door ajar for 2–3 hours. Move to a warm place until dry.*

SEEDS

Collect ripe seed pods, capsules, or flowering stems in late summer before the seeds have been scattered.

For seeds that are very small, hang small bunches of seed heads upside down over a paper-lined tray, as here, or place in a paper bag. Allow to dry and gently shake. Remove larger seeds by hand when dry.

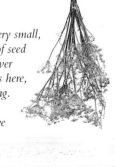

SAP & GEL

Harvest sap only from trees in your own garden. Collect sap in the spring as it rises or as it falls in the autumn. Trees such as silver birch (*Betula pendula*, p. 176) produce huge quantities of sap if tapped, although this reduces the tree's vitality. Bore a deep hole into the trunk of the tree – no more than a quarter of the diameter of the trunk – and place a collecting cup under the mouth of the hole. In spring, quarts of sap may be produced, and it is essential to stop the hole with resin or wood filler once about a quart of fluid has been removed. Collect milky juices or latex from plants such as dandelion (*Taraxacum officinale*, p. 140) by squeezing the stems over a bowl. Wear gloves since latex or sap can be corrosive. The gel from aloe vera (*Aloe vera*, p. 57) is scraped out after slicing the leaf lengthwise and peeling back the edges (*see* below).

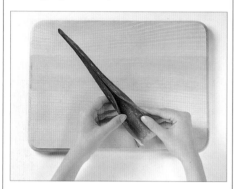

1 *With the fingers and thumb of each hand, carefully slice along the length of an aloe vera leaf and peel back the edges.*

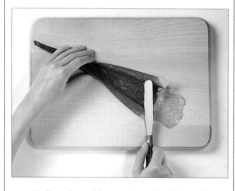

2 *Collect the gel by scraping the blunt edge of a knife along the inside of the leaf. Use aloe vera gel immediately; it cannot be saved.*

BARK

Harvest bark only from your own shrubs or trees since it carries the risk of losing the whole plant through overstripping or "ringing" (removing a whole band of bark). It is far better to collect bark from outlying branches, which can then be pruned back. If stripping bark from a plant, gather it in autumn when the sap is falling. Remove insects, lichen, and moss from the bark; cut it into small pieces and place on a tray to dry.

OTHER WAYS TO PRESERVE HERBS

Apart from simply air-drying herbs, there are a number of other ways to preserve their medicinal benefits.

DEHUMIDIFYING

An effective but expensive way to dry herbs is to use a dehumidifier, which literally sucks water out of the plant. The dehumidifier should be placed in a more or less sealed small room where the herbs are hung in loose bunches or placed on mesh trays. Herbs will dry quickly with this method and, since no heat is used, there is little deterioration or decay.

FREEZE-DRYING

Freeze-drying retains color and flavor but is more suited to culinary than to medicinal herbs. Whole sprigs of herbs such as parsley (*Petroselinum crispum*, p. 244) or sage (*Salvia officinalis*, p. 130) can be frozen in plastic freezer bags. There is no need to defrost before use since the leaves crumble easily when still frozen. Chickweed (*Stellaria media*, p. 270) can also be frozen and used topically for itchy and weeping skin conditions. Many plants may be juiced (*see* p. 296), then frozen as ice cubes and thawed as required.

MICROWAVING

It is possible to dry herbs in a microwave oven. The cut parts should be spread out on paper towels and dried according to the temperature guidelines provided by the manufacturer. This should take about 2–3 minutes, but progress should be checked every 30 seconds and the parts rearranged to ensure even drying.

BUYING DRIED HERBS

Dried herbs are usually available from herbal suppliers, some of which offer a mail order service. Buying from shops is more convenient since the herbs can be examined before purchasing, but mail order companies often have a much higher rate of turnover and may supply better-quality, fresher herbs as a result. To gain the best medicinal effect, good-quality produce is essential. Shop around and bear in mind the following points before buying:

■ Herbs should not be stored in clear glass jars or in direct sunlight since this causes oxidation, which affects their efficacy.
■ Good-quality aromatic herbs should have a distinct scent and taste.
■ Check for signs of infestation due to poor drying techniques or of adulteration. The latter can sometimes be recognized by the inclusion of dried grass or other non-medicinal material in the jar.
■ Herbs lose their color as they age. Look for bright material that has been well dried and stored, and that is not too old. Calendula

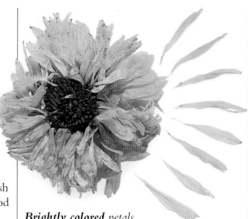

Brightly colored petals indicate high levels of active constituents.

flowers (*Calendula officinalis*, p. 69) that are a vivid yellow/orange color are likely to make good medicine. If they have been sitting on a shelf for 18 months, they will probably look drab and pale.

STORING HERBS

It is vital to store dried herbs properly or they will not last. Leaves, flowers, roots, and other parts should be stored in sterilized dark glass containers with airtight lids. They may also be stored in new brown paper bags that must be kept dry and away from light. Metal and plastic containers are inadvisable because they may contaminate the herb. If stored in a cool dark place, herbs can be kept for about 12 months after harvesting. Herbs frozen in freezer bags can be used for up to 6 months. Make sure the container you use is labeled with the herb, source, strength of preparation if appropriate, and date of harvesting. Keep a sharp eye out for insect infestation. If this occurs, place all affected material in a sealed plastic bag and discard. Sterilize the container and check all other herbs for contamination.

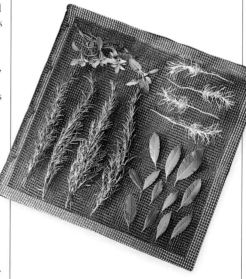

A drying rack for herbs can be simply made by covering a wooden frame with wire mesh.

MAKING HERBAL REMEDIES

IN THE PAST, medicinal herbs have been made into an extraordinary variety of formulations – not only infusions, decoctions, and tinctures but also preparations such as oxymels and elixirs. The following pages give simple step-by-step instructions for making common herbal preparations. Making most types of herbal medicine is not difficult, but it can be time-consuming – if you lack time or equipment, buy ready-made remedies from an herbal supplier (see *Over-the-Counter Remedies*, p. 299).

IDENTIFICATION

Before using medicinal plants that have been collected from the wild, it is essential that they are correctly identified. If in doubt, do not use the herb. Many cases of poisoning have occurred from the mistaken identification of herbs. Foxglove leaves (*Digitalis purpurea*, p. 199) are often mistaken for comfrey (*Symphytum officinale*, p. 136).

UTENSILS

Use glass, enamel, or stainless steel pots and pans, wooden or steel knives and spatulas, and plastic or nylon sieves. A wine press is useful for making tinctures. Never use aluminum utensils; this element is potentially toxic and easily absorbed by herbs.

STERILIZATION

All utensils used to make herbal remedies should be sterilized for at least 30 minutes in a well-diluted sterilizing solution, such as the type used for a baby's bottle. After soaking, rinse thoroughly with boiled water and dry in a hot oven or wash in a dishwasher. Proper sterilization maintains hygiene and prevents remedies, especially creams and syrups, from becoming moldy.

WEIGHTS & MEASURES

For most purposes, ordinary kitchen scales are suitable, although electronic scales are more accurate. Metric measurements of grams and liters are generally much easier to use than imperial measures when making remedies. If it is difficult to weigh a small quantity, such as 10 g, on your scales, measure double the weight, i.e., 20 g, then halve the quantity. Liquids can be measured in a kitchen measuring jug, although conical or straight-sided glass measures are more accurate. Very small volumes of liquid can be measured in drops (see *Measuring Remedies*, right).

STORAGE

Different preparations may be kept for varying periods of time before they begin to lose their medicinal properties. Infusions should be made fresh each day, and decoctions must be consumed within 48 hours. Store both in a refrigerator or cool place. Tinctures and other liquid preparations, such as syrups and essential oils, need to be stored in dark glass bottles in a cool environment away from sunlight, but can be kept for a number of months or years. Ointments, creams, and capsules are best kept in dark glass jars, although plastic containers can also be used. See also *Storing Herbs*, p. 288.

MEASURING REMEDIES

1 ml	= 20 drops
5 ml	= 1 teaspoon
10 ml	= ½ tablespoon
20 ml	= 1 tablespoon
70 ml	= 1 sherry glass
150 ml	= 1 cup or wine glass

Never exceed the quantity of herbs used or the recommended dosage. Although these measurements are approximate, they are accurate enough for most purposes and are used as standard throughout this book. The number of drops to 1 ml depends on the caliber of the pipette (or size of the dropper tip) being used. This can be checked by counting the number of drops required to fill a 5-ml measuring spoon (this book assumes that 100 drops is equal to 5 ml) and then adjusting the dosage as necessary.

THE BASIC FIRST-AID KIT

ADDING HERBAL REMEDIES to the conventional first-aid kit in your home increases the options available to you and your family when accidents happen or illness strikes. The 13 remedies in this first-aid kit can usually be found in pharmacies, herbal stores, and health food stores. Alternatively, some can be homemade, as detailed on the following pages. *Check any cautions for each herb before use.*

BANDAGE

THERMOMETER

ADHESIVE BANDAGE

FEVERFEW (*Tanacetum parthenium*, p. 139) capsules for headaches and migraine

SLIPPERY ELM (*Ulmus rubra*, p. 144) powder for coughs and digestive upsets

ECHINACEA (*Echinacea* spp., p. 90) capsules for colds, flu, and infections

LAVENDER (*Lavandula officinalis*, p. 107) essential oil for insect bites and stings, burns, and headaches

TEA TREE (*Melaleuca alternifolia*, p. 110) essential oil is antiseptic and antifungal

VALERIAN (*Valeriana officinalis*, p. 146) tablets for stress and insomnia

COMFREY (*Symphytum officinale*, p. 136) ointment for bruises and sprains, and for healing fractures

CALENDULA (*Calendula officinalis*, p. 69) cream for inflamed or minor wounds, skin rashes, and sunburn

MYRRH (*Commiphora molmol*, p. 84) tincture for sore throats and acne

THYME (*Thymus vulgaris*, p. 142) syrup for coughs, colds, and chest infections

WITCH HAZEL (*Hamamelis virginiana*, p. 100) distilled water for healing cuts and scrapes

ARNICA (*Arnica montana*, p. 170) cream for painful bruises and muscle pain

GARLIC (*Allium sativum*, p. 56) capsules for infections; the oil from the capsules for earache

INFUSIONS

AN INFUSION IS the simplest way to prepare the more delicate aerial parts of plants, especially leaves and flowers, for use as a medicine or as a revitalizing or relaxing drink. It is made in a similar way to tea, using either a single herb or a combination of herbs, and may be drunk hot or cold.

The medicinal value of many herbs lies chiefly in their volatile oils, which will disperse into the air if a lid is not used. This is especially important in the case of German chamomile (*Chamomilla recutita*, p. 76). Use a teapot, or place a lid or saucer over a cup if making a small quantity. Use water that has just boiled.

Popular herbal teas, such as German chamomile, are often taken as much for their refreshing taste as for their medicinal value and can be safely consumed in quantities of up to 5 or 6 cups a day. Some herbs, however, such as yarrow (*Achillea millefolium*, p. 54), are significantly stronger and must be taken in less frequent doses. Other herbs, such as feverfew (*Tanacetum parthenium*, p. 139), are so strong that they are not suitable for use in infusions. Always check the recommended dosage and quantity of herb, since infusions have medicinal actions and can produce unwanted effects at the wrong dosage.

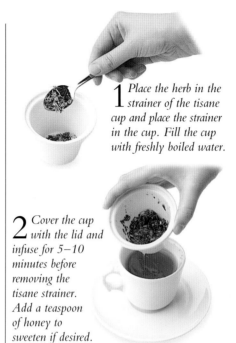

1 *Place the herb in the strainer of the tisane cup and place the strainer in the cup. Fill the cup with freshly boiled water.*

2 *Cover the cup with the lid and infuse for 5–10 minutes before removing the tisane strainer. Add a teaspoon of honey to sweeten if desired.*

STANDARD QUANTITY
CUP 1 tsp (2–3 g) dried or 2 tsp (4–6 g) fresh herb (or mixture of herbs) to a cup of water (this makes 1 dose)
POT 20 g dried herb or 30 g fresh herb (or a mixture of different herbs) to 500 ml of water
STANDARD DOSAGE
Take 3–4 doses (500 ml) each day.
STORAGE
Store in a covered jug in a refrigerator or cool place for up to 24 hours.

POT INFUSION
Warm the pot, then add the herb. Pour in water that has just boiled, replace the lid, and infuse for 10 minutes. Strain some of the infusion into a cup. A teaspoon of honey may be added if desired.

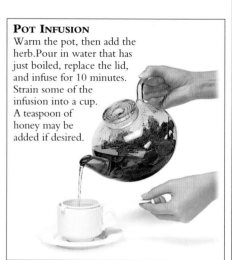

DECOCTIONS

ROOTS, BARK, TWIGS, and berries usually require a more forceful treatment than leaves or flowers to extract their medicinal constituents. A decoction involves simmering these tougher parts in boiling water. Fresh or dried plant material may be used and should be cut or broken into small pieces before decocting. Like infusions, decoctions can be taken hot or cold.

Decoctions are usually made using roots, bark, and berries, but sometimes leaves and flowers may be included. Add these more delicate parts of a plant once the heat has been turned off and the decoction has finished simmering and is beginning to cool. Then strain and use as required.

CHINESE DECOCTIONS
In traditional Chinese medicine, decoctions are the main way in which herbal medicines are prepared. Large quantities of herbs are often used to produce a highly concentrated liquid, or the decoction is further reduced so that there is only 200 ml of liquid remaining. This increases the preparation's concentration. This process is useful for astringent barks such as babul (*Acacia arabica*, p. 156) and common oak (*Quercus robur*, p. 258), which may be used externally to tighten gums or wash weeping skin rashes. (Do not take internally.)

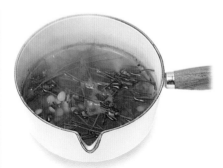

1 *Place the herbs in a saucepan. Cover with cold water and bring to a boil. Simmer for about 20–30 minutes, until the liquid is reduced by about one-third.*

2 *Strain the liquid through a sieve into a jug. Pour the required amount into a cup, then cover the jug and store in a cool place.*

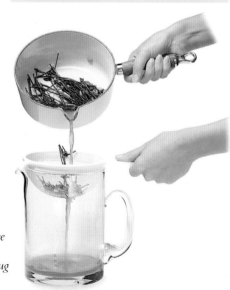

STANDARD QUANTITY
20 g dried or 40 g fresh herb (or mixture of herbs) to 750 ml cold water, reduced to about 500 ml after simmering (this makes 3–4 doses)
STANDARD DOSAGE
Take 3–4 doses (500 ml) each day.
STORAGE
Store in a covered jug in a refrigerator or cool place for up to 48 hours.

TINCTURES

TINCTURES ARE MADE by soaking an herb in alcohol (vodka or rum). This encourages the active plant constituents to dissolve, giving tinctures a relatively stronger action than infusions or decoctions. They are convenient to use and last up to two years. Tinctures can be made using a jug and a jelly bag, instead of a wine press. Although mainly used in European, American, and Australian herbal medicine, tinctures play a part in most herbal traditions.

Tinctures are strong preparations, and it is essential to check the recommended dosage. Never use industrial alcohol, methylated spirits (methyl alcohol), or rubbing alcohol (isopropyl alcohol) in tinctures.

ALCOHOL-REDUCED TINCTURES
Alcoholic tinctures should sometimes be avoided – for example, during pregnancy or a gastric inflammation. Adding 5 ml of tincture to a small glass of almost boiling water and leaving it for 5 minutes allows the alcohol to evaporate. To make nonalcoholic tinctures, replace the alcohol with vinegar or glycerol.

TINCTURE RATIOS
Tinctures are made in different strengths, expressed as ratios. In this book, a 1:5 ratio (1 part herb to 5 parts alcohol) is used, unless otherwise stated.

STANDARD QUANTITY
200 g dried or 300 g fresh herb chopped into small pieces to 1 liter alcohol – vodka of 35–40% alcohol is ideal, although rum hides the taste of bitter or unpalatable herbs

STANDARD DOSAGE
Take 5 ml (1 tsp) 2–3 times a day diluted in 25 ml of water or fruit juice.

STORAGE
Store in sterilized dark glass bottles in a cool dark place for up to 2 years.

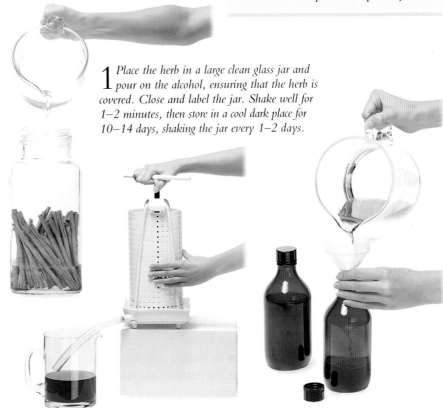

1 *Place the herb in a large clean glass jar and pour on the alcohol, ensuring that the herb is covered. Close and label the jar. Shake well for 1–2 minutes, then store in a cool dark place for 10–14 days, shaking the jar every 1–2 days.*

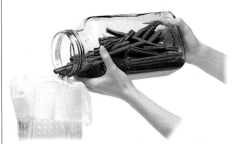

2 *Set up the wine press, placing a muslin or nylon mesh bag securely inside. Pour in the mixture and collect the liquid in the jug.*

3 *Slowly close the wine press, extracting the remaining liquid from the herbs until no more drips appear. Discard the leftover herbs.*

4 *Pour the tincture into clean dark glass bottles using a funnel. When full, stopper with a cork or screw top and label the bottles.*

CAPSULES & POWDERS

POWDERED HERBS ARE most easily taken as capsules but can be sprinkled on food or taken with water. Externally, they can be applied as a dusting powder to the skin or mixed with tinctures as a poultice (*see* p. 294).

Reputable herbal suppliers are the best place to buy powdered herbs and, in general, the finer the powder, the better the grade and quality. Gelatin or vegetarian capsule cases are also available from specialty outlets. Powdered slippery elm (*Ulmus rubra*, p. 144) makes a useful base for poultices (*see* p. 294), and astringents such as witch hazel (*Hamamelis virginiana*, p. 100) may be applied to weeping skin or mixed into ointments (*see* p. 294) for hemorrhoids and varicose veins.

MAKING CAPSULES

STANDARD QUANTITY
Fill size 00 capsules which contain approximately 250 mg of powdered herb

STANDARD DOSAGE
Take 2–3 capsules twice a day.

STORAGE
Store in airtight, dark glass containers in a cool place for up to 3–4 months.

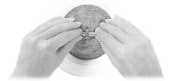

1 *Pour the powder into a saucer and slide the capsule halves toward one another, scooping up the powder (or use a capsule-making tray).*

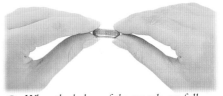

2 *When the halves of the capsule are full of powder, slide them together without spilling the powder and store.*

OINTMENTS

OINTMENTS CONTAIN OILS or fats heated with herbs and, unlike creams, contain no water. As a result, ointments form a separate layer on the surface of the skin. They protect against injury or inflammation of damaged skin and carry active medicinal constituents, such as essential oils, to the affected area. Ointments are useful in conditions such as hemorrhoids or where protection is needed from moisture, as in chapped lips and diaper rash.

STANDARD QUANTITY
60 g dried or 150 g fresh herb
(or mixture of herbs) to 500 g
of petroleum jelly or soft paraffin wax
STANDARD APPLICATION
Apply a little 3 times a day.
STORAGE
Store in sterilized dark glass jars with lids

Ointments can be made with dozens of bases, and they vary in consistency, depending on the constituents and proportions used. The simplest way to make a soft all-purpose ointment is to use petroleum jelly or soft paraffin wax (other methods are explained below). Petroleum jelly is impermeable to water and provides a protective barrier for the skin. Single herbs or mixtures of herbs may be used as required, provided that they are finely cut, and essential oil can be stirred into the ointment just before straining.

DIFFERENT CONSISTENCIES

A solid and relatively grease-free ointment will spread easily and is useful for preparations such as lip balms. This may be made by using alternatives to mineral oils. Melt 140 g of coconut oil with 120 g of beeswax and 100 g of powdered herb. Simmer gently for 90 minutes in a glass bowl set in a pan of boiling water, or a double boiler, then strain and pour into jars.

A less solid ointment, for conditions such as skin rashes, may be made by combining olive oil and beeswax. Melt 60 g of beeswax with 500 ml of olive oil and 120 g of dried or 300 g of fresh herb in a glass bowl. Cover and place in a warm oven for 3 hours, then remove, strain, and pour into jars. This ointment can also be made by combining 500 ml of hot infused oil (*see* p. 293) with 60 g of melted beeswax.

1 *Melt the petroleum jelly or wax in a glass bowl set in a pan of boiling water, or use a double boiler. Add the finely cut herb and simmer for 15 minutes, stirring continuously.*

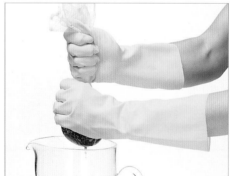

2 *Pour the herb mixture into a jelly bag secured to the rim of a jug with string, and allow the liquid to filter through.*

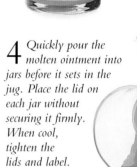

4 *Quickly pour the molten ointment into jars before it sets in the jug. Place the lid on each jar without securing it firmly. When cool, tighten the lids and label.*

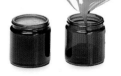

3 *Wearing rubber gloves, squeeze as much of the hot herb mixture as possible through the bag into the jug.*

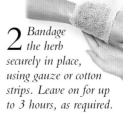

POULTICES

A POULTICE IS a mixture of fresh, dried, or powdered herbs that is applied to an affected area. Poultices are used to ease nerve or muscle pains, sprains, or broken bones, and to draw pus from infected wounds, ulcers, or boils.

STANDARD QUANTITY
Sufficient herb to cover the affected area
STANDARD APPLICATION
Apply a new poultice every 2–3 hours.
Repeat as often as required.

A poultice of self-heal (*Prunella vulgaris*, p. 122) relieves sprains and fractures, while St. John's wort (*Hypericum perforatum*, p. 104) can help ease muscle or nerve pains.

DRAWING BOILS & INFECTED WOUNDS

Slippery elm powder (*Ulmus rubra*, p. 144) mixed with calendula (*Calendula officinalis*, p. 69) tincture or myrrh (*Commiphora molmol*, p. 84) tincture makes a useful poultice for drawing boils and wounds.

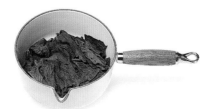

1 *Simmer the herb for 2 minutes. Squeeze out any excess liquid, rub some oil on the affected area to prevent sticking, and apply the herb while hot.*

2 *Bandage the herb securely in place, using gauze or cotton strips. Leave on for up to 3 hours, as required.*

CREAMS

MAKING A CREAM involves combining oil or fat and water in an emulsion. If the process is rushed, the oil and water may separate. Unlike ointments, creams blend with the skin and have the advantage of being cooling and soothing while at the same time allowing the skin to breathe and sweat naturally. They can, however, deteriorate quite quickly and are best stored in dark airtight jars in a refrigerator.

Small quantities of additional ingredients such as tinctures, powders, and essential oils can be added to a cream before or after it is put in jars. Adding an essential oil, such as 1 ml of tea tree (*Melaleuca alternifolia*, p. 110) to 100 ml of cream, counters mold growth and lengthens shelf-life, as does 5 ml of borax. Other recipes for making cream use infusions, tinctures, or infused oils.

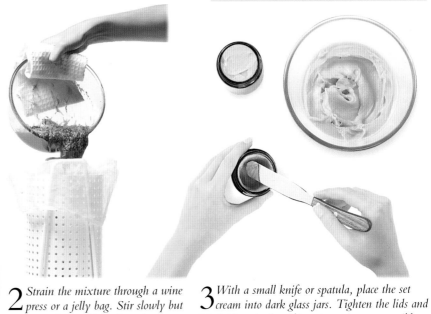

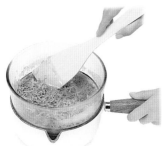

1 *Melt the emulsifying wax in a glass bowl set in a pan of boiling water or a double boiler. Add the glycerine, water, and herb while stirring, and simmer for 3 hours.*

2 *Strain the mixture through a wine press or a jelly bag. Stir slowly but continuously until it cools and sets.*

3 *With a small knife or spatula, place the set cream into dark glass jars. Tighten the lids and label. Store in the refrigerator as soon as possible.*

COMPRESSES & LOTIONS

LOTIONS ARE WATER-BASED herbal preparations such as infusions, decoctions, or diluted tinctures that are used to bathe inflamed or irritated skin. Compresses are cloths soaked in a lotion and held against the skin. Both lotions and compresses are simple ways to use herbs externally, and can be very effective in relieving swelling, bruising, and pain, soothing inflammation and headaches, and cooling fevers.

After an accident or sports injury, bruising and swelling can often be reduced or prevented if a hot compress is swiftly applied, provided that the skin is unbroken. Cold compresses are particularly useful in soothing inflammation, cooling fevers, and easing headaches. Both hot and cold compresses should be frequently soaked and reapplied for maximum benefit.

APPLYING A LOTION

As specified, make an infusion or decoction (*see* p. 290), and strain it well. Alternatively, dilute a tincture with water. Soak a clean cloth in the lotion and wring it out thoroughly. Then gently bathe the affected area with the cloth (rather than laying it on the skin as you would a compress).

APPLYING A COMPRESS

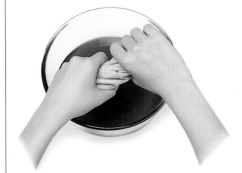

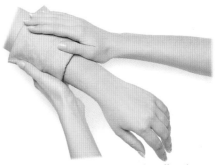

1 *Wash your hands thoroughly and soak a soft cloth or clean washcloth in the lotion. Wring out the excess liquid. Before applying, rub some oil on the affected area to prevent sticking.*

2 *Place the compress against the affected area. For pain and swellings, secure the compress with plastic wrap or plastic and safety pins, and leave for up to 2 hours. Reapply as required.*

OTHER PREPARATIONS

DIFFERENT HERBAL PREPARATIONS suit different ailments. Most of the following preparations provide localized relief. Steam inhalations, for example, help clear various respiratory complaints; gargles and mouthwashes soothe sore throats and canker sores; massage oils can ease aching muscles; and skin washes relieve inflamed skin conditions.

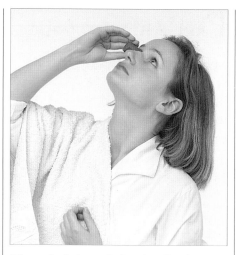

The eyebath is applied to the affected eye and the head is tilted well back.

STEAM INHALATIONS

Steam inhalations are an effective way to clear congestion, and relieve sinusitis, hay fever, and bronchial asthma. The combination of steam and antiseptic ingredients clears the airways throughout the respiratory system.

To make Pour 1 liter of water that has just boiled into a large bowl, add 5–10 drops of essential oil, and stir well. Alternatively, make an infusion of 25 g of herb to 1 liter of water, brew for 15 minutes, and pour into a bowl. Cover the head and bowl with a towel, close the eyes, and inhale the steam for about 10 minutes or until the preparation cools. After a steam inhalation, it is advisable to stay in a warm room for 30 minutes to allow the airways to adjust and any mucus to clear.

Inhalations using essential oil relieve many respiratory complaints.

GARGLES & MOUTHWASHES

Gargles and mouthwashes usually contain astringent herbs that tighten the mucous membranes of the mouth and throat. Astringent herbs, such as rhatany (*Krameria triandra*, p. 223) and myrrh (*Commiphora molmol*, p. 84), can be made more palatable and more effective for sore throats by adding a little licorice (*Glycyrrhiza glabra*, p. 99) or a pinch of cayenne pepper (*Capsicum frutescens*, p. 70) to the preparation. Since gargles and mouthwashes are made from infusions, decoctions, or diluted tinctures, they can usually be swallowed for internal treatment. Make sure that you do not exceed the daily internal dose of an herb.

To make Make an infusion (*see* p. 290), but allow it to stand for 15–20 minutes in

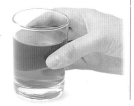

Infusions made with antiseptic herbs make useful gargles and mouthwashes for sore throats and canker sores.

order to increase its astringency. Strain, then gargle, or rinse the mouth with a cupful. Alternatively, use a decoction (to make, p. 290) or dilute about 5 ml of tincture in 100 ml of hot water and use in the same way. Repeat as often as required unless specified.

SUPPOSITORIES

Suppositories are waxy pellets containing essential oil or fine powder. They are used when oral medicine is likely to be broken down during digestion before reaching its intended site. Suppositories are inserted into the vagina or the anus where they melt at body temperature. The herb is quickly absorbed into the bloodstream, providing fast relief. It is best to buy ready-made suppositories.

To make suppositories Use a suppository mold or make 24 molds from cooking foil shaped around a thimble. Mix 10 g of soft soap, 50 ml of glycerine, and 40 ml of methylated spirits, and pour into the molds. Leave for a few minutes to coat the molds, then pour out the excess and leave to harden. Melt 20 g of cocoa butter, remove from the heat, and add 30 drops of essential oil or 5 g of powder. Pour into the shells and leave to set for 3 hours before removing the suppositories. Store in a cool place in a pot lined with greaseproof paper for up to 3 months.

ESSENTIAL OILS

Essential oils can be used in massage to soothe minor aches and pains. Before use, they should be diluted with a carrier oil since they can irritate the skin. Essential oils deteriorate rapidly after dilution, so it is best to mix small quantities as you need them.

For massage Mix 5–10 drops of essential oil with 1 tbsp of carrier oil, such as wheat germ or almond oil, and massage gently into the skin.

Oil burner Use 5–10 drops of neat essential oil mixed with water. Burn for 30 minutes.

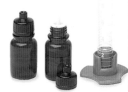

Essential oils are used in baths, oil burners, and in massage to relieve tension and stress.

BATHS & SKIN WASHES

Herbal baths and skin washes can relieve many conditions, including aching limbs and stuffy sinuses. They are made from diluted essential oils or infusions. Eyebaths soothe sore, inflamed, or irritated eyes.

To make an herbal bath Add 500 ml of strained infusion (*see* p. 290) or 5–10 drops of essential oil to a running bath.

To make a skin wash Make an infusion, strain it, and bathe the affected area.

To make an eyebath Make a small quantity of an infusion or use an herbal teabag. Strain the liquid carefully into a sterilized eyebath. Alternatively, add 2–3 drops of a tincture to an eyebath filled with water that has just boiled. Allow to cool and place the eyebath firmly over the eye. Tip the head back and bathe the eye by continuously blinking. Repeat up to 3 times a day.

General cautions Eyebaths should be very weak so as not to sting the eyes. Always use boiled cooled water in a sterilized container. Do not bathe eyes over a period of more than 2–3 weeks at a time. If bathing eyes frequently, add a tiny pinch of salt to each eyebath to counter leaching of salts and minerals from the eye.

COLD MACERATIONS

Heat destroys the active constituents of some herbs, and a cold maceration is more appropriate than a decoction.

To make Pour 500 ml of cold water over 25 g of herb and leave to stand overnight. Strain and use as you would a decoction.

JUICES

The juices extracted from many herbs can be taken internally or applied externally.

To make Pulp the plant, preferably using a mechanical juicer. Otherwise use a food processor. Squeeze the pulp through a jelly bag to collect the juice. Some herbs need to be cooked in order to extract their juice.

PLANTS THAT PREVENT ILLNESS

MEDICINAL HERBS DO not have to be used only when things go wrong with your health. Although many herbs are primarily used to treat illness, a great number act as cleansing "spring tonics" and nourishing foods. They can be taken when you are fit and well, and, in this way, they maintain health and prevent illness.

HERBS FOR HEALTH

All traditions of herbal medicine have aimed to maintain health rather than treat illness. Unlike today, in the past the spiritual aspect of health and "dis-ease" was considered as important as the physical aspect. However, herbal medicines can only help to maintain health as part of a lifestyle that includes a balanced diet, appropriate exercise, and a positive and relaxed attitude to life and its everyday stresses. Herbal medicine can often help sustain health into ripe old age. Tonic herbs, such as ginseng (*Panax ginseng*, p. 116), improve the body's ability to cope with physical and mental stress, while thyme (*Thymus vulgaris*, p. 142) appears to slow down the aging process. In this way, many of the plants in this book (*see pp. 54–281*) help support the body and mind in adapting to life's unpredictable demands.

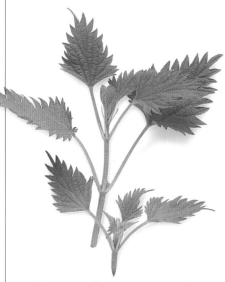

Nettle is an excellent spring tonic and is even richer in iron than spinach. The leaves can be cooked as a vegetable and added to soups.

Early growing, green leafy herbs, such as nettle (*Urtica dioica*, p. 145), were traditional "spring tonics" after the winter months. Herbs such as this are nourishing, and they also help cleanse waste products from the body. Today, some herbs are readily available all year, providing a continuous source of vital nutrients and helping form an important part of a balanced diet.

VITAMINS & MINERALS

All plants contain trace amounts of vitamins and minerals, and many have special medicinal properties as well. Some plants have such high levels of vitamins, minerals, or other nutrients that they are considered "natural food supplements." Watercress (*Nasturtium officinale*, p. 237) is an example. It contains vitamins A, B_1, B_2, C, and E, as well as iodine, iron, and phosphorus. It also has antibiotic constituents that make it especially useful. Other herbs that are rich in vitamins and minerals are listed below.

VITAMINS
Pro-vitamin A (carotene) & vitamin A carrot (*Daucus carota*, p. 198), yellow dock (*Rumex crispus*, p. 126), apricots (*Prunus armeniaca*, p. 254)
Vitamins B_1 and B_2 lycium fruit (*Lycium chinense*, p. 109)
Vitamin B_6 soybean (*Glycine max*, p. 215), potato (*Solanum tuberosum*, p. 269)
Vitamin B_{12} Chinese angelica (*Angelica sinensis*, p. 60)
Vitamin C parsley (*Petroselinum crispum*, p. 244), lemon (*Citrus limon*, p. 81)
Vitamin E seed oils, especially butternut (*Juglans cinerea*, p. 222)
Vitamin K alfalfa (*Medicago sativa*, p. 232)

MINERALS
Calcium sesame seeds (*Sesamum indicum*, p. 268), celery (*Apium graveolens*, p. 61), rose hips (*Rosa canina*, p. 261)
Copper cocoa (*Theobroma cacao*, p. 274)
Germanium garlic (*Allium sativum*, p. 56)
Iodine seaweeds, including kelp (*Fucus vesiculosus*, p. 211)
Iron all green herbs – for example parsley (*Petroselinum crispum*, p. 244), cabbage (*Brassica oleracea*, p. 178), nettle (*Urtica dioica*, p. 145)
Manganese soybean (*Glycine max*, p. 215)
Phosphorus watercress (*Nasturtium officinale*, p. 237), celery seed (*Apium graveolens*, p. 61)
Potassium dandelion (*Taraxacum officinale*, p. 140), cornsilk (*Zea mays*, p. 152)
Selenium garlic (*Allium sativum*, p. 56)
Silica horsetail (*Equisetum arvense*, p. 202), nettle (*Urtica dioica*, p. 145)
Zinc pumpkin seeds (*Cucurbita pepo*, p. 194), coltsfoot (*Tussilago farfara*, p. 277)

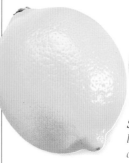

Watercress is a vitamin and mineral supplement in its own right. It has a "bite" to its taste, which indicates its antibiotic abilities.

FLAVOR & COLOR IN COOKING

Most plants that lend zest to the taste or appearance of food have some medicinal value. For example, rosemary (*Rosmarinus officinalis*, p. 125), a traditional and aromatic accompaniment to red meat in European cookery, is an effective aid to digestion. Lemon (*Citrus limon*, p. 81), much used in cookery the world over, has a strongly antiseptic action, which, medicinally, makes it a useful remedy for colds and stomach infections. It also helps to reduce the incidence of food poisoning.

Sharp-tasting lemon protects against colds and infection.

In China, there is no meaningful difference between something that is a "food" and a "medicine." "Medicinal food" is simply what is constitutionally good for you. Strong-acting tonic herbs, such as Chinese angelica (*Angelica sinensis*, p. 60), ginkgo fruit (*Ginkgo biloba*, p. 98), and American ginseng (*Panax quinquefolium*, p. 241), are flavorful and regularly used ingredients in Chinese recipes. Throughout southern Asia and Africa, herbs and hot spices give color, piquancy, and medicinal value to food. The herbs turmeric (*Curcuma longa*, p. 88), cardamom (*Elettaria cardamomum*, p. 91), and ginger (*Zingiber officinale*, p. 153), which are all used in cooking, protect against gastrointestinal discomfort and infection.

REMEDIES FOR COMMON AILMENTS

HERBAL KNOWLEDGE IS continuing to grow as more people choose herbs as an alternative to pharmaceutical drugs. The following remedies are safe and effective treatments for a range of common ailments but, like all medicines, they must be treated with respect. The suggestions given here are mostly quite straightforward. However, if you are unsure about what to do, always seek professional advice (*see* p. 320). For instructions on how to make herbal preparations, *see* pp. 289–296.

ESSENTIAL INFORMATION

Before using remedies read the following.

DOSAGE

■ Except in *Infants & Children* (*see* p. 318), all dosages given are for adults.

■ Never exceed the stated dose; doubling it will *not* make the medicine twice as effective.

■ Before taking a remedy, check the cautions in the relevant herb entry (*see* pp. 54–281).

■ Do not take more than two internal remedies at any one time or more than one internal and one external remedy for the same complaint, unless specified. Alternative remedies using different herbs are divided by a leaf symbol. Where different forms of a remedy are given (e.g., take tincture or infusion), the first is preferable.

HOW LONG TO TAKE REMEDIES

Take remedies until symptoms disappear. If there is no improvement within 2–3 weeks, if the condition worsens, or if in doubt, consult a professional practitioner (*see* p. 320).

PROFESSIONAL ADVICE

■ Advice is given on when to seek professional help. Consult a professional if taking a remedy for over 3 weeks.

INFANTS & CHILDREN

■ Do not give babies under 6 months any internal herbal (or other) medicine without professional advice.

■ *Infants & Children* (p. 318) gives children's dosages. Remedies elsewhere can be used for children under 12, but the dose must be reduced as follows:

■ 6–12 months old – 1/10 adult dose
■ 1–6 years old – 1/3 adult dose
■ 7–12 years old – 1/2 adult dose

THE ELDERLY

The elderly, because of their slower metabolism, may require less than the full adult dose. People over 70 should take 3/4 of the adult dose.

PREGNANCY

■ During the first 3 months of pregnancy, avoid all medicines, herbal or otherwise, unless absolutely essential.

■ Avoid alcoholic tinctures in pregnancy.

■ The herbs in *Pregnancy* (*see* p. 317) are safe to use. Many of the remedies elsewhere are also safe, *but always check the cautions for the remedy and in the relevant herb entry (see pp. 54–281).*

■ Herbs in this section to avoid are: arbor vitae (*Thuja occidentalis*, p. 274); black cohosh (*Cimicifuga racemosa*, p. 78); buchu (*Barosma betulina*, p. 67); Chinese angelica (*Angelica sinensis*, p. 60); Chinese rhubarb (*Rheum palmatum*, p. 124); *dan shen* (*Salvia miltiorrhiza*, p. 129); devil's claw (*Harpagophytum procumbens*, p. 101); elecampane (*Inula helenium*, p. 105); feverfew (*Tanacetum parthenium*, p. 139); ginseng (*Panax ginseng*, p. 116); juniper (*Juniperus communis*, p. 223); licorice (*Glycyrrhiza glabra*, p. 99); motherwort (*Leonurus cardiaca*, p. 225); myrrh (*Commiphora molmol*, p. 84); pennyroyal (*Mentha pulegium*, p. 233); prickly ash (*Zanthoxylum americanum*, p. 151); senna (*Cassia senna*, p. 72); shepherd's purse (*Capsella bursa-pastoris*, p. 181); vervain (*Verbena officinalis*, p. 147); white peony (*Paeonia lactiflora*, p. 115); wild yam (*Dioscorea villosa*, p. 89); wormwood (*Artemisia absinthium*, p. 63); yarrow (*Achillea millefolium*, p. 54); yellow dock (*Rumex crispus*, p. 126).

■ Avoid medicinal doses of angelica (*Angelica archangelica*, p. 166), anise (*Pimpinella anisum*, pp. 246–247), cayenne (*Capsicum frutescens*, p. 70), celery (*Apium graveolens*, p. 61), and sage (*Salvia officinalis*, p. 130). Cautions appear where relevant.

■ Essential oils to avoid include German chamomile (*Chamomilla recutita*, p. 76) and thyme (*Thymus vulgaris*, p. 142).

PRESCRIPTION MEDICINE

Some herbs interact with pharmaceutical drugs. If you are taking a prescribed medicine, consult a professional practitioner before taking an herbal remedy, and do not discontinue any medicine without prior approval.

HERBAL PREPARATIONS

■ All quantities given are for dried herbs unless specified.

■ Where more than one part of a herb is used, the instructions specify which part to use. Only use that part. Do not use seeds sold for horticultural purposes.

■ Unless specified otherwise, preparations are made with standard quantities of herb, as follows:

Infusions Use a teaspoon of herb to a cup of water, or, make enough for 3–4 doses using 25 g herb to 500 ml of water. Use a covered container to retain the herb's valuable volatile oils. To make, *see* p. 290.

Decoctions Use 25 g herb to 500 ml of water. To make, *see* p. 290.

Inhalations Add 25 g herb or 5–10 drops essential oil to 1 liter of steaming hot water. To make, *see* p. 296.

Lotions Use 500 ml infusion or decoction, or 25 ml tincture diluted in 500 ml of water. To make, *see* p. 296.

Tablets or capsules Many herbs are available over the counter in both forms. Take according to the instructions on the packet. To make capsules, use 250 mg powdered herb per capsule (*see* p. 292).

Tinctures Make with 1 part herb to 5 parts alcohol. To make, *see* p. 296. Some tinctures are available ready-made. Take tinctures with cold water unless specified.

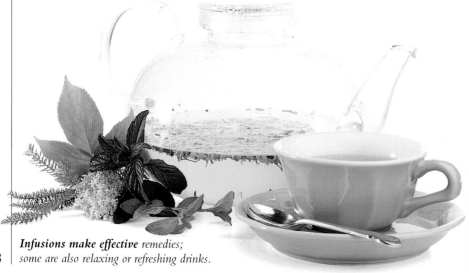

Infusions make effective remedies; *some are also relaxing or refreshing drinks.*

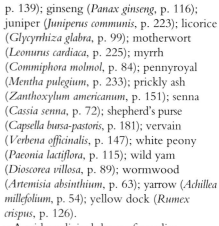

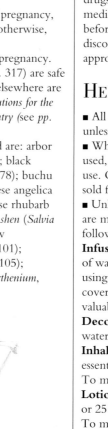

MEASUREMENTS

1 ml	= 20 drops
5 ml	= 1 tsp
20 ml	= 1 tbsp
70 ml	= 1 sherry glass
150 ml	= 1 cup or wine glass

ESSENTIAL OILS

Do not take essential oils internally unless directed to do so by a professional practitioner. For external use, dilute essential oils with a carrier oil, such as sunflower or almond, in a ratio of 1 part essential oil to 20 parts carrier oil, e.g., 5 drops essential oil to 1 tsp (5 ml) carrier oil. For a bath, add 5 drops of neat essential oil to the running water. To use essential oils in massage, *see p. 296*.

OTHER INFORMATION

For other preparations, weighing & measuring, and equipment, *see pp. 290–296*.

SELF-HELP

Lifestyle, diet, and exercise advice is given throughout this section. In general, these suggestions do not provide a "quick fix" solution and need to be followed over the long term to be effective. They should be used in addition to the herbal remedy that is recommended. By ensuring that your body has the right nutrition and level of fitness, you protect yourself against many ailments such as infections and circulatory problems as well as increasing your chances of a speedy and effective recovery. Herbs containing high levels of vitamins and minerals are listed on p. 297.

Fennel & lemon balm infusion relieves indigestion.

OVER-THE-COUNTER REMEDIES

The number of stores and mail order companies selling ready-made preparations is growing. It is usually most convenient to buy tablets, essential oils, suppositories, ointments, and perhaps tinctures, and to make your own infusions, decoctions, and syrups. Belladonna plasters should be bought, not made. Before buying an herbal medicine, always carefully read the list of contents on the label. (In certain countries some herbal medicines have a product license number.) Follow the instructions on the label; do not exceed the recommended dosage. If buying preparations or dried herbs, use a reputable supplier and brand name. Many essential oils that are commercially produced use synthetic ingredients, which have little or no medicinal value. See also *Buying Dried Herbs*, p. 288, and *Useful Addresses*, p. 336.

AILMENTS INDEX

See the pages listed for remedies for the following ailments.

Chest rubs provide relief for respiratory complaints.

ALLERGIES

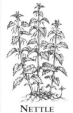

NETTLE
(*Urtica dioica*)

ALLERGIES OFTEN DEVELOP when the body's immune system overreacts to an external irritant such as pollen, insect stings, and certain plants, or internal substances such as chemicals and foods. The allergens trigger a reaction in those who have a built-in or natural sensitivity. In the long term, allergies are treated by both reducing contact with allergens (if known) and working to reduce the body's oversensitivity. Herbal remedies can bring relief to some allergic states and are helpful in gradually reducing allergic reactions. See also *Skin Rashes*, p. 303.

SEEK IMMEDIATE PROFESSIONAL ADVICE FOR

- Life-threatening allergies such as asthma. Consult a professional practitioner prior to taking any herbal remedies for such conditions
- Any allergy that shows signs of deterioration after taking an herbal remedy

ALLERGIC RHINITIS, INCLUDING HAY FEVER

ALLERGIC RHINITIS IS an umbrella term for allergic reactions to irritants such as pollution, dust, or pollen. It may occur throughout the year, while hay fever is usually caused by seasonal grass or pollens. Symptoms include sneezing, copious nasal mucus, sinus congestion, watery, irritated eyes, and even asthmalike wheezing. Self-treatment will help relieve mild conditions, but, for severe outbreaks, consult a professional practitioner who can prescribe herbs such as ephedra (*Ephedra sinica*, p. 93). See also *Congestion, Sinus Problems & Earache*, p. 312.

DIET
Reduce your intake of or cut out mucus-forming foods such as dairy products, eggs, sugar, white flour, fatty foods, and alcohol.

GENERAL REMEDIES
Herbs Nettle (*Urtica dioica*, p. 145), elderflower (*Sambucus nigra*, p. 131)
Remedy Make a nettle infusion. Take 3–4 cups a day for 3 months at a time. Alternatively, make an infusion with 1 tsp of each herb to 2 cups of water and take daily for 3 months at a time.

Herb Baical skullcap (*Scutellaria baicalensis*, p. 133)
Remedy Make a decoction and take 2 cups a day.

HAY FEVER
Herb Elderflower (*Sambucus nigra*, p. 131)
Remedy Make an infusion and take 2–3 cups a day. Take for a few months before, as well as during, the hay fever season.

ALLERGIC RHINITIS WITH MUCUS
Herbs Eyebright (*Euphrasia officinalis*, p. 208), plantain (*Plantago major*, p. 249), goldenrod (*Solidago virgaurea*, p. 269), boneset (*Eupatorium perfoliatum*, p. 206)
Remedy Make an infusion with one or a mixture of all of the herbs and drink up to 3 cups a day.
NOTE Use this remedy especially for copious, watery mucus.

Herbs Echinacea (*Echinacea* spp., p. 90), marsh mallow (*Althaea officinalis*, p. 163), elderflower (*Sambucus nigra*, p. 131), thyme (*Thymus vulgaris*, p. 142)
Remedy Take 1 tsp of equal parts of each tincture 3 times daily with warm water.
NOTE Use this remedy especially for thick yellow/green mucus and sinus congestion.

ECZEMA

CHARACTERIZED BY RED inflamed skin, eczema causes irritation, flaking, scaling, and tiny blisters. Although it is often the result of an allergic reaction to certain substances, eczema can also be inherited, result from prolonged contact with an irritant, or it may simply appear for an unknown reason. It is advisable to consult a professional practitioner since eczema is difficult to self-treat. However, the following remedies, taken for at least a week, can bring relief. Two remedies may be used at once. Chickweed reduces soreness or itchiness, and oats can be used to impart a soothing, emollient effect to bathwater. See also *Skin Rashes*, p. 303.

SELF-HELP
To avoid scratching, cover the affected area with an absorbent nonirritating material such as cotton.

General caution If there is no improvement, or if the condition deteriorates, seek professional advice.

GENERAL REMEDIES
Herbs Peppermint (*Mentha* x *piperita*, p. 112), chickweed (*Stellaria media*, p. 270)
Remedy 1 Make peppermint lotion by infusing 1 tsp of herb to 1 cup of water. Leave for 10 minutes, then strain and cool. Use to wash gently over the affected skin 2–3 times a day.
Remedy 2 Apply chickweed ointment, cream, or freshly squeezed juice up to 5 times a day.
Option Add 2 drops of peppermint oil to 1 tsp of any of the chickweed preparations.

Herb Gotu kola (*Centella asiatica*, p. 74)
Remedy Dust the affected area with powder 2–3 times a day. Alternatively, mix the powder with enough water to make a thick paste and spread over the affected area 1–2 times a day.

ECZEMA WITH WEEPING SKIN
Herb Witch hazel (*Hamamelis virginiana*, p. 100)
Remedy Apply lotion or cream up to 5 times a day (the lotion is preferable). Alternatively, make a decoction with 2 tsp of leaves to 1 cup of water, leave for 15 minutes, strain, and cool. Use as a wash up to 5 times a day.

Herb German chamomile (*Chamomilla recutita*, p. 76)
Remedy Make an infusion using 50 g of herb to 750 ml of water. Apply directly to the itchy area when cool, or add the hot infusion to a warm bath and soak in it for at least 20 minutes.

Herb Oats (*Avena sativa*, p. 172)
Remedy Fill a muslin (or similar) bag with milled oats and place under a hot tap while running a bath. Relax in the bath for 5–10 minutes.

MILD ASTHMA, WHEEZING & SHORTNESS OF BREATH

ASTHMA IS USUALLY prompted by an allergic reaction to substances such as pollen, dust, animal hair, or certain foods, but may also be related to an infection. The listed remedies will relieve immediate symptoms, but in order to find the cause of your ailment, or for long-term treatment, it is best to consult an herbalist. All the herbal remedies that are suggested here can be taken along with conventional treatment. Herbs such as nettle, thyme, crampbark, and echinacea help to ease breathing, while essential oil of German chamomile reduces inflammation.

General cautions Seek professional help for asthma. Do not stop using steroidal or other inhalants suddenly. Their use should be phased out gradually and only with professional guidance.

WHEEZING & SHORTNESS OF BREATH
Herbs Nettle (*Urtica dioica*, p. 145), thyme (*Thymus vulgaris*, p. 142)
Remedy Make an infusion using 15 g of each herb to 750 ml of water and drink throughout the day.

Herb German chamomile (*Chamomilla recutita*, p. 76)
Remedy Make an infusion with 2 heaping tsp of the herb to 1 cup of water and leave to stand for 10 minutes in a covered saucepan. Remove the lid, inhale the steam, and strain and drink the tea.
Option Use the essential oil in a steam inhalation, or inhale 2 drops of undiluted oil placed on a handkerchief.

Herb Baical skullcap (*Scutellaria baicalensis*, p. 133)
Remedy Make a decoction and take up to 2 cups a day.

BREATHING DIFFICULTY & TIGHT CHEST
Herb Crampbark (*Viburnum opulus*, p.148)
Remedy Take 1 tsp of tincture with water up to 8 times a day for 3 days, then reduce the dose to a maximum of 1 tsp 3 times a day for 7 days.

MILD BRONCHIAL ASTHMA FROM COLDS & CHEST INFECTIONS
Herb Echinacea (*Echinacea* spp., p. 90)
Remedy Take tablets or capsules, or ½ tsp of tincture with water 2–3 times a day.

CIRCULATORY PROBLEMS

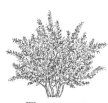

WITCH HAZEL
(*Hamamelis virginiana*)

TO MAINTAIN GOOD health, the body's three trillion cells need to be bathed in fluid that brings them vital nutrients and removes waste products. When this process is undermined by poor circulation, the body may react with conditions such as raised blood pressure, which places a long-term strain on the heart. A low-fat, high-fiber diet and regular aerobic exercise help keep the heart and arteries active and clear of fatty deposits that can "fur up" their linings. A number of herbs act preventively to sustain good circulation – none more so than garlic (*Allium sativum*, p. 56).

SEEK IMMEDIATE PROFESSIONAL ADVICE FOR

- Severe chest pain
- Palpitations lasting several minutes
- Hot, swollen, or ulcerated tender veins, or dark red discoloration of the skin or veins
- Fainting or dizziness with weakness, numbness, or tingling in any part of the body

ANEMIA

THERE ARE SEVERAL types of anemia. Iron deficiency anemia, caused by blood loss from a wound or menstrual bleeding, can be countered with herbs. Bitter herbs, such as gentian, improve the absorption of nutrients and nettle contains plenty of iron. Increase your intake of other herbs that contain iron; see *Vitamins & Minerals*, p. 297.

General caution Seek professional advice to determine the type of anemia you have before home treatment.

GENERAL REMEDIES
Herbs Gentian (*Gentiana lutea*, p. 97), wormwood (*Artemisia absinthium*, p. 63)
Remedy Take 2–5 drops of either tincture with water, half an hour before meals.
Caution Do not take wormwood during pregnancy.

Herb Chiretta (*Swertia chirata*, p. 135)
Remedy Take 5–10 drops of tincture with water 3 times a day before meals.

ANEMIA DUE TO HEAVY MENSTRUAL BLEEDING
Herb Nettle (*Urtica dioica*, p. 145)
Remedy Make an infusion using 25 g of herb to 750 ml of water. Sip the whole dose at intervals throughout the day.
See also *Heavy Menstrual Bleeding – Four Things Soup* remedy, p. 315.

HIGH BLOOD PRESSURE & ARTERIOSCLEROSIS

MILD CASES OF high blood pressure and arteriosclerosis (hardening of the arteries) can benefit from herbs. Garlic thins the blood, reduces fatty deposits, and lowers blood pressure; buckwheat and ginkgo aid circulation, reduce blood pressure, and prevent arteriosclerosis; and ginger improves circulation, especially to the capillaries.

General caution Seek professional advice, especially if already taking medication for a circulatory condition.

GENERAL REMEDIES
Herbs Garlic (*Allium sativum*, p. 56), buckwheat (*Fagopyrum esculentum*, p. 208)
Remedy Take either herb in tablet form, or eat 1–2 fresh garlic cloves each day.
NOTE Garlic is most effective when used as a regular preventative, rather than a remedy.

Herb Ginkgo (*Ginkgo biloba*, p. 98)
Remedy Take tablets or ½ tsp of fluid extract with water twice a day for 2–3 months at a time.

Herb Ginger (*Zingiber officinale*, p. 153)
Remedy Grate ¼ tsp of fresh ginger into your food each day.

301

PALPITATIONS & PANIC ATTACKS

PALPITATIONS OCCUR WHEN the heart suddenly beats faster or irregularly. They can result from stress, anxiety, and nervous tension; however, they may also be caused simply by drinking too much caffeine (in tea, coffee, and cola drinks). In rare cases, palpitations indicate a heart problem. They are a key symptom of panic attacks, which are characterized by sudden acute feelings of fear and anxiety. Linden flowers and valerian root are especially relaxing and calming to the nervous system, specifically helping to reduce underlying anxiety.

General caution Seek immediate professional advice if palpitations last for several minutes.

PALPITATIONS
Herb Linden (*Tilia* spp., p. 275)
Remedy Make an infusion with up to 20 g of linden to 750 ml of water. Divide into 3–4 doses and drink throughout the day.

Herb Dan shen (*Salvia miltiorrhiza*, p. 129)
Remedy Make a decoction and take 3–4 doses during the day for up to 1 week. Alternatively, take half the daily dose for up to 2–3 weeks.

Cautions Do not take *dan shen* with anticoagulant or antiplatelet drugs, or during pregnancy.

PANIC ATTACKS
Herbs Linden (*Tilia* spp., p. 275), valerian (*Valeriana officinalis*, p. 146)
Remedy Make an infusion using 1 tsp of linden and ½ tsp of powdered valerian to 1 cup of water. Drink 4 cups a day.

Herbs Motherwort (*Leonurus cardiaca*, p. 225), linden (*Tilia* spp., p. 275)
Remedy Make an infusion of motherwort or make an infusion using ½ tsp of each herb to 1 cup of water. Drink up to 4 cups of either remedy a day.

Caution Do not take motherwort during pregnancy.

COLD EXTREMITIES & CHILBLAINS

POOR CIRCULATION CAN cause discomfort and painful chilblains (sores caused by poor local blood flow) on the fingers and toes. By stimulating the circulation and getting more "warmth" into the system with herbs and exercise, the peripheral blood flow to the hands and feet is improved. Hot acrid herbs, such as cayenne or ginger, stimulate the flow of blood through the arteries, helping to prevent the development of chilblains.

EXERCISE
Aerobic exercise is often the key to improving this condition.

General caution Seek professional advice if fingers and toes frequently become cold and numb.

**POOR CIRCULATION
TO THE HANDS & FEET**
Herb Cayenne (*Capsicum frutescens*, p. 70)
Remedy Take cayenne tablets in winter.
Option Add a pinch of cayenne powder or chili sauce to every main meal.

Caution Do not take tablets during pregnancy.

Herbs Crampbark (*Viburnum opulus*, p. 148), prickly ash (*Zanthoxylum americanum*, p. 151)
Remedy 1 Make a decoction using 15 g of crampbark to 750 ml of water, and take 3 doses each day.
Remedy 2 Mix 5 g of prickly ash and 10 g of crampbark, and make a decoction using 750 ml of water. Take 3 doses each day.

Caution Do not take prickly ash during pregnancy.

CHILBLAINS
Herbs Ginger (*Zingiber officinale*, p. 153), lemon (*Citrus limon*, p. 81), echinacea (*Echinacea* spp., p. 90)
Remedy (Internal) Grate ¼ tsp of fresh ginger into your food each day. Alternatively, drink a sherry glass of ginger wine each day.
Remedy (External) Apply either fresh ginger, undiluted lemon juice, or neat echinacea tincture to unopened chilblains twice a day.
NOTE The external remedy helps to prevent blistering and weeping. Once the blister opens you can continue to apply, but it will sting on contact.

VARICOSE VEINS & HEMORRHOIDS

VARICOSE VEINS RESULT from a weakness, or increased pressure, in the veins. This causes the thin supporting walls of the veins to bulge out, resulting in distended veins and the pooling of blood. Hemorrhoids are usually caused by constipation. Many herbs can be of use in relieving these conditions. Distilled witch hazel is an excellent astringent, and yarrow has astringent, healing, and anti-inflammatory properties.

SELF-HELP
Home treatment should aim to relieve pressure on the veins. Varicose vein sufferers should avoid tight clothing around the waist or legs. Try to maintain regular bowel movements to ease hemorrhoids (see *Constipation & Diarrhea*, p. 307).

General caution Do not massage or rub varicose veins.

VARICOSE VEINS
Herbs Witch hazel (*Hamamelis virginiana*, p. 100), calendula (*Calendula officinalis*, p. 69)
Remedy Gently apply distilled witch hazel, or witch hazel cream or ointment to the affected area 1–2 times a day, or combine equal parts of the creams of both herbs and apply 1–2 times a day.
NOTE This remedy is particularly effective on painful varicose veins.

Herb Yarrow (*Achillea millefolium*, p. 54)
Remedy (External) Wash varicose veins in a cool infusion, or apply the ointment 1–2 times a day.
Remedy (Internal) Make an infusion and leave for 10 minutes. Take 1–2 cups a day for up to 10 weeks.

Caution Do not take yarrow during pregnancy.

HEMORRHOIDS
Herbs Witch hazel (*Hamamelis virginiana*, p. 100), lesser celandine (*Ranunculus ficaria*, p. 258), common oak (*Quercus robur*, p. 258), calendula (*Calendula officinalis*, p. 69)
Remedy 1 Apply either distilled witch hazel or witch hazel ointment, or lesser celandine ointment 1–2 times a day.
Remedy 2 Mix 1 tsp of common oak bark powder with 2½ tbsp of calendula ointment and apply 1–2 times a day.

**DIFFICULT PASSAGE OF THE STOOL &
PAINFUL HEMORRHOIDS**
Herb Slippery elm (*Ulmus rubra*, p. 144)
Remedy Take either slippery elm "food" (see *Acidity & Indigestion*, p. 307) or tablets.

Herb Psyllium (*Plantago* spp., p. 120)
Remedy Take 1–2 tsp of seeds soaked in 1 cup of water overnight, twice a day.

SKIN PROBLEMS

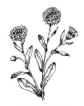

CALENDULA
(Calendula officinalis)

THE LARGEST ORGAN of the body, the skin protects against heat, cold, infection, and trauma from the outside world. Although continuously shedding its surface, the skin needs regular cleansing and nourishing to remain healthy. Its ability to resist injury and recover from damage largely depends on the health of the body as a whole. Although many minor skin problems respond promptly to simple external remedies, severe or chronic skin conditions need internal treatment and usually require professional advice. See also *Eczema*, p. 300.

> ### SEEK IMMEDIATE PROFESSIONAL ADVICE FOR
>
> - Changes to freckles, moles, or warts
> - Sudden swelling or allergic reaction
> - Nonminor burns, including sunburn
> - Shingles or suspected shingles
> - Boils that do not disperse or burst
> - Serious wounds, scrapes, bruises, bites, and stings

MINOR BITES, STINGS & SWELLINGS

INFLAMED SWOLLEN AREAS of skin are a common reaction to bites and stings. Although they can be very uncomfortable, most only cause local itching and inflammation that usually subside within a few hours. All the remedies listed will help to ease irritation and soreness. For the most effective relief, use both an external and internal remedy. Lavender relieves irritation as well as being an insect repellent, aloe vera is soothing and healing, and both calendula and St. John's wort reduce inflammation. Echinacea stimulates the immune system, and nettle is antiallergic.

General cautions Seek immediate professional attention if prone to, or if there are signs of, extreme allergic reactions, or if there is a sting in the mouth and the throat starts to swell. Some stings and animal bites are poisonous and may need inoculations and immediate medical attention.

EXTERNAL REMEDIES
Herb Lavender (*Lavandula officinalis*, p. 107)
Remedy Rub fresh leaves, neat tincture, or essential oil on and around the bite or sting.
OTHER USES This will also repel insects.

Herbs Sweet basil (*Ocimum basilicum*, p. 238), holy basil (*Ocimum sanctum*, p. 114), sage (*Salvia officinalis*, p. 130), thyme (*Thymus vulgaris*, p. 142)
Remedy Apply freshly squeezed juice from the leaves of one of the herbs.

Herbs Aloe vera (*Aloe vera*, p. 57), calendula (*Calendula officinalis*, p. 69), St. John's wort (*Hypericum perforatum*, p. 104)
Remedy Apply either aloe vera gel, calendula ointment, cream, lotion, or tincture, or St. John's wort oil. To make the calendula lotion, infuse 2 heaped tbsp of calendula in 1 cup of water. Strain, cool, then apply.
Option Add 5 drops each of lavender (*Lavandula officinalis*, p.107) and German chamomile (*Chamomilla recutita*, p. 76) essential oils to 1 tsp of one of the above preparations.
Caution Do not apply chamomile oil in pregnancy.
TIP Apply neat lemon juice (*Citrus limon*, p. 81) if there is nothing else available.

INTERNAL REMEDIES
Herb Nettle (*Urtica dioica*, p. 145)
Remedy Make an infusion, and drink 3 cups a day, or take 1 tsp of tincture with water 3 times a day for up to 3 days.

Herb Echinacea (*Echinacea* spp., p. 90)
Remedy Take tablets or capsules.

SKIN RASHES, MINOR BURNS & SUNBURN

MORE ANNOYING THAN debilitating, skin rashes and minor burns, including sunburn, usually clear up without assistance, although herbal treatment can speed recovery.
Nettle rash (urticaria) is usually caused by an allergic reaction but can also be triggered by heat, cold, or sunlight. It only lasts for a few hours but will often recur. For the most effective relief, apply chickweed cream and take one of the internal remedies.
Skin rashes have many causes, such as allergy, infection, irritation, bites, stings, and temperature changes. Use these remedies to alleviate itchiness and swelling.
Small-scale burns usually respond well to herbal medicine, but even small burns may be deep and can quickly become infected. Before using a remedy, bathe the burned area in clean cold water, and keep the area cool for at least 3 hours with a clean cotton cloth that has been soaked in cold water.

General caution If there is any sign of infection, seek professional advice.

NETTLE RASH (URTICARIA)
Herbs Nettle (*Urtica dioica*, p. 145), heartsease (*Viola tricolor*, p. 280), calendula (*Calendula officinalis*, p. 69)
Remedy (Internal) Drink an infusion of 5 g of each herb and 750 ml of water regularly during the day. Repeat for one week. If symptoms persist, take for another week.

Herbs Dandelion (*Taraxacum officinale*, p. 140), yellow dock (*Rumex crispus*, p. 126), burdock (*Arctium lappa*, p. 62)
Remedy (Internal) Make a decoction with 5 g of each root to 750 ml of water. Drink 2 cups a day and repeat for at least 1 week.
Caution Do not take yellow dock in pregnancy.

Herb Chickweed (*Stellaria media*, p. 270)
Remedy (External) Apply cream as required.

INFLAMED SKIN RASHES
Herbs Calendula (*Calendula officinalis*, p. 69), comfrey (*Symphytum officinale*, p. 136)
Remedy Apply calendula or comfrey ointment, cream, or lotion to troubled areas 2–4 times a day. For the lotion, make an infusion, strain, cool, and then apply.
Caution Do not apply comfrey to broken skin.

WEEPING SKIN
Herbs Aloe vera (*Aloe vera*, p. 57), witch hazel (*Hamamelis virginiana*, p. 100)
Remedy Apply aloe vera gel or distilled witch hazel or witch hazel ointment to the affected area 2–4 times a day.

MINOR BURNS & SUNBURN
Herbs Aloe vera (*Aloe vera*, p. 57), lavender (*Lavandula officinalis*, p. 107)
Remedy Apply aloe vera gel or neat lavender essential oil to the affected area as needed.

Herb Calendula (*Calendula officinalis*, p. 69)
Remedy Infuse 1 heaping tbsp of herb in 1 cup of water. Strain, cool, and then apply as a lotion to the affected area as required.

303

MINOR WOUNDS & BRUISES

MINOR WOUNDS, BRUISES, and scrapes are part of everyday life, and the remedies listed are effective home treatments.

Witch hazel is a very good astringent for minor scrapes, bruises, and swellings, protecting and soothing the damaged area. Arnica can be used to relieve bruising, pain, and swelling, and it combines well with witch hazel. Wounds can be cleansed with aloe vera gel which, like comfrey, is an excellent wound healer. Comfrey ointment is also helpful in clearing old scars. See also *Sprains & Fractures*, p. 312.

General caution Seek immediate medical attention for serious or deep wounds, bruises, or scrapes, especially if the pain has not lessened considerably after 24 hours.

CLEANSING WOUNDS
Herb Yarrow (*Achillea millefolium*, p. 54)
Remedy Make a yarrow lotion, then allow to cool, and use as a wash.

Herb Calendula (*Calendula officinalis*, p. 69)
Remedy Make a calendula lotion with 2 heaping tsp of herb to 1 cup of water, or use the tincture neat or diluted in water. Apply either preparation to the wound.
NOTE Calendula tincture will sting strongly, but it has a greater antiseptic action.

Herb Aloe vera (*Aloe vera*, p. 57)
Remedy Cleanse the wound with the gel and cover with a dressing soaked in gel. Change as required.

Herb Witch hazel (*Hamamelis virginiana*, p. 100)
Remedy Apply distilled witch hazel (available over the counter) to the affected area 2–3 times a day.

HEALING WOUNDS
Herbs Comfrey (*Symphytum officinale*, p. 136), aloe vera (*Aloe vera*, p. 57)
Remedy Apply comfrey ointment around the edges of the wound or, once a scab has formed, use a comfrey poultice. Also use aloe vera gel to cleanse the wound (*see left*).
Caution Do not use comfrey on an open wound.

BRUISES
Herbs Arnica (*Arnica montana*, p. 170), witch hazel (*Hamamelis virginiana*, p. 100)
Remedy Apply arnica ointment to bruises and swellings 2–3 times a day or use distilled witch hazel, as above.
Caution Do not use arnica on broken skin.

COLD SORES, CHICKEN POX, SHINGLES & WARTS

HERBAL MEDICINE CAN help all these viral infections that affect the skin.

Cold sores are caused by the herpes simplex virus, and usually occur when the body has an infection or has been exposed to sunshine or wind. Tiny blisters form, mainly around the nostrils and lips.

Shingles and chicken pox are the result of a similar virus, causing sores to form all over the body. Shingles are a sign that the nervous system is run down and open to infection, so herbs that support the nerves and the immune system as a whole are as important as ones that work topically.

Warts are caused by the papilloma virus and can be difficult to clear. With persistence, the remedies here are often effective.

General cautions Always consult a professional practitioner if you have, or suspect you have, shingles. Take professional advice if you notice a sudden change to a wart.

COLD SORES, CHICKEN POX & SHINGLES
Herbs Echinacea (*Echinacea* spp., p. 90), St. John's wort (*Hypericum perforatum*, p. 104)
Remedies Take ½ tsp of tincture of either herb with water 2–3 times a day. Alternatively, take echinacea tablets or capsules, or make an infusion of St. John's wort and drink up to 1 cup a day.

Herbs Garlic (*Allium sativum*, p. 56), ginger (*Zingiber officinale*, p. 153), lemon (*Citrus limon*, p. 81)
Remedy (Internal) Eat 1–2 cloves of garlic and 1–2 slices (1 g) of fresh ginger a day.
Remedy (External) Apply either fresh ginger, half a clove of garlic, or lemon juice to unopened cold sores, shingles, or pox marks up to 6 times a day.

Herb Lemon balm (*Melissa officinalis*, p. 111)
Remedy (Internal) Make an infusion and drink up to 5 cups a day.
Remedy (External) Make a lotion by infusing 1½ tbsp of fresh or 3 tsp of dried leaves in 1 cup of water for 10 minutes. Strain and dab onto spots 3–5 times a day.

WARTS
Herb Aloe vera (*Aloe vera*, p. 57)
Remedy Apply the gel directly to the wart 2–3 times a day for up to 3 months.

Herb Arbor vitae (*Thuja occidentalis*, p. 274)
Remedy Apply neat tincture to the wart 1–2 times a day for up to 3 months.

FUNGAL SKIN INFECTIONS, INCLUDING ATHLETE'S FOOT

FUNGAL SKIN INFECTIONS are easily picked up through physical contact, and can be hard to clear. Athlete's foot is a fungus (tinea) that grows in the skin between and under the toes, causing it to split and peel away. This itchy, sore condition can be difficult to treat at home.

SELF-HELP
Keep feet dry and clean, and do not wear synthetic socks or tightly fitting shoes.

GENERAL REMEDIES
Herb Comfrey (*Symphytum officinale*, p. 136)
Remedy Make a poultice and firmly apply to the affected area for 1–2 hours each day.
Caution Do not use comfrey on broken skin.

Herbs Tea tree (*Melaleuca alternifolia*, p. 110), clove (*Eugenia caryophyllata*, p. 95), calendula (*Calendula officinalis*, p.69), thyme (*Thymus vulgaris*, p. 142)
Remedy Mix 5 drops of tea tree, clove, or thyme essential oil with 1 tsp of calendula ointment. Apply 1–2 times a day.
Caution Do not use thyme oil during pregnancy.

Herb Garlic (*Allium sativum*, p.56)
Remedy Rub on ½ clove 2–3 times a day.

ATHLETE'S FOOT
Herbs Turmeric (*Curcuma longa*, p. 88), calendula (*Calendula officinalis*, p. 69)
Remedy Mix ½ tsp of turmeric powder with 15 ml of calendula ointment. Rub in between and under the toes each day.

ACNE & BOILS

ACNE AND BOILS are the result of local infection, hormonal imbalance, or internal toxicity, which cause inflammation of the hair follicles and, with acne, sebaceous glands. They should be treated on the surface of the skin as well as internally.

Acne generally occurs during the teenage years and results in whiteheads, pustules, and cysts, usually on the face and back.

Boils are large, pus-filled areas of skin. They either disperse or burst within a week. Since boils are often the body's way of expelling toxins, recurrent boils may indicate a weakened immune system, or they can suggest diabetes or a deep-seated bacterial infection.

Herbs such as tea tree and garlic are antiseptic and antibiotic. Calendula and comfrey promote healing.

SELF-HELP
Increase intake of vitamin C and garlic.

General cautions Do not squeeze boils or acne pimples because the infection might spread. Seek professional advice for recurrent boils.

EXTERNAL REMEDIES
Herbs Tea tree (*Melaleuca alternifolia*, p. 110), clove (*Eugenia carophyllata*, p. 95), garlic (*Allium sativum*, p. 56)
Remedy Dab 1 drop of neat tea tree or clove essential oil on the pus-filled head of a boil or spot twice a day. Alternatively, cut a clove of garlic in half and rub over the area twice a day.

Herb Calendula (*Calendula officinalis*, p. 69)
Remedy Apply ointment or cream, or dab undiluted tincture onto the pus-filled area twice a day.

Herb Comfrey (*Symphytum officinale*, p. 136)
Remedy Apply comfrey ointment or cream to the pus-filled area twice a day.
Caution Do not use comfrey on broken skin.

Herb Lemon (*Citrus limon*, p. 81)
Remedy Dab pure lemon juice onto the pus-filled area, or dilute 1 tsp of lemon juice with 1 tbsp of water and use as a skin wash twice a day.

Herbs Slippery elm (*Ulmus rubra*, p. 144), calendula (*Calendula officinalis*, p. 69), myrrh (*Commiphora molmol*, p. 84), echinacea (*Echinacea* spp., p. 90)
Remedy Mix 1 level tsp of slippery elm powder with sufficient calendula, myrrh, or echinacea tincture to make a thick, smooth paste. Place on and around the boil, and bandage securely. Remove after 1–2 hours.
NOTE This remedy is especially useful for drawing painful boils and splinters.

INTERNAL REMEDIES
Herbs Dandelion (*Taraxacum officinale*, p. 140), burdock (*Arctium lappa*, p. 62)
Remedy Make a decoction using 5 g of burdock root and 10 g of dandelion root with 750 ml of water. Divide into 3 doses and drink during the day.

Herb Echinacea (*Echinacea* spp., p. 90)
Remedy Take echinacea tablets or capsules, or make a decoction of 10 g of root to 750 ml of water and drink during the day.

DIGESTIVE DISORDERS

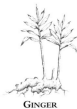
GINGER
(*Zingiber officinale*)

EVERYONE FALLS PREY to certain digestive problems and, for those with a weak or unsettled digestion, life can be a misery. Poor digestive health usually results from insufficient or excessive digestive secretions, infections (such as gastroenteritis), candida, stress, and anxiety. Herbal medicines can improve the complex functioning of the digestive organs, helping to relieve acidity, nausea, and bloating. Eating simple wholesome food can be beneficial, but it is difficult to generalize about diet. Some conditions may require fasting while, in other cases, a certain type of food might need to be avoided.

SEEK IMMEDIATE PROFESSIONAL ADVICE FOR

- Difficulty in swallowing
- Severe pain
- Vomiting blood
- Blood in the stool

IMPORTANT NOTE
For continuing or recurrent digestive problems, seek professional advice to determine the cause.

STOMACHACHE

CRAMPING PAIN IS a sign that the stomach and intestines are overtightening. This is normally due to poor digestion of food, excessive nervous tension and stress, food poisoning, or infection. Stomachache may occur on its own or lead to vomiting and diarrhea (in which case, use the remedies on p. 306). Garlic and calendula are both antiviral and will help clear digestive infections. Relaxing herbs, such as German chamomile and crampbark, relieve stomach spasms. For maximum benefit, they are mixed with carminative herbs to relieve gas.

General cautions Seek professional advice if stomach pain is severe or recurrent. All species of mint (*Mentha* spp.) are unsuitable for children under 5.

STOMACH SPASM
Relaxing herbs German chamomile (*Chamomilla recutita*, p. 76), lemon balm (*Melissa officinalis*, p. 111), crampbark (*Viburnum opulus*, p. 148)
Carminative herbs Anise (*Pimpinella anisum*, p. 246), fennel (*Foeniculum vulgare*, p. 210), mint (*Mentha* spp., p. 232), angelica (*Angelica archangelica*, p. 166)
Remedy Mix 3 parts of a relaxing herb to 1 part of a carminative herb and make an infusion. For the carminative herbs, use fennel seeds, anise, mint leaves, or angelica root. Drink up to 5 cups a day.

DIGESTIVE INFECTIONS
Herb Garlic (*Allium sativum*, p. 56)
Remedy Eat 1–2 fresh cloves a day.

Herb Calendula (*Calendula officinalis*, p. 69)
Remedy Infuse 2 tsp of herb in 750 ml of water and drink up to 5 cups a day.

Herbs Yarrow (*Achillea millefolium*, p. 54), peppermint (*Mentha* x *piperita*, p. 112), catnip (*Nepeta cataria*, p. 237)
Remedy Mix equal parts of each herb. Make an infusion using 2 tsp of the herb mixture to 1 cup of water. Drink 2 cups a day.
Caution Do not take yarrow in pregnancy.

BEFORE TAKING ANY HERBAL REMEDIES, SEE PAGES 289 & 298
Digestive Disorders continued on page 306

NAUSEA & VOMITING, INCLUDING MOTION SICKNESS

NAUSEA AND VOMITING can occur for numerous reasons, including food poisoning, infections, fever, migraine, stress or emotional problems, as well as motion sickness.
For short-term conditions, there are many effective herbs that reduce or relieve the unpleasant, empty, gnawing symptoms of nausea and vomiting. Most of the herbs listed are also very useful for motion sickness, especially ginger and related species.
Ginger, in particular, and other close relatives such as galangal and turmeric, are widely used for nausea and vomiting, helping to "warm" and settle the digestion.
Chiretta strengthens a weak digestion and relieves nausea.
Lemon is an excellent cleansing remedy for a weak and sluggish digestion.
If you are pregnant, or suspect you may be pregnant, see *Morning Sickness*, p. 317, before taking any of these remedies.

General cautions Seek professional advice if nausea is severe or is recurrent. All types or species of mint (*Mentha* spp.) are unsuitable for children under 5.

NAUSEA & MOTION SICKNESS
Herbs Ginger (*Zingiber officinale*, p. 153), galangal (*Alpinia officinarum*, p. 58), turmeric (*Curcuma longa*, p. 88)
Remedy Make an infusion with one of the herbs using about 1–2 slices (0.5 g) of fresh root or ¼–½ tsp of dried, powdered, or grated root to 1 cup of water. Use the fresh root if possible. Infuse for at least 5 minutes and sip while hot. Drink up to 5 cups a day. Add 1–2 cloves (*Eugenia carophyllata*, p. 95) if desired.
Option Use the remedy under *Nausea with Headache*.
TIP For motion sickness, take the infusion in a flask or chew crystallized ginger.

WEAK DIGESTION
Herbs Chiretta (*Swertia chirata*, p. 135), centaury (*Erythraea centaurum*, p. 204)
Remedy Take 2–4 drops of one of the tinctures on the tongue each hour.

Herb Lemon (*Citrus limon*, p. 81)
Remedy Drink the freshly squeezed juice of a lemon, neat or diluted, each morning.

NAUSEA DUE TO EMOTIONAL PROBLEMS
Herb Lemon balm (*Melissa officinalis*, p. 111)
Remedy Make an infusion with the dried herb or use 2 tsp of fresh herb per cup of water. Drink up to 5 cups a day.

VOMITING WITH DIZZINESS & VERTIGO
Herb Black horehound (*Ballota nigra*, p. 174)
Remedy Make an infusion and drink up to 5 cups a day.

Caution Seek professional advice if symptoms do not immediately improve.

NAUSEA WITH HEADACHE
Herbs Peppermint (*Mentha* x *piperita*, p. 112), pennyroyal (*Mentha pulegium*, p. 233), *bo he* (*Mentha haplocalyx*, p. 232)
Remedy Make an infusion with 1 level tsp of one herb per cup of water. Drink up to 4–5 cups a day.
OTHER USES This remedy combats abdominal fullness, and helps improve the appetite and digestion.

Cautions Do not give these herbs to children under 5. Do not take pennyroyal during pregnancy.

LOSS OF APPETITE & VOMITING
Herb Codonopsis (*Codonopsis pilosula*, p. 82)
Remedy Make a decoction and sip 50 ml every 2–3 hours until the vomiting stops or the dose has been taken over 2 days.
OTHER USES For anorexia add 5 g of licorice (*Glycyrrhiza glabra*, p. 99) or *gan cao* (*Glycyrrhiza uralensis*, p. 215).

Caution Do not take licorice during pregnancy.

GAS & BLOATING

GAS AND BLOATING are common digestive problems. As a preventative, take bitter herbs, such as centaury and gentian, to improve the digestion. Infusions of aromatic plants such as fennel, cardamom, anise, lemon verbena, or peppermint are effective remedies. All the herbs listed under *General Remedies* can be combined by adjusting the measurements of each herb using the same proportion to water.

General cautions Bitters are generally unsuitable and unpalatable for children under 5. All types or species of mint (*Mentha* spp.) are unsuitable for children under 5.

PROTECTION & PREVENTION
Herbs Centaury (*Erythraea centaurum*, p. 204), gentian (*Gentiana lutea*, p. 97)
Remedy Take 5–10 drops of tincture 3 times a day with water.

GENERAL REMEDIES
Herbs Fennel (*Foeniculum vulgare*, p. 210), anise (*Pimpinella anisum*, p. 246)
Remedy Make an infusion with ¼ – ½ tsp of fennel or anise seeds per cup of water and drink up to 5 cups a day.

Herb Cardamom (*Eletteria cardamomum*, p. 91)
Remedy Make an infusion with the crushed seeds of 2 cardamoms per cup of water. Drink up to 5 cups a day.

Herb Lemon verbena (*Lippia citriodora*, p. 227)
Remedy Make an infusion using 1 tsp of dried or 2 tsp of fresh leaves per cup of water and take up to 5 cups a day.

Herb Peppermint (*Mentha* x *piperita*, p. 112)
Remedy Make an infusion, and drink up to 5 cups a day. (See *General cautions*, left.)

CANKER SORES & GUM PROBLEMS

MANY ASTRINGENT HERBS can be used to treat canker sores, and tighten up weak gums and loose teeth. Sage is particularly effective since it also disinfects the mouth. Myrrh tincture will sting, but it speeds up the rate of healing.

GENERAL REMEDIES
Herb Myrrh (*Commiphora molmol*, p. 84)
Remedy Dab pure tincture on canker sores and infected gums once every hour.

Herb Sage (*Salvia officinalis*, p. 130)
Remedy Use an infusion as a mouthwash, or rub gums with leaves or powder.

MOUTH & TONGUE ULCERS
Herbs Myrrh (*Commiphora molmol*, p. 84), echinacea (*Echinacea* spp., p. 90), licorice (*Glycyrrhiza glabra*, p. 99)
Remedy Mix equal parts of the tinctures and apply neat or diluted (1 part tincture to 5 parts water) every hour.

CONSTIPATION & DIARRHEA

HERBS HELP BOTH constipation and diarrhea by gently restoring normal bowel function. Constipation often results from insufficient intake of fruit, vegetables, and whole grains, while diarrhea is usually caused by intestinal infection or inflammation, such as food poisoning. Irritable bowel syndrome gives rise to alternating bouts of constipation and diarrhea, and spastic constipation results from tension and muscle spasm in the colon.

HERBS

Dandelion root, licorice, and yellow dock are mild laxatives.
Senna is a strong laxative and should only be taken when other herbs have failed.
Psyllium seeds and husks cleanse the colon and encourage normal bowel habits.
Crampbark has antispasmodic properties and can help spastic constipation.
Agrimony, bael, bistort, and black catechu are astringent herbs that dry and tighten the bowel lining. Only take in the short term since they impair absorption of food. They are taken mixed with soothing, demulcent herbs, such as psyllium or marsh mallow, for diarrhea.

DIET FOR CONSTIPATION

Fruit acts as a gentle laxative within the large bowel. Eat plenty of fresh fruit every day, such as figs (*Ficus carica*, p. 209), apples, or tamarind (*Tamarindus indica*, p. 272), which also counter vomiting, gas, and indigestion.

General caution Seek professional advice for persistent constipation or diarrhea.

CONSTIPATION

Herbs Yellow dock (*Rumex crispus*, p. 126), Chinese rhubarb (*Rheum palmatum*, p. 124)
Remedy Make a decoction using 1 tsp of either herb to 1 cup of water and take last thing at night.
NOTE Yellow dock is one of the mildest laxatives and should be tried first. If this has no effect, take a single dose of Chinese rhubarb each day. This has a stronger action than yellow dock.
Cautions Do not take Chinese rhubarb or yellow dock during pregnancy.

PERSISTENT CONSTIPATION

Herbs Dandelion (*Taraxacum officinale*, p. 140), licorice (*Glycyrrhiza glabra*, p. 99), yellow dock (*Rumex crispus*, p. 126)
Remedy 1 Make a decoction using 20 g of dandelion root to 750 ml of water and drink each day, or use the ground root to make an infusion and drink 3–4 cups a day.
Remedy 2 Mix 3 tsp of dandelion root and yellow dock and 1 tsp of licorice. Use the mixture to make a decoction with 750 ml of water and drink 1–2 cups a day.
Cautions Do not take yellow dock or licorice during pregnancy.

❧

Herbs Senna (*Cassia senna*, p. 72), ginger (*Zingiber officinale*, p. 153)
Remedy Steep 3–6 senna pods and 2–3 slices (1 g) of fresh ginger in 150 ml of warm water. Alternatively, take senna tablets. Take either preparation for up to 10 days at a time.
NOTE This is the strongest laxative listed.
Cautions Senna is a strongly stimulant laxative, and long-term use is harmful. Do not give to children under 5. Do not take during pregnancy.

SPASTIC CONSTIPATION

Herb Crampbark (*Viburnum opulus*, p. 148)
Remedy Make a decoction using 15 g of the root to 750 ml of water and take 1–2 cups a day, or take 2 tsp of tincture with water once per day.

DIARRHEA

Herbs Agrimony (*Agrimonia eupatoria*, p. 160), sage (*Salvia officinalis*, p. 130), bael (*Aegle marmelos*, p. 159), bistort (*Polygonum bistorta*, p. 251), black catechu (*Acacia catechu*, p. 157)
Remedy The above herbs are listed in ascending order of astringency. Make a decoction using 1 heaping tsp of one herb to 1½ cups of water and simmer for 15–20 minutes. Take up to 3 cups a day for no longer than 3 days.
NOTE If using bistort or black catechu (the most astringent herbs), mix with demulcents such as psyllium seeds (*Plantago* spp., p. 120) or marsh mallow root (*Althaea officinalis*, p. 163). Add 1 tsp, plus a pinch of peppermint (*Mentha* x *piperita*, p. 112) or other mint (*Mentha* spp., p. 232–3), per 1½ cups of decoction.
Cautions Do not take for more than 3 days at a time, and do not take again for 3 days. If there is no improvement, seek professional advice. Do not take sage during pregnancy. Do not give mint to children under 5.

CHRONIC DIARRHEA & IRRITABLE BOWEL SYNDROME

Herb Psyllium (*Plantago* spp., p. 120)
Remedy Take 1 heaping tsp of seeds and husks with at least 1 cup of water, 2–3 times daily, or mix with food, and then drink at least 1 cup of water. Seeds may be soaked in cool water overnight before taking.

ACIDITY & INDIGESTION

INDIGESTION, CAUSED BY too much acid production, suggests a poor or inappropriate diet. To coat the inner lining of the stomach and intestines and protect them from excess acidity, take slippery elm, arrowroot, or Iceland moss, which are sticky mucilaginous herbs when soaked in water. Meadowsweet strengthens the lining of the stomach and reduces acidity, while chamomile is amazingly versatile for a number of gastrointestinal problems.

DIET

Cut out acidic foods, such as oranges, red meat, spinach, and tomatoes, as well as alcohol and tobacco.

GENERAL REMEDIES

Herbs Slippery elm (*Ulmus rubra*, p. 144), arrowroot (*Maranta arundinacea*, p. 231), Iceland moss (*Cetraria islandica*, p. 184)
Remedy 1 Make an infusion with 2 heaping tsp of one of the herbs to 100 ml of water. Leave for 15 minutes. Take 100 ml up to 4 times a day.
Remedy 2 Make slippery elm "food" by mixing 1 heaping tsp of powder and 3 tsp of cold water. Stir in 250 ml of boiling water. Add a pinch of cinnamon (*Cinnamomum verum*, p. 80) or nutmeg (*Myristica fragrans*, p. 113) to taste. Take 250 ml 3 times a day.

❧

Herbs Fennel (*Foeniculum vulgare*, p. 210), galbanum (*Ferula gummosa*, p. 209), anise (*Pimpinella anisum*, p. 246), or any one of the *Nausea & Vomiting* herbs on p. 306.
Remedy Make an infusion using 1 heaping tsp of fennel or anise seeds, or galbanum to 750 ml of water. Drink during the day.

INDIGESTION, ABDOMINAL PAIN, BLOATING & HICCUPS

Herb German chamomile (*Chamomilla recutita*, p. 76)
Remedy Make an infusion in a covered container. Drink up to 5 cups a day.

ACIDITY WITH GASTRITIS

Herb Meadowsweet (*Filipendula ulmaria*, p. 96)
Remedy Make an infusion with the flowering tops. Drink up to 5 cups a day.

BEFORE TAKING ANY HERBAL REMEDIES, SEE PAGES 289 & 298

NERVE & STRESS-RELATED PROBLEMS

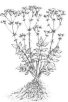

VALERIAN
(*Valeriana officinalis*)

MOST OF US HAVE little opportunity to escape from daily pressures, and consequently the nervous system is unable to recover its natural vitality. Long-term stress can lead to anxiety, nervousness, depression, insomnia, palpitations, and irritability. Herbal medicines can be wonderfully effective for nourishing the nervous system, calming and relaxing the mind, and gently stimulating or sedating the body. Headaches and migraine respond well to treatment with herbs, as can conditions directly affecting the nerves, such as neuralgia.

SEEK IMMEDIATE PROFESSIONAL ADVICE FOR

- Severe nerve, chest, or head pain
- Headache or pain that does not improve within 48 hours despite self-medication
- Loss of sensation or loss of movement
- Double vision
- Severe depression

ANXIETY, DEPRESSION & TENSION

MANY PEOPLE HAVE experienced lack of well-being and feelings of powerlessness that develop as stress, anxiety, and tension take hold. There is no instant answer, but a remarkable number of herbs can reduce these symptoms and, by supporting the nervous system, gradually restore health.

Lemon balm, skullcap, and damiana are all calming herbs that ease physical tension and help maintain a balanced mental and emotional state. Lemon balm alleviates stress-related digestive problems, skullcap combats panic attacks, and damiana acts as a gentle "pick-me-up."

Valerian has tranquilizing qualities.

Ginseng and Siberian ginseng are excellent for coping with stressful events such as competitive sports, examinations, or moving a household.

Withania is a supportive tonic herb, strengthening and encouraging recovery from long-term stress or chronic illness.

LIFESTYLE

When emotionally stressed, it is important to eat well, exercise regularly, and allow time for relaxation. Yoga and tai chi can be particularly helpful.

GENERAL REMEDIES

Herbs Lemon balm (*Melissa officinalis*, p. 111), damiana (*Turnera diffusa*, p. 143), skullcap (*Scutellaria lateriflora*, p. 134)

Remedy Make an infusion using one of the herbs. Drink up to 4 cups a day.

Herb St. John's wort (*Hypericum perforatum*, p. 104)

Remedy Take tablets or make an infusion and drink up to 4 cups a day.

NOTE This remedy may take 2–3 weeks before there is a noticeable effect.

DIGESTIVE PROBLEMS DUE TO STRESS

Herb Lemon balm (*Melissa officinalis*, p. 111)

Remedy Make an infusion with a handful of fresh leaves and 150 ml water, or make an infusion with the dried herb. Drink up to 5 cups a day, or add the daily dose to a bath.

NOTE This remedy also calms palpitations and encourages sleep.

PANIC ATTACKS & HEADACHES

Herb Skullcap (*Scutellaria lateriflora*, p. 134)

Remedy Make an infusion and drink up to 5 cups a day.

CHRONIC ANXIETY & HYPERACTIVITY

Herb Valerian (*Valeriana officinalis*, p. 146)

Remedy Take 10 drops of tincture in water every hour for up to 2 weeks at a time.

NERVOUS EXHAUSTION, MUSCLE TENSION & HEADACHES

Herb Codonopsis (*Codonopsis pilosula*, p. 82)

Remedy Make a decoction and drink in equal doses during the day, or cook up to 25 g of the root a day in a soup or stew.

SHORT-TERM STRESS

Herbs Ginseng (*Panax ginseng*, p. 116), Siberian ginseng (*Eleutherococcus senticosus*, p. 92)

Remedy Either take ginseng tablets, chew 0.5–1 g of root a day, or use it in cooking. Alternatively take 2–3 g of Siberian ginseng capsules up to 3 times a day.

Cautions Do not take for more than 6 weeks at a time. Do not give to children under 12. Do not take during pregnancy. Avoid drinks that contain caffeine.

LONG-TERM STRESS & CONVALESCENCE

Herb Withania (*Withania somnifera*, p. 150)

Remedy Make an decoction using 1 g of root to 1 cup of water, and take during the day, or chew the same amount of root.

NEURALGIA (NERVE PAIN)

NEURALGIA IS THE pain caused by an irritated, damaged, or pinched nerve. It usually occurs in brief, severe bouts and can be felt shooting along the nerve. Although it is difficult to treat, the following remedies may bring relief to minor problems. St. John's wort is analgesic and antiviral, helping to relieve sciatica (pain caused by a pinched spinal nerve) and head pain. Cloves have an anesthetic effect, and peppermint eases pain. Try also the St. John's wort oil rub (see *Back Pain*, p. 313).

General caution Seek professional advice if there is fever, or swelling of the gums with toothache.

GENERAL REMEDIES

Herbs St. John's wort (*Hypericum perforatum*, p. 104), lavender (*Lavandula officinalis*, p. 107), clove (*Eugenia carophyllata*, p. 95)

Remedy Apply neat St. John's wort infused oil to painful areas, or add 20 drops each of clove and lavender essential oil to 50 ml of St. John's wort infused oil and then apply every 2–3 hours as required.

Herb Peppermint (*Mentha x piperita*, p. 112)

Remedy Make an infusion with 25 g herb to 750 ml of water and bathe the affected area. Alternatively, dilute 20 drops of essential

oil in 50 ml of carrier oil and gently massage into the painful area.

Caution Do not use on children under 5.

HEAD PAIN

Herb Clove (*Eugenia carophyllata*, p. 95)

Remedy Mix ½ tsp of powder with water to make a thick paste and apply to the head.

TOOTHACHE

Herb Clove (*Eugenia carophyllata*, p. 95)

Remedy Chew a clove or rub 1–2 drops of neat essential oil onto the affected tooth 2–3 times a day for up to 3 days.

HEADACHES & MIGRAINE

HEADACHES AND MIGRAINE can be very debilitating, especially when they occur frequently.

Headaches are caused by many factors, including toothache, neck tension, eyestrain, and hangovers. It is important to diagnose and treat the underlying cause, which could mean visiting a dentist, optician, or osteopath in the first instance. Herbal medicine can be very helpful for headaches, although choosing the right herbs can be difficult. The following remedies contain relaxing herbs that alleviate headaches triggered by stress as well as other more specific factors. Lavender is soothing, while vervain is a tonic and relaxing herb for nervous exhaustion. Peppermint is effective for headaches linked to indigestion.

Migraine is a more specific problem. The remedies aim both to prevent the onset of a migraine and to treat the symptoms.

Hangovers are not a nerve problem in a direct sense, but they should be treated in the same way as any other type of mild poisoning that requires detoxification and headache relief. Make sure you also drink plenty of water.

General caution For migraine or recurrent headaches, consult a professional practitioner to diagnose and treat the underlying cause.

GENERAL REMEDY
Herb Lavender (*Lavandula officinalis*, p. 107)
Remedy Rub a few drops of neat essential oil on the temples.

TENSION & SINUS HEADACHES
Herb Linden (*Tilia* spp., p. 275)
Remedy Make an infusion using 1 heaping tsp of linden to 1 cup of water, or use teabags. Drink up to 5 cups a day.

NERVOUS EXHAUSTION & OVERACTIVITY
Herbs Vervain (*Verbena officinalis*, p. 147), valerian (*Valeriana officinalis*, p. 146)
Remedy Make an infusion of vervain, and drink up to 4 cups a day. Alternatively, mix ½ tsp of each tincture, and take with water up to 3 times a day.
Caution Do not take vervain during pregnancy.

DIGESTIVE HEADACHES & BILIOUSNESS
Herbs Peppermint (*Mentha* x *piperita*, p. 112), pennyroyal (*Mentha pulegium*, p. 233)
Remedy Make an infusion of either herb in a covered container, using either a teabag, a small handful of fresh leaves, or 1 level tsp of dried herb per cup of water. Drink up to 5 cups a day for up to 1 week, or up to 4 cups a day if taking for 2–3 weeks.
Cautions Do not give to children under 5. Do not take pennyroyal during pregnancy.

MIGRAINE PREVENTION
Herb Feverfew (*Tanacetum parthenium*, p. 139)
Remedy At the first sign of an impending attack, take tablets or 10 drops of tincture with water. Alternatively, place a fresh leaf between slices of bread and eat as a sandwich.
Cautions Do not repeat the dose. Do not give to children under 12. Do not take during pregnancy.

MIGRAINE
Herb Skullcap (*Scutellaria lateriflora*, p. 134)
Remedy Make an infusion using 1 heaped tsp of dried herb to 1 cup of water. Drink up to 5 cups a day.

Herb Rosemary (*Rosmarinus officinalis*, p. 125)
Remedy Make an infusion using 1 level tsp of dried herb per cup of water, and take up to 4 cups each day.

DETOXIFICATION FOR HANGOVER
Herb Dandelion (*Taraxacum officinale*, p. 140)
Remedy Make a decoction using 15 g of root to 750 ml of water. Take the decoction in small quantities at frequent intervals throughout the day.

INSOMNIA

DIFFICULTY IN SLEEPING affects everyone at one time or another. Herbs can provide a safe and gentle solution to this problem.

Sedative herbs such as German chamomile, linden, lavender, hops, and passionflower are relaxing and, unlike some herbs, are most likely to prove effective against insomnia when taken at night. Hops is excellent when the mind refuses to "switch off."

Stimulant herbs are effective when the body suffers from nervous exhaustion and feels, paradoxically, too tired for sleep. Oats and ginseng encourage a good night's sleep, especially for people suffering from nervous tension and fatigue.

Herbal sleeping pills, containing combinations of valerian, hops, passionflower, and similar herbs, are often helpful in overcoming mild sleep problems and in reducing feelings of anxiety and stress.

GENERAL REMEDIES
Herbs German chamomile (*Chamomilla recutita*, p. 76), linden (*Tilia* spp., p. 275), lavender (*Lavandula officinalis*, p. 107), passionflower (*Passiflora incarnata*, p. 117)
Remedy The above herbs are listed in ascending order of strength. Start with the weakest, German chamomile, and if it does not help, try the next strongest. Make an infusion in a covered container using 1–2 heaping tsp per cup of water. Take prior to sleeping. Alternatively, take 1 tsp of tincture with water up to 3 times a night.

Herbs Valerian (*Valeriana officinalis*, p. 146), hops (*Humulus lupulus*, p. 102), passionflower (*Passiflora incarnata*, p. 117)
Remedy 1 Take tablets containing one or more of the herbs.
Remedy 2 Make a sachet with dried hops (*see* p. 102) and place inside your pillow.
Caution Do not take hops internally if feeling low or depressed.

OVERACTIVE MIND
Herb Hops (*Humulus lupulus*, p. 102)
Remedy Take the tincture with water at night. Start with 10 drops up to a maximum of 40 drops each night.
Caution Do not take hops internally if feeling low or depressed.

POOR SLEEP & NERVOUS EXHAUSTION
Herb Oats (*Avena sativa*, p. 172)
Remedy Eat oats daily – for example, as a hot cereal – and take 1 tsp of oat straw tincture with water 3 times a day.

Herbs Ginseng (*Panax ginseng*, p. 116), Siberian ginseng (*Eleutherococcus senticosus*, p. 92)
Remedy Take 0.5–1 g of ginseng or 2–3 g of Siberian ginseng up to 3 times during the day. Either chew the root, or cook it in a soup. Alternatively, take tablets.
Cautions Take ginseng only during the day, and do not take with caffeine. Do not take continuously for more than 6 weeks. Do not take during pregnancy. Do not give to children under 12.

BEFORE TAKING ANY HERBAL REMEDIES, SEE PAGES 289 & 298

RESPIRATORY TRACT PROBLEMS

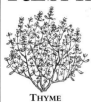

THYME
(*Thymus vulgaris*)

THE RESPIRATORY SYSTEM stretches from the lining of the eyes and sinuses to the base of the lungs, and is constantly exposed to dust, dirt, and organisms in the air. It is no surprise that in our ever more polluted world we often face problems such as sinus congestion and asthma. Herbal remedies aim to protect the linings of the eyes, ears, sinuses, nose, and throat, as well as the respiratory "tree" of the lungs by countering infection, clearing mucus, soothing the mucous membranes, and relieving inflammation or allergy.

SEEK IMMEDIATE PROFESSIONAL ADVICE FOR

- Difficulty in breathing or chest pain
- Cough that lasts for more than 2 weeks
- Severe pain in the respiratory tract
- Coughing up blood
- Fever of 102°F (39°C) or more
- Heavy nosebleed lasting longer than 1 hour

COUGHS & BRONCHITIS

THE ACT OF coughing is usually a reaction to irritant particles in the bronchial tubes. It is worthwhile considering the type of cough you have and where it is centered. Herbal remedies can then be chosen to work effectively to clear or ease the cough.
Productive, chesty coughs may produce white, yellow, or green phlegm.
Unproductive coughs are dry and irritant, and often take a long time to clear.
Bronchitis occurs when the lining of the lungs' airways becomes inflamed, resulting in a chesty cough, possible breathlessness, and a raised temperature. Use both an external and an internal remedy.
Thyme is an effective antiseptic for the whole system. Licorice acts as a soothing expectorant for persistent coughs and makes any remedy more palatable. Take plenty of garlic to fight bronchitis.

General caution Seek professional advice if a cough lasts for more than 1 week without a cold or infection.

GENERAL REMEDY
Herb Thyme (*Thymus vulgaris*, p. 142)
Remedy Take 5 cups of infusion a day.

DRY COUGHS IN THE THROAT & CHEST
Herbs Balm of Gilead (*Populus* **x** *candicans*, p. 252), thyme (*Thymus vulgaris*, p. 142), licorice (*Glycyrrhiza glabra*, p. 99)
Remedy Make an infusion using equal parts of thyme, balm of Gilead buds, and licorice powder. Take ½ cup 6 times a day, or mix equal parts of each tincture and take 1 tsp up to 5 times a day with water. Reduce the dosage as the cough eases.
Cautions Seek professional advice if no improvement occurs after 1 week. Do not take licorice if pregnant.

CHESTY COUGHS & BRONCHITIS
Herbs Elecampane (*Inula helenium*, p. 105), eucalyptus (*Eucalyptus globulus*, p. 94), licorice (*Glycyrrhiza glabra*, p. 99)
Remedy (Internal) Make a decoction of elecampane and take 2–3 cups a day. Add 5 g of licorice powder to the decoction to improve the flavor if desired.
NOTE For acute bronchitis and coughs, add 5 g of eucalyptus leaf to the decoction.
Caution Do not take elecampane during pregnancy.

Herbs Echinacea (*Echinacea* spp., p. 90), garlic (*Allium sativum*, p. 56)
Remedy (Internal) Take ½ tsp of echinacea tincture with water 2–3 times a day, or take tablets. In addition, eat 2 garlic cloves daily.

Herbs Thyme (*Thymus vulgaris*, p. 142), cajuput (*Melaleuca leucadendron*, p. 232), eucalyptus (*Eucalyptus globulus*, p. 94)
Remedy (External) Mix 5 drops each of eucalyptus and thyme essential oils with 2 tsp of olive or sunflower oil. Massage over the chest and back, up to twice a day. Alternatively, burn 5–10 drops of one of the oils in a burner for 30 minutes.
Caution Do not apply thyme oil during pregnancy.

NOSEBLEEDS

MANY HERBS ARE reputed to stop nosebleeds, and most are effective. Using an herb as snuff is a traditional way of staunching a nosebleed.

Caution If the nosebleed continues for some hours or is very heavy, seek immediate professional advice.

PREVENTION OF NOSEBLEEDS
Herbs Eyebright (*Euphrasia officinalis*, p. 208), nettle (*Urtica dioica*, p. 145)
Remedy Make an infusion using 25 g of either herb to 750 ml of water. Take up to 4 cups a day.

NOSEBLEEDS
Herb American cranesbill (*Geranium maculatum*, p. 214)
Remedy First, pinch the nostrils and tilt back the head. Then sniff ½ tsp of the powdered herb.

EYE PROBLEMS

RATHER THAN TREATING the eyes themselves, these remedies benefit the mucous tissue lining the eyes, which is contiguous with the nose and throat. Problems affecting the linings of the eyes often respond well to local treatment with herbal remedies, but care must be taken not to irritate the eyes with particles of herbs left in the lotion.

SORE & TIRED EYES
Herbs German chamomile (*Chamomilla recutita*, p. 76), ju hua (*Chrysanthemum morifolium*, p. 77)
Remedy Make a compress by infusing a chamomile teabag for 5 minutes, or make a poultice with 15 g of either herb to 250 ml of water. Cool, squeeze out excess liquid, and place teabag or poultice over the eye.

CONJUNCTIVITIS
Herbs Eyebright (*Euphrasia officinalis*, p. 208), cornflowers (*Centaurea cyanus*, p. 183)
Remedy Make an infusion with either herb and strain. While warm, but not hot, place in an eyebath and bathe eyes well (*see* p. 296). Do not use more than twice a day.

Caution If there is no improvement in 3–4 days, seek professional advice.

COLDS, FLU & FEVERS

THE COMMON COLD, with which most of us are only too familiar, is a viral infection normally affecting the nose and throat. Flu is considerably more debilitating and may include fever, headache, muscular pain, nausea, and vomiting. Both have a habit of striking when we are stressed or run down. Herbal home treatment is especially suitable for these familiar "self-limiting" ailments since it enables us to make life more comfortable, control fever, and improve the body's recovery rate.

Garlic, ginger, and lemon combine to create the classic flu remedy that can also be used to relieve colds, sore throats, and tonsillitis.

Ginger, cinnamon, cloves, and cayenne have heating properties and stimulate sweating. This helps to lower the body's temperature during fever.

Yarrow and elderflower also stimulate sweating and astringe the mucous membranes of the nose and throat, thereby reducing the production of mucus.

Boneset and cayenne are particularly helpful for respiratory infections.

Wormwood and gentian are bitter herbs that cool the body and combat high fever.

DIET
For all these problems, eat lightly. Fruit and vegetables are best, the latter perhaps in a soup. Avoid greasy, fatty, sugar-rich food and dairy products.

SELF-HELP
Reduce fever and temperature by washing with cool or cold water and drinking plenty of liquid, especially when sweating.

General cautions Remember that in the very young and very old, even a common cold can develop into pneumonia. Always seek professional advice if symptoms persist or suddenly worsen.

GENERAL REMEDIES
Herbs Garlic (*Allium sativum*, p. 56), ginger (*Zingiber officinale*, p. 153), lemon (*Citrus limon*, p. 81)
Remedy Crush a medium-sized garlic clove, grate a similarly sized piece of fresh ginger, and squeeze the juice from 1 lemon. Mix together with 1 tsp of honey. Add 1 cup of warm water and stir. Drink up to 3 cups a day while symptoms last.

Herbs Thyme (*Thymus vulgaris*, p. 142), boneset (*Eupatorium perfoliatum*, p. 206)
Remedy Make an infusion using ½ tsp of each herb with 1 cup of water and drink 3–4 cups a day.
NOTE This remedy is very effective if thick green mucus and nasal congestion occur.

COLDS
Herbs Lemon (*Citrus limon*, p. 81), cinnamon (*Cinnamomum verum*, p. 80)
Remedy Drink the freshly squeezed juice of 1 lemon, neat or diluted in warm water.
Option Add 1 tsp of honey to the juice and ½ tsp of cinnamon powder.

Herb Ginger (*Zingiber officinale*, p. 153)
Remedy Infuse 2–3 slices (1 g) of fresh ginger with 1 cup of water for 5 minutes. Take up to 5 cups a day.

HIGH FEVER
Herbs Yarrow (*Achillea millefolium*, p. 54), boneset (*Eupatorium perfoliatum*, p. 206), cayenne (*Capsicum frutescens*, p. 70)
Remedy Make an infusion using 1 tsp each of yarrow and boneset, with a pinch of cayenne, to 1 cup of water. Brew for 5 minutes and drink hot. Take up to 4 cups a day.
Options Add 1 or 2 of the following herbs: 2–3 cloves (*Eugenia carophyllata*, p. 95),

½ tsp of powdered or grated fresh ginger (*Zingiber officinale*, p. 153), ½ tsp of chopped or powdered cinnamon bark (*Cinnamomum verum*, p. 80), 1–2 crushed cardamom seeds (*Eletteria cardamomum*, p. 91), 2–3 crushed peppercorns (*Piper nigrum*, p. 248).
Caution Do not take yarrow during pregnancy.

Herbs Wormwood (*Artemisia absinthium*, p. 63), gentian (*Gentiana lutea*, p. 97).
Remedy Take 10 drops of either tincture with water 3 times a day in addition to the above remedy.
Caution Do not take wormwood during pregnancy.

MILD FEVER
Herbs Yarrow (*Achillea millefolium*, p. 54), elderflower (*Sambucus nigra*, p. 131)
Remedy Make an infusion with ½ tsp of each herb in 100 ml water. Brew for 10 minutes and drink up to 4 cups a day.
Caution Do not take yarrow during pregnancy.

Herb Onion (*Allium cepa*, p. 162)
Remedy Bake a large onion at 200°C (400°F) for 40 minutes. Remove, and mix the juice with an equal amount of honey. Take 1–2 tsp an hour up to 8 times a day.

FLU WITH MUSCLE ACHES & PAINS
Herbs Thyme (*Thymus vulgaris*, p. 142), lemon balm (*Melissa officinalis*, p. 111), elderflower (*Sambucus nigra*, p. 131)
Remedy Make an infusion using 5 g of each herb to 750 ml of water. Brew for 10 minutes and drink up to 5 cups a day.

Herb Echinacea (*Echinacea* spp., p. 90)
Remedy Take tablets or capsules, or up to ½ tsp of tincture with water twice a day. Alternatively, make a decoction with 5 g of root to 750 ml of water and drink 2–4 cups a day.

SORE THROATS & TONSILLITIS

THE GARLIC, GINGER, and lemon mixture listed under *General Remedies* for *Colds, Flu & Fevers* (*see* above) can alleviate the symptoms of both sore throats and tonsillitis. The brave can slowly chew a clove of garlic; sage and echinacea are also strongly antiseptic. All these herbs will relieve symptoms and aid in a speedy recovery.

General caution Always seek professional advice and treatment for children under 5 suffering from tonsillitis.

SORE THROATS
Herbs Tamarind (*Tamarindus indica*, p. 272), lemon (*Citrus limon*, p. 81)
Remedy Gargle with either a decoction of tamarind fruit or 20 ml of lemon juice either neat or diluted in warm water.

Herbs Rosemary (*Rosmarinus officinalis*, p. 125), sage (*Salvia officinalis*, p. 130), myrrh (*Commiphora molmol*, p. 84), echinacea (*Echinacea* spp., p. 90)
Remedy 1 Dilute 1 tsp of equal parts of all tinctures in 5 tsp of warm water and gargle. Swallow the mixture (except if pregnant).

Remedy 2 Make a sage infusion, brew for 10 minutes, and allow to cool a little. Gargle, then swallow. Add 5 ml of vinegar and 1 tsp of honey to strengthen its action.
Caution Do not swallow sage during pregnancy.

TONSILLITIS
Herbs Echinacea (*Echinacea* spp., p. 90), all herbs listed under *Sore Throats*
Remedy Take echinacea (see *Flu with Muscle Aches & Pains* above), or use one of the gargles listed under *Sore Throats*.

Caution Seek professional advice if there is no improvement after 2 days.

311

BEFORE TAKING ANY HERBAL REMEDIES, SEE PAGES 289 & 298
Respiratory Tract Problems continued on page 312

CONGESTION, SINUS PROBLEMS & EARACHE

EXCESSIVE NASAL CONGESTION is not always easy to treat and suggests poor air quality, inappropriate diet, or an allergy. The shape of the nose and sinuses (the air-filled cavities in the bones around the nose) can also play a role in this condition. Sinuses can become blocked with fluid, causing painful pressure. Earache may be caused by local infection – in which case garlic is particularly effective – or mucous congestion. Lavender is helpful in soothing the pain of all types of earache.

DIET
As a first step, reduce foods thought to increase mucus production, such as dairy products, eggs, fried and fatty food, sugar, and refined carbohydrates, such as white flour, as well as alcohol.

General caution Seek professional advice for earache, especially in children.

GENERAL REMEDY
Herb Eucalyptus (*Eucalyptus globulus*, p. 94)
Remedy Make a steam inhalation by infusing 15 g of herb or 5–10 drops of essential oil in 750 ml of water. Inhale for 10 minutes.

ALLERGIC STATES WITH EXCESSIVE NASAL CONGESTION, SUCH AS HAY FEVER
Herb German chamomile (*Chamomilla recutita*, p. 76)
Remedy Make a steam inhalation by infusing 15 g of herb or put 5–10 drops of essential oil in 750 ml water. Inhale for 10 minutes.

EARACHE
Herb Lavender (*Lavandula officinalis*, p. 107)
Remedy Place 2 drops of neat lavender oil on a cotton ball and plug into the ear.

EARACHE CAUSED BY INFECTION
Herb Garlic (*Allium sativum*, p. 56)
Remedy Break open a garlic oil capsule, place 2 drops on a cotton ball, and plug into the affected ear. Alternatively, crush a large clove of garlic and soak in 1 tbsp of sunflower or olive oil for at least 24 hours. Strain the oil and warm it to body temperature. Then place 2 drops on a cotton ball and plug into the ear.

EARACHE DUE TO CHRONIC CONGESTION
Herbs Echinacea (*Echinacea* spp., p. 90), thyme (*Thymus vulgaris*, p. 142), marsh mallow (*Althaea officinalis*, p. 163), elderflower (*Sambucus nigra*, p. 131)
Remedy Mix equal parts of each tincture and take 1 tsp 3 times a day with water.

COPIOUS LIQUID MUCUS & SINUS CONGESTION
See *Allergic rhinitis*, p. 300.

SINUS HEADACHES
See *Tension & Sinus Headaches*, p. 309.

MUSCULOSKELETAL PROBLEMS

CRAMPBARK
(*Viburnum opulus*)

WHETHER CAUSED BY accident, sports injury, or simple wear and tear, musculoskeletal problems can lead to a significant deterioration in quality of life. Manipulation is often the primary treatment, but herbal remedies can reduce pain and inflammation, relax muscles, detoxify the body, and speed up the rate of healing. External treatments soothe back muscles and joints, and sprained or sore limbs. Persevering with the simple home treatments given below can bring about a marked improvement of many problems.

SEEK IMMEDIATE PROFESSIONAL ADVICE FOR
- Severe pain
- Significant or sudden joint swelling
- Broken or suspected broken bones
- Any injury that may need an X ray

Caution Only give external remedies to children. Seek professional advice before giving internal remedies to them.

SPRAINS & FRACTURES

MINOR DAMAGED AREAS benefit from herbs such as arnica and comfrey, which soothe bruising and speed up the healing process. Apply as soon as possible after treatment.

General caution Always seek professional treatment for broken bones, fractures, and severe sprains.

SPRAINS
Herb Arnica (*Arnica montana*, p. 170)
Remedy Apply ointment or cream to the damaged area and gently massage into the skin at least 3 times a day.
Caution Do not use arnica on broken skin.

FRACTURES
Herb Comfrey (*Symphytum officinale*, p. 136)
Remedy Gently apply ointment, cream, or infused oil to the area at least 3 times a day.
Caution Do not use comfrey on broken skin.

MUSCLE ACHES & CRAMPS

MUSCLE ACHES AND cramps are entirely normal, particularly after strenuous activity, and the pain should lessen in time. Meanwhile, rubs and ointments containing soothing herbs, such as arnica, thyme, and crampbark, can alleviate aching muscles. Rheumatism is a general term for muscle or joint pain and stiffness, and the remedies listed here and under *Joint Pain & Stiffness*, p. 313, are appropriate for this condition.

TIRED & ACHING MUSCLES
Herb Arnica (*Arnica montana*, p. 170)
Remedy Apply cream or ointment.
Caution Do not use arnica on broken skin.

Herbs Thyme (*Thymus vulgaris*, p. 142), rosemary (*Rosmarinus officinalis*, p. 125)
Remedy Make an infusion with 25 g of one herb to 750 ml water. Brew for 10 minutes. Strain into a bathtub; soak for 20 minutes.

Option Try also the rub containing St. John's wort oil, listed under *General Remedies* for *Back Pain*, p. 313.

CRAMPS & MUSCLE SPASMS
Herb Crampbark (*Viburnum opulus*, p. 148)
Remedy (Internal) Take 1 tsp of tincture with water up to 3 times a day.
Remedy (External) Rub neat tincture firmly into the affected area.

JOINT PAIN & STIFFNESS, INCLUDING ARTHRITIS & GOUT

THE MOST COMMON ailment characterized by joint pain and stiffness is arthritis, which is caused by inflammation of the joints. Aging or wear and tear may be the cause, but some arthritic conditions, and other joint problems such as gout, are due to the build-up of waste products in the joints.

Devil's claw is anti-inflammatory, relieving swollen and inflamed joints.

Lemon juice reduces acidity in the body.

White willow relieves inflammation and pain and, when combined with other herbs, can lead to significant improvement in mild to moderate arthritis.

Meadowsweet and celery combine well to reduce acidity. All the herbal remedies here can be safely taken for 1–2 months.

SELF-HELP

Improving posture, managing anxiety, and using herbal remedies to help the body eliminate toxins can all help control these conditions. Avoid acid-forming foods such as red meat, spinach, tomatoes, and oranges. Regular, but not excessive, exercise is beneficial, as is a relaxed positive attitude.

General cautions For severe arthritis, consult a professional practitioner. Do not take devil's claw, black cohosh, or celery during pregnancy.

ARTHRITIS & INFLAMED JOINTS

Herb Devil's claw (*Harpagophytum procumbens*, p. 101)
Remedy Take tablets (see *General cautions*).

Herb Lemon (*Citrus limon*, p. 81)
Remedy Squeeze the juice from a lemon and drink neat or diluted in water each morning.

Herb White willow (*Salix alba*, p. 128)
Remedy Take tablets, or make a decoction using 10 g of root to 750 ml water. Take in 3 doses over 1–2 days as required.

Herbs Devil's claw (*Harpagophytum procumbens*, p. 101), celery (*Apium graveolens*, p. 61), white willow (*Salix alba*, p. 128)
Remedy Make a decoction with 8 g of each herb to 750 ml of water, divide into 4 doses, and take 2–3 doses a day; or mix equal parts of the tinctures and take 1 tsp with water 3 times a day (see *General cautions*).
Option If arthritis develops during menopause, replace devil's claw with 8 g of black cohosh (*Cimicifuga racemosa*, p. 78)

Herb Deadly nightshade (*Atropa belladonna*, p. 66)
Remedy Apply belladonna plasters in addition to one of the above remedies.

ARTHRITIS ASSOCIATED WITH
ACID INDIGESTION OR PEPTIC ULCER

Herbs Meadowsweet (*Filipendula ulmaria*, p. 96), celery (*Apium graveolens*, p. 61)
Remedy Make an infusion with meadowsweet and drink up to 5 cups a day, or mix 2 parts meadowsweet tincture with 1 part celery tincture and take ½ tsp with water 2–3 times a day (see *General cautions*).

STIFF & ACHING JOINTS

Herbs St. John's wort (*Hypericum perforatum*, p. 104), comfrey (*Symphytum officinale*, p. 136), lavender (*Lavandula officinalis*, p. 107)
Remedy Mix 2½ tbsp of St. John's wort or comfrey infused oil with 20–40 drops of lavender essential oil and gently massage into the affected area.
Option Try the rub containing St. John's wort infused oil under *General Remedies* for *Back Pain* below.

GOUT

Herb Celery (*Apium graveolens*, p. 61)
Remedy Take tablets, or make a decoction with the seeds. Divide into 3 doses and drink during the day or add 25 g of seeds to food per day (see *General cautions*).

BACK PAIN

ABOVE ALL, BACK problems require a specialist's attention and plenty of rest. Herbal remedies contribute to overall improvement by alleviating pain and muscle tension, and helping to make life more comfortable.

Crampbark and prickly ash are warming relaxing herbs, which when rubbed into the affected area help to "unknot" taut muscles.

Lavender and St. John's wort are useful herbs when nervous tension is contributing to the problem.

Devil's claw and crampbark have effective anti-inflammatory properties and help reduce swollen joints.

Passionflower encourages sleep, particularly when back pain is accompanied by nervous tension.

Sciatica (a painful condition caused by a pinched spinal nerve) and neuralgia can both be relieved by using an external rub containing St. John's wort infused oil.

General cautions Back problems need a specialist's care. For chronic or severe back pain, seek the advice of a professional practitioner to gain the most benefit from herbal medicine.

GENERAL REMEDIES

Herbs Crampbark (*Viburnum opulus*, p. 148), prickly ash (*Zanthoxylum americanum*, p. 151)
Remedy Make a decoction using 15 g of crampbark and 5 g of prickly ash bark to 750 ml of water. Strain and rub into the affected area, or use 1 tbsp of tincture and apply in the same way.
NOTE Use especially for tense neck and lumbar regions.

Herb Thyme (*Thymus vulgaris*, p. 142)
Remedy Make an infusion using 25 g of herb to 750 ml of water and strain into a bath. Soak for 20 minutes.

Herbs St. John's wort (*Hypericum perforatum*, p. 104), lavender (*Lavandula officinalis*, p. 107), pepper (*Piper nigrum*, p. 248), crampbark (*Viburnum opulus*, p. 148)
Remedy Take 2 tbsp of sunflower oil or St. John's wort infused oil, add 20 drops of lavender essential oil, 10 drops each of rosemary and pepper essential oil, and 1 tsp of crampbark tincture. Shake and rub into tense areas, either after a bath or having

first warmed the area with a hot towel.
OTHER USES Use for sciatica and other back problems that cause neuralgia, as well as for stiff joints and chronic muscle ache.

BACK PAIN DUE TO JOINT INFLAMMATION

Herbs White willow (*Salix alba*, p. 128), crampbark (*Viburnum opulus*, p. 148), devil's claw (*Harpagophytum procumbens*, p. 101)
Remedy Mix equal parts of each root and make a decoction. Divide into 6 doses and take over 2 days. If there is no improvement after 7 days, divide the decoction into 3 doses and take daily for up to a week.
Caution Do not take devil's claw during pregnancy.

SLEEPLESSNESS DUE TO BACKACHE

Herbs Passionflower (*Passiflora incarnata*, p. 117), valerian (*Valeriana officinalis*, p. 146), crampbark (*Viburnum opulus*, p. 148)
Remedy Make a decoction using 8 g each of passionflower, valerian, and crampbark to 750 ml of water, and drink 1–2 cups at night (the decoction is sufficient for 2 days).

URINARY & FUNGAL INFECTIONS

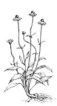

ECHINACEA
(*Echinacea* spp.)

INFECTIONS SIGNAL THAT the body's resistance to disease has become weakened, particularly if they are long-lasting or recurrent. Minor infections affecting the kidneys and urinary system are common and, despite being hard to shake off, can be treated by boosting the body's natural defenses. Fungal infections can also be difficult to clear and may require professional treatment, although herbs such as garlic (*Allium sativum*, p. 56) and tea tree (*Melaleuca alternifolia*, p. 110) are highly antifungal. If the infection is chronic, it will often be necessary to support the immune system as a whole with herbs such as echinacea (*Echinacea* spp., p. 90).

> ### SEEK IMMEDIATE PROFESSIONAL ADVICE FOR
>
> - Infections that show no signs of improvement or that deteriorate after taking an herbal remedy
> - Temperatures above 102°F (39°C)
> - Pain in the kidneys
> - Blood in the urine

URINARY INFECTIONS

CYSTITIS (AN INFECTION of the bladder and urinary tubules) can be a serious problem if it spreads to the kidneys. Mild cystitis and other urinary infections can be cured with a mixture of antiseptic herbs such as buchu and soothing herbs such as marsh mallow. Taking echinacea or garlic at the same time improves the body's resistance to infection. Bilberry and cranberry are both excellent for urinary infections.

General cautions Seek immediate professional help if cystitis is severe or recurrent, or if there is blood in the urine, or pain around the kidneys or small of the back.

GENERAL REMEDIES
Herbs Buchu (*Barosma betulina*, p. 67), cornsilk (*Zea mays*, p. 152), marsh mallow (*Althaea officinalis*, p. 163)
Remedy Make an infusion with 5 g of each herb to 750 ml of water. Divide into 4 doses and drink throughout the day.
Option Substitute juniper (*Juniperus communis*, p. 223) or goldenrod (*Solidago virgaurea*, p. 269) for buchu.

Caution Do not take juniper or buchu in pregnancy.

Herb Bilberry (*Vaccinium myrtillus*, p. 278)
Remedy Make a decoction of the berries and drink 3–4 cups a day.
TIP Cranberry juice may be substituted for bilberry decoction.

Herbs Garlic (*Allium sativum*, p. 56), echinacea (*Echinacea* spp., p. 90)
Remedy Take either or both herbs in capsule or tablet form.
NOTE Take in addition to other remedies.

FUNGAL INFECTIONS

FUNGAL INFECTIONS ARE common and can be hard to treat. Vaginal yeast infections are increasingly found as a side effect of conventional antibiotic treatment. Calendula can be helpful in treating this troublesome condition. Candidiasis can cause considerable problems, but mild cases may be helped with antiseptic and antifungal herbs, such as garlic. All types of fungal infections can be helped with herbs that boost the immune system, such as echinacea, as well as by applying an external remedy to the affected area.

DIET
Diet is an important factor when treating fungal problems. Cut out or reduce intake of bread, alcohol, and other foods containing yeast or sugar.

SELF-HELP
Candidiasis sufferers can take acidophilus capsules or live yogurt to help the growth of beneficial bacteria in the intestines. For yeast infections, live yogurt can be inserted into the vagina.

General caution Seek professional advice for candidiasis. It is often a difficult condition to treat.

GENERAL REMEDIES
Herbs Echinacea (*Echinacea* spp., p. 90), thyme (*Thymus vulgaris*, p. 142)
Remedy Mix 2 parts echinacea tincture to 1 part thyme tincture and take 1 tsp twice a day with water.

Herb Garlic (*Allium sativum*, p. 56)
Remedy Take 1–2 garlic cloves a day, crushed and swallowed with water or mixed with food.

VAGINAL YEAST INFECTIONS
Herb Calendula (*Calendula officinalis*, p. 69)
Remedy Make an infusion and allow to cool. Strain and use as a douche or wash.
Option Add the infusion to a bath and soak for 20 minutes.

Herb Tea tree (*Melaleuca alternifolia*, p. 110)
Remedy Use suppositories or place 1–2 drops of essential oil diluted with 3 drops of olive oil on a tampon and insert into the vagina (this may sting). Remove after 2–3 hours and only use once a day.

Caution During pregnancy, use these suppositories and tampons only with professional advice.

ORAL THRUSH
Herbs Licorice (*Glycyrrhiza glabra*, p. 99), myrrh (*Commiphora molmol*, p. 84), echinacea (*Echinacea* spp., p. 90)
Remedy Mix equal parts of the tincture of each herb. Take 1 tsp as a mouthwash with water every 3–4 hours, as required.

CANDIDIASIS
Herbs Elderflower (*Sambucus nigra*, p. 131), calendula (*Calendula officinalis*, p. 69), thyme (*Thymus vulgaris*, p. 142)
Remedy Make an infusion with 8 g of each herb to 750 ml water and drink 2–3 cups each day.

Herb Lapacho (*Tabebuia* spp., p. 138)
Remedy Make a decoction with 12 g of bark to 750 ml of water. Divide into 3–4 doses and drink throughout the day. Alternatively, take capsules or ½ tsp of tincture with water up to 3 times a day.

FUNGAL SKIN INFECTIONS, INCLUDING ATHLETE'S FOOT
See p. 304.

Reproductive & Menstrual Problems

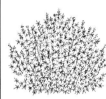

AGNUS CASTUS
(*Vitex agnus-castus*)

WOMEN HAVE ALWAYS tended to use herbal medicine more than men, traditionally in their role as healers in the home and now, in part, due to the proven effects of many herbs on the reproductive system. Herbs such as agnus castus contain constituents similar to the female sex hormones, estrogen and progesterone, which can help regulate the menstrual cycle, increase or decrease fertility, and support the body through menopause. Common menstrual problems, such as cramps, premenstrual tension, and heavy bleeding, respond well to self-treatment. However, chronic conditions or infertility in either women or men require professional attention.

SEEK IMMEDIATE PROFESSIONAL ADVICE FOR

- Severe pain in the abdomen or pelvis
- Significant or sudden change in menstruation, such as prolonged, heavy, or irregular periods

IMPORTANT NOTE

For the best treatment, consult an herbalist. Seek professional advice before taking a remedy if you believe that you may be pregnant. See *Pregnancy*, p. 317.

MENSTRUAL PROBLEMS

THE MENSTRUAL CYCLE can be disturbed for many reasons, most of them relating to hormonal imbalances. Other causes include stress, too much or too little exercise, weight problems, food sensitivity or allergy, steroids, the contraceptive pill, chronic illness, vitamin and mineral deficiency, and even excess caffeine, alcohol, or smoking. To determine the underlying cause, it is important to consult a professional practitioner.

Taking remedies for menstrual problems. The remedies listed should all be taken at the appropriate point in the cycle for 2–3 cycles.

The normal menstrual cycle lasts about 28 days. If this cycle varies greatly from one period to another without reason, it could be termed irregular.

Premenstrual syndrome (PMS) and menstrual pain are caused by many factors and are experienced at some stage by most women. Breast tenderness, sore nipples, and fluid retention are common symptoms.

Heavy periods can result in anemia. If your period lasts longer than 5 days or if you have to change your protection every 2 hours, your periods may be too heavy. Nettle (*Urtica dioica*, p. 145) is an excellent tonic, especially for heavy bleeding, since it contains more iron than spinach and can be eaten as a nourishing vegetable.

SELF-HELP

Combine herbal remedies with a diet high in fresh vegetables and fruit, and low in fatty foods, sugar, and alcohol. Try to avoid smoking. Regular exercise, particularly of the waist and pelvis, is helpful, as is a relaxed attitude to life. All reproductive problems will benefit from this simple approach.

General caution For any chronic menstrual problem, it is wise to seek professional attention, especially if your periods are very heavy or painful.

IRREGULAR CYCLE

Herb Agnus castus (*Vitex agnus-castus*, p. 149)
Remedy Take tablets, or take 1.5–2 ml of tincture with water each morning on awakening for at least 2 months.

Herb Motherwort (*Leonurus cardiaca*, p. 225)
Remedy Make an infusion and take 1–2 cups a day for up to 3 monthly cycles.
Caution Do not take if menstrual bleeding is heavy.

PREMENSTRUAL TENSION

Herbs Vervain (*Verbena officinalis*, p. 147), linden (*Tilia* spp., p. 275)
Remedy (Internal) Make an infusion using either herb (or an equal mix of both) and drink up to 5 cups throughout the day.

Herb Valerian (*Valeriana officinalis*, p. 146)
Remedy (Internal) Take tablets containing valerian, or take 20–40 drops of tincture with water up to 5 times a day.

Herb Rosemary (*Rosmarinus officinalis*, p. 125)
Remedy (External) Make an infusion with 1 tbsp of dried or 2 tbsp of fresh leaves to 1 liter of water and strain into a warm bath each morning. Alternatively, add 5–10 drops of essential oil to a bath.
NOTE Also try the agnus castus remedy under *Irregular Cycle* above.

BREAST TENDERNESS & SORE NIPPLES

Herb German chamomile (*Chamomilla recutita*, p. 76)
Remedy Make a compress with an infusion of 50 g of herb and 250 ml of water. Place gently over the breasts. Repeat as often as required.

Herb Calendula (*Calendula officinalis*, p. 69)
Remedy Apply calendula ointment to the nipples. If breast-feeding, wipe off the ointment before feeding.

FLUID RETENTION

Herb Dandelion (*Taraxacum officinale*, p. 140)
Remedy Make an infusion with the leaves and drink up to 3 cups a day.

HEAVY MENSTRUAL BLEEDING

Herbs Chuang xiong (*Ligusticum wallachii*), white peony (*Paeonia lactiflora*, p. 115), Chinese angelica (*Angelica sinensis*, p. 60), rehmannia (*Rehmannia glutinosa*, p. 123)
Remedy Mix equal parts of each root and make a decoction using 15 g of the mixture to 750 ml of water. Drink in 3 equal doses throughout the day.
NOTE Any of these herbs will help, but they are best together, in which form they are known as *Four Things Soup*.

Herbs Shepherd's purse (*Capsella bursa-pastoris*, p. 181), nettle (*Urtica dioica*, p. 145)
Remedy Make an infusion using 7.5 g of each herb (or 15 g of shepherd's purse only) to 750 ml of water. Divide into 3–4 doses and drink throughout the day.

MENSTRUAL PAIN

Flavor the decoctions with 1 heaping tsp of caraway seeds (*Carum carvi*, p. 182). Mix before decocting.
Herbs Wild yam (*Dioscorea villosa*, p. 89), crampbark (*Viburnum opulus*, p. 148), black haw (*Viburnum prunifolium*, p. 279)
Remedy Make a decoction using 15 g of one root to 750 ml of water. Sip small amounts during the day; or take 2 tsp of tincture with water 3–4 times a day for up to 3 days, then reduce the dose to 1 tsp a day for 5 days, or take tablets.

Herb White peony (*Paeonia lactiflora*, p. 115)
Remedy Make a decoction using 20 g of root to 750 ml of water. Sip throughout the day.

315

FERTILITY PROBLEMS IN WOMEN

ALTHOUGH MUCH MORE research is needed, herbal medicine does appear to increase fertility in women who are trying to conceive, especially if the problem is related to hormonal imbalances, age, or the amount of mucus produced by the cervix. Where there appears to be no physical problem preventing conception – for example, a blocked fallopian tube, ovarian cysts, or internal scarring – herbal medicines are well worth trying. Diet, exercise, and lifestyle may also play a significant role in improving fertility.

AIDING CONCEPTION
Herb Agnus castus (*Vitex agnus-castus*, p. 149)
Remedy Take tablets or take 20–40 drops of tincture with water each morning for a maximum of 3 months at a time.

❧

Herb Chinese angelica (*Angelica sinensis*, p. 60)
Remedy Take tablets or make a decoction using 12 g of root to 750 ml of water and drink each day for up to 3 months.
Caution Discontinue if you become pregnant.

LOW SEX DRIVE
Herb Schisandra (*Schisandra chinensis*, p. 132)
Remedy Soak 5 g (a small handful) of berries in water overnight. Strain the berries and make a decoction with 250 ml of water. Brew for 15 minutes and take the dose each day.
NOTE Traditionally, this remedy is taken for 100 days to raise sexual energy and vitality. (It is safe to take it for this period.)

FERTILITY PROBLEMS IN MEN

IMPOTENCE IN MEN is a common problem, and herbal medicine has been used throughout history to help restore healthy sexual function. A low sperm count, which is a common cause of infertility, is often related to lifestyle and general state of health.
Saw palmetto is a tonic herb that increases stamina. It benefits the male sexual organs and is reputed to increase potency.
Withania is an all-round tonic that is not as stimulating as ginseng, but is nonetheless helpful in restoring normal vitality after a long-term illness or stress.

GENERAL VITALITY
Herb Withania (*Withania somnifera*, p. 150)
Remedy Take 2 g of the dried root a day, either by chewing it or taking it in powder form mixed with honey and, if required, water. Take for up to 6 weeks.

IMPOTENCE & PREMATURE EJACULATION
Herb Ginseng (*Panax ginseng*, p. 116)
Remedy Take 0.5–1 g up to 3 times a day for 6 weeks at a time, either by chewing the root, cooking it in a soup or stew, or taking it in tablet form.
NOTE Ginseng is the best-known remedy for this condition. However, schisandra (*Schisandra chinensis*, p. 132) berries also benefit male sexuality. Take as listed above in *Fertility Problems in Women* under *Low Sex Drive* for up to 6 weeks.
Caution Do not take caffeine while taking ginseng.

❧

Herb Saw palmetto (*Sabal serrulata*, p. 127)
Remedy Take ½ tsp of tincture with water up to 3 times a day for up to 6 weeks.

MENOPAUSAL PROBLEMS

MENOPAUSE IS defined as the cessation of menstruation. It usually takes place between the ages of 45 and 55. After two years without having a period, you can be sure that the "change of life" has occurred.
Both estrogen and progesterone levels decline during menopause despite opinion to the contrary. Herbs such as agnus castus, that have a progesterogenic effect, are as important as those that support estrogen levels, since both hormones appear to help maintain bone density, reducing the risk of osteoporosis.
Maintaining vitality is important during menopause, since many problems result as much from being run-down and tired as from hormonal changes. If you feel low and exhausted, some of these remedies may help to raise vitality and spirits. St. John's wort is an excellent medicine for depression.
Hot flashes and night sweats are principally caused by hormonal changes. However, nervous exhaustion increases the occurrence of these conditions.

General caution Seek professional advice if there is prolonged or irregular menstrual bleeding.

DECREASED ESTROGEN & PROGESTERONE LEVELS
Herb Agnus castus (*Vitex agnus-castus*, p. 149)
Remedy Take tablets, or 20–40 drops of tincture with water each morning.

❧

Herb Helonias (*Chamaelirium luteum*, p. 75)
Remedy It is best to take tablets. Alternatively take 20 drops of tincture with water 2–3 times a day.

❧

Herb Black cohosh (*Cimicifuga racemosa*, p. 78)
Remedy Take tablets, or take 25 drops of tincture with water 3 times a day.
Option Black cohosh combines well with helonias. Mix equal parts of each tincture and take 1.5–2 ml with water 3 times a day.

DEPRESSION & DECREASED VITALITY
Herb St. John's wort (*Hypericum perforatum*, p. 104)
Remedy Take ½ tsp of tincture with water 3 times a day.

❧

Herb Oats (*Avena sativa*, p. 172)
Remedy Eat 25–50 g of oats as a breakfast cereal or with other food.
Option In addition, make an infusion with oat straw. Divide into 3 doses and drink throughout the day.

HOT FLASHES & NIGHT SWEATS
Herb Sage (*Salvia officinalis*, p. 130)
Remedy Make an infusion and drink 3 cups, either during the day or mainly at night, if this is when the problem usually occurs.

❧

Herbs White willow (*Salix alba*, p. 128), black cohosh (*Cimicifuga racemosa*, p. 78)
Remedy Take one of the above herbs, either in tablet form or take 1 tsp of tincture with water at night.

❧

Herb White peony (*Paeonia lactiflora*, p. 115)
Remedy Make a decoction with 20 g root to 750 ml of water. Sip throughout the day.

PREGNANCY

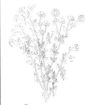

CHAMOMILE
(*Chamomilla recutita*)

ALTHOUGH IN MANY cultures herbs have traditionally been taken throughout pregnancy, it is wise to take herbs medicinally only when essential. Some herbs such as German chamomile (*Chamomilla recutita*, p. 76), linden (*Tilia* spp., p. 275), and cornsilk (*Zea mays*, p. 152) are very useful and can be taken safely for 2–3 weeks at a time during pregnancy. Other herbs should be avoided altogether since they have constituents that stimulate the muscles of the womb and, in large doses, could cause a miscarriage (see *Essential Information*, p. 298). It is safe to continue using herbs in cooking throughout pregnancy.

SEEK IMMEDIATE PROFESSIONAL ADVICE FOR

- Prolonged nausea causing an inability to eat properly and frequent vomiting leading to dehydration.
- Frequent urination lasting for more than 3 days (or with pain after 2 days).
- Breast pain with swollen glands under the arms or fever.
- Fluid retention that has not decreased after 3 days.

GENERAL AILMENTS

PREGNANCY IS A time of great change for the body. Many minor ailments can be relieved by homemade herbal remedies.

Morning sickness (sensations of nausea) need not be restricted to the morning. Generally starting in the 4th–6th week and lasting until the 14th–16th week, morning sickness has many causes, including hormone fluctuations, low blood pressure, low sugar levels, food allergies, poor diet, and stress.

Edema (fluid retention and bloating) is extremely common during pregnancy. Water seeps from the blood vessels into the surrounding tissue, causing puffiness. The ankles and calves are mostly affected.

Constipation often occurs as pregnancy develops. Pressure increases on the lower bowel, impeding circulation.

Heartburn (pain in the center of the chest) may also be caused by increased pressure within the body.

Stretch marks sometimes appear as the body swells. They can be minimized by rubbing aloe vera gel or olive oil into the skin to maintain its elasticity.

Childbirth can be helped by drinking raspberry leaf tea, a traditional remedy that prepares the uterine muscles for labor and giving birth.

HERBS DURING PREGNANCY

- For the first 3 months avoid all herbal remedies, including essential oils, unless professionally prescribed.
- The following herbs are particularly dangerous and should on no account be taken during pregnancy: blue cohosh (*Caulophyllum thalictroides*, p. 73), goldenseal (*Hydrastis canadensis*, p. 103), juniper (*Juniper communis*, p. 223), pennyroyal (*Mentha pulegium*, p. 233), yarrow (*Achillea millefolium*, p. 54), and therapeutic doses of sage (*Salvia officinalis*, p. 130). *See* p. 298 for herbs included on pp. 300–319 that should also be avoided.

MORNING SICKNESS & NAUSEA

The following remedies are an exception and can be taken during the first 3 months of pregnancy.

Herb German chamomile (*Chamomilla recutita*, p. 76)
Remedy Make an infusion in a covered container. Sip small quantities during the day. Do not drink more than 5 cups a day.

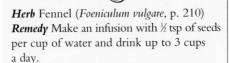

Herb Ginger (*Zingiber officinale*, p. 153)
Remedy Make an infusion with ½–1 tsp of grated fresh ginger per cup of water. Sip small amounts frequently throughout the day, rather than drinking a whole cup at a time. Take a maximum of 3 cups a day.

Herb Fennel (*Foeniculum vulgare*, p. 210)
Remedy Make an infusion with ½ tsp of seeds per cup of water and drink up to 3 cups a day.

EDEMA
Herb Cornsilk (*Zea mays*, p. 152)
Remedy Make an infusion and drink up to 5 cups a day.

CONSTIPATION
Herbs Psyllium (*Plantago* spp., p. 120), linseed (*Linum usitatissimum*, p. 226)
Remedy Take 1–2 tsp of either of the seeds with a large glass of water each day or soak them in cold water overnight before taking.
NOTE Eat more dried fruit, especially figs.

HEARTBURN
Herb Meadowsweet (*Filipendula ulmaria*, p. 96)
Remedy Make an infusion and drink 1–2 cups a day.

HEADACHE & NERVOUS TENSION
Herb Linden (*Tilia* spp., p. 275)
Remedy Make an infusion and drink 3–4 cups a day.

PREPARING FOR CHILDBIRTH
Herb Raspberry (*Rubus idaeus*, p. 262)
Remedy Make an infusion using 1 tsp of the chopped fresh or dried leaf per cup of water. Brew for 5–6 minutes and drink 1–2 cups a day during the last 10 weeks of pregnancy.

Cautions Do not leave the infusion to brew for more than 5–6 minutes. Do not take until the last 10 weeks of pregnancy.

STRETCH MARKS
Herbs Aloe vera (*Aloe vera*, p. 57), olive (*Olea europaea*, p. 239)
Remedy Rub aloe vera gel over the affected areas or massage olive oil firmly into the skin 1–2 times a day.

POOR SLEEP
See *Insomnia* (the German chamomile, linden, lavender, and passionflower remedy under *General Remedies*), p. 309.

ANEMIA & HIGH BLOOD PRESSURE
See *Circulatory Problems*, p. 301.

HEMORRHOIDS
See *Varicose Veins & Hemorrhoids*, p. 302 and *Constipation & Diarrhea*, p. 307.

BACKACHE
See *Back Pain*, p. 313.

VARICOSE VEINS
See *Varicose Veins & Hemorrhoids*, p. 302.

VAGINAL YEAST INFECTIONS
See *Fungal Infections*, p. 314.

BLADDER & KIDNEY INFECTIONS
See *Edema*, left.

HEALING AFTER CHILDBIRTH
See *Cleansing Wounds & Healing Wounds*, p. 304.

INFANTS & CHILDREN

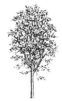

SLIPPERY ELM
(*Ulmus rubra*)

THE FOLLOWING HERBS are considered particularly suitable for children, easing symptoms and speeding recovery. Most of the remedies are best given as infusions and can be given in a bottle. Infusions can be flavored with honey (see *Cautions* right) or maple syrup if necessary, but they are better given unsweetened. The dosages given are for 1–6-year-olds, but they can be adjusted to suit other age groups (*see* below). Many of the remedies listed in other sections are also suitable for babies and children; herbs that are not appropriate are clearly identified (*see* p. 298 for dosage requirements before administering any adult remedies).

GENERAL AILMENTS

INFANTS AND CHILDREN are susceptible to a wide array of ailments.

Digestive upsets that result in diarrhea and constipation can be the result of food intolerance or allergy in infants, especially when foods such as dairy products are being introduced into the diet. Other minor digestive upsets due to infection or inflammation can cause loss of appetite.

Colic is a spasm of the gut causing cramping pain in the abdomen. It usually occurs during the first 3 months of life, particularly after feeding in the evening, when the digestion may not be working so well.

Diaper rash occurs when urine, moisture, and irritants in the diaper cause the baby's skin to become red, sore, and damp. It is essential to clean the baby thoroughly at each diaper change. Make sure that cloth diapers are thoroughly rinsed; avoid leaving a wet chafing diaper on the baby; and remove the diaper whenever possible.

Cradle cap is a thick yellow-brown encrustation on the baby's scalp, caused by overactivity of the sebum oil glands.

Headaches, colds, and chesty coughs are common problems in childhood and respond well to herbal treatment.

Insomnia is a common childhood problem even though children require more sleep than adults and should sleep with ease. Overexcitement, teething, a wet diaper, or being too hot or cold may interfere with sleep patterns. Herbs such as linden will encourage a relaxed night's sleep.

DOSAGE
The dosages on this page are for 1- to 6-year-olds. For other ages, adapt the dose as follows:

6–12 months old – ⅓ dose
7–13 years old – 1½ dose
To adapt remedies from elsewhere in the book for children, *see* p. 298.

DIGESTIVE UPSETS, GAS & COLIC
The following infusions are suitable for infants over 6 months. For those under 6 months, the infusions can be taken by breast-feeding mothers.

Herb Ginger (*Zingiber officinale*, p. 153)
Remedy Give ¼ level tsp of powder with ½ cup of hot water 1–2 times a day.

Herb German chamomile (*Chamomilla recutita*, p. 76)
Remedy Make an infusion with 1 level tsp to 1 cup of water. Give up to 3 cups a day.

Herbs Anise (*Pimpinella anisum*, p. 246), fennel (*Foeniculum vulgare*, p. 210)
Remedy Make an infusion with 1 level tsp of either of the seeds to 1 cup of water. Give up to 2 cups a day.

Herb Slippery elm (*Ulmus rubra*, p. 144)
Remedy Mix 1 tsp of powder with hot water to make a paste, then blend with cold or warm water as required and flavor with honey, cinnamon, or maple syrup. Give up to 50 g powder in doses during the day.

CONSTIPATION
Herbs Linseed (*Linum usitatissimum*, p. 226), slippery elm (*Ulmus rubra*, p. 144)
Remedy Give 1 tsp of linseed or slippery elm with a large glass of water each day.

DIARRHEA
Herbs Agrimony (*Agrimonia eupatoria*, p. 160), common plantain (*Plantago major*, p. 249)
Remedy Make an infusion using 15 g of either herb to ½ liter of water and give up to 2 cups each day.

HEADACHES
Herbs Linden (*Tilia* spp., p. 275), lemon balm (*Melissa officinalis*, p. 111)
Remedy Make an infusion using either herb and give 1–2 cups a day.

DIAPER RASH & INFLAMED SKIN RASHES
Herb Chickweed (*Stellaria media*, p. 270)
Remedy Apply ointment 1–2 times a day.

Herb Calendula (*Calendula officinalis*, p. 69)
Remedy Apply ointment or cream to clean dry skin at each diaper change.
NOTE For diaper rash, the ointment is best.

Herbs Calendula (*Calendula officinalis*, p. 69), nettle (*Urtica dioica*, p. 145)
Remedy Make an infusion with 1 level tsp of each herb to 1 cup of water. Give 1–2 cups a day.

CRADLE CAP
Herb Olive (*Olea europea*, p. 239)
Remedy Apply olive oil to the affected area 1–2 times a day.

COLDS, CONGESTION, & CHESTY COUGHS
Herb Thyme (*Thymus vulgaris*, p. 142)
Remedy Make an infusion with 1 level tsp herb to 1 cup of water. Give 1–2 cups a day.

EARACHE
Herb Garlic (*Allium sativum*, p. 56)
Remedy Break open a garlic oil capsule, put 1 drop on a cotton ball, and plug into the ear.

TEETHING
Herbs German chamomile (*Chamomilla recutita*, p. 76), slippery elm (*Ulmus rubra*, p. 144)
Remedy Give German chamomile infusion (see *Digestive Upsets*) or make a paste from slippery elm powder and the infusion, and rub on the gums.

DIFFICULTY IN SLEEPING
Herbs German chamomile (*Chamomilla recutita*, p. 76), linden (*Tilia* spp., p. 275)
Remedy Make an infusion using either herb and give 1–2 cups before bedtime.

OLD AGE/THIRD AGE

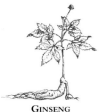

GINSENG
(*Panax ginseng*)

TRADITIONALLY, AS WE AGE, the "fire" or *qi* within us glows less brightly and our vitality slowly weakens. Many herbal medicines are ideally suited to treating the health problems that begin when people reach their late fifties, such as circulatory problems, weak digestion, and poor memory. The herbs recommended here can help to maintain good health, preventing or reducing the severity of symptoms that are often accepted as an inevitable consequence of aging. Self-treatment for other problems often experienced later in life, such as arthritis, is suggested in earlier sections.

IMPORTANT NOTE

- If taking conventional medication, tell your doctor if you intend to take an herbal remedy. This is especially important for the elderly.
- All remedies on this page need to be taken for up to 3 months continuously.
- If you are over 70 years of age, take ¾ of the stated dose for remedies given on other pages.

MAINTAINING VITALITY

THERE ARE MANY herbs that help to maintain vitality.

Thyme is a much underrated herb. Recent research has found it to have antiaging and tonic properties that maintain vitality, and reduce the chance of catching colds, flu, and other respiratory infections.

Withania is an alternative to ginseng and is considered a tonic herb that prevents or slows aging. It is particularly helpful for regaining strength after a long illness, and is reputed to prevent hair turning gray.

Ginseng is taken by the elderly in China to help cope with the harsh winters. It is an excellent tonic for old age, improving vitality and resistance to stress and infection. Take for long-term stress and convalescence.

GENERAL REMEDY
Herb Thyme (*Thymus vulgaris*, p. 142)
Remedy Make a standard infusion. Take 2–3 cups a day.

STRESS OR CONVALESCENCE
Herb Withania (*Withania somnifera*, p. 150)
Remedy Take 1 g of root 2–3 times a day, either by chewing it or chopping it and mixing with a little water.

Herb Ginseng (*Panax ginseng*, p. 116)
Remedy Take 1 g 1–2 times a day for up to 3 months. Chew the fresh or dried root, cook it in a soup, or take it in tablet form. Wait 3–4 weeks before taking it again.
Caution Do not take caffeine while taking ginseng.

Option If ginseng is too stimulating, take 3 g of codonopsis (*Codonopsis pilosula*, p. 82) a day in the same way as ginseng. This has a milder, but nonetheless tonic and strengthening, effect.

NERVOUS EXHAUSTION & STRESS
Herb Oats (*Avena sativa*, p. 172)
Remedy Eat 25 g of oats each day (for example, as a hot cereal). Alternatively, take ½ tsp of the tincture twice a day.

GENERAL CONDITIONS

CONDITIONS THAT ARISE through aging need patient, long-term treatment.

Ginkgo is the oldest tree on the planet. Its leaves maintain good circulation to the head and brain, improving memory, concentration, and energy levels. Evidence suggests it may reduce the risk of a stroke.

Garlic has great value as a long-term dietary supplement, helping to maintain healthy circulation, balance blood sugar levels, reduce high blood pressure and fat levels in the blood, and improve resistance to infection, especially bronchitis.

Rehmannia, a Chinese tonic herb with strengthening and mildly stimulant properties, appears to lower blood pressure and blood fat levels. It is suitable for people who have a weak liver and metabolism.

Gentian, a bitter herb, helps the absorption of food by maintaining digestive secretions, which diminish with age. Aperitifs, usually flavored with bitter herbs such as gentian, are a traditional way of preparing a weak digestion for a heavy or rich meal.

FAILING MEMORY & CONCENTRATION
Herb Ginkgo (*Ginkgo biloba*, p. 98)
Remedy Take ginkgo tablets. These need to be taken regularly for at least 3 months before there is a noticeable improvement.

POOR CIRCULATION & HIGH BLOOD PRESSURE
Herb Garlic (*Allium sativum*, p. 56)
Remedy Take 1–2 raw cloves a day with food, or take garlic tablets or capsules on a regular basis.

Herb Buckwheat (*Fagopyrum esculentum*, p. 208)
Remedy Make a standard infusion and drink up to 2 cups a day.

CHRONIC INFECTIONS
Herbs Garlic (*Allium sativum*, p. 56), echinacea (*Echinacea* spp., p. 90)
Remedy Take 1–2 raw cloves of garlic each day with food, or take either herb in tablet or capsule form on a regular basis.

WEAKENED LIVER & METABOLISM
Herb Rehmannia (*Rehmannia glutinosa*, p. 123)
Remedy Chew 5 g of the root 1–3 times a day, or make a decoction with 5 g of root to 250 ml of water and take 1–3 times a day.

WEAKENED DIGESTION
Herb Gentian (*Gentiana lutea*, p. 97)
Remedy Take 5–10 drops of tincture with water 30 minutes before eating, 3 times a day.
Caution Do not take gentian if you suffer from acid indigestion or a peptic ulcer.

ARTHRITIC PAIN & RHEUMATISM
See *Joint Pain & Stiffness, Including Arthritis & Gout*, p. 313.
NOTE Take one of the remedies for a maximum of 2–3 weeks. If there is no improvement, consult an herbal practitioner.

BEFORE TAKING ANY HERBAL REMEDIES, SEE PAGES 289 & 298

CONSULTING AN HERBAL PRACTITIONER

Many common health problems, such as colds and indigestion, do not require a professional consultation and can be successfully treated using herbs at home. However, persistent or more serious ailments, such as stomach ulcers and shingles, require professional advice and treatment from a qualified herbal practitioner.

WHAT DOES HERBAL MEDICINE TREAT BEST?

It is difficult to state exactly which ailments best respond to herbal medicine, since almost no research has been undertaken with this question in mind. Nevertheless, the experience of herbal practitioners and their patients suggests that many chronic and some acute illnesses readily improve with herbal medicine. Conditions that are commonly treated by herbalists include allergies, arthritis, chronic or infrequent infections, circulatory problems, liver disease, menstrual and gynecological problems, skin disorders, and stress-related complaints, such as headaches, insomnia, and palpitations.

CHOOSING AN HERBALIST

Herbal practitioners tend to treat ill health more effectively as they gain greater experience. Anyone with a serious illness, such as rheumatoid arthritis or cancer, should seek an experienced practitioner. Nevertheless, herbalists newly launched into practice often bring a more flexible approach to treatment, having the time and enthusiasm for patients that may be lacking in their more senior counterparts. That said, a trusting relationship is as important as the treatment itself – always find a practitioner with whom you feel confident. The best way to find a herbalist is by recommendation. Otherwise, consult the American Association of Acupuncture and Oriental Medicine (*see* p. 336) for a list of practitioners in your area.

THE CONSULTATION

On visiting a herbalist you should be made to feel welcome, receiving an attentive and sympathetic ear. The first consultation takes about an hour, so there is ample time for the practitioner to gain a rounded view of your health problems and life as a whole.

You will probably be asked about family traits, diet, lifestyle, levels of stress, and any particular anxieties that you may have. If appropriate, a physical examination will take place, and the practitioner will explain as far as possible what may be wrong and how much improvement can be expected. Clinical tests may include urine analysis or measuring hemoglobin levels from a single drop of blood.

The herbalist will then recommend appropriate treatment, usually involving a herbal prescription, dietary advice, and a suggested exercise regime. If you are already undergoing conventional treatment, the herbalist will advise you on its compatibility with herbal medicine and, if necessary, devise a program to discontinue pharmaceutical medicines gradually.

Subsequent consultations generally last about 30 minutes and are likely to take place every 4 to 6 weeks for a period of 3 months. Of course, this may vary, depending on the nature of the treatment.

SAFETY OF HERBS

Although herbal medicine is extremely safe, the fact that it is natural does not necessarily mean it is harmless. In fact, a national study undertaken between 1983 and 1991 by the UK National Poisons Unit found 49 instances of side-effects (including one fatality) associated with herbal medicines and vitamin supplements. The best guarantee against poor treatment is to consult a well-trained practitioner who belongs to a recognized professional association and prescribes high quality herbal medicines.

Herbalism is in the paradoxical position of experiencing a flowering of interest, yet having few educational avenues to explore. The US is one of the very few countries where medical herbalism is not legally recognized, thereby making professional training a true challenge!

A move to change this anachronistic state of affairs has been started by the American Herbalists Guild. A professional body dedicated to promotion of excellence in herbalism, it is committed to the development of high educational and ethical standards in the practice and integration of herbalism into community health care. The guild provides a list of practitioners and herbal education throughout the US and Canada. For more information, contact The American Herbalist Guild, P.O. Box 1683, Soquel, CA 95073.

TRAINING

Traditionally herbalists learned their craft by apprenticeship. Nicholas Culpeper (1616–1654), for example, was apprenticed as an apothecary for 10 years. Today, herbal practitioners are generally trained at college or university, acquiring their clinical skills in herbal and, in some cases, hospital clinics. Such training attempts to honor and retain the best of traditional herbal medicine, while incorporating the benefits of medical, pharmacological, and clinical science.

Since there is no governmental licensing body, no degree-giving schools of herbal medicine currently exist in the US. The best herbal education and training is offered by schools that are educationally unorthodox. Such places have developed where herbalists live, rather than where the demand is. They are generally on a small scale and, on the whole, excellent. Since they are expressions of the vision, skills, and wisdom of the herbalists involved, they have their unique strengths and weaknesses. Some of the schools offer full-time training, while others are based on workshop formats or correspondence courses. For more information, see *Useful Addresses*, p. 336.

ALTERNATIVE TREATMENT

Western medical herbalism is the traditional form of herbal medicine practiced in Britain and the US. However, the Chinese and Ayurvedic traditions, among others, are becoming more popular and are raising their standards of training. The Register of Traditional Chinese Medicine is currently seeking to establish a BS degree course in this discipline. If you wish to consult a Chinese or Ayurvedic herbalist, it is strongly recommended that you select a member of the associations listed on p. 336.

REGULATIONS WORLDWIDE

The regulation of medical herbalism varies considerably around the world. In the Far East, practitioners and hospitals offer herbal medicine, acupuncture, and other traditional healing practices side-by-side with Western medicine. In contrast, in some states of the US, the practice of herbal medicine is illegal.

Medical herbalists in continental Europe are known as phytotherapists, and are usually conventional medical practitioners who have studied plant medicine at post-graduate level.

In Australia, the National Herbalists' Association of Australia (NHAA) is the leading professional body of herbal practitioners.

In other parts of the world, herbal medicine is unregulated. For this reason, caution is strongly advised in pursuing any course of treatment.

GLOSSARY

Many plant constituents and their actions are explained in *How Medicinal Plants Work*, pp. 10–15.

MEDICAL

Abortifacient Causes abortion

Adaptogenic Helps the body adapt to stress and supports normal function

Anabolic Promotes tissue growth

Analgesic Reduces pain

Anaphrodisiac Inhibits libido and sexual activity

Anesthetic Numbs perception of external sensations

Anorexia Lack of appetite

Anthelmintic Expels or destroys parasitic worms

Anthraquinones Irritate the intestinal wall causing a bowel movement

Antibiotic Destroys or inhibits micro-organisms

Anticoagulant Prevents blood clotting

Antifungal Combats fungal infections

Anti-inflammatory Reduces inflammation

Antimicrobial Destroys or inhibits micro-organisms

Antioxidant Prevents oxidation and breakdown of tissues

Antiseptic Destroys or inhibits micro-organisms that cause infection

Antispasmodic Relieves muscle spasm, or reduces muscle tone

Antitussive Soothes and relieves coughing

Aperient Mild laxative

Aphrodisiac Excites libido and sexual activity

Aseptic Free from contamination by harmful bacteria, viruses or other micro-organisms

Astringent Tightens mucous membranes and skin, reducing secretions and bleeding from abrasions

Autonomic nervous system Part of the nervous system responsible for the control of bodily functions that are not consciously directed, e.g., sweating, beating of the heart

Ayurveda Traditional Indian system of medicine, see pp. 34–37

Bitter Stimulates secretions of saliva and digestive juices, increasing appetite

Carcinogenic Causes cancer

Cardiotonic Improves heart function

Carminative Relieves digestive gas and indigestion

Carrier oil Oil such as wheatgerm, to which essential oils are added in order to dilute them for use

Cathartic A drastic purgative

Circulatory stimulant Increases blood flow, usually to a given area, e.g., hands and feet

Colic Abdominal pain produced by strong contractions of intestines or bladder

Compress A cloth pad soaked in a hot or cold herbal extract and applied to the skin

Counterirritant Superficial irritant used to relieve more deep-seated pain or discomfort

Cream A mixture of water and fat or oil that blends with the skin

Decoction Water-based preparation of bark, roots, berries, or seeds simmered in boiling water

Demulcent Coats, soothes and protects body surfaces such as the gastric mucous membranes

Depurative Detoxifying agent

Detoxification The process of aiding removal of toxins and waste products from the body

Diaphoretic Induces sweating

Diuretic Stimulates urine flow

Doctrine of Signatures Theory that the appearance of a plant reveals its medicinal properties

Eclectic Popular system of herbal medicine in 19th- and early 20th-century North America

Edema Fluid retention

Elixir A liquid herbal preparation with a pleasant taste, due to the addition of honey or sugar

Emetic Causes vomiting

Emmenagogue Stimulates menstrual flow

Emollient Softens or soothes the skin

Essential oil Distillation of volatile oils derived from aromatic plants

Estrogenic With a similar action to estrogen in the body, supporting and maintaining the female reproductive organs.

Expectorant Stimulates coughing and helps clear phlegm from the throat and chest

Febrifuge Reduces fever

Fixed oil A non-volatile oil (plant constituent). An oil produced by hot or cold infusion (preparation)

Galenical A medicine, in a standard formula, prepared from plants

Hallucinogenic Causes visions or hallucinations

Hemostatic Stops or reduces bleeding

Hepatic Affects the liver

Hepatoprotective Protects the liver

Humor An important body fluid in traditional European or Indian medicine

Hypertension High blood pressure

Hypnotic Induces sleep

Hypoglycemic Lowers blood glucose levels

Hypotension Low blood pressure

Immune stimulant Stimulates the body's immune defences to counter infection

Infusion Water-based preparation in which flowers, leaves or stems are brewed in a similar way to tea

Inhalation Breathing of medicinally infused steam or liquid through the nasal passages

Intermittent fever A fever that recurs regularly, e.g., malaria

Laxative Promotes evacuation of the bowels

Liniment External medication applied by rubbing

Mydriatic Dilates the pupil of the eye

Narcotic Causes drowsiness or stupor and relieves pain

Nervine Restores the nerves; relaxes the nervous system

Neuralgia Pain resulting from irritation or inflammation of a nerve

Ointment A blend of fats or oils that form a protective layer over the skin

Oxytocic Induces contractions of the uterus

Parasiticide Kills parasites

Parasympathetic nervous system Part of the nervous system involved in vegetative functions, especially digestion

Pectoral Acts on the lungs

Photosensitive Heightened sensitivity to sunlight

Physiomedicalism 19th- and 20th-century American and British system of herbal medicine

Poultice Herbal preparation usually applied hot to affected area to alleviate pain and reduce swelling

Prostaglandins Chemicals in plants and the human body that have a hormonal action affecting a wide range of conditions, including pain and inflammation

Purgative A very strong laxative

Qi Vital energy force in Chinese philosophy, see pp. 22–23

Rubefacient Stimulates blood flow to skin, causing reddening and warming

Sedative Reduces activity and nervous excitement

Simple A herb used on its own

Spasmolytic Relaxes muscles

Steroids Active chemicals, of animal and plant origin, with powerful hormonal actions

Stimulant Increases rate of activity and nervous excitement

Stomachic Eases stomach pain or increases stomach activity

Styptic Stops bleeding when applied topically

Sympathetic nervous system Part of the nervous system involved in maintaining arousal, alertness and muscle tone

Systemic Affecting the body as a whole rather than individual organs

Terpenes Molecules that form the base of most constituents of volatile oils

Tincture Plant medicine prepared by macerating herb in water and alcohol

Tonic Exerts a restorative or nourishing action on the body

Tonify Strengthens and restores body systems

Topical Application of herbal remedy to body surface

Vasoconstrictor Contracts and narrows blood vessels

Vasodilator Relaxes and widens blood vessels

Vermifuge Expels intestinal worms

Volatile oil Plant constituent distilled to produce essential oil

Vulnerary Heals wounds

Yin and yang Complementary opposites in Chinese philosophy, see pp. 38–39

BOTANICAL

Aerial parts Parts of plant growing above ground

Annual Plant that completes its life cycle in a year

Aril Secondary covering over the seed in certain plants

Aromatic Plant with high levels of volatile oil

Axil Upper angle formed by leaf stem and supporting stem or branch

Basal leaves Leaves growing from the base of the stem

Biennial Plant that completes its life cycle in 2 years, generally flowering in the second year

Capsule Dry fruit that splits open when ripe to scatter seeds

Composite flowers Flowers of plant of the *Compositae* family, typically having ray or disk flowers, or both

Compound Leaves or flowers made up of many individual small flowers or leaflets

Cordate Having heart-shaped leaves

Corm Bulblike, underground storage organ formed by a swollen stem base

Corolla Collective term for the petals of a flower

Deciduous Plant that sheds its leaves each year

Dioecious Species with male and female parts on separate plants

Herbaceous Plant that dies down at the end of the growing season

Insectivorous Traps and digests insects and other small animals

Lanceolate Lance-shaped

Latex Milky fluid found in various plants and trees

Panicle A branched cluster of flowers on stalks in a pyramid-shaped arrangement

Perennial Plant that lives for at least 3 seasons

Pinnate A compound leaf with leaflets growing in 2 rows on each side of its mid-rib

Rhizome Underground storage stem

Stamen Male fertilizing organ of a flowering plant

Stigma Female organ of a flower

Succulent Plant with thick, fleshy leaves and/or stems

Trifoliate Plant with 3 leaves or leaflets

Tuber Thickened part of underground stem

Umbel Umbrella-like arrangement of flowers with all flower stems arising from the same point

Whorl Ring of leaves or flowers radiating out horizontally from a central point

Wildcrafting Harvesting herbs from the wild

ADDITIONAL READING & BIBLIOGRAPHY

This selected listing of references is provided as a guide to those interested in learning more about the history, science, and present-day practice of herbal medicine.

HERBAL MEDICINE

Barnard, J. & M.
Healing Herbs of Edward Bach
(Hereford, UK, Flower Remedy Programme, 1988)

Bartram, T.
Encyclopedia of Herbal Medicine
(Bournemouth, UK, British Herbal Medicine Association, 1995)

Beinfield, H. & Korngold, E.
Between Heaven and Earth: A Guide to Chinese Medicine
(New York, NY, Ballentine Books, 1991)

Bensky, D.
& Gamble, A.
Chinese Herbal Medicine Materia Medica
(Seattle & Washington, Eastland Press, 1993)

Bergner Communications
Medical Herbalism
(Portland, OR)

Bown, D.
The Encyclopedia of Herbs & Their Uses
(New York, DK Pub., Inc., 1995)

Bremness, L.
Herbs
(New York, DK Pub., Inc., 1994)

Bruneton, J.
Pharmacognosy and Phytochemistry of Medicinal Plants
(Andover, Hampshire, UK, Intercept, 1995)

Bryant, B.
Cancer and Consciousness
(Boston, MA, Sigo Press, 1990)

The Burton Goldberg Group
Alternative Medicine: The Definitive Guide
(Fife, WA, Future Medicine Publishing Inc., 1993)

Castleman, M.
The Healing Herbs
(Emmaus, PA, Rodale Press, 1991)

Chevallier, A.
Herbal First Aid
(Christchurch, Dorset, UK, Amberwood, 1993)

Chopra, D.
Ageless Body, Timeless Mind
(New York, NY, Harmony Books, 1993)

Chopra, D.
Perfect Health
(New York, NY, Harmony Books, 1991)

Collinge, W.
Recovering from Chronic Fatigue Syndrome: A Guide to Self-Empowerment
(New York, Puttnam/Perigee, 1993)

Conrow, B. & Hecksel, A.
Herbal Pathfinders
(Santa Barbara, CA, Woodbridge Press, 1984)

Dharmananada, S.
A Bag of Pearls (Zhen Zhu Nang); Chinese Herbal Therapies for Immune Disorders; Foundations of Chinese Herb Prescribing; The Golden Mirror of Chinese Medicine
(available from Eastwind Books & Arts Inc., 633 Vallejo St., San Francisco, CA 94133)

Eisenberg, D.
Encounters with Qi: Exploring Chinese Medicine
(New York, W. W. Norton & Co., 1985)

Environmental Protection Agency
Toxics in the Community: 1988 National and Local Perspectives
(Washington, DC, USEPA, 1990)

Forest History Society
Forest Pharmacy – Medicinal Plants in American Forests
(Durham, NC, Duke University Press, 1995)

Foster, S. & Chongxi Y.
Herbal Emmisaries – Bringing Chinese Herbs to the West
(Rochester, VT, Healing Arts Press, 1992)

Fratkin, J.
Chinese Herbal Patent Formulas: A Practical Guide
(available from Eastwind Books & Arts Inc., 633 Vallejo St., San Francisco, CA 94133)

Frawley, D.
Ayurvedic Healing: A Comprehensive Guide
(Salt Lake City, Passage Press, 1989)

Fulder, S.
The Book of Ginseng
(Rochester, Vermont, Arts Press, 1993)

Grieve, M. (ed. Leyel, C. F.)
A Modern Herbal
(London, Penguin, 1980)

Hoffman, D.
The New Holistic Herbal
(Shaftesbury, Dorset, UK, Element, 1990)

Hoffman, D.
Welsh Herbal Medicine
(Abercastle, Pembrokeshire, UK, Abercastle Publishing, 1978)

Keville, K.
The Illustrated Herb Encyclopedia
(New York, NY, Mallard Press, 1992)

Leung, A. Y.
Chinese Herbs & Foods
(Glen Rock, NJ, AYSL Corp., 1995)

Murray, M. &

Pizzorno, J.
Encyclopedia of Natural Medicine
(Rocklin, CA, Prima Publishing, 1991)

Ody, P.
The Complete Medicinal Herbal
(New York, DK Pub., Inc., 1993)

Ody, P.
Home Herbal
(New York, DK Pub., Inc., 1994)

Peterson Field Guide Series
A Field Guide to Medicinal Plants of the Eastern and Central United States
(New York, NY, Houghton Mifflin, 1990)

Peterson Field Guide Series
A Field Guide to Venomous Animals and Poisonous Plants of North America, North of Mexico
(New York, NY, Houghton Mifflin, 1994)

Phillips, R.
& Foy, N.
Herbs
(London, Pan, 1990)

Reid, D. P.
Chinese Herbal Medicine
(available from Eastwind Books & Arts Inc., 633 Vallejo St., San Francisco, CA 94133)

Rogers, C.
The Woman's Guide to Herbal Medicine
(London, Hamish Hamilton, 1995)

Romanucci-Ross, L., et al
The Anthropology of Medicine: from Culture to Method
(Massachusetts, Bergin & Garvey, 1983)

Svoboda, R.
Ayurveda: Life, Health and Longevity
(London, Arkana, 1992)

Tierra, L.
The Herbs of Life: Health and Healing using Western and Chinese Techniques
(Freedom, CA, Crossing Press, 1992)

Wagner, H. et al. (ed.)
Economic and Medicinal Plant Research (vols. 1–5)
(London, Sangam, 1993)

Warrier, P. et al. (ed.)
Indian Medicinal Plants (vols. 1–5)
(London, Sangam, 1993)

Weil, A.
Health and Healing
(Boston, Houghton Mifflin, 1988)

Werbach, M.
Nutritional Influences on Illness (2nd edition)
(Tarzana, CA, Third Line Press, 1988)

Wren, R. C.
Potter's New Cyclopaedia of Botanical Drugs and Preparations
(Saffron Walden, Essex, UK, C. W. Daniel, 1988)

HISTORY OF HERBAL MEDICINE

Culpeper, N.
The English Physitian Enlarged
(London, George Sawbridge, 1653)

Gerard, J.
The Herball or General History of Plants
(London, John North, 1597)

Gunther, R.
The Greek Herbal of Dioscorides
(Oxford University Press, 1934)

ab Ithel, W. (ed.)
The Physicians of Myddafai
(London, Longman, 1861)

K'Eogh, J. (ed. Scott, M.)
An Irish Herbal
(Wellingborough, UK, Aquarian Press, 1986)

Pliny the Elder (ed. Healey, J.)
Natural History: A Selection
(London, Penguin, 1991)

Unschuld, P.
Medicine in China
(University of California Press, 1985)

Vogel, V.
American Indian Medicine
(University of Oklahoma Press, 1970)

Weiner, M.
Weiner's Herbal
(Mill Valley, CA, Quantum Books, 1990)

JOURNALS

Alternative Medicine Digest
American Aromatherapy Association Newsletter
American Herb Association Quarterly
American Herbalist Guild Newsletter
American Horticulturalist
Australian Journal of Medical Herbalism
British Medical Journal
Canadian Journal of Herbalism
Fitotherapia, The Journal of Research & Applications of Medicinal Plants
Harrowsmith
HerbalGram
The Herbalist
The Herb Companion
The Herb Magazine
The Herb Quarterly
Herbs, Spices and Medicinal Plant Digest
Journal of Alternative and Complementary Medicine
Journal of Ethno-Pharmacology
Journal of Natural Products
Journal of Naturopathic Medicine
Journal of the Ontario Herbalists Association
Journal of Traditional Chinese Medicine
Lancet
Medical Herbalism
Mother Jones
Natural Health
Phytotherapy Research
Planta Medica
Protocol Journal of Botanical Medicine
Review of Aromatic and Medicinal Plants

CD-ROM/DATABASE

Herbalism
Medline
Napralert
New Scientist

GENERAL INDEX

Bold page numbers refer to main plant entries in *Key Medicinal Plants* and *Other Medicinal Plants*. Ailments for which there is a self-help treatment are in **bold**.

INDEX OF HERBS BY AILMENT

This index includes a wide range of ailments, listing key herbs used to treat each one. Page numbers in **bold** denote a self-help use.

USEFUL ADDRESSES

UNITED STATES

PROFESSIONAL ORGANIZATIONS & TRAINING COURSES

Academy of Chinese Culture & Health Sciences
1601 Clay St., Oakland, CA 94612

American Aromatherapy Association
Box 606, San Rafael, CA 94915

American Association of Acupuncture and Oriental Medicine
433 Front Street, Catasauqua, PA 18032-2526

American Association of Naturopathic Physicians
2366 Eastlake Avenue East, Ste. 322, Seattle, WA 98102

American Herb Association
PO Box 1673, Nevada City, CA 95959

American Herbalists Guild
Box 1683, Soquel, CA 95073

American Holistic Medical Association
4101 Lake Boone Trail, Ste. 201, Raleigh, NC 27607

Association of Natural Medicine Pharmacists
8369 Champs d'Elysses, Forestville, CA 95436

Bastyr University
14500 Juanita Dr., NE Bothew, WA 98011

California School of Herbal Studies
PO Box 39, Forestville, CA 95476

Herb Research Foundation
1007 Pearl St., Ste. 200, Boulder, CO 80302

National College of Naturopathic Medicine
11231 SE Market St., Portland OR 97216

National College of Phytotherapy
122 Tulane SE, Albuquerque, NM 87106

Southwest College of Naturopathic Medicine & Health Sciences
6535 East Osborne Rd., Ste. 703 Scottsdale, AZ 85251

HERBAL SUPPLIERS

China Herb Company
633 Wayne Avenue, Philadelphia, PA 19144

East Coast Herbs
118 16th Street South, Ste. 200, Nashville, TN 37203

Electic Institute
11231 SE Market St., Portland, OR 97216

Ethical Nutrients
21020 N. Rand Rd., #AB, Lake Zurich, Il 60074-3942

Gaia Herbs
62 Old Littleton Road, Harvard, MA 01451

Herb-Pharm
347 East Fork Road, Williams, OR 97544

Herbalist & Alchemist Inc.,
PO Box 553, Broadway, NJ 08808

Herbs Etc.
1340 Rufina Circle, Santa Fe, NM 87501

Kiehls Pharmacy
109 Third Avenue, New York, NY 10009

Nature's Way Products Inc.,
10 Mountain Springs Parkway, PO Box 2233, Springville, UT 84663

Planetary Formulas
PO Box 533, Soquel, CA 95073

The Body Shop by Mail
43 Horsehill Road, Cedar Knolls, NJ 07927

EQUIPMENT SUPPLIERS

Wine presses, etc.
Kedco Wine Storage Systems
475 Underhill Blvd., Syosset, NY 11791

Milan Home Wine and Beer
57 Spring Street, New York, NY 10012

CANADA

PROFESSIONAL ORGANIZATIONS & TRAINING COURSES

Canadian Association of Herbal Practitioners
921–17th Avenue Southwest, Calgary, Alta., T2T 0A4

Dominion Herbal College
7527 Kingsway, Burnaby, B.C., V3N 3C1

International College of Traditional Chinese Medicine
301-1847 West Broadway, Vancouver, B.C., V6J 1Y6

Ontario Herbalists Association
11 Winthrop Place, Stoney Creek, Ont., L8G 3M3

Wild Rose College
400–1228 Kensington Road Northwest, Calgary, Alta., T2N 4P9

CONSUMER ASSOCIATION

Health Action Network Society
202-5262 Rumble St., Burnaby, BC V5J 2B6

HERBAL SUPPLIERS

Gaia Garden Herbal Apothecary
2672 West Broadway, Vancouver, BC, V6K 2G3

Herboristerie Desjardins Inc.,
3383 St. Catherine Street East, Montreal, Que., H1W 2C5

International Herbs Co.,
31 St. Andrews, Toronto, Ont., M5T 1K7

The Body Shop by Mail
33 Kern Road, Don Mills, Ont., M3B 1S9

EQUIPMENT SUPPLIERS

wine presses
Vinothèque Products
2142 Trans-Canada Highway, Dorval, Que., H9P 2N4

Capsule-making machines, containers, ointment bases, glycerine, cocoa butter, fixed oils, paraffin waxes, and other supplies are available from pharmacies and medical supplies companies.

ACKNOWLEDGMENTS

AUTHOR'S ACKNOWLEDGMENTS

Without the unfailing good humor and commitment of the team at Dorling Kindersley this book would not have been possible. My sincere and heartfelt thanks to Penny Warren, Valerie Horn, Spencer Holbrook, Christa Weil, and Rosie Pearson. The responsibility for faults or omissions in this encyclopedia is entirely mine, though I have been greatly helped in compiling sections of this book by Anne McIntyre MNIMH, Noel Rigby MNHAA and Eve Rogans MRTCM. Many other fellow medical herbalists and colleagues have contributed in discussion or ideas, whether knowingly or not, to the writing of this book. In particular I would like to thank Richard Adams MNIMH, Celia Bell PhD, Christopher Hedley MNIMH, Michael McIntyre FNIMH, Ellis Snitcher MD, Christine Steward MNIMH, Midge Whitelegg PhD MNIMH, and John Wilkinson PhD. Above all, I am indebted to those who kept the fires of herbal medicine burning in the mostly chill and dispiriting winds of the mid-twentieth century. Without their commitment and love for herbal medicine, the current renaissance in plant medicine would not be taking place. Lastly, to Maria, Leon and Tamara for whom I have had so little time while writing, my deepest thanks for your patience, love and understanding.

PUBLISHER'S ACKNOWLEDGMENTS

Dorling Kindersley would like in particular to thank Ruth Midgley for her editorial expertise and Colin Nicholls MNIMH for his expert advice. Many thanks also to Tracey Beresford, Joanna Chisholm, Charlotte Evans, Fay Franklin, Fred Gill, Nell Graville, Constance Novis, Blanche Sibbald, Linda Sonntag, and Clare Stewart for editorial assistance; to Tracey Clarke who contributed to the original design and to Maxine Chung for design assistance; to Raquel Leis and Ana Pedro for help with finding plants;

and to Kathie Gill for the index. Dorling Kindersley are particularly grateful to Duncan Ross of Poyntzfield Herb Nursery; to Fiona Crumley and the staff of the Chelsea Physic Garden and to Dr. Yongfeng Wang at Aston University and Dr. Y. Wong at Hosten University. Many thanks also to Jacqueline Horn, Professor Shouming Zhong of East West Herbs; Noel Rigby and Woods & Woods in Australia; Neal's Yard in Covent Garden; Anthony Lymon-Dixon of Arne Herbs; Hambledon Herbs and Iden Croft Herbs of Kent. Grateful thanks also to Deni Bown, and to James Morley and the staff of the Royal Botanic Gardens Kew for their expertise. Also: University of Oklahoma Press, University of California Press, and Arkana.

DK Publishing would like to thank Leah Kennedy, Keri Manfield and the AAOM staff, Michael Wise, and Phoebe Todd-Taylor.